CLINICAL DIAGNOSIS AND MANAGEMENT OF ALZHEIMER'S DISEASE

Other Titles by Serge Gauthier

1. Clinical Diagnosis and Management of Alzheimer's Disease. Gauthier S (Ed). Martin Dunitz, London, 1996.
2. Slide Kit and Companion Document to Clinical Diagnosis and Management of Alzheimer's Disease. Gauthier S. Martin Dunitz, London, 1996.
3. Alzheimer's Disease in Primary Care. Gauthier S, Burns A, Pettit W. Martin Dunitz, London, 1997.
4. La Enfermedad de Alzheimer en Aencion Primaria. Gauthier S, Burns A, Pettit W, Bernejo F. Martin Dunitz, London, 1997.
5. La Malattia di Alzheimer: Une Guida per il Medico di Base. Gauthier S, Amaducci L, Burns A, Pettit W. Martin Dunitz, London, 1997.
6. Alzheimer – Demenz in der Primärversorgung. Gauthier S, Burns A, Pettit W, Kurz A. Martin Dunitz, London, 1997.
7. La Maladie d'Alzheimer en Médecine Générale. Gauthier S, Burns A, Pettit W. Martin Dunitz, London, 1997.
8. Birinci Basamak Salik Hizmetlerinde Alzheimer Hastaligi. Gauthier S, Burns A, Pettit W. Martin Dunitz, London, 1997.
9. Pharmacotherapy of Alzheimer's Disease. Gauthier S (Ed). Martin Dunitz, London, 1998.
10. Alzheimer's Disease in Primary Care. Gauthier S. Martin Dunitz, London, 1999 (2nd edition).
11. Clinical Diagnosis and Management of Alzheimer's Disease. Gauthier S (Ed). Martin Dunitz, London, 1999 (2nd edition).
12. Alzheimer Hastaliginin farmakoterapisi. Gauthier S (Ed). Martin Dunitz, London, Yelkovan Yaymcilik, Istanbul, 2000.
13. Alzheimer's Disease and Related Disorders Annual. Gauthier S, Cummings J (Eds). Martin Dunitz, London, 2000.
14. Clinical Diagnosis and Management of Alzheimer's Disease. Gauthier S (Ed). Martin Dunitz, London, 2001 (2nd edition, revised).
15. Management of Dementia. Lovestone S, Gauthier S. Martin Dunitz, London, 2001.
16. Alzheimer's Disease and Related Disorders Annual 2001. Gauthier S, Cummings J (Eds). Martin Dunitz, London, 2001.
17. Aging: culture, health, and social change. Weisstub DN, Thomasma DC, Gauthier S, Tomossy GF (Eds). International Library of Ethics, Law, and the New Medicine, Vol 10, Kluwer Academic Publishers, Boston, 2002.
18. Aging: caring for our elders. Weisstub DN, Thomasma DC, Gauthier S, Tomossy GF (Eds). International Library of Ethics, Law, and the New Medicine, Vol 11, Kluwer Academic Publishers, Boston, 2002.
19. Aging: decisions at the end of life. Weisstub DN, Thomasma DC, Gauthier S, Tomossy GF (Eds). International Library of Ethics, Law, and the New Medicine, Vol 12, Kluwer Academic Publishers, Boston, 2002.
20. Vascular Cognitive Impairment. Erkinjuntti T, Gauthier S (Eds). Martin Dunitz, London, 2002.
21. Alzheimer's Disease and Related Disorders Annual 2002. Gauthier S, Cummings J (Eds). Martin Dunitz, London, 2002.
22. Alzheimer's Disease and Related Disorders Annual 2004. Gauthier S, Scheltens, P, Cummings J (Eds). Martin Dunitz, London, 2004.
23. Alzheimer Disease. Neuropsychology and Pharmacology. Emilien G, Durlach C, Minaker KL, Winblad B, Gauthier S, Maloteaux JM. Birkäuser Publishers Ltd, Basel, 2004.
24. Alzheimer's Disease and Related Disorders vol 5. Gauthier S, Scheltens, P, Cummings J (Eds). Taylor & Francis, London, 2005.
25. Trial designs and outcomes in dementia therapeutic research. Rockwood K, Gauthier S. Taylor & Francis, 2005.

CLINICAL DIAGNOSIS AND MANAGEMENT OF ALZHEIMER'S DISEASE

Third Edition

Edited by

SERGE GAUTHIER MD FRCPC
Professor and Director
Alzheimer's Disease Research Unit
McGill Centre for Studies in Aging
Douglas Hospital
Verdun, QC
Canada

Professeur titulaire et Directeur
Unité de recherche sur la maladie d'Alzheimer
Le Centre McGill d'études sur le vieillissement
Hôpital Douglas
Verdun, QC
Canada

Foreword by
Zaven S Khachaturian PhD

informa
healthcare

© 2007 Informa UK Limited

First and Second Edition published in the United Kingdom in 1996 and 1999 by Martin Dunitz Ltd

Third Edition published in 2006 by Informa Healthcare, 4 Park Square, Milton Park, Abingdon, Oxon OX14 4RN. Informa Healthcare is a trading division of Informa UK Ltd, Registered Office: 37/41 Mortimer Street, London W1T 3JH. Registered in England and Wales Number 1072954.

Tel: +44 (0)20 7017 6000
Fax: +44 (0)20 7017 6699
E-mail: info.medicine@tandf.co.uk
Website: www.informahealthcare.com

A CIP record for this book is available from the British Library.

Library of Congress Cataloging-in-Publication Data

Data available on application

ISBN-10: 0 415 37299 2
ISBN-13: 978 0 415 37299 2

Distributed in North and South America by
Taylor & Francis
6000 Broken Sound Parkway, NW, (Suite 300)
Boca Raton, FL 33487, USA

Within Continental USA
Tel: 1 (800) 272 7737; Fax: 1 (800) 374 3401
Outside Continental USA
Tel: (561) 994 0555; Fax: (561) 361 6018
E-mail: orders@crcpress.com

Distributed in the rest of the world by
Thomson Publishing Services
Cheriton House
North Way
Andover, Hampshire SP10 5BE, UK
Tel: +44 (0)1264 332424
E-mail: tps.tandfsalesorder@thomson.com

Composition by J&L Composition, Filey, North Yorkshire
Printed and bound in India by Replika Press Pvt Ltd

Contents

III NATURAL EVOLUTION

IV MEDICAL MANAGEMENT

V COMMUNITY AND INSTITUTIONAL MANAGEMENT

VI ETHICAL AND QUALITY OF LIFE ISSUES

Contributors

Emmanuel Barbeau MD
Service de Neurologie et de Neuropsychologie
AP-HM Timone
Marseille
France

Frederik Barkhof MD PhD
Department of Radiology and Image Analysis Center
VU University Medical Center
Amsterdam
The Netherlands

Stéphanie Bélanger MD
McGill Centre for Studies in Aging
Douglas Hospital Research Center and Department
of Psychiatry
Montréal, QC
Canada

Sylvie Belleville PhD
Centre de Recherche
Institut Universitaire de Gériatrie de Montréal
Montréal, QC
Canada

Karen Berman MB BCh
Academic Department for Old Age Pyschiatry
Prince of Wales Hospital
Randwick, NSW
Australia

Rémi W Bouchard MD MSc FRCP
Professeur Agrégé de Clinique (Neurologie)
Directeur de la clinique de mémoire

Université Laval
Centre Hospitalier *Affilié* Universitaire de Québec
Hôpital de l'Enfant-Jesus
Québec City, QC
Canada

Henry Brodaty MD BS FRACP FRANZCP
Academic Department for Old Age Psychiatry
School of Psychiatry
University of New South Wales
Randwick, NSW
Australia

Nicole Caza PhD
Centre de Recherche
Institut Universitaire de Gériatrie de Montréal
Montréal, QC
Canada

Richard Camicioli MD FRCPC
Associate Professor
Department of Medicine (Neurology)
University of Alberta
Edmonton, AB
Canada

Howard Chertkow MD
Bloomfield Centre for Research in Aging
Lady Davis Institute for Medical Research
Sir Mortimer B Davis-Jewish General Hospital
McGill University
Montreal, QC
Canada

Jeffrey L Cummings MD
Augustus Rose Professor of Neurology
UCLA Alzheimer's Disease Center
David Geffen School of Medicine at UCLA
Los Angeles, CA
USA

Laura E Dreer PhD
Department of Physical Medicine and
Rehabilitation
University of Alabama at Birmingham
Birmingham, AL
USA

Bruno Dubois MD
INSERM E 007 and Centre de Neuropsychologie
Fédération de Neurologie
Hôpital de la Salpêtrière
Paris
France

David Edvardsson RN PhD
Senior Lecturer at the Department of Nursing
Umeå University
Sweden

Howard Feldman MD
Professor and Head
Division of Neurology Clinic for Alzheimer's
Disease and Related Disorders
University of British Columbia
Vancouver Coastal Health Line
Vancouver, BC
Canada

Douglas Galasko MD
Department of Neurosciences
University of California, San Diego
and
Neurology Service, VA Medical Center, San Diego
San Diego, CA
USA

Serge Gauthier MD FRCPC
Professor and Director
Alzheimer's Disease Research Unit
McGill Centre for Studies in Aging
Douglas Hospital
Verdun, QC
Canada

Isabelle Gélinas PhD
Associate Professor
School of Physical and Occupational Therapy
McGill University
Montreal, QC
Canada

Brigitte Gilbert PhD
Service de Neuropsychologie
Institut Universitaire de Gériatrie de Montréal
Montréal, QC
Canada

Nathan Herrmann MD FRCPC
Professor of Psychiatry
University of Toronto
and
Head, Division of Geriatric Psychiatry
Sunnybrook and Women's College Health
Sciences Centre
Toronto, ON
Canada

Nikki Horne MD
INSERM E 007 and Fédération de Neurologie
Hôpital de la Salpêtrière
Paris
France

Yves Joanette PhD
Director
Centre de Recherche
Institut Universitaire de Gériatrie de Montréal
Montréal, QC
Canada

Steve Joncas PhD
Service de Neuropsychologie
Institut Universitaire de Gériatrie de Montréal
Montréal, QC
Canada

Roy Jones MB BSc (Hons) FRCP FFPM DipPharmMed
Director, The Research Institute for the
Care of the Elderly (RICE)
St Martin's Hospital
Bath
Professor of Clinical Gerontology
School for Health
University of Bath
Bath
UK

Sven Joubert PhD
Centre de Recherche
Institut Universitaire de Gériatrie de Montréal
Montréal, QC
Canada

Jason Karlawish MD
University of Pennsylvania
Institute on Aging
Philadelphia, PA
USA

Lilly Katofsky BA BSW MSW PSW

António J Bastos Leite MD
Department of Radiology and Image Analysis Center
VU University Medical Center
Amsterdam
The Netherlands

Lenore J Launer PhD
Laboratory of Epidemiology, Demography and
Biometry
Intramural Research Program
National Institute on Aging
Bethesda, MD
USA

Simon Lovestone MD
Professor of Old Age Psychiatry
Departments of Old Age Psychiatry and
Neuroscience
Institute of Psychiatry
London
UK

Daniel C Marson JD PhD
Department of Neurology
University of Alabama at Birmingham
Birmingham, AL
USA

John C Morris MD
Harvey and Dorismae Hacker Friedman
Distinguished Professor of Neurology, Professor of
Pathology and Immunology, Professor of Physical
Therapy and Director of the Memory and Aging
Project, the Memory Diagnostic Center and the
Center for Aging
Washington University
St Louis, MO
USA

Agneta Nordberg MD PhD
Karolinska Institutet
Department NEUROTEC
Division of Molecular Neuropharmacology
Huddinge University Hospital
Stockholm
Sweden

Vanessa Pearson MD
McGill Centre for Studies in Aging
Douglas Hospital Research Centre and
Department of Psychiatry
Montréal, QC
Canada

Judes Poirier MD
Director, McGill Centre for Studies in Aging
Montréal, QC
Canada

Constant Rainville PhD
Centre de Recherche
Institut Universitaire de Gériatrie de Montréal
Montréal, QC
Canada
and
Centre de Recherche Interdisciplinaire
en Réadaptation du Montréal Métropolitain
Hôpital Juif de Réadaptation
Chomedey
Laval, QC
Canada

Kenneth Rockwood MD FRCPC
Professor of Medicine (Geriatric Medicine and
Neurology) and Kathryn Allen Weldon
Professor of Alzheimer Research
Dalhousie University
Halifax, NS
Canada

Martin N Rossor MA MD FRCP
Professor of Clinical Neurology
Dementia Research Group
The National Hospital for Neurology and
Neurosurgery
London
UK

A Dessa Sadovnick MD
Professor, Department of Medical Genetics and
Faculty of Medicine
Division of Neurology
University of British Columbia
Vancouver, BC
Canada

Sam Salek MD
Director
Centre for Socioeconomic Research
Welsh School of Pharmacy
Cardiff University
Cardiff
UK

Per-Olof Sandman RN DMSci
Professor at the Department of Nursing
Umeå University
Sweden

Marie Sarazin MD
INSERM E 007 and Fédération de Neurologie
Hôpital de la Salpêtrière
Paris
France

Philip Scheltens MD PhD
Department of Neurology/Alzheimer Center
VU University Medical Center
Amsterdam
The Netherlands

Bernadette Ska PhD
Centre de Recherche de l'Institut Universitaire de
Gériatrie de Montréal
Montréal, QC
Canada

Cornelis J Stam MD
Professor of Clinical Neurophysiology
Department of Clinical Neurophysiology and
MEG Center
VU University Medical Center
Amsterdam
The Netherlands

Edmond Teng MD PhD
Department of Neurology
David Geffen School of Medicine at UCLA
Los Angeles, CA
USA

Leon L Thal MD
Professor and Chairman
Department Neurosciences, Neurology Services
University of California, San Diego and
Veterans Affairs Medical School
San Diego, CA
USA

Lilian Thorpe BSc MSc MD FRCP
Professor (Clinical) of Psychiatry
University of Saskatchewan
Chair, Section on Geriatric Psychiatry
Canadian Psychiatric Association
Chair, Geriatric Grand Rounds Committee, SHR
Geriatric Assessment Program
Saskatoon City Hospital
Saskatoon, SK
Canada

Ladislav Volicer MD PhD
School of Aging Studies
University of South Florida
Tampa, FL
USA

Mel Walker MD
Research Fellow
Centre for Socioeconomic Research
Welsh School of Pharmacy
Cardiff University
Cardiff
UK

Bengt Winblad MD PhD
Professor at the Department of Geriatrics
Karolinska Institutet
Stockholm
Sweden

Michael Woodward MD
Associate Professor in Geriatric Medicine
University of Melbourne
Aged and Residential Care
Austin Health
Heidelberg, VIC
Australia

Foreword

Although Alzheimer's disease was described as a clinical neuropathologic entity one hundred years ago by Alois Alzheimer, the preponderance of knowledge on the disease has accumulated since the 1970s, propelling the disease from near obscurity to the forefront of modern biomedical science. The remarkable transformation of this field of study is reflected by the exponential increase in the numbers of investigators, publications, and funded projects. The current preeminence of dementia research is largely due to the increasing numbers and quality of significant breakthroughs in understanding the molecular neurobiology of the disease. Multiple promising leads now have created an atmosphere of optimism about the prospects of discovering effective interventions to delay the progression of the disease. Some of the key factors that influenced the pace of progress and helped to change the 'status' of dementia research were: (a) recruitment of new scientific talent and perspectives from different disciplines; (b) convergence of know-how and technologies from both basic and clinical research; (c) several crucial discoveries in molecular neurobiology of dementia; and (d) establishment of several nationwide networks of collaborating interdisciplinary research teams, programs and shared resources, e.g. Alzheimer's Disease Centers [ADCs], Alzheimer Disease Clinical Studies [ADCS], European Alzheimer's Disease Consortium [EADC], Alzheimer's Disease Neuroimaging Initiative [ADNI], Clinical and Genetic National Databases, etc.

This volume on *Clinical Diagnosis and Management of Alzheimer's Disease* by Serge Gauthier through its third and current edition reflects the advances in evidence-based clinical knowledge and the remarkable improvements in the accuracy of the clinical diagnosis. During the last two decades, the procedures for clinical assessment have steadily advanced toward well-validated algorithms for identification of positive clinical phenotypes of the disease. Twenty years ago what would have been considered 'mild' dementia, now more likely would be staged as 'moderate' dementia. Capabilities for early diagnosis and the prospects for even earlier detection of the disease has been one of the most important clinical accomplishments, with profound implications for: more accurate assessment of the true prevalence of AD, initiating treatments with optimal benefit, and better understanding the biology of the disease. The efforts to improve algorithms for distinguishing early stages from non-demented people, including attempts to define or characterize border-zone conditions and the introduction of *mild cognitive impairment* (MCI) concept as a potential precursor of the disease were significant accomplishment.

This work sets the stage for the next important step: exploration of biomarkers.

Advances in molecular neurobiology and emerging imaging technologies promise to provide early markers of the asymptomatic stages of AD. The individual chapters in *Clinical Diagnosis and Management of Alzheimer's Disease* reflect how rapidly the classification of degenerative dementias is moving, not just toward diagnostic and prognostic biomarkers, but toward antecedent biomarkers; a system of categorization based on combined behavioral and biological abnormalities.

Recent advances in neuroimaging technologies offer the potential to detect and follow longitudinally the clinical course of the disease. The potential value of structural and functional neuroimaging for early diagnosis is that, in the future, it may be possible to monitor more direct monitoring of some biological phenotypes of the disease (e.g. brain metabolic changes, Aβ, Tau, synapse loss or cell death). The prospects are promising that validated molecular and biochemical markers may soon complement clinical approaches in making early and valid diagnoses. In the future the combination of neuropsychological measurements with well-validated imaging measurements could allow clinicians to follow the more proximal brain changes associated with disease progression. However, prior to use as a routine clinical tool, any potential biomarker must detect a fundamental biological feature of the disease and must be validated in neuropathologically confirmed cases. At present, none of the putative biomarkers have been validated in adequately powered investigations; the Alzheimer's Disease Neuroimaging Initiative (ADNI) study is a first attempt to address this need.

The current edition of *Clinical Diagnosis and Management of Alzheimer's Disease* documents how much has been learned about the pathogenesis, diagnosis, treatment and management of dementia-neurodegeneration. At the publication of the first edition the idea of a 'cure' was inconceivable and the concept of 'prevention' was a remote possibility. People at risk for the disease were not easy to identify and clinical trials to delay the symptoms were not well developed. In contrast, this edition describes novel intervention strategies that are being developed on multiple fronts, from basic science to genetics to drug therapy to care giving.

In summary, the third edition of *Clinical Diagnosis and Management of Alzheimer's Disease* edited by Serge Gauthier provide an excellent overview of the remarkable advances in understanding the cause, diagnosing, treating, and caring for patients with Alzheimer and shows how dramatically the prospect of discovering disease modifying therapies have improved in the course a few short years.

Zaven S Khachaturian PhD
Editor-in-Chief, Alzheimer's and Dementia:
Journal of the Alzheimer's Association
President and CEO, Keep Memory Alive
Foundation for the Lou Ruvo Alzheimer Institute
Las Vegas, NV
USA

Preface to Third Edition

There has been steady progress in our understanding of the natural history, prognostic factors and treatments for Alzheimer's disease since the first edition of this textbook was published in 1996. The authors are happy to share their knowledge with all interested readers who care for someone afflicted by this condition. The chapters deal with the full spectrum of populations at risk, persons in prodromal stages, and patients from mild to severe and even terminal stages. Quality of life for patients and families is paramount in our thoughts and hopes for the future.

SG

I Introduction to the disease process

1

Definitions and diagnostic criteria

Jeffrey L Cummings

Alzheimer's disease (AD) is a progressive neurodegenerative disorder with characteristic clinical and pathological features. Alzheimer's disease is aetiologically heterogeneous and can be produced by mutations of chromosomes 21, 14 and 1 as well as by as yet unrecognized causative factors. Clinical variations are common including differences in age at onset, rate of progression, pattern of neuropsychological deficits, and occurrence of non-cognitive neuropsychiatric symptoms.[1] Except in rare cases of identifiable mutations in presymptomatic individuals, there are currently no biological markers available for AD that allow preclinical detection or definitive premorbid diagnosis. Pathologically, characteristic findings include neuronal loss, neurofibrillary tangles, neuritic plaques and amyloid angiopathy; the severity of each of these changes differs considerably among individual patients. Thus, AD exhibits aetiological, clinical and pathological heterogeneity. This diversity makes accurate diagnosis more difficult. Correct diagnosis is critical to advancing research in AD, implementing treatment of AD and identifying non-AD causes of dementia. This introductory chapter reviews current clinical definitions of AD, discusses strengths and weaknesses of the three major definitional approaches, describes disorders with features that overlap with those of AD and makes recommendations for improving diagnostic precision.

Detection of AD early in its clinical course has proven to be an elusive goal despite the fact that the disease was described almost 100 years ago. Although there have been substantial research advances in the past 20 years, there is still no generally accepted biological marker for the disease that allows early diagnosis or facilitates differential diagnosis. Mild cognitive impairment (MCI) is increasingly recognized as a transitional state denoting the earliest stages of a dementia, but not all patients with MCI progress to AD or dementia. AD must be distinguished from other dementing illnesses such as vascular dementia, frontotemporal dementias, movement disorders with dementia and many others. Clinical criteria must allow for clinical variability in symptoms based on the patient's intelligence, language and memory skills, social and cultural background, presence of non-cognitive emotional disorders and differences in how the disease affects the brain (e.g. differences in symmetry and rate of brain involvement).

Diagnostic accuracy has been improved through the development of specific criteria for dementia, AD and other causes of dementia, but the sensitivity and specificity of these criteria are imperfect and errors continue to occur. Definitive diagnoses can be achieved through a combination of clinical and pathological studies but the relationship between clinical and histological changes is also incompletely defined: patients with advanced dementia and limited cellular changes as well as patients with little or no dementia and marked AD-type pathology at autopsy are observed. It is increasingly recognized that AD is heterogeneous and the different etiologic contributions may lead to different clinicopathological relationships. Many aspects of AD including clinical manifestations, risk factors and response to therapeutic agents, are influenced by this heterogeneity. Despite the causative diversity of AD, the evidence suggests that there is activation of a similar cascade of events by different processes, eventually leading to cell dysfunction, loss of synapses and neuronal death. An ideal biological marker would allow detection of the occurrence of the earliest steps in this cascade, would be inexpensive and would be non-invasive.[2] Until such a marker is available, the clinician must rely on the careful application of clinical diagnostic criteria; this chapter reviews these criteria and provides a perspective on their utility.

DEFINITIONS OF ALZHEIMER'S DISEASE

There are three widely used criteria-based approaches to the diagnosis of AD: the International Classification of Diseases, 10th revision (ICD-10),[3] the Diagnostic and Statistical Manual of Mental Disorders, 4th edition (DSM-IV)[4,5] and the National Institute of Neurological and Communicative Disorders and Stroke–Alzheimer's Disease and Related Disorders Association (NINCDS-ADRDA)[6] Work Group criteria. Not surprisingly, the three definitions share many common features. Table 1.1 compares the principal features of the three approaches.

Three common misconceptions regarding AD – that it is a global disorder, that it is a diagnosis of exclusion and that it can be diagnosed only at autopsy – are all eschewed by the three diagnostic frameworks.

All require that attention be sufficiently intact to exclude delirium as the cause of the mental status changes, whereas a global disorder would include attentional abnormalities. All the definitions specify expected findings (memory impairment, absence of focal findings), thus utilizing inclusionary criteria in the diagnosis rather than approaching the disorder as a diagnosis of exclusion. All are predicated on the feasibility of clinical diagnosis and most series find autopsy-confirmed, accuracy rates of 85–90 per cent based on these criteria.[7,8]

ICD-10 criteria

The ICD-10[3] defines dementia as a disorder with deterioration in both memory and thinking which is sufficient to impair personal activities of daily living. The impair-

---

Table 1.1 Comparison of three commonly used criteria for the diagnosis of Alzheimer's disease

Characteristics	ICD-10	DSM-IV	NINCDS-ADRDA Probable AD
Memory decline	+	+	+
Thinking impairment	+	−	−
Aphasia, apraxia, agnosia or disturbed executive function	−	+	−
Impairment of at least one non-memory intellectual function	+	+	+
Dementia established by questionnaire	−	−	+
Dementia confirmed by neuropsychological testing	−	−	+
ADL impairment	+	−	−
Social or occupational impairment	−	+	−
Decline from previous level	+	+	+
Onset between age 40 and 90	−	−	+
Insidious onset	+	+	−
Slow deterioration	+	−	+
Continuing deterioration	−	+	+
Absence of clinical or laboratory evidence of another dementing disorder	+	+	+
Absence of sudden onset	+	−	+
Absence of focal neurological signs	+	−	+
Absence of substance abuse	−	+	−
Deficits not limited to delirious period	+	+	+
Absence of another major mental disorder	−	+	−

ICD-10 – International Classification of Diseases, 10th revision; DSM-IV – Diagnostic and Statistical Manual of Mental Disorders, 4th edition; NINCDS-ADRDA – National Institute of Neurological and Communicative Disorders and Stroke–Alzheimer's Disease and Related Disorders; AD – Alzheimer's Disease; ADL – activities of daily living.

ment of memory is noted to typically affect the registration, storage and retrieval of new information. The definition requires that the patient have deficits in thinking and reasoning in addition to the memory disturbance.

The diagnostic guidelines for AD include the presence of dementia, insidious onset and slow deterioration of cognition, absence of clinical or laboratory evidence of a systemic illness or brain disease that can induce a dementia and absence of a history of sudden onset of neurological signs indicative of focal brain injury. Early-onset (before age 65) and late-onset subtypes are recognized as well as atypical and mixed types (i.e. mixed AD–vascular dementia).

DSM-IV criteria

The DSM-IV[4] and DSM-IV Text Revision[5] define dementia as a syndrome characterized by the development of multiple cognitive deficits including memory impairment and at least one of the following cognitive disturbances: aphasia, apraxia, agnosia or a disturbance in executive functioning. The deficits must be sufficiently severe to cause impairment in occupational or social functioning and must represent a decline from a previously higher level of functioning.

AD is defined as a dementia syndrome that has a gradual onset and continuing cognitive decline. Other neurological disorders, systemic conditions or substance abuse sufficient to induce dementia must be excluded. The deficits must not occur exclusively during a delirium and must not be attributable to a major psychiatric disorder such as depression or schizophrenia. Subtypes of AD recognized in DSM-IV include early-onset (at age 65 or below) and late-onset types as well as AD with delirium, with delusions or with depressed mood. Behavioural subtypes are noted.

NINCDS-ADRDA criteria

The NINCDS-ADRDA criteria[6] take a somewhat different approach; definite, probable and possible AD are defined. Differences between definite, probable and possible reflect the available information (clinical and pathological versus clinical only) and how closely the patient's syndrome resembles classic AD. Criteria for definite AD require that the patient has met clinical criteria for probable AD while living and has histopathological evidence of AD obtained by biopsy or autopsy. This is a radical departure from earlier formulations in requiring that both clinical and pathological criteria be present to establish a diagnosis of AD. Abandoning the earlier approach that gave diagnostic pre-eminence to the pathologist, these criteria prohibited the identification of AD on the basis of

pathological examination alone; both clinical observations and pathological information were required.

Probable AD is characterized by the presence of dementia established by a questionnaire and confirmed by neuropsychological testing, deficits in two or more areas of cognition, progressive worsening of memory and other cognitive functions, no disturbance of consciousness, onset between ages 40 and 90 and absence of systemic disorders or brain diseases that could account for the memory and cognitive deficits. Dementia is defined in these criteria by decline in memory and other cognitive functions in comparison with one's previous level of function. Features that support the diagnosis of AD but are not required for diagnosis include: progressive deterioration of specific functions such as language (aphasia), motor skills (apraxia) and perception (agnosia); impaired activities of daily living and altered patterns of behaviour; family history of similar disorders, particularly if confirmed neuropathologically; normal routine cerebrospinal fluid studies; normal or non-specific changes on EEG and evidence of cerebral atrophy on computerized tomography (CT) with progression documented by serial observation. Clinical features that are consistent with the diagnosis of AD (but not required for diagnosis) include: plateaus in the course of the illness; associated symptoms such as depression, insomnia, incontinence, delusions, hallucinations, catastrophic outbursts, sexual disorders and weight loss; motor signs such as increased muscle tone, myoclonus or gait disturbances, especially late in the course of the illness; seizures in advanced stages of disease and CT that is normal for age.

Features that make the diagnosis of probable AD uncertain or unlikely include sudden onset, focal neurological findings or seizures or gait disturbances early in the course of the illness.

Possible AD is diagnosed when: (a) the patient has a dementia syndrome with no apparent cause but there are variations in the onset, presentation or clinical course compared with typical AD; (b) the patient has a second brain disorder or systemic illness that is sufficient to produce dementia but is not considered to be *the* cause of the dementia and (c) the patient has a single gradually progressive deficit in the absence of any other identifiable cause. The latter could indicate MCI.

Comment on current definitions

These three commonly used definitions of AD – ICD-10, DSM-IV, NINCDS-ADRDA – have similar features. They all require that the patient exhibit a dementia syndrome and that memory loss be a major feature of the clinical presentation; they require that the patient show impairment in at least one non-memory cognitive domain and they require that other potential causes of dementia be excluded. All require the absence of delirium if dementia is identified as the sole cause of the intellectual decline, although some note that delirium and dementia can occur together. All address the gradually progressive course expected in AD, although slightly different terms are used – insidious onset, progressive deterioration or continuing intellectual decline. The ICD-10 and DSM-IV criteria require that the patient have deficits in activities of daily living or occupational or social function, whereas the NINCDS-ADRDA approach notes that disturbances in activity of daily living are supportive but not necessary for the diagnosis of AD. The ICD-10 and NINCDS-ADRDA criteria emphasize that focal neurological findings or an abrupt onset exclude the diagnosis of AD or make it unlikely. The DSM-IV criteria exclude patients who have substance abuse, depression or schizophrenia.

The DSM-IV criteria for dementia are most inclusive and the ICD-10 criteria least inclusive. Erkunjuntti[9] and colleagues found that, of a large population of elderly individuals, 13.7 per cent were identified as demented by DSM-IV criteria and 3.1 per cent by ICD-10 criteria. Since a diagnosis of dementia is closely related to a diagnosis of AD, similar discrepancies are likely when the criteria for AD are applied.

CLINICOPATHOLOGICAL STUDIES OF DIAGNOSTIC CRITERIA

The critical test of diagnostic criteria is the extent to which they provide accurate premortem identification of pathological features found at autopsy. There have been no comparative studies of the diagnostic accuracy of the three sets of criteria based on pathological confirmation of the clinical diagnoses. Kukull et al[10] compared the sensitivity and validity of the DSM-III[4] criteria, which closely resemble those of DSM-IV, with the NINCDS-ADRDA criteria in a retrospective study of pathologically studied cases. They found that DSM-III criteria had better specificity (0.80) but lower sensitivity (0.76) compared to the NINCDS-ADRDA approach (specificity 0.65, sensitivity 0.92). The authors concluded that clinicians desiring the highest diagnostic accuracy should use the DSM criteria, whereas clinicians desiring to limit the number of undetected patients should use the NINCDS-ADRDA approach. The retrospective design of this study limits the conclusions that can be drawn regarding the prospective application of the criteria.

Clinicopathological studies of patients diagnosed using NINCDS-ADRDA criteria support the generally acceptable but not outstanding level of diagnostic precision associated with these definitions. In a study employing the prospective application of DSM-III criteria, Alafuzoff et al[11] found that only 63 per cent of patients with a pathological diagnosis of AD were accurately diagnosed in life.[11] Tierney et al[7] found that the NINCDS-ADRDA criteria accurately predicted a pathological diagnosis of AD in 81–88 per cent of 57 cases, depending on the pathological criteria applied. Many of the cases had some degree of ischaemic injury, and the criteria demonstrated a sensitivity of 64–86 per cent in predicting pure AD, depending on the severity of the ischaemic changes accepted as 'normal'. Specificity ranged from 89 to 91 per cent. Boller et al[12] applied NINCDS-ADRDA criteria retrospectively to 54 demented patients with pathologically established diagnoses and reported that two clinicians agreed on the correct diagnosis of AD in 63 per cent of cases. The authors concluded that the criteria did not allow accurate clinical diagnosis of AD. Risse et al[13] reported that 68 per cent of patients who met clinical criteria for AD based on either DSM-III or NINCDS-ADRDA criteria met neuropathological criteria for AD at autopsy. Misdiagnosis was highest in patients with onset of dementia before age 65. Galasko et al[8] found that NINCDS-ADRDA criteria had 90 per cent accuracy in predicting the presence of AD-type pathology in a series of 137 autopsied cases of dementia, although only 78 per cent of patients with pure AD were diagnosed clinically as suffering from probable AD. The criteria were least successful in identifying AD with co-existing Lewy bodies (see discussion below) and AD with vascular lesions. Gearing et al[14] reported that the diagnostic accuracy of the clinical diagnosis of probable AD was 87 per cent among 106 autopsied patients who had been studied as part of the Consortium to Establish a Registry for Alzheimer's Disease (CERAD). Twenty-eight per cent of the patients had vascular lesions and 21 per cent had co-existent Parkinson's disease. Similarly, pathological verification studies of patients assessed prospectively in the Honolulu-Asia Aging Study showed that 65 per cent of individuals diagnosed with AD using NINCDS-ADRDA criteria met pathological criteria for probable AD.[15]

McDaniel et al[16] described eight patients clinically diagnosed as having AD and found at autopsy to have non-AD diagnoses. Retrospective rigorous application of the NINCDS-ADRDA criteria revealed that seven of the eight had exclusionary features that disqualified them for a diagnosis of probable AD. Focal neurological findings, gait abnormalities, motor speech changes and extrapyramidal features indicated the presence of a non-AD disorder. In a review of 20 studies in which there was a clinical diagnosis of AD with pathological confirmation, Cummings[17] found that Parkinson's disease was the disorder most frequently misidentified in life as AD. A smaller number of patients with vascular dementia (VaD) were inaccurately identified as having AD. Rasmusson and colleagues[18] found in a clinico-pathological study that NINCDS-ADRDA criteria were highly predictive of a pathological diagnosis of AD; errors in diagnosis arose when patients had prominent behavioural disturbances or other atypical features.

Together, these studies indicate that substantial gains have been made in developing criteria that allow an accurate clinical diagnosis of AD. Clinico-pathological studies, however, reveal that accuracy rates vary between 63 and 90 per cent in academic medical centres. Thus, there is still an undesirable amount of variability in the predictive value of the criteria, and there is a definite need to continue to seek means of improving diagnostic approaches.

LIMITATIONS OF THE CURRENT CRITERIA

Several limitations of the current criteria can be discerned. The criteria are not operationalized and exactly how they are to be applied is not described. How the presence of extrapyramidal signs is to impact on diagnosis is not specified and remains problematic. How to distinguish syndromes that share many features with AD, such as the frontotemporal dementias (FTDs), is inadequately addressed, and how to identify mixed syndromes with AD plus a comorbid condition is unclear.

Lack of operationalization of definitions

One of the major shortcomings of existing criteria is the lack of operationalization of the criteria. Among all three sets of criteria, only one aspect of one set is described so that it is known exactly how the criteria are to be applied. Establishment of the presence of dementia is specified in the NINCDS-ADRDA criteria to be based on questionnaires such as the Mini-Mental State Examination[19] and confirmed by neuropsychological assessment. Cut-off scores are established for these tests and can be used to determine when an abnormality is present. No other aspects of the criteria have definitions or anchor points to guide the clinician in determining how to evaluate the patient, how to establish the presence of an abnormality or how severe the deficit must be before it is accepted as suffi-

cient to fulfil the criterion. For example, the degree of memory impairment, the severity of language disturbances or the degree of occupational disability necessary to warrant a diagnosis is unspecified. The lack of operationalization makes the criteria largely subjective and dependent on clinician expertise.

Extrapyramidal signs

How extrapyramidal signs are to be regarded is ambiguous in all three sets of criteria. The NINCDS-ADRDA criteria specify that early gait changes make a diagnosis of AD unlikely, but also indicate that increased muscle tone is consistent with a diagnosis of AD. Both the NINCDS-ADRDA and ICD-10 approaches indicate that focal neurological signs militate against a diagnosis of AD but neither addresses whether parkinsonism, an indication of focal basal ganglia dysfunction, is to be regarded as evidence of focal brain impairment. Extrapyramidal signs have been reported in AD,[20,21] but these were not autopsy-confirmed diagnoses. The demonstration that early gait changes[16] or parkinsonism[17] are often indicative of non-AD diagnoses at post mortem suggests that the presence of an extrapyramidal syndrome should cause scepticism with regard to the diagnosis of AD. Diagnosing patients with dementia and extrapyramidal syndromes as AD will result in inclusion of occasional patients with Parkinson's disease, progressive supranuclear palsy, striatonigral degeneration, corticobasal degeneration, dementia with Lewy bodies (DLB) and multisystem atrophy in the sample.

The status of DLB is controversial. Whether it is a variant of AD or a separate condition is currently debated, but in either circumstance identifying the disorder clinically seems warranted since it may differ from classic AD in terms of heredity, course, clinical manifestations or treatment response. Table 1.2 presents recent criteria for DLB.[22] The past versions of the criteria have been shown to have high validity and reliability and variable sensitivity.[23,24]

Frontotemporal dementias

Another aspect of all the definitions relates to the need to exclude other brain disorders capable of producing a dementia syndrome. FTDs such as Pick's disease may have clinical features resembling those of AD, and clinicians unfamiliar with characteristics that distinguish the two disorders may misidentify FTD as AD. In a clinicopathological study of FTD by Mendez et al,[25] 19 of 21 patients (90 per cent) were misdiagnosed

---

Table 1.2 Criteria for diagnosis of dementia with Lewy bodies[22]

(1) Central feature (essential for a diagnosis of possible or probable DLB):
- dementia defined as progressive cognitive decline of sufficient magnitude to interfere with normal social or occupational function;
- prominent or persistent memory impairment may not necessarily occur in the early stages but is usually evident with progression;
- deficits in test of attention, executive function and visuospatial ability may be especially prominent.

(2) Core features (two features are sufficient for a diagnosis of probable DLB, one for possible DLB):
- fluctuating cognition with pronounced variations in attention and alertness;
- recurrent visual hallucinations that are typically well formed and detailed;
- spontaneous features of parkinsonism.

(3) Suggestive features (If one or more of these is present in the presence of one or more core features, a diagnosis of probable DLB can be made. In the absence of any core features, one of more suggestive features is sufficient for possible DLB. Probable DLB should not be diagnosed on the basis of suggestive features alone.):
- REM sleep behaviour disorder;
- low dopamine transporter uptake in basal ganglia demonstrated by SPECT or PET imaging.

(4) Supportive features (commonly present but not proven to have diagnostic specificity):
- repeated fall and syncope;
- transient, unexplained loss of consciousness;
- severe autonomic dysfunction, e.g. orthostatic hypotension, urinary incontinence;
- hallucinations in other modalities;
- systematized delusions;
- depression;
- relative preservation of medial temporal lobe structures on CT/MTI scan;
- generalized low uptake on SPECT/PET perfusion scan with reduced occipital activity;
- abnormal (low uptake) MIBG myocardial scintigraphy;
- prominent slow wave activity on EEG with temporal lobe transient sharp waves.

(5) A diagnosis of DLB is less likely:
- in the presence of cerebrovascular disease evident as focal neurological signs or on brain imaging;
- in the presence of any other physical illness or brain disorder sufficient to account in part or in total for the clinical picture;
- if parkinsonism only appears for the first time at a stage of severe dementia.

(6) Temporal sequence of symptoms:
- DLB should be diagnosed when dementia occurs concurrently with parkinsonism (if it is present). The term Parkinson Disease Dementia (PDD) should be used to describe dementia that occurs in the context of well-established Parkinson's disease. In a practice setting the term that is most appropriate to the clinical situation should be used and generic terms such as LB disease are often helpful. In research studies in which distinction needs to be made between DLB and PDD, the existing 1-year rule between the onset of dementia and parkinsonism DLB continues to be recommended. Adoption of the other time periods will simply confound data pooling or comparison between studies. In other research settings that may include clinicopathological studies and clinical trials, both clinical phenotypes may be considered collectively under categories such as LB disease or alpha-synucleinopathy.

---

clinically as suffering from AD. This study demonstrated that among patients whose brains were referred for evaluation to a brain bank, an accurate antemortem diagnosis of FTD was unusual and most were erroneously considered to have AD. Table 1.3 presents the ICD-10 criteria for Pick's disease. DSM-IV does not provide specific diagnostic criteria for Pick's disease but does provide a description of the

Table 1.3 ICD-10 criteria[3] for Pick's disease

(1) Progressive dementia.

(2) A predominance of frontal lobe features with euphoria, emotional blunting and coarsening of social behaviour, disinhibition and with apathy or restlessness.

(3) Behavioural manifestations, which commonly precede frank memory impairment.

(4) Frontal lobe features are more marked than temporal and parietal, unlike in Alzheimer's disease.

typical behavioural changes associated with fronto-temporal degenerations. The description contains many of the same elements as the ICD-10 criteria.

A group of disorders related to FTD and presenting a challenge to the clinical diagnosis of AD are the focal atrophies. Pathologically, these disorders tend to exhibit the same histological changes as the FTDs, although a few of the patients have AD. Clinically, they manifest gradually progressive neuropsychological disturbances that are largely confined to a single intellectual domain. Primary progressive aphasia, progressive visuospatial deficits, progressive amusia and aprosodia and progressive apraxia are examples of reported focal cortical atrophies.[26–29] When the limited nature of their deficit is recognized clinically, the patients meet criteria for possible AD; if memory is affected secondarily, they would meet criteria for a diagnosis of probable AD, despite the observation that they do not typically show Alzheimer-type pathology at autopsy.

Vascular dementia

There is little consensus about the best clinical criteria to identify VaD and hence substantial opportunity to misdiagnose VaD as AD. Table 1.4 compares the DSM-IV, ICD-10 and National Institute of Neurological Diseases and Stroke–Association Internationale pour l'Enseignement en Neurosciences (NINDS-AIREN)[30] diagnostic criteria for VaD. The DSM-IV criteria for VaD emphasize the presence of dementia (defined identically to the dementia of AD) in conjunction with focal neurological signs and symptoms or laboratory evidence of cerebrovascular dementia. Historical findings such as an abrupt onset or stepwise deterioration, traditionally considered characteristic of VaD, are not included in the criteria. Neuroimaging is not required for the diagnosis if focal

neurological signs or symptoms are identified. The ICD-10 criteria incorporate more of the conventional criteria for VaD, including uneven impairment of cognitive function, focal neurological signs, preservation of insight and judgment, abrupt onset and stepwise deterioration and neuroimaging abnormalities. A reliability study of the NINDS-AIREN criteria based on a retrospective review of charts of patients with VaD indicated moderate to good reliability.[31] Comparative studies show that the diagnostic criteria for VaD are not readily interchangeable. In an autopsy-based study, Gold et al[32] found that DSM-IV criteria had a sensitivity of 0.50, NINDS-AIREN criteria sensitivity was 0.55 and ICD-10 sensitivity was 0.20. The specificity was 0.84, 0.84 and 0.94, respectively.

Mixed dementia syndromes

Alzheimer's disease is increasingly common among the elderly and is particularly frequent among the old-old.[33] Very aged individuals also have higher rates of other medical and neurological disorders, creating the conditions for common co-occurrence of AD with other diseases. How best to identify mixed syndromes and distinguish them from pure AD or from pure alternative aetiologies such as cerebrovascular disease is a major clinical challenge.

The co-existence of ischaemic brain injury and AD is particularly common. It may take the form of co-occurring VaD and AD, or the presence of more limited ischaemic brain injury may 'expose' the presence of AD by allowing it to become symptomatic with plaque and tangle burdens below those usually associated with clinical symptoms. In a study of nuns with AD, those with brain infarctions had more evidence of dementia and worse cognitive function than those without concomitant cerebrovascular disease.[34] Diagnostic errors in these circumstances may lead to the overdiagnosis of VaD or the underappreciation of ischaemic changes in AD that may have prognostic, functional and treatment implications. The currently available criteria for AD and VaD are best at identifying patients with 'pure' aetiological syndromes; the presence of mixed pathologies has a deleterious effect on the positive predictive value of the criteria.[35]

Criteria facilitating the diagnosis of mixed cerebrovascular–AD syndromes are needed. Such criteria might include: (1) the presence of cognitive impairment prior to the occurrence of cerebrovascular events; (2) a gradual decline in intellectual function between cerebrovascular events; (3) disproportionately severe dementia compared to the severity of ischaemic brain injury revealed by neuroimaging;

Table 1.4 Comparison of DSM-IV, ICD-10, and NINDS-AIREN criteria for vascular dementia

	DSM-IV	ICD-10†	NINDS-AIREN Probable VaD
Memory impairment	+	+	+
Aphasia, agnosia, apraxia, or executive dysfunction	+	−	−
Impairment of two or more cognitive domains	−	−	+
Intellectual impairment	−	+	−
Insight and judgment preserved	−	+	−
Decline from previous level of function	+	−	+
Impaired social or occupational function	+	−	−
Focal neurological signs and symptoms	+*	+	−
Abrupt onset or stepwise deterioration	−	+	+
Onset of dementia within 3 months of stroke	−	−	+
Laboratory evidence of cerebrovascular disease	+*	−	+
Computerized tomography	−	+	+
Deficits not limited to delirium	+	−	+
Subtypes			
With delirium	+	−	−
With delusions	+	−	−
With depressed mood	+	−	−
Uncomplicated	+	−	−
With behavioural disturbance	+	−	−
VaD of acute onset	−	+	−
Multi-infarct dementia	−	+	+
Subcortical VaD	−	+	−
Mixed cortical and subcortical VaD	−	+	+
Other VaD	−	+	+
VaD, unspecified	−	+	−
Strategic single infarct dementia	−	−	+
Small vessel disease with dementia	−	−	+
Hypoperfusion	−	−	+
Haemorrhagic dementia	−	−	+

† Given as 'guidelines' rather than as criteria; * one but not both required.

(4) the presence of the AD phenotype with amnestic type memory impairment in a patient with evidence of cerebrovascular disease; (5) the presence in patients with evidence of cerebrovascular disease of reduced parietal metabolism or perfusion on single photon emission computed tomography (SPECT) or positron emission tomography (PET) in the absence of relevant ischaemic brain injury; (6) the presence in patients with evidence of cerebrovascular disease of the apolipoprotein E (apoE)-4 genotype; (7) the presence of elevated cerebrospinal fluid tau or phosphatau and decreased levels of amyloid beta-protein in patients with dementia and cerebrovascular disease.

DEMENTIA EVALUATION

Accurate diagnosis of AD and exclusion of other types of dementia is aided by a comprehensive diagnostic evaluation. The Quality Standards Subcommittee of the American Academy of Neurology[36] recommended that the assessment of demented patients include: complete blood count, serum electrolytes (including calcium), glucose, BUN/creatinine, liver function tests, free thyroid index and thyroid stimulating hormone, serum vitamin B_{12} and neuroimaging. Optional tests to be considered under specific circumstances included syphilis serology, sedimentation rate, serum folate, human immunodeficiency virus testing, chest x-ray, urinalysis, 24-hour urine collection for heavy metals, toxicology screen, lumbar puncture, electro-encephalography, PET and SPECT. Whether structural neuroimaging should be included as a part of the routine dementia evaluation is controversial but is recommended by most expert diagnosticians[37] and the Academy guidelines.[36] This comprehensive assessment will identify nearly all systemic conditions and toxic encephalopathies but will not help distinguish among the degenerative disorders. Unless neuroimaging is performed, the evaluation may not reliably detect evidence of VaD.

The role of apolipoprotein E (apoE) genotyping in the assessment of dementia patients is controversial. The apoE4 genotype increases the risk of AD. However, patients without the apoE4 genotype may develop AD, and those with the genotype may live to advanced ages without developing AD. Thus, genotyping cannot be used as a prognostic test in asymptomatic individuals.[38] The presence of the apoE4 genotype in individuals with dementia increases the likelihood that the dementia is due to AD.[39,40] Thus, genotyping may be useful in patients with atypical or mixed syndromes.

RECOMMENDATIONS FOR IMPROVED CLINICAL DIAGNOSIS

Review of the criteria employed for clinical diagnosis of AD reveals that the diagnostic accuracy of the existing criteria has limitations when assessed in clinicopathological studies. In addition, there has been relatively little research into the diagnosis of mixed AD–VaD dementias, and the dementias associated with extrapyramidal syndromes continue to pose unresolved challenges for AD diagnosis. One potential resolution of this problem is to use different types of criteria for different types of studies. For example, if a research question requires study of pure AD, then very

stringent criteria would be used and the criteria would be rigorously operationalized. A specific storage-type memory deficit would be required, patients with any evidence of extrapyramidal dysfunction would be excluded and imaging would be employed to exclude evidence of ischaemic brain injury. On the other hand, studies of the efficacy of cholinergic agents might allow patients whose clinical syndrome suggests the presence of cortical Lewy bodies, since this disorder is known to have a cholinergic deficiency comparable to or greater than that of AD.[41] Phase III clinical trials of antidementia agents might use lenient criteria allowing inclusion of patients thought to have AD but with modest associated cerebrovascular disease or mild extrapyramidal dysfunction, since this will more closely mimic the application of the agent if released for general use. Pharmacological studies should carefully specify modifying factors that may affect or predict treatment response, including age, age at onset, gender, neuropsychiatric disturbances, apolipoprotein genotype, presence of an extrapyramidal syndrome and family history of dementia.

Future studies should strive to define the precise neuropsychological correlates or the range of types of neuropsychological deficits observed with different types of dementia, particularly AD. These should be related to stage of the disease, and the influence of age, education, gender and other clinical variables on their expression should be determined. Moreover, the specificity of non-cognitive neuropsychiatric disturbances – depression, psychosis, anxiety, apathy, etc. – in different types of dementia has received little investigation and should be explored. These studies would help in the development of more precise criteria for diagnosing AD and would aid in distinguishing AD from other dementias.

SUMMARY

The diagnostic accuracy of current clinical criteria for identification of AD is acceptable but can be improved. Operationalizing the definitions and their criteria would strengthen them. Excluding patients with extrapyramidal signs and prominent evidence of frontal lobe dysfunction would help eliminate non-AD patients from samples where high diagnostic accuracy is desired, and use of neuroimaging is the best means of identifying patients with VaD or mixed AD–VaD. Future studies of the neuropsychological and neuropsychiatric manifestations of autopsy-proven AD patients will aid in refining the diagnostic criteria. Different levels of diagnostic specificity might be considered for different types of research.

ACKNOWLEDGEMENTS

This project was supported by a National Institute on Aging Alzheimer's Disease Core Center grant (P50 AG16570), an Alzheimer's Disease Research Center of California grant to UCLA and the Sidell-Kagan Foundation.

REFERENCES

1. Cummings JL. Cognitive and behavioral heterogeneity in Alzheimer's disease: seeking the neurological basis. Response to commentaries. Neurobiol Aging 2000; 21: 845–861.
2. The Ronald and Nancy Reagan Research Institute of the Alzheimer's Association at NIoAWG. Consensus report of the Working Group on: molecular and biochemical markers of Alzheimer's disease. Neurobiol Aging 1998; 19:109–116.
3. World Health Organization. The ICD-10 Classification of Mental and Behavioural Disorders: Clinical Descriptions and Diagnostic Guidelines. Geneva: World Health Organization 1992.
4. American Psychiatric Association. Diagnostic and Statistical Manual of Mental Disorders: DSM-IV, 4th edn. Washington, DC: American Psychiatric Association 1994.
5. American Psychiatric Association. Diagnostic and Statistical Manual of Mental Disorders Fourth Edition Revised: DSM-IV-TR, 4th edn. Washington, DC: American Psychiatric Association 2000.
6. McKhann G, Drachman D, Folstein M, et al. Clinical diagnosis of Alzheimer's disease: report of the NINCDS-ADRDA Work Group under the auspices of Department of Health and Human Services Task Force on Alzheimer's Disease. Neurology 1984; 34:939–944.
7. Tierney MC, Fisher RH, Lewis AJ, et al. The NINCDS-ADRDA Work Group criteria for the clinical diagnosis of probable Alzheimer's disease: a clinicopathologic study of 57 cases. Neurology 1988; 38:359–364.
8. Galasko D, Hansen LA, Katzman R, et al. Clinical–neuropathological correlations in Alzheimer's disease and related dementias. Arch Neurol 1994; 51:888–895.
9. Erkinjuntti T, Ostbye T, Steenhuis R. The effect of different diagnostic criteria on the prevalence of dementia. N Engl J Med 1997; 337:1667–1674.
10. Kukull WA, Larson EB, Reifler BV, et al. The validity of 3 clinical diagnostic criteria for Alzheimer's disease. Neurology 1990; 40:1364–1369.
11. Alafuzoff I, Iqbal K, Friden H, et al. Histopathological criteria for progressive dementia disorders: clinical–pathological correlation and classification by multivariate data analysis. Acta Neuropathol (Berl) 1987; 74:209–225.
12. Boller F, Lopez OL, Moossy J. Diagnosis of dementia: clinicopathologic correlations. Neurology 1989; 39:76–79.
13. Risse SC, Raskind MA, Nochlin D, et al. Neuropathological findings in patients with clinical diagnoses of probable Alzheimer's disease. Am J Psychiatry 1990; 147:168–172.
14. Gearing M, Mirra SS, Hedreen JC, et al. The consortium to establish a registry for Alzheimer's disease (CERAD). Part X. Neuropathology confirmation of the clinical diagnosis of Alzheimer's disease. Neurology 1995; 45:461–466.
15. Petrovitch H, White LR, Ross GW, et al. Accuracy of clinical criteria for AD in the Honolulu-Asia Aging Study, a population-based study. Neurology 2001; 57:226–234.
16. McDaniel LD, Lukovits T, McDaniel KD. Alzheimer's disease: the problem of incorrect clinical diagnosis. J Geriatr Psychiatry Neurol 1993; 6:230–234.
17. Cummings J. Accuracy of the clinical diagnosis of Alzheimer's disease: review of clinicopathological investigations. Bull Clin Neurosci 1991; 56:5–16.
18. Rasmusson DX, Brandt J, Steele C, et al. Accuracy of clinical diagnosis of Alzheimer disease and clinical features of patients with non-Alzheimer disease neuropathology. Alzheimer Dis Assoc Disord 1996; 10:180–188.
19. Folstein MF, Folstein SE, McHugh PR. 'Mini-Mental State': a practical method for grading the cognitive state of patients for the clinician. J Psychiatr Res 1975; 12:189–198.
20. Chui HC, Teng EL, Henderson VW, et al. Clinical subtypes of dementia of the Alzheimer type. Neurology 1985; 35:1544–1550.
21. Mayeux R, Stern Y, Spanton S. Heterogeneity in dementia of the Alzheimer type: evidence of subgroups. Neurology 1985; 35:453–461.
22. McKeith IG, Dickson DW, Lowe J, et al. Diagnosis and management of dementia with Lewy bodies: third report of the DLB Consortium. Neurology 2005; 65:1863–1872.
23. McKeith IG, Perry RH, Fairburn AF, et al. Operational criteria for senile dementia of Lewy body type (SDLT). Psychol Med 1992; 22:911–922.
24. McKeith IG, Fairbairn AF, Bothwell RA, et al. An evaluation of the predictive validity and inter-rater reliability of clinical diagnostic criteria for senile dementia of the Lewy body type. Neurology 1994; 44:872–877.
25. Mendez MF, Selwood A, Mastri AR, et al. Pick's disease versus Alzheimer's disease: a comparison of clinical characteristics. Neurology 1993; 43:289–292.
26. Abe K, Yorifuji S, Tanabe H, et al. Progressive perceptual-motor impairment without generalized dementia: a type of cortical degenerative syndrome. Behav Neurol 1994; 7:83–86.
27. Caselli RJ, Jack CR, Jr, Petersen RC, et al. Asymmetric cortical degenerative syndromes: clinical and radiologic correlations. Neurology 1992; 42:1462–1468.
28. Confavreux C, Croisile B, Garassus P, et al. Progressive amusia and aprosody. Arch Neurol 1992; 49:971–976.
29. Weintraub S, Rubin N, Mesulam MM. Primary progressive aphasia, longitudinal course, neuropsychological profile, and language features. Ann Neurol 1990; 31:174–183.
30. Roman GC, Tatemichi TK, Erkinjuntti T, et al. Vascular dementia: diagnostic criteria for research studies: Report of the NINDS-AIREN international workshop. Neurology 1993; 43:250–260.
31. Lopez OL, Larumbe MR, Becker JT, et al. Reliability of NINDS-AIREN clinical criteria for the diagnosis of vascular dementia. Neurology 1994; 44:1240–1245.
32. Gold G, Bouras C, Canuto A, et al. Clinicopathological validation study of four sets of clinical criteria for vascular dementia. Am J Psychiatry 2002; 159:82–87.
33. Evans DA, Funkenstein HH, Albert MS, et al. Prevalence of Alzheimer's disease in a community population of older persons: higher than previously reported. JAMA 1989; 262:2551–2556.
34. Snowden DA, Greiner LH, Mortimer JA, et al. Brain infarction and the clinical expression of Alzheimer disease: the Nun Study. JAMA 1997; 277:813–817.
35. Holmes C, Cairns N, Lantos P, et al. Validity of current clinical criteria for Alzheimer's disease, vascular dementia and dementia with Lewy bodies. Br J Psychiatry 1999; 174:45–50.
36. Knopman DS, DeKosky ST, Cummings JL, et al. Practice parameter: diagnosis of dementia (an evidence-based

review). Report of the Quality Standards Subcommittee of the American Academy of Neurology. Neurology 2001; 56:1143–1153.

37. Corey-Bloom J, Thal LJ, Galasko D, et al. Diagnosis and evaluation of dementia. Neurology 1995; 45:211–218.

38. American College of Medical Genetics/American Society of Human Genetics Working Group on ApoE and Alzheimer disease. Statement on use of apolipoprotein E testing for Alzheimer disease. JAMA 1995; 274:1627–1629.

39. Roses AD. Apolipoprotein E genotyping in the differential diagnosis, not prediction, of Alzheimer's disease. Ann Neurol 1995; 38:6–14.

40. Mayeux R, Saunders AM, Shea S, et al. Utility of the apolipoprotein E genotype in the diagnosis of Alzheimer's disease. N Engl J Med 1998; 338:506–511.

41. Langlais PJ, Thal L, Hansen L, et al. Neurotransmitters in basal ganglia and cortex of Alzheimer's disease with and without Lewy bodies. Neurology 1993; 43: 1927–1934.

2

Pathophysiology: a neurochemical perspective

Stéphanie Bélanger, Vanessa Pearson and Judes Poirier

Epidemiological studies suggest that a variety of factors contribute to the occurrence of Alzheimer's disease (AD), particularly late-onset AD. Table 2.1 summarizes the most general categories of disease mechanisms that are believed to have a role in the aetiology of AD as well as their presumed order of importance. One 'risk factor', such as genetics, may be chosen as primary, and the others may be considered as contributing or permissive.[1,2] On the other hand, choosing one risk factor over the others cannot be supported objectively. The least arbitrary assumption is that a variety of factors can contribute to the clinical-pathological syndrome of AD – that is, that AD itself is often a convergence syndrome, particularly in its later-onset forms. In the following discussion, demen-

tia of the Alzheimer's type is assumed to be a syndrome rather than a single disease with a single, discrete aetiology. A multifactorial model is used in which a variety of environmental and genetic mechanisms can converge to cause the type of scarring of the brain that characterizes the clinical-pathological syndrome of AD. Pathophysiology is discussed under three broad headings: aetiological 'risk' factors, molecular neuropathology and brain–behaviour relationships.

ANALYSIS OF EPIDEMIOLOGY AND RISK FACTORS

A number of factors have been firmly established as contributing to the development of AD (Table 2.1).

Age

Age is clearly the most important risk factor for AD.[3,4] Alzheimer originally described this disorder as a form of accelerated ageing invoking the concept of excessive wear and tear. The changes that accompany ageing, especially ageing of the brain, are subjects too extensive to be discussed in detail in this chapter. No specific age-related change has been established as mechanistically important in the causation of AD. 'Error theories' of ageing postulate that ageing is caused by an accumulation of damage. Random events have also been postulated to be the trigger for activating 'age' or 'killer' genes. These ideas support the concept of a multifactorial model of AD in which a variety of harmful events can potentially contribute to the development of the syndrome. Age-related cell loss is certainly a subject of controversy as it is unclear whether neurons die or exhibit reduced size in selected

Table 2.1 List of proposed mechanisms underlying the pathophysiology of Alzheimer's disease	
Category	**Proposed mechanisms (in order of importance)**
Degenerative (wear and tear)	Age – as a risk factor
Genetic	Chromosome 19, 21, 14 and 1 (possibly 12)
Vascular	Cerebrovascular amyloidosis
Toxic	Copper/glutamate derivatives
Traumatic	Head injuries
Inflammatory	Acute phase reactants
Metabolic lesions	Decreased mitochondrial metabolism/integrity
Infectious	Slow virus-like/herpes simplex

areas of the brain. Furthermore, it appears that compensatory synaptic remodelling associated with cell loss is somehow reduced during ageing and is markedly compromised in AD,[5] sometime as a function of specific genotypes.[6,7]

Genetics

Family history of AD is one of the most consistent risk factors, increasing disease risk by approximately 4-fold at any age.[8] Statistical corrections for cases 'censored' as a result of death from other causes have suggested that as many as 75 per cent of AD cases may be familial. The familial disease occurs in a pattern consistent with autosomal dominant inheritance; 50 per cent of individuals surviving to the age of risk are affected.

Familial clustering need not be genetic in origin. In monozygotic pairs of twins, the concordance rates for AD have varied between 31 and 83 per cent around the world. Only one co-twin control study in twins discordant for AD has been published.[9–11] Even in concordant twins, the time of disease onset may vary by a decade or more, clearly implicating environmental factors. At present, a conservative position is that genetics plays a variable role in the causation of AD. In other families, a genetic aberration may predispose members to the development of the disease, but the clinical expression will depend on environmental factors. The genetic aberration in the latter case is not an inborn error of late clinical onset, but rather an inborn predisposition. In some individuals with 'sporadic' AD, genetics may represent a secondary contributing factor. While in some families, genetic abnormality plays a dominant role, leading to the disease in essentially any environment, genetic aberration in other families may rather predispose members to the development of the disease and the clinical expression will depend on environmental factors. It is noteworthy, however, that the familial form of AD only accounts for 5–10 per cent of all cases worldwide, whereas the sporadic form of AD represents 90–95 per cent of the remaining cases, and is believed to be of late onset, occurring generally after 65 years of age. Within affected families, early-onset familial AD (FAD) shows an autosomal dominant transmission of rare and penetrant mutations in different genes, while late-onset FAD presents no obvious familial segregation but is rather explained by common variants (polymorphisms with low penetrance) that increase the risk without directly causing the disease. However, the discovery of apolipoprotein E type 4 (apoE4) allele as a marker of both familial and sporadic late-onset AD raises the possibility of a genetic role in sporadic subjects.[12,13]

So far, over 120 AD candidate genes have been analysed worldwide and only four of them have been proven to play a direct role in the pathogenesis of AD or to consistently increase the risk of the disease. The first genetic link between AD and an abnormal gene came from the observation that almost all individuals with Down's syndrome's (DS) trisomy 21 invariably began to develop the characteristics of senile plaques and tau tangles in their 30s and 40s.[14] Only a decade later, it became apparent that a region on chromosome 21 coding for the amyloid-beta (Aβ) precursor protein (APP) overlaps with the region for DS.[15,16] To date, 23 mutations have been reported in the APP gene and most of them are associated with an overproduction of toxic Aβ peptide. Although these APP mutations invariably cause AD, they only account for a minimal fraction of all FAD cases, therefore opening the way for the identification of other genes.

A year after the discovery of APP mutation, the most common genetic abnormality in FAD was identified on chromosome 14 at 14q24.3, referred as the PS1 gene.[17,18] This gene encodes the presenilin 1 (PS1) protein, a member of the γ-secretase complex and essential for the activity of the latter so that it can perform a proper processing of APP.[19] Consequently, mutations in PS1 gene are believed to affect APP processing through modulation of γ-secretase activity, thus affecting the generation of toxic Aβ peptides. To date, a total of 140 rare mutations in this gene are reported to be linked to AD (AD mutation database at http://www.alzforum.org/res/com/mut/default.asp).

Accounting for the smallest fraction of FAD cases, 10 AD-causing mutations in the PS2 gene located on chromosome 1 are currently known.[20] Despite a high homology between presenilin 2 (PS2) and PS1 proteins, a mutation in the PS2 gene seems to present a later age of onset and slower progression of the disease compared to APP or PS1 mutations. Even though these familial mutations have been well established and create no doubt for their genetic risk factor, together they only account for about 50 per cent of all the FAD cases, suggesting that additional genetic factors remain to be identified for this rare form of the disease.

Apolipoprotein E4

A susceptibility locus, particularly in late-onset FAD, has been identified on 19q13.2.[21] The gene for apolipoprotein E is located within this region, and the allele frequency of the E4 allele in patients with familial and sporadic late-onset AD has been reported[12,13] to be nearly three times higher than in unrelated age-matched controls.

Apolipoproteins are protein components of lipoprotein particles. The latter are macromolecular complexes that carry lipids such as cholesterol and phospholipids from one cell to another within a tissue or between organs. Apolipoproteins regulate extracellular enzymatic reactions related to lipid homeostasis or act as ligands for cell surface receptors that mediate lipoprotein uptake into cells and their subsequent metabolism.

ApoE is a component of several classes of plasma and cerebrospinal fluid lipoproteins. It was shown to be synthesized and secreted by glial cells, predominantly astrocytes.[22,23] Several cell surface receptors for apoE are known to be expressed on one or many of the different cell types that constitute the brain parenchyma. These receptors are members of a single family and include the low-density lipoprotein (LDL) receptor, the very low-density (VLDL) receptor, the apoER2 receptor, the LDL receptor-related protein (LRP) and the megalin/gp330 receptor.

The importance of apoE in lipid homeostasis in the brain is underscored by the fact that major plasma apolipoproteins such as apoB and apoA-I are not synthesized in the central nervous system (CNS). Animal lesion paradigms such as sciatic nerve crush[24] and entorhinal cortex lesioning[25] indicate that apoE plays a strategic role in the coordinated storage and redistribution of cholesterol and phospholipids among cells within the remodelling area. ApoE is now believed to play an important role not only in reactive synaptogenesis by delivering lipids to remodelling and sprouting neurons in response to tissue injury, but also in physiological ongoing synaptic plasticity and maintenance of neuronal integrity, as well as in cholinergic activity.[26]

Three alleles (ε2, ε3, and ε4) at a single gene locus on the long arm of chromosome 19 code for the common isoforms of apoE, namely apoE2, apoE3 and apoE4. This allelic heterogeneity gives rise to a protein polymorphism at two positions: (residues 112 and 158 on the mature protein). The presence of either a cysteine or an arginine at these polymorphic sites leads to a charge difference detectable by isoelectric focusing. The most common apoE allele is ε3 and its frequency is greater than 60 per cent in all populations. Allelic distribution in a typical aged Caucasian population is approximately 8 per cent for ε2, 78 per cent for ε3 and 14 per cent for ε4.[27] Relative allelic frequencies for other ethnic groups, such as African Americans, Hispanics and Japanese, were reported to be quite similar in the elderly population.[27]

Recently, the apoE4 allele was found to be overrepresented in groups of both familial and sporadic cases of late-onset AD, which accounts for ~99 per cent of all AD cases. The ε4 allele frequency was shown to be significantly higher (~3-fold i.e. 40–50 per cent) in the Alzheimer population. Interestingly, a sharp decline in the prevalence of the ε4 allele was observed in very old subjects (>85 years), suggesting the presence of a late-late-onset form of AD and consistent with the increased risk of coronary heart disease in apoE4 carriers.[28] The effect of the more uncommon ε2 allele would be to decrease the risk and increase the age of onset compared to the common ε3 allele; therefore the ε2 allele is said to be protective.[29]

Increasing the dose of ε4 allele is also associated with an earlier age of onset of AD. In families with late-onset AD, the mean age of onset was reported to decrease from 84 to 68 years as the ε4 allele dose increased from 0 to 2. Likewise, a decrease in average ages of onset (from 78 to 70 years) as a function of ε4 allele copy number was found in sporadic cases.[12]

The use of subjects populations, homogeneous with respect to age of onset, severity and duration of disease, allowed monitoring of disease progression by reducing intrinsic variability due to non-linear decline of function in AD patients. When such populations enrolling in clinical drug trials (patients' mean age 75 years) were analysed, the placebo arm revealed a clear difference in the rate of progression as monitored by variation in the Alzheimer's Disease Assessment Scale – cognition (ADAS-cog) over a period of 6 months[30] in mild-to-moderate AD. Similar apoE4 genotype influence was recently published in so-called mild cognitively impaired (MCI), non-AD subjects. In that particular case, it is the rate of conversion from MCI status to clinically diagnosed AD which was shown to be greatly influenced by the presence of the ε4 allele.

In addition to its effect on increasing risk and lowering age of onset, increasing the number of ε4 alleles is also known to correlate with an increase in the number of senile plaque and neurofibrillary tangles (NFT) in the brains of sporadic late-onset subjects, though the latter association is more controversial and could be attributed to the correlation existing between NFT and duration of illness associated with apoE4 carriers.[31,32] Immunochemical localization of apoE to extracellular amyloid deposits, including vascular deposits, and to neurons containing neurofibrillary tangles suggested that apoE is involved in the pathogenesis of common AD. These results led to studies on the interactions of apoE3 and apoE4 with the main constituent of senile plaque deposits, the Aβ peptide, and with microtubule-associated protein tau. Studies revealed isoform-specific differences in the in vitro affinity of apoE for amyloid and for tau. However, discrepancies between the results obtained from these studies make it difficult to explain the above correlations between the ε4 copy number and the histopathological marker density. Although the importance of apoE in triggering Aβ peptide deposition in brains of amyloid precursor protein transgenic mice has been clearly demonstrated,[33] the pathogenicity of the protein interaction as the primary cause or the consequence of dying neurons is still debated.

Brain levels of cholesterol and choline, a precursor for the neurotransmitter acetylcholine, were shown to be reduced in AD patients. Moreover, losses of cholinergic neurons and/or choline acetyltransferase (ChAT) activity are other well-known features of AD. It is interesting to note that ApoE4 allele copy number shows an inverse relationship with residual brain ChAT activity and nicotinic receptor binding sites in both the hippocampal formation and the temporal cortex of AD subjects.[6,7,34] Furthermore, the density of cholinergic neurons in the basal forebrain, which represents the primary cholinergic input to these areas, was significantly reduced in ε4 allele carriers when compared to non-ε4 AD cases or control subjects.[6,7] The fact that the ratio between the loss of cholinergic markers in the projecting areas and the loss of cholinergic neurons in the basal forebrain is lower in non-ε4 carriers suggests that the brain of these individuals can compensate to a certain extent for the loss of synapses by producing more acetylcholine and/or by sprouting. Increased cholinergic neuron vulnerability and reduced plasticity in ε4 carriers would support the hypothesis of a less efficient delivery of cholesterol and phospholipids (including donor intermediates of choline) to cells in the central nervous system as a consequence of lower apoE expression in these subjects.

The role of apoE polymorphisms as potent pharmacogenetic markers has been validated by several independent groups which have shown the presence or absence of the ε4 allele (in combination with gender) in a given subject markedly affect the drug response of several antidementia drugs such as tacrine,[7,35] metrifonate,[36] S12024[37] and more recently rivastigmine.[30,38]

The emerging field of the pharmacogenetics of AD is bound to have a striking impact on the development of the next generation of antidementia drugs. These new drugs will have to be tested in genetically distinct populations of patients in order to assess the pharmacogenetic contribution of each of the apoE alleles as well as the contribution of novel genetic variants such as the presenilins, butyrylcholinesterase and α_1-antichimotrypsin, which have already been associated with sporadic AD.

In other words, AD may be one of the first diseases, if not the first one, to be treated in the context of molecular medicine where genetic information will have to be combined with rigorous clinical assessment to carefully individualize treatment.

Gender

Meticulous epidemiological studies have established that being a woman is an independent risk factor for common AD in Europe[39,40] and Asia, but apparently not in the US.[41] Most prevalence studies have corrected for the increased proportion of women in the older, at-risk population that results from their increased longevity. In addition, they have allowed for potential diagnostic artifacts caused by the higher prevalence of cerebrovascular disease among men and the resulting difficulty in confidently diagnosing AD in older men. The higher prevalence of AD in women is not yet entirely understood. Possible explanations include unrecognized environmental influences, unspecified hormonal effects (including late effects of menopause, low testosterone levels), the presence of one or more predisposing genes on the X chromosome, longer disease duration and the higher incidence of the apoE4 allele in women.[12] Several epidemiological studies have found a female-to-male prevalence ratio in AD of 2:1, raising the possibility that a contributing gene acts as an X-linked dominant. These findings have now been challenged by a more recent incidence study from Canada and the US. In the familial form of AD discussed above, the disorder is clearly inherited as an autosomal dominant, including transmission from father to son.

Trauma

Head trauma has been reported as a risk factor for AD in several, but not all, studies considering its potential role in the disease.[42,43] In dementia pugilistica, repeated head trauma leads to dementia with the accumulation of neuropathological abnormalities associated with AD, including many neurofibrillary tangles and diffuse Alzheimer amyloid. Head trauma can contribute to the development of clinically significant dementia, including the presence of tangles and probably amyloid, as well. The assumption that trauma can also contribute to dementia in individuals predisposed to AD is also quite reasonable. Mayeux and his colleagues showed in population-based studies that head injury is a significant risk factor for AD only in apoE4 carriers,[44] illustrating the possible interplay between genetic and environmental factors in triggering AD.

Toxins

Until recently, little attention was given by neuroscientists to the neurometabolism of metals. However, since evidence has linked metals to many neurodegenerative diseases, increased emphasis has been placed on studies aimed at determining their mechanisms of neurotoxicity. Consequently, it has been postulated that disruption of iron and copper metabolism may have a role to play in the pathogenesis of AD. Indeed, it has become apparent that iron accumulates in the AD brain and invades cells associated with senile plaques and neurofibrillary tangles.[45] Furthermore, since iron and copper are transition metals involved in the formation of hydroxyl radicals, it strongly supports the idea that abnormal accumulation of iron participates in the induction of oxidative stress promoting neurodegeneration in AD. Some studies have suggested that iron promotes the Aβ protein neurotoxicity by facilitating its aggregation whereas other have argued that, by binding iron, Aβ might rather protect the surrounding neurons from oxidative stress.[46] The discovery of recent genetic mutations linked to iron overload in the brain will help to delineate the molecular mechanisms through which misregulation of iron metabolism can lead to neuro-degeneration. Similarly, the addition of trace amounts of copper to the drinking water of cholesterol-fed rabbits induces a marked accumulation of Aβ in the brain, concomitant with formation of senile plaque-like structures and significant retardation of the rabbit's ability to learn difficult tasks.[47]

Additional studies are planned to investigate the mechanisms of metal-mediated neurotoxicity and their individual contribution to the pathogenesis of sporadic AD and Parkinson's disease (PD).

Aluminium (Al) is another metal which had been proposed to play a role in the pathogenesis of AD. The exact mechanism of Al toxicity is not known, but evidence suggests that it can slightly potentiate oxidative stress by enhancing iron-induced oxidation[48] and indirectly inflammatory events. However, multiple epidemiological and aetiological research studies have failed to show a direct link between aluminium, amyloid deposition and AD.

Vascular disease

The prevalence and incidence of degenerative and vascular dementias increase almost exponentially with age, from 70 years onward. In view of the increasing longevity of humans, both varieties have progressively evolved into a major public health problem worldwide. The integrity of the cerebral vasculature is crucial to the maintenance of cognitive function during ageing. Prevailing evidence suggests that cerebrovascular function declines during normal ageing, with pronounced effects in AD. The cause of this change remains largely unknown. While previous studies recorded age-related impairments, such as atherosclerosis and loss of innervation in basal surface arteries of the brain, it has only recently been realized that a number of subtle alterations in both intracranial resistance vessels and smaller capillaries is apparent in both ageing animals and humans. Abnormalities entail profound irregularities in the course of microvessels, unexplained inclusions in the basement membrane and changes in unique proteins and membrane lipids associated with the blood–brain barrier. Brain imaging and permeability studies show no clear functional evidence to support the structural and biochemical anomalies, but it is plausible that focal and transient breaches of the blood–brain barrier in ageing, and more notably in AD, occur in the early stages of the disease. Vascular diseases per se are now considered to be significant contributing risk factors for AD.[49,50] Previous myocardial infarction has been reported to increase the risk of probable AD by 5-fold in elderly women. In addition, coronary artery disease at autopsy, with or without myocardial infarction, was found to be associated with a 6-fold increase in the proportion of older patients with significant amyloid deposits in the brain. Brun and Englund[51] reported that 60 per cent of patients with autopsy-proven AD also had white matter changes of the type usually associated with compromised circulation. Neuroradiological studies indicate that white matter abnormalities consistent with vascular damage to the brain occur in 15–30 per cent of neurologically intact elderly persons, 30–60 per cent of patients with AD and most patients with vascular dementia. In recent years, both epidemiological and neuropathological studies have suggested an association between common AD and specific vascular risk factors, such as hypertension, inheritance of the apoE4 allele, atherosclerosis, myocardial infarction, diabetes mellitus, ischaemic white matter lesions, generalized atherosclerosis and, more recently, high consumption of animal fat with a 2-fold range in risk. These findings may reflect an over-diagnosis of AD in individuals with silent cerebrovascular disease or that cerebrovascular disease may affect the clinical expression and onset of AD. Further possibilities include that AD may increase the risk of vascular disease or that vascular disease may silently stimulate the disease process. Similar mechanisms may also be involved in the pathogenesis of both disorders, such as disturbances in lipid homeostatic processes or abnormal cholesterol transport and distribution.

MOLECULAR NEUROPATHOLOGY

The anatomical pathology of AD, including ultrastructure, has been extensively reviewed in the past. The following discussion concentrates on the molecular neuropathology and emphasizes more recent findings.

Amyloid

Amyloid has a key role in AD.[52] By definition, the one neuropathological abnormality required for the diagnosis of definite AD is an adequate number of amyloid plaques.[53] In the absence of amyloid plaques, the diagnosis of AD is not made, even in the presence of atrophy and a large number of neurofibrillary tangles, as is found in dementia pugilistica. Any description of the pathophysiology of AD must explain the amyloidosis.

Amyloid metabolism is widely believed to play a central role in the pathogenesis of AD. Amyloid-β protein arises from a precursor protein called APP, which is identical to the previously described protein α_2-nexin.[54] The APP gene located on chromosome 21, its promoter, four major splicing variants, the distribution of these entities in tissues and within the brain, the processing of APP and the formation of fibrils from the amyloidogenic fragment have all been intensively studied (for a review, see Selkoe and Schenk[55]).

The strongest evidence for a key and early role of amyloid in the pathogenesis of AD is the genetic evidence from the families with APP mutations. These disease-causing mutations imply that an abnormality in APP is sufficient to lead to the full clinical-pathological picture of AD. Accepting this implication poses at least two problems, however.

First, it would be surprising if conservative mutations in a non-amyloidogenic region of APP led to significantly altered processing, and the available data do not suggest that they do so. Second, and perhaps most important, the association of a mutation in APP with AD in the few families in whom such mutations have been found does not imply that APP is the initiating factor in most forms of AD.

Other genetic evidence is based on patients with C21 trisomy or Down's syndrome. Patients with C21 trisomy express the APP gene at 150 per cent of nor-

mal throughout their life, and essentially all of them develop the typical neuropathological lesions of AD by age 40 years, including both amyloid plaques and neurofibrillary tangles.[56] On the other hand, a progressive decline in intellect from young adult baseline levels may occur in less than half of these patients, even among the rare Down's syndrome patients who live into their eighth decade. These observations suggest that amyloid accumulation may be enough to cause the neuropathology but not the syndrome. AD itself is not associated with a generalized overexpression of APP, and earlier studies suggested that the mRNA for APP is usually sequentially normal in AD. Patients with C21 trisomy overexpress other genes as well. According to conventional criteria, elderly mentally retarded people without Down's syndrome have also been reported to develop the neuropathology of AD. This has been observed in 70 per cent of subjects between the ages of 66 and 75 years, and in 87 per cent of subjects older than 75 years.

Experimental studies appear to support a role of amyloid in the pathogenesis of AD. Amyloidogenic fragments of APP left in tissue culture medium for periods sufficient to allow aggregation appear to be toxic to neurons in culture. Thus, the deposits of dense amyloid in the AD brain may damage the surrounding nerve endings. Extensive studies of the effects on brain cells of amyloid and other fragments of APP are underway, including studies of APP fragments not found in AD. Some of these fragments are ampophilic, requiring that controls include other peptides with equivalent detergent properties. Results in transgenic mice do not yet allow firm conclusions. While no convincing pathology has been detected in mice overexpressing amyloid or analogous proteins,[57,58] the second generation of transgenic mice carrying the 717 human mutation or the combined presenilin/amyloid mutations clearly show extensive accumulation of amyloid staining in the neuropil of hippocampal and cortical structures.[59,60] Mild or no significant behavioural alterations have been reported in these particular animal models nor any evidence of ongoing neuronal cell loss.

Evidence for a pathogenetic role of Aβ in AD provided by neuropathological studies is equivocal at best. Quantitative studies using radioimmunoassay indicate that the amount of soluble APP in AD brains is equal to that in brains from non-AD controls of the same age, casting doubt on a pathogenetic role of APP itself. Dense amyloid made up of the beta amyloid peptide (β/A4) peptide is insoluble and, therefore, harder to quantitate reliably, making it more difficult to come to conclusions about its relationship with the clinical disorder. Dense plaques accumulate with age, even in people without cognitive impairment.

Neurofibrillary tangles and cytoskeletal abnormalities

The second neuropathological hallmark of AD is the neurofibrillary tangle. NFTs are one of a number of cytoskeletal abnormalities characteristic of AD.[61] They are not, however, specific for AD and are found in a variety of neurodegenerative disorders. NFTs are intracellular fibrillar structures composed of aggregations of paired helical filaments (PHFs), which appear to be formed primarily from abnormal accumulation of hyperphosphorylated tau proteins.[62] Tau proteins belong to the group of microtubule-associated proteins (MAPs); these proteins associate with polymerized tubulin, altering the properties of microtubules and thus the shape of cells. So far, no specific function is attributed to tau, although it has been shown to play a role in neurite extension and axonal transport.[63,64] Accordingly, tau and MAP2 double knockout transgenic mice show defects in axonal elongation and neuronal migration.[65,66] A prevailing hypothesis suggests that hyperphosphorylated tau loses its capacity to bind microtubules and they accumulate in the cell body as PHF-tau. In turn, this could compromise microtubule stability and function, causing a decrease in axonal and dendritic transport.

However, the importance of tau filaments for neurodegeneration is controversial, since overexpression of human APP, PS1 or PS2 mutants, known to directly cause AD, failed to produce significant tau pathology in these transgenic mice.[59] On the other hand, relevant links between Aβ accumulation and changes in tau have been demonstrated. Among others, studies have shown that tau expression is required for the neurotoxicity of Aβ and that Aβ accumulation in APP transgenic mice is not sufficient to cause a progressive cognitive impairment.[67] Based on co-expression studies, it is believed that Aβ deposition influences tau tangle formation, whereas neurodegeneration results from tau filament accumulation. In other words, the Aβ neurotoxicity together with abnormal changes in tau proteins definitively modulates the progressive neurodegeneration observed in AD. Moreover, the discovery of tau mutations leading to non-AD tauopathies, which are distinct from AD by the absence of APP, Aβ and presenilin involvement, demonstrated that tau accumulation alone is sufficient to lead to neurodegeneration and memory loss.[68]

Although the exact mechanism that triggers tau filament assembly and aggregation is still unclear, phosphorylation has been proposed as the primary modification that alters tau proteins. A number of kinases have been reported to act on tau to induce abnormalities associated with PHF. Which of these kinases, or combination of kinases, plays a significant role in the formation of PHF in the AD brain is not yet known. However, glycogen synthase kinase-3 (GSK-3), cyclin-dependent protein kinase-5 (cdk5) and mitogen-activated protein (MAP) kinase ERK 1/2 have been shown to phosphorylate tau at the same sites where tau is abnormally hyperphosphorylated in AD.[69] Even though numerous factors contribute to the clinico-pathological syndrome of AD, several lines of evidence have strongly suggested that tau filaments are a key component in this disease and the only contributor so far to be linked to neurodegeneration and dementia.

Acute phase reactants/inflammation

The possibility of an autoimmune or other inflammatory component in AD has been considered for some time. However, the lack of strong evidence of increased levels of circulating anti-brain specific antibodies and the absence of classic inflammatory cell exudates have worked against that possibility.[61] A variety of studies during the past 13 years have documented the presence of a localized inflammatory reaction in AD brains.[70–72] More specifically, inflammatory molecules and activated products of the complement system are associated with amyloid plaques in different brain areas affected by AD. Immunocytochemistry with specific antibodies demonstrated elements of the classic but not the alternative complement pathway on senile plaques, dystrophic neurites, neuropil threads and some NFTs.[71] The factors that precipitate the inflammatory reaction have not yet been identified. No evidence for an effect of prions or typical viruses has been found. However, the finding that Aβ can activate the complement system and potentiate cytokine secretion[73] has strongly suggested that Aβ peptide itself can induce a local inflammatory response. Like inflammation in other tissues, inflammatory response may be a physiological reaction to remove the products of chronic degeneration.

In turn, an excessive inflammatory reaction stimulated by complement activators such as Aβ may overtake the physiological role of inflammation and, instead, release highly toxic products such as oxygen free radicals, reactive nitrogen species or inflammatory cytokines that can be cytotoxic and cause the death of adjacent neurons. Epidemiological studies have previously indicated that prolonged use of non-steroidal anti-inflammatory drugs (NSAIDs) diminishes the risk of AD, delays dementia and reduces cognitive impairment.[74] Interestingly, a variety of studies in transgenic mice encoding the familial AD mutation has demonstrated that a chronic use of NSAIDs, such as ibuprofen, flurbiprofen or indomethacin, suppresses inflammation and reduces Aβ deposition in brain.[75,76] On the other hand, when these drugs were pre-clinically and clinically tested they did not demonstrate any significant effects on cognition improvement.[77–79] However, the marked side effects associated with the use of conventional NSAIDs may have affected these studies. Some NSAID derivatives producing fewer side effects are now available, thus clinical investigations on them will be necessary in order to demonstrate whether or not they can have benefits for AD.

Loss of neurons and synapses

Loss of brain substance has been considered a pathological hallmark of AD since Alzheimer's original report. Studies over the past 20 years, notably those of Terry and colleagues, have permitted the nature and extent of the anatomical damage to be explained more precisely. Although the weight of AD brains statistically tends to be less than that of brains of age- and sex-matched cognitively intact controls, the overlap is so large that gross atrophy has little diagnostic value in AD patients older than age 65 or 70 years. Certain populations of neurons tend to be lost selectively, notably large neurons of association cortices and certain subcortical nuclei, including the cholinergic cells of the nucleus basalis complex and the serotonergic cells of the raphe nucleus. Terry et al[80] used quantitative densitometry after immunocytochemical analysis with antibodies to synaptophysin or other synaptic proteins. DeKofsky and Scheff[81] measured synapse density by electron microscopy in biopsies of AD brains. The density of synapses in the frontal lobe correlated with scores on the Mini-Mental State Examination with a coefficient of 0.73 in the studies of Terry et al[80] and a coefficient of 0.77 in the study of DeKofsky and Scheff.[81] Terry proposed that synapse loss is likely to have a more immediate relationship to the dementia in AD than does Aβ accumulation.[82] Independent neuropathological studies[83,84] support a similar view.

According to this analysis, a critical issue is identifying the insult in AD that leads to the formation of distended neurites containing swollen vesicles, dense bodies and abnormal mitochondria.

FORMULATION OF PATHOPHYSIOLOGY

The list of AD risk factors and abnormalities at the anatomical, cellular and molecular levels supports the view that a variety of different mechanisms may contribute to the characteristic brain damage, which is itself the basis of the clinical disability. A conservative formulation that is in accord with the available AD data is that these different causes of brain damage can contribute, in varying combinations, to the particular type of scarring that characterizes AD; i.e. AD is a convergence syndrome.

The mechanisms of brain damage that have been linked to AD are not mutually exclusive. No compelling evidence indicates that these mechanisms are mutually dependent. In some patients, a particular mechanism may play a major role, while in others it may not. Amyloid is key at least in the sense that, according to pathological criteria, definitive diagnosis is not made without it, even if other abnormalities characteristic of AD are present.[53] Patients with dementia, loss of neurons and synapses and an inflammatory response are classified as having a form of motor neuron disease. Dementia pugilistica, in which all of these changes and numerous NFTs are found, is not considered a form of AD even in an elderly person and even though head injury is an established a risk factor for AD,[85] it is the presence of the apoE4 allele with the head injury that most significantly enhances the risk of developing the disease in both elderly boxers and football players.[86–88]

The changes that appear to be found almost invariably in AD include loss of neurons and particularly of synapses in vulnerable areas, cytoskeletal abnormalities typically including NFTs, a localized inflammatory reaction and Aβ accumulation. Table 2.2 depicts relationships among these factors, indicating that a variety of genetic and environmental abnormalities can contribute to the brain damage in AD.

The increasingly important role of apoE4 in familial and sporadic AD raises some new fundamental questions regarding the pathophysiology of AD and the role of cholesterol homeostasis in this disease. What is the role of the interaction between apoE4, cholesterol and Aβ? Why do senile plaques tend to

Table 2.2 Genetic contribution to the pathophysiology of Alzheimer's disease: correlational association and biochemical relevance

Category	Neuropathological markers (in order of prevalence)	Genetic contribution to the extent of the pathology
Plaques (senile/amyloid)	Amyloid peptides and apoE (plus some 70 additional components)	Density is enhanced by APP mutations, presenilin mutations and apoE polymorphisms
Tangles	Hyperphosphorylated-tau and ApoE	Density is enhanced apoE polymorphisms and tau mutations
Gliosis	Astrocytic and microglial (proliferation and hypertrophy)	N/A
Neuronal cell loss	Widespread (extensive damage of the cholinergic system)	Severity is enhanced by apoE polymorphisms
Synaptic loss	Widespread (cortical and subcortical)	Density is reduced by APP mutations and apoE polymorphisms
Inflammatory response	Acute phase reactants and complement activation	Response is enhanced by APP mutations, presenilin mutations and apoE polymorphisms

accumulate more heavily in apoE4 carriers? Why do middle aged men who died with high blood cholesterol levels exhibit amyloid deposition commonly found in the AD brain? Why are cholinergic neurons and synapses selectively lost in apoE4 carriers? How is apoE4 modulating age of onset in mutated-APP, presenilin 1 and presenilin 2 families? Why do traditional cardiovascular risk factors such as diabetes, high blood cholesterol, hypertension and apoE4 appear as significant risk factors for common AD in recent epidemiological and clinical studies?

In many patients, cholesterol metabolism dysfunction may have a key mechanistic role by reducing the ability of neurons to maintain their viability and ability to sustain synaptic integrity and remodelling in the face of a variety of stressors.[26] The resulting dysregulation of this core metabolism was shown to lead to cytoskeletal abnormalities,[89] including accumulation of PHFs and NFTs, and an inflammatory reaction, including complement-mediated cell damage and amyloidosis. The apoE4 allele, in which two cysteine residues are replaced by arginines, is more subject to oxidation than are the apoE2 or apoE3 alleles. More importantly, it appears to be directly involved in the transport and distribution of lipid-soluble antioxidants such as vitamin E and beta carotene in the brain.[90,91] In a subpopulation of patients with early-onset AD, genetic abnormalities in the APP gene appear to be the dominant factor causing the disease. The mechanisms leading to the inflammatory reaction are not known, and no clear evidence is available to determine whether it is primarily a result of brain damage or primarily a contributor to brain damage or both.

The formulation that AD is a convergence syndrome has implications for therapeutics. For example, it was shown that AD subjects carrying apoE4 respond quite differently to cholinomimetic drugs such as tacrine, rivastigmine, galantamine (acetylcholine esterase inhibitors[7,30,38,92]) and xanomeline (an M1-agonist drug) when compared to non-ε4 AD subjects. While the conversion rate of mildly cognitively impaired (MCI) elderly subject to probable/possible AD is greatly influenced by the apoE4 allele, the clinical response to donepezil and galantamine was shown to be apoE4 dependent in MCI patients.[93]

The disease is not likely to be cured or prevented by controlling one factor. Instead, the implication is that the presence of multiple mechanisms provides multiple sites for therapy, including, specifically, therapy directed at the cholinergic system, lipid homeostasis and at the inflammatory/amyloidogenic component. These therapies are not likely to be mutually exclusive. Therefore, many of the medications now in development or clinical trial may have a place in the treatment of AD. This formulation also implies that biologically important subgroups of AD patients may respond differently to different treatments. An example is the effect of apoE status on response to cholinomimetic therapy. A butyrylcholinesterase K variant, which was first described as a potent genetic risk factor for common AD,[94,95] was also recently shown to modulate the clinical efficacy of cholinergic[38] symptomatic therapies in a multicentre, randomized parallel group study in moderate-to-severe AD subjects.

Since disease stabilizing therapies for this syndrome are now emerging, an important aim of research into clinical and laboratory diagnosis will be to develop means to target specific treatments to specific subgroups of patients with AD. For this reason, one has now to consider molecular diagnostic as part of the therapeutic strategy of today's clinical practice.

REFERENCES

1. van Duijn CM, Hendriks L, Cruts M, et al. Amyloid precursor protein gene mutation in early-onset Alzheimer's disease [letter]. Lancet 1991; 337:978.
2. Hardy J. New insights into the genetics of Alzheimer's disease. Ann Med 1996; 28:255–258.
3. Katzman R. Alzheimer's disease as an age-dependent disorder. Ciba Found Symp 1988; 134:69–85.
4. Mann DM, Yates PO, Marcynuik B. Age and Alzheimer's disease. Lancet 1984; 1:281–282.
5. Flood DG, Buell SJ, Horwitz GJ, Coleman PD. Dendritic extent in human dentate gyrus granule cells in normal aging and senile dementia. Brain Res 1987; 402:205–216.
6. Arendt T, Schindler C, Bruckner MK, et al. Plastic neuronal remodeling is impaired in patients with Alzheimer's disease carrying apolipoprotein epsilon 4 allele. J Neurosci 1997; 17:516–529.
7. Poirier J, Delisle MC, Quirion R, et al. Apolipoprotein E4 allele as a predictor of cholinergic deficits and treatment outcome in Alzheimer disease. Proc Natl Acad Sci USA 1995; 92:12260–12264.
8. Tanzi RE, Bertram L. New frontiers in Alzheimer's disease genetics. Neuron 2001; 32:181–184.
9. Gatz M, Fratiglioni L, Johansson B, et al. Complete ascertainment of dementia in the Swedish Twin Registry: the HARMONY study. Neurobiol Aging 2005; 26:439–447.
10. Gatz M, Pedersen NL, Berg S, et al. Heritability for Alzheimer's disease: the study of dementia in Swedish twins. J Gerontol A Biol Sci Med Sci 1997; 52:M117–M125.
11. Raiha I, Kaprio J, Koskenvuo M, Rajala T, Sourander L. Alzheimer's disease in twins. Biomed Pharmacother 1997; 51:101–104.
12. Poirier J, Davignon J, Bouthillier D, Kogan S, Bertrand, Gauthier S. Apolipoprotein E polymorphism and Alzheimer's disease [see comments]. Lancet 1993; 342:697–699.
13. Strittmatter WJ, Saunders AM, Schmechel D, et al. Apolipoprotein E: high-avidity binding to beta-amyloid and increased frequency of type 4 allele in late-onset familial Alzheimer disease. Proc Natl Acad Sci USA 1993; 90:1977–1981.
14. Heston LL, Mastri AR, Anderson VE, White J. Dementia of the Alzheimer type. Clinical genetics, natural history, and associated conditions. Arch Gen Psychiatry 1981; 38:1085–1090.
15. Robakis NK, Wisniewski HM, Jenkins EC, et al. Chromosome 21q21 sublocalisation of gene encoding beta-amyloid peptide in cerebral vessels and neuritic (senile) plaques of people with Alzheimer disease and Down syndrome. Lancet 1987; 1:384–385.
16. Goldgaber D, Lerman MI, McBride OW, Saffiotti U, Gajdusek DC. Characterization and chromosomal localization of a cDNA encoding brain amyloid of Alzheimer's disease. Science 1987; 235:877–880.
17. Schellenberg GD, Bird TD, Wijsman EM, et al. Genetic linkage evidence for a familial Alzheimer's disease locus on chromosome 14. Science 1992; 258:668–671.
18. St George-Hyslop P, Haines J, Rogaev E, et al. Genetic evidence for a novel familial Alzheimer's disease locus on chromosome 14. Nat Genet 1992; 2:330–334.
19. Marjaux E, Hartmann D, De SB. Presenilins in memory, Alzheimer's disease, and therapy. Neuron 2004; 42:189–192.
20. Sherrington R, Rogaev E, Liang Y, et al. Cloning of a gene bearing missense mutations in early-onset familial Alzheimer's disease. Nature 1995; 375:754–760.
21. Schellenberg GD, Boehnke M, Wijsman EM, et al. Genetic association and linkage analysis of the apolipoprotein CII locus and familial Alzheimer's disease. Ann Neurol 1992; 31:223–227.
22. Diedrich JF, Minnigan H, Carp RI, et al. Neuropathological changes in scrapie and Alzheimer's disease are associated with increased expression of apolipoprotein E and cathepsin D in astrocytes. J Virol 1991; 65:4759–4768.
23. Poirier J, Hess M, May PC, Finch CE. Cloning of hippocampal poly(A) RNA sequences that increase after entorhinal cortex lesion in adult rat. Brain Res Mol Brain Res 1991; 9:191–195.
24. Boyles JK, Zoellner CD, Anderson LJ, et al. A role for apolipoprotein E, apolipoprotein A-I, and low density lipoprotein receptors in cholesterol transport during regeneration and remyelination of the rat sciatic nerve. J Clin Invest 1989; 83:1015–1031.
25. Poirier J, May PC, Osterburg HH, Geddes J, Cotman C, Finch CE. Alterations of gene expression in rat hippocampus after entorhinal cortex lesioning. Proc Natl Acad Sci USA 1990; 87:303–307.
26. Poirier J. Apolipoprotein E and cholesterol metabolism in the pathogenesis and treatment of Alzheimer's disease. Trends Mol Med 2003; 9:94–101.
27. Farrer LA, Cupples A, Haines JL, et al. Effects of age, sex and ethnicity on the association between apolipoprotein E genotype and Alzheimer disease. A meta-analysis. JAMA 1997; 278:1349–1356.
28. Davignon J, Gregg RE, Sing CF. Apolipoprotein E polymorphism and atherosclerosis. Arteriosclerosis 1988; 8:1–21.
29. Corder EH, Saunders AM, Strittmatter WJ, et al. Gene dose of apolipoprotein E type 4 allele and the risk of Alzheimer's disease in late onset families [see comments]. Science 1993; 261:921–923.
30. Farlow M, Lane R, Kudaravalli S, He Y. Differential qualitative responses to rivastigmine in APOE epsilon 4 carriers and noncarriers. Pharmacogenomics J 2004; 4:332–335.
31. Beffert U, Poirier J. Apolipoprotein E, plaques, tangles and cholinergic dysfunction in Alzheimer's disease. Neurobiol Alzheimer's Dis 1996; 777:166–174.

32. Schmechel DE, Saunders AM, Strittmatter WJ, et al. Increased amyloid beta-peptide deposition in cerebral cortex as a consequence of apolipoprotein E genotype in late-onset Alzheimer disease. Proc Natl Acad Sci USA 1993; 90:9649–9653.

33. Bales KR, Verina T, Cummins DJ, et al. Apolipoprotein E is essential for amyloid deposition in the APP(V717F) transgenic mouse model of Alzheimer's disease. Proc Natl Acad Sci USA 1999; 96:15233–15238.

34. Soininen H, Kosunen O, Helisalmi S, et al. A severe loss of choline acetyltransferase in the frontal cortex of Alzheimer patients carrying apolipoprotein epsilon 4 allele. Neurosci Lett 1995; 187:79–82.

35. Farlow MR, Lahiri DK, Poirier J, et al. Treatment outcome of tacrine therapy depends on apolipoprotein genotype and gender of the subjects with Alzheimer's disease. Neurology 1998; 50:669–677.

36. Poirier J, Sevigny P. Apolipoprotein E4, cholinergic integrity and the pharmacogenetics of Alzheimer's disease. J Neural Trans 1998; 53 (Suppl):199–207.

37. Richard F, Helbecque N, Neuman E, et al. APOE genotyping and response to drug treatment in Alzheimer's disease [letter]. Lancet 1997; 349:539.

38. Bullock R, Touchon J, Bergman H, et al. Rivastigmine and donepezil treatment in moderate to moderately-severe Alzheimer's disease over a 2-year period. Curr Med Res Opin 2005 21:1317–1327.

39. Corso EA, Campo G, Triglio A, et al. Prevalence of moderate and severe Alzheimer dementia and multiinfarct dementia in the population of southeastern Sicily. Ital J Neurol Sci 1992; 13:215–219.

40. Manubens JM, Martinezlage JM, Lacruz F, et al. Prevalence of Alzheimer's disease and other dementing disorders in Pamplona, Spain. Neuroepidemiology 1995; 14:155–164.

41. Rocca WA, Cha RH, Waring SC, Kokmen E. Incidence of dementia and Alzheimer's disease: a reanalysis of data from Rochester, Minnesota, 1975–1984. Am J Epidemiol 1998; 148:51–62.

42. Chandra V, Kokmen E, Schoenberg BS, Beard CM. Head trauma with loss of consciousness as a risk factor for Alzheimer's disease. Neurology 1989; 39:1576–1578.

43. Gedye A, Beattie BL, Tuokko H, Horton A, Korsarek E. Severe head injury hastens age of onset of Alzheimer's disease. J Am Geriatr Soc 1989; 37:970–973.

44. Mayeux R, Ottman R, Maestre G, et al. Synergistic effects of traumatic head injury and apolipoprotein-epsilon 4 in patients with Alzheimer's disease [see comments]. Neurology 1995; 45:555–557.

45. Levine SM, Chakrabarty A. The role of iron in the pathogenesis of experimental allergic encephalomyelitis and multiple sclerosis. Ann NY Acad Sci 2004; 1012:252–266.

46. Perry G, Cash AD, Smith MA. Alzheimer Disease and Oxidative Stress. J Bromed Biotechnol 2002; 2:120–123.

47. Sparks DL, Lochhead J, Horstman D, Wagoner T, Martin T. Water quality has a pronounced effect on cholesterol-induced accumulation of Alzheimer amyloid beta (Abeta) in rabbit brain. J Alzheimers Dis 2002; 4:523–529.

48. Campbell A. The potential role of aluminium in Alzheimer's disease. Nephrol Dial Transplant 2002; 17:17–20.

49. Sparks DL, Scheff SW, Hunsaker JC III, et al. Induction of Alzheimer-like beta-amyloid immunoreactivity in the brains of rabbits with dietary cholesterol. Exp Neurol 1994; 126:88–94.

50. Skoog I. Vascular aspects in Alzheimer's disease. J Neural Transm Suppl 2000; 59:37–43.

51. Brun A, Englund E. A white matter disorder in dementia of the Alzheimer type: a pathoanatomical study. Ann Neurol 1986; 19:253–262.

52. Hardy J, Allsop D. Amyloid deposition as the central event in the aetiology of Alzheimer's disease. Trends Pharmacol Sci 1991; 12:383–388.

53. Khachaturian ZS. Diagnosis of Alzheimer's disease. Arch Neurol 1985; 42:1097–1105.

54. Van Nostrand WE, Wagner SL, Farrow JS, Cunningham DD. Immunopurification and protease inhibitory properties of protease nexin-2/amyloid beta-protein precursor. J Biol Chem 1990; 265:9591–9594.

55. Selkoe DJ, Schenk D. Alzheimer's disease: molecular understanding predicts amyloid-based therapeutics. Annu Rev Pharmacol Toxicol 2003; 43:545–584.

56. Thase ME, Tigner R, Smeltzer DJ, Liss L. Age-related neuropsychological deficits in Down's syndrome. Biol Psychiatry 1984; 19:571–585.

57. Sandhu FA, Salim M, Zain SB. Expression of the human beta-amyloid protein of Alzheimer's disease specifically in the brains of transgenic mice. J Biol Chem 1991; 266:21331–21334.

58. Ohuchi K, Matsuda A, Maeda S, Shimada K, Miyakawa T. A transgenic mouse line developed to express human amyloidogenic transthyretin cDNA in the brain. Biochem Int 1991; 23:809–817.

59. Games D, Adams D, Alessandrini R, et al. Alzheimer-type neuropathology in transgenic mice overexpressing V717F beta-amyloid precursor protein [see comments]. Nature 1995; 373:523–527.

60. Borchelt DR, Thinakaran G, Eckman CB, et al. Familial Alzheimer's disease-linked presenilin 1 variants elevate Abeta1-42/1-40 ratio in vitro and in vivo. Neuron 1996; 17:1005–1013.

61. Terry RD, Katzman R. Senile dementia of the Alzheimer type. Ann Neurol 1983; 14:497–506.

62. Kosik KS. Tau protein and Alzheimer's disease. Curr Opin Cell Biol 1990; 2:101–104.

63. Drubin DG, Caput D, Kirschner MW. Studies on the expression of the microtubule-associated protein, tau, during mouse brain development, with newly isolated complementary DNA probes. J Cell Biol 1984; 98:1090–1097.

64. Stamer K, Vogel R, Thies E, Mandelkow E, Mandelkow EM. Tau blocks traffic of organelles, neurofilaments, and APP vesicles in neurons and enhances oxidative stress. J Cell Biol 2002; 156:1051–1063.

65. Takei Y, Teng J, Harada A, Hirokawa N. Defects in axonal elongation and neuronal migration in mice with disrupted tau and map1b genes. J Cell Biol 2000; 150:989–1000.

66. Teng J, Takei Y, Harada A, et al. Synergistic effects of MAP2 and MAP1B knockout in neuronal migration, dendritic outgrowth, and microtubule organization. J Cell Biol 2001; 155:65–76.

67. Savonenko AV, Xu GM, Price DL, Borchelt DR, Markowska AL. Normal cognitive behavior in two distinct congenic lines of transgenic mice hyperexpressing mutant APP SWE. Neurobiol Dis 2003; 12:194–211.

68. Arriagada PV, Growdon JH, Hedley-Whyte ET, Hyman BT. Neurofibrillary tangles but not senile plaques parallel duration and severity of Alzheimer's disease. Neurology 1992; 42:631–639.

69. Pei JJ, Braak H, An WL, et al. Up-regulation of mitogen-activated protein kinases ERK1/2 and MEK1/2 is associated

with the progression of neurofibrillary degeneration in Alzheimer's disease. Brain Res Mol Brain Res 2002; 109: 45–55.

70. Rogers J, Mufson EJ. Demonstrating immune-related antigens in Alzheimer's disease brain tissue. Neurobiol Aging 1990; 11:477–479.

71. McGeer PL, McGeer EG, Kawamata T, Yamada T, Akiyama H. Reactions of the immune system in chronic degenerative neurological diseases. Can J Neurol Sci 1991; 18(3 suppl): 376–379.

72. Johnson SA, Lampert-Etchells M, Pasinetti GM, Rozovsky I, Finch CE. Complement mRNA in the mammalian brain: responses to Alzheimer's disease and experimental brain lesioning. Neurobiol Aging 1992; 13:641–648.

73. Rogers J, Cooper NR, Webster S, et al. Complement activation by beta-amyloid in Alzheimer disease. Proc Natl Acad Sci USA 1992; 89:10016–10020.

74. Rich JB, Rasmusson DX, Folstein MF, et al. Nonsteroidal anti-inflammatory drugs in Alzheimer's disease. Neurology 1995; 45:51–55.

75. Eriksen JL, Sagi SA, Smith TE, et al. NSAIDs and enantiomers of flurbiprofen target gamma-secretase and lower Abeta 42 in vivo. J Clin Invest 2003; 112:440–449.

76. Yan Q, Zhang J, Liu H, et al. Anti-inflammatory drug therapy alters beta-amyloid processing and deposition in an animal model of Alzheimer's disease. J Neurosci 2003; 23: 7504–7509.

77. Reines SA, Block GA, Morris JC, et al. Rofecoxib: no effect on Alzheimer's disease in a 1-year, randomized, blinded, controlled study. Neurology 2004; 62:66–71.

78. Aisen PS, Schafer KA, Grundman M, et al. Effects of rofecoxib or naproxen vs placebo on Alzheimer disease progression: a randomized controlled trial. JAMA 2003; 289: 2819–2826.

79. Scharf S, Mander A, Ugoni A, Vajda F, Christophidis N. A double-blind, placebo-controlled trial of diclofenac/misoprostol in Alzheimer's disease. Neurology 1999; 53:197–201.

80. Terry RD. Normal aging and Alzheimer's disease: growing problems. Monogr Pathol 1990; 32:41–54.

81. DeKosky ST, Scheff SW. Synapse loss in frontal cortex biopsies in Alzheimer's disease: correlation with cognitive severity. Ann Neurol 1990; 27:457–464.

82. Terry RD, Masliah E, Salmon DP, et al. Physical basis of cognitive alterations in Alzheimer's disease: synapse loss is the major correlate of cognitive impairment. Ann Neurol 1990; 30:572–580.

83. Tabaton M, Mandybur TI, Perry G, et al. The widespread alteration of neurites in Alzheimer's disease may be unrelated to amyloid deposition. Ann Neurol 1989; 26: 771–778.

84. DeKosky ST, Scheff SW, Styren SD. Structural correlates of cognition in dementia: Quantification and assessment of synapse change. Neurodegeneration 1996; 5:417–421.

85. Roberts GW, Allsop D, Bruton C. The occult aftermath of boxing. J Neurol Neurosurg Psychiatry 1990; 53:373–378.

86. Jordan BD, Relkin NR, Ravdin LD, et al. Apolipoprotein E epsilon4 associated with chronic traumatic brain injury in boxing. JAMA 1997; 278:136–140.

87. Kutner KC, Erlanger DM, Tsai J, Jordan B, Relkin NR. Lower cognitive performance of older football players possessing apolipoprotein E epsilon 4. Neurosurgery 2000; 47: 651–657.

88. Chiang MF, Chang JG, Hu CJ. Association between apolipoprotein E genotype and outcome of traumatic brain injury. Acta Neurochir (Wien) 2003; 145:649–653.

89. Meske V, Albert F, Richter D, Schwarze J, Ohm TG. Blockade of HMG-CoA reductase activity causes changes in microtubule-stabilizing protein tau via suppression of geranylgeranylpyrophosphate formation: implications for Alzheimer's disease. Eur J Neurosci 2003; 17:93–102.

90. Ramassamy C, Krzywkowski P, Averill D, et al. Impact of apoE deficiency on oxidative insults and antioxidant levels in the brain. Brain Res Mol Brain Res 2001; 86:76–83.

91. Pussinen PJ, Lindner H, Glatter O, et al. Lipoprotein-associated alpha-tocopheryl-succinate inhibits cell growth and induces apoptosis in human MCF-7 and HBL-100 breast cancer cells. Biochim Biophys Acta 2000; 1485: 129–144.

92. Poirier J. Apolipoprotein E: a pharmacogenetic target for the treatment of Alzheimer's disease. Mol Diagn 1999; 4:335–341.

93. Petersen RC, Thomas RG, Grundman M, et al. Vitamin E and donepezil for the treatment of mild cognitive impairment. N Engl J Med 2005; 352:2379–2388.

94. Lehmann DJ, Johnston C, Smith AD. Synergy between the genes for butyrylcholinesterase K variant and apolipoprotein E4 in late-onset confirmed Alzheimer's disease. Hum Mol Genet 1997; 6:1933–1936.

95. Wiebusch H, Poirier J, Sevigny P, Schappert K. Further evidence for a synergistic association between APOE epsilon4 and BCHE-K in confirmed Alzheimer's disease. Hum Genet 1999; 104:158–163.

3

Pathophysiology: an epidemiological perspective

Lenore J Launer

INTRODUCTION

Frequency

Dementia is the most common neurological disease in the elderly. From studies based on large populations it is estimated that 2.5 cases of dementia develop per 1000 persons/year among 65-year-olds; by 90 years of age the number of new cases increases to 85.6 cases per 1000. Alzheimer's disease (AD), followed by vascular dementia (VaD) are the most common subtypes of dementia.[1]

Diagnosis

Currently AD and VaD are classified as different diseases. Globally, AD is clinically characterized by progressive brain atrophy, loss of cognitive function including memory, orientation and language, and exclusion of any other cause of dementia. The basis of AD pathology is considered to be neuritic plaques (NPs), and neurofibrillary tangles (NFTs) and marked brain atrophy. VaD has a more heterogeneous course: it is characterized by impairment of executive functions such as attention, speed of processing and planning and, variously, by memory impairment, motor impairment, mood changes and urinary incontinence.[2] Most typically VaD is a sequale of small or large vessel disease.

In epidemiological studies, dementia and subtypes are diagnosed according to international guidelines. The most commonly used research criteria to diagnose dementia are the DSM-IV[3] (or earlier versions) and ICD-10 guidelines,[4] the NINDS-ADRDA guidelines[5] are used to diagnose AD. These guidelines are operationalized with relatively good reliability.[6] There is less agreement about the guidelines used to diagnose

vascular dementia. The most commonly used are the ADDTC[7] and NINDS-AIREN[8] criteria. However, the validity and reliability of these guidelines have not been as well tested as those for dementia and AD; efforts are underway to better define diagnostic guidelines for vascular dementia (see Chapter 1).

Disease characteristics

Mixed clinical presentation

There is substantial overlap in structural and functional characteristics of AD and VaD.[9,10] For instance, a recent meta-analysis[11] suggested that changes in episodic memory are generally predictive of AD when persons are in the pre-clinical stage of the disease. However, persons who develop AD also perform poorly on tests of subcortical function, which is usually impaired in vascular related cognitive impairment.[12] Another example of overlapping clinical symptoms is the frequently used magnetic resonance image (MRI) marker of hippocampal atrophy. Atrophy in this critical brain region has been found more often in AD cases compared to controls,[13] but other subtypes of dementia may also be accompanied by atrophy in this region.[14] Conversely, typical VaD features are also found in AD cases including large and small infarcts[15] and white matter lesions.[10]

Distinguishing between AD and VaD has proven difficult given the overlap in the symptoms. There are no generally accepted sensitive and specific markers of AD or VaD. There is a new initiative to identify functional, biological or image-based biomarkers of AD.[16]

Prevalence of mixed neuropathology

In neuropathological specimens, cerebrovascular disease in both AD and VaD has been described, including disruption of the endothelium, basement membranes and blood–brain barrier, focal necrosis and blood vessels that are elongated, tortuous and have thickened walls, with evidence of lipohyalinosis.[2,9,15]

Dementia cases occurring in late age often have mixed pathology. A study in a large United Kingdom population-based autopsy series of 209 persons showed that 46 per cent of the dementia cases and 33 per cent of the non-demented participants had multiple vascular lesions, most of which constituted small vessel disease.[17] In the Honolulu Asia Aging Study (HAAS) autopsy study of 333 Japanese American men (mean age 78 years), only 9 per cent had no AD or vascular lesions, 31 per cent had only AD lesions and 68 per cent had mixed pathology.[18] Together, the epidemiological, clinical and neuropathological data suggest that AD is phenotypically heterogeneous and can at a minimum be subclassified based on the extent of mixed pathology.

Hypothesized disease mechanisms

Amyloid cascade
One of the central mechanisms hypothesized to contribute to AD is the beta-amyloid (β-amyloid) cascade. According to this hypothesis, amyloid precursor protein (APP) processing is altered to form modified proteins (i.e., β-amyloid 40–42) that lose normal function and become neurotoxic.[19] The production of these proteins leads to the extracellular accumulation and deposition of β-amyloid 40–42 oligomers. This sets off a cascade that leads to the formation of neuritic plaques, microglia activation, oxidative stress and possibly hyperphosphorolation of tau and neurofibrillary tangles.

Vascular
Because of the heterogeneity in the anatomical substrate of vascular lesions that may impair cognition, there are several pathophysiological mechanisms that could lead to neurodegeneration. For example, atherosclerosis, thrombosis and haemodynamic disturbances can all contribute to vascular lesions and subsequent hypoperfusion to the brain, generation of an inflammatory response and oxidative stress,[20,21] leading to neuronal death.

Disease mechanisms common to AD and VaD
There are several pathophysiological processes that are common to vascular disease and AD and that may underlie the observed associations. These include oxidative stress,[22,23] inflammation,[24,25] glucose dysregulation,[26] impaired lipid metabolism[21] and genetic

susceptibility factors. Many of these pathways are inter-related: for instance, pro- and anti-inflammatory events are stimulated by triggers such as β-amyloid toxicity,[27] as well as by vascular injury and ischaemia caused by hypertension, atherosclerosis and hypercholesterolemia;[21] oxidative stress may modulate inflammatory pathways[24] and glucose dysregulation may generate an inflammatory response.[28]

Associations between vascular factors and AD have been reported for clinical presentation and risk. Several studies show more severe clinical presentation in cases with both AD and vascular disease compared to those with no vascular disease.[29,30] An association between AD and cardiovascular risk factors and disease has also been reported.[31-33] Much of this evidence is based on cohorts from the community that were diagnosed as demented with standardized protocols applied to the total sample. With this approach a wide range of mild to severe cases with a spectrum of clinical symptoms can be identified, giving a different mix of cases than those identified in specialized clinic settings. This makes it possible to detect associations that are more prevalent in the general population compared to selected clinic populations. Here we will review the epidemiological evidence for an association of cardiovascular risk factors and disease.

RISK FACTORS

Based on cardiovascular disease epidemiology, four levels of risk factors can be conceptualized: non-modifiable factors, modifiable life style factors, physiological factors and disease.

Non-modifiable risk factors

Genes
To date, the mutations in the amyloid pre-processing protein, presenilin 1 and presenilin 2 have been identified in large families with early onset (i.e., <65 years of age) AD. These mutations have provided evidence for a role of amyloid processing in AD, but reflect monogenic disorders that are very rare, probably explaining less than 0.5 per cent of all AD cases. It is likely that the 'typical' AD cases, such as those detected in older community dwelling men and women, are not only phenotypically heterogeneous, but also genetically heterogeneous, with multiple genes making small contributions to the disease.[34]

Considerable effort is going into identifying genes for AD. To date the only major susceptibility gene that has been identified is the apolipoprotein E polymorphism; out of the three alleles, the ε4 increases the risk for AD. The allele frequency varies by ethnic group, and the risk associated with the ε4 allele varies by age, with a peak at about 60–65 years of age.[35] Based on simulation[36] and empirical studies there is evidence that other genes exist, but these have proven difficult to identify.

In addition to specific genes modulating amyloid or tau, genetic susceptibility may also be conferred by clusters of genes that are involved in such diseases as hypertension, diabetes and in processes such as the inflammatory response and oxidative stress. For example, studies have found associations of AD with polymorphisms of the ACE gene (which is involved in blood pressure regulation[37]) and with polymorphisms regulating Il-1 cytokine levels.[38] However, in general, the associations between such candidate genes and AD have not been as consistently replicated, as has the finding on apoE polymorphism, in different AD case groups defined by age of onset, ethnicity and family history.

Genetic factors undoubtedly play an important role in determining one's susceptibility for AD, but other factors are important, and increase in importance as a person ages.[39]

Gender differences

Despite the publication of numerous studies, it is still unclear whether men and women have a different risk for AD. Some studies have found an increased risk for AD in women compared to men,[40,41] while others have not.[42–44] Many of these studies are based on small population sizes, particularly at older ages when the incidence of dementia increases exponentially. In the largest study published on this question, with 525 incident cases of dementia, women had a higher risk for AD, particularly over the age of 85 years, and the same risk for VaD as men.[41] The expression of disease may also vary by sex. In a neuropathological study of religious order members, women had a greater probability of being diagnosed with AD during life, especially among the men and women with relatively a high number of NFTs and NPs.[45]

Early education

The link between early educational attainment and the risk for AD was one of the first risk factors to be extensively studied. There have been several prospective studies linking low educational level to an increased risk for AD,[46–48] although some studies do not find an association[49] or find an association only in a subgroup of the cohort, such as women.[50]

Biological, social and methodological hypotheses have been put forward to explain how education may directly or indirectly modify the risk for AD.

Methodological explanations include inadequate control for cardiovascular risk factors that might be more prevalent in those with lower education, systematic non-participation in higher educated persons at risk for AD[50] and screening bias such that those with lower education fall more often below cognitive score cut-points used to select subjects for further dementia work-up. Other hypotheses relate to the life circumstances of people with lower education. For instance, education may reflect early life experiences or low socio-economic status accompanied by stress-related increases in cortisol, which has been shown to impair hippocampal function.[51,52]

A hypothesis of current interest relates to education as a proxy for 'cognitive reserve'. This concept reflects the 'quantity and quality' of functional brain matter and an individual's capacity to use it to manage impairment and adapt performance in the presence of disease.[53,54] The concept of cognitive reserve has been illustrated in studies showing that, compared to subjects with lower education, those with higher education have greater metabolic deficits when they finally reach the clinical threshold of dementia. Education may also be a marker for engagement in cognitively stimulating activities.[55] Experimental studies suggest that exposure to an enriched environment may be accompanied by an increase in cortical thickness and number of synapses.[56]

Lifestyle factors

Smoking

There are several pathways through which smoking can contribute to both neuropathological and vascular disease. Smoking has well-known effects on the cardiovascular system that increase the risk for coronary and cerebral disease.[57] Cigarette smoke contains free radicals,[58] thereby increasing the risk for oxidative stress, activating phagocytes and generating more oxidative damage.[59] Compared with non-smokers, smokers also have a lower dietary intake of antioxidants[60] and therefore may have even less defence against oxidative stress.

Data from early case-control studies suggested smoking was associated with a reduced risk for AD.[61] Indeed, experimental studies show nicotine has neuroprotective effects.[62] Recent prospective cohort studies, however, have repeatedly indicated smokers have an increased risk of AD,[1,63–65] particularly those with no apoE ε4 allele. There is evidence that middle-aged smokers with the ε4 die disproportionately early,[66] so the effect only in non-ε4 carriers may reflect a mortality bias of ε4s who were at risk for AD. This needs further study. Smoking has also been shown to increase the risk for cognitive decline in middle age, when mortality is much lower.[67]

Physical activity

Physical activity (PA) may increase brain neurotropins, specifically brain-derived neurotrophic factors, which in animals improve performance in cognitive-related activities.[68] PA also has several benefits related to improved vascular health and reduced risk for cardiovascular disease.[69] There have been a few studies published on the relationship of PA to risk for dementia. Some studies show a reduced risk for dementia in those with increased levels of PA.[70] However, others show a reduced risk for dementia only in subsamples, such as those who carry the apoE ε4 allele,[71] and other studies show no effect.[55] Additional studies on PA are needed to better understand the association.

Diet

Diet may be another modifiable risk factor for AD. Several dietary constituents have been investigated including saturated fat, hypothesized to increase atherosclerosis,[72] polyunsaturated fatty acids, hypothesized to reduce atherosclerosis and inflammation,[73] alcohol, moderate intake of which may reduce cardiovascular risk,[74] and folate and B12 in their role as homocysteine intermediaries.[75] Antioxidants, in their role against oxidative stress, have been the most frequently studied.

Frequently consumed antioxidants include carotenoids (beta-carotene), ascorbic acid (vitamin C), tocopherols (vitamin E) and flavonoids. Prospective studies reported a reduced risk for AD associated with increased intake of dietary antioxidants,[76–78] but the same benefits were not found in vitamin supplement users.[76,78–80] Possibly, too high a level of antioxidant intake leads to a paradoxical increase in oxidative stress,[81] but additional research is needed. Another aspect that needs to be taken into account when interpreting these studies is the difficulty of obtaining valid and reliable dietary data in studies of older persons, some of whom may have incipient dementia.[82] Midlife antioxidant dietary intake was not associated with late-life dementia.[83]

Trials investigating the effects of antioxidant vitamins on cognitive function and dementia have also had inconsistent results. Compared to placebo, treatment with vitamin E for 2 years in 341 cases of moderate severe probable AD was beneficial in slowing the progression of disease, but no improvement in cognitive test scores was detected.[84] In the MRC/BHF Heart Protection Study, 20 536 individuals were randomized to receive either antioxidant vitamin supplements (vitamins E and C, and beta-carotene) or placebo; no difference was observed between groups in the percentage identified as cognitively impaired or in mean cognitive scores after 5 years of treatment.[85] In addition, no difference was observed in the number of individuals who developed dementia during follow-up. A large randomized trial is underway to test the effects of gingko biloba, an alternative medicine with antioxidant properties, on the occurrence of dementia in persons 75 years and older (http://NCCAM.nih.gov).

Physiological risk factors

Blood pressure

Several metabolic events associated with hypertension have been implicated in neuronal death as well as vascular damage.[86] Elevated levels of blood pressure (BP) may destroy the blood–brain barrier integrity around capillaries and result in hylination.[20] Cerebral blood flow is reduced, which impairs the delivery to the brain of nutrients. Hypertension may also increase free radical damage through an imbalance in nitric oxide production caused by endothelial damage.[87] High BP may modulate pathways that regulate cellular calcium homeostasis and related excitotoxic and oxidative reactions.[88] Further, experimental studies suggest that the extracellular accumulation of APP and cleavage to β-amyloid does occur under extreme hypoxic conditions[89] caused by vessel damage. Hypertension is also a risk factor for atherosclerosis.[90] At the other end of the spectrum, animal studies suggest hypotension can lead to ischaemic conditions that promote neuronal death.[91]

The dementing disease process may also affect BP. For example, vasoconstrictive properties of circulating serum β-amyloid in pre-clinical stages of AD may lead to increased BP,[92] although typically BP decreases in the period prior to diagnosis.[33] Early neurodegeneration in areas such as the hypothalamus can lead to impaired blood pressure regulation.

High BP has been associated with the risk for late-life cognitive impairment,[93] white matter lesions,[94,95] hippocampal atrophy,[96] clinical dementia,[33,97] and neuropathological markers of AD.[98] Data from the HAAS[97] and the Finnish Kuopio study[99] showed that the risk for late-life AD increased with increasing BP measured in mid-life, more than 20 years prior.

Some studies have not shown a significantly increased risk for brain ageing associated with elevated BP.[100,101] These mixed findings have intensified the debate about whether or not older persons should be treated for hypertension.[102] There is some concern that older persons already adapted to high BP would not be able to sufficiently perfuse their brains if their BP was lowered. However, the duration of follow-up, age at baseline and history of treatment with antihypertensives may explain much of the discrepancy among the studies. In particular, the timing of the BP measure relative to dementia assessment is an important factor modifying the association of BP with dementia, as BP declines with incipient dementia.[33]

Several observational studies suggest that persons using antihypertensive medication have a lower risk for AD.[103,104] In the HAAS study the hypertensive men never treated with antihypertensives constituted the group at the highest risk for dementia.[97] In the Kungsholmen study of persons older than 75 years of age, use of diuretics was associated with a lower risk for AD.[103]

As yet, there are limited data from clinical trials informing on the efficacy of controlling BP to reduce the incidence of dementia in older persons. Clinical trials, such as the MRC trial,[105] the SHEP trial,[106] the Syst-Eur trial[107] and the SCOPE trial[108] have reported no or moderately beneficial effects (and not harmful) of antihypertensive treatment on cognitive function or dementia. There are several trials in progress to test this question.[109]

However, there are several design features of the trials that weaken the power to detect a significant effect of treatment on the risk for AD. For instance, in many trials the entry age of the trial participants was about 60 years,[106,107] well before the age when incidence of dementia increases. The trials were conducted on specific patient populations, with relatively short treatment periods. One aspect of treatment that cannot be examined in these trials is the question as to whether long-term treatment of high BP through to late age reduces the risk of dementia.

Inflammation

To better understand the role of inflammation in dementia, identify relevant biomarkers for dementia and select individuals who may have an 'inflammation-related' genetic susceptibility to dementia, several different measures of inflammation and inflammatory response have been explored in epidemiological studies.

Non-steroidal anti-inflammatory medications

Consumption of non-steroidal anti-inflammatory medications (NSAIDs) has been used in many epidemiological studies as a marker of 'dampened inflammatory response'. In a recent review of incidence studies, the pooled effect size of the association of NSAID use and incident AD was estimated to be

0.79 (0.68–0.92).[110] Based on pharmacy records of NSAID use, risk has been shown to decrease in a dose-dependent way, with increasing use of NSAIDs.[111]

Serum markers of inflammation

A study based on the HAAS[112] suggested a raised level of mid-life CRP significantly increased the risk 25 years later for dementia, including AD with or without cardiovascular disease contributing to the dementia. The risk estimates were moderately reduced after controlling for cardiovascular risk factors, suggesting these factors partially explain the association of mid-life CRP and late-life AD. The Rotterdam Study investigated the risk for AD and late-life markers of inflammation. They found α_1 antichymotrypsin and interleukin (Il)-6, and CRP to a lesser extent, were associated with an increased risk for dementia.[113]

Randomized clinical trials

Randomized clinical trials to test the benefits of NSAIDs have been conducted for relatively short periods of time in patients who were already diagnosed with AD.[114] To date, none of these trials have demonstrated efficacy of NSAIDs in this patient group.

Diabetes

Dysregulation in glucose metabolism has been shown in in vitro and in vivo studies to cause vascular[115] and neuronal damage.[116] Hyperglycaemia leads to advanced glycated end products (AGEPs), which have been shown to impair vascular and endothelial function, damage proteins, DNA and mitochondrial and increase free radicals and inflammatory responses. AGEPs have been found to co-localize with amyloid deposition.[117] Further, receptors on AGEPs may mediate amyloid toxicity to microglia and astrocytes.[118,119] Hyperglycaemia also alters glucose metabolism, thereby reducing the production of the memory-regulating neurotransmitter acetylcholine. On the other hand, diabetics are at increased risk for hypoglycaemic events, which disturb the delivery of nutrients to the brain and increase the amount of glutamate, a neurotoxin, in the brain.

Diabetes increases the risk for cognitive decline,[120] AD-like and vascular brain changes measured on MRI,[121,122] and neuropathological changes, including neuritic plaques and cerebral amyloid angiopathy.[123]

There are now several large population-based cohort studies in which diabetics were estimated to have a 2–3 times increased risk for AD compared to normoglycaemic subjects. This is a fairly robust finding as the studies are based on different ethnic/race/lifestyle groups, including Japanese-American men,[123] a mixed ethnic/race cohort,[124] European Caucasians[125,126] and religious order members.[127] The results of four of these studies suggest diabetics are at higher risk for AD, and in particular AD combined with cerebrovascular disease.

Besides diabetes, co-morbidities including hypertension (reviewed above), high cholesterol and hyperinsulinaemia have also been reported to increase the risk for AD.

Other co-morbid conditions with diabetes: hypercholesterolaemia

The transport of cholesterol out of degenerating cells and to regenerating cells contributes to cell viability; disturbed cholesterol transport may alter membrane composition, leading to neurodegeneration.[128] Cholesterol may also be involved in the deposition of β-amyloid, perhaps through cleavage of the amyloid precursor protein (APP)[129] to β-amyloid fragments. Cholesterol has been associated with levels of the APP metabolites, Aβ.[40–42,130]

Multiple studies have examined the association of mid-life cholesterol levels with dementia. In settings such as Finland, where very high levels of cholesterol are characteristic of the population, a positive association between total cholesterol level and late-life cognitive impairment[99] and dementia[131] has been reported. However, these findings have not been replicated in other cohorts.[132] Unlike BP, there is no consistent relationship of the interval between cholesterol measure and cognition and the strength of the association. More basic research is needed to understand the role of cholesterol and lipoproteins in brain ageing. In addition, there are questions about the interpretation of the epidemiological association that need to be raised. Many studies have demonstrated that cholesterol levels are lower in persons with certain medical conditions,[133] including occult illness, such as cancer, inflammation, weight loss or change in diet that might follow events such as myocardial infarction. Grouping individuals with low cholesterol due to illness with individuals who have always had low cholesterol will make it more difficult to find a relationship, if it exists.

In a pilot randomized trial of 63 Alzheimer's patients, atorvastatin reduced circulating cholesterol levels and was associated with reduced depression symptomatology and less decline on the Alzheimer's Disease Assessment Scale – cognitive subscale at 6 months.[134] Additional trials with larger sample sizes are on-going.

Other co-morbid conditions with diabetes: hyperinsulinaemia

Insulin may prevent hyperphosphorylation of tau, thus inhibiting the formation of neurofibrillary tangles.[135] Impairment in insulin metabolism in the brain or ensuing glucose dysregulation could affect neurons directly.[26] AD cases may have impaired insulin regulation.[136] On the other hand, insulin may act as a neurotropic factor[137] and modulator of neurotransmittor activity.[138] High insulin levels have been reported as a risk factor for dementia in some epidemiological studies.[139-141]

CONCLUSION

Many lines of investigation suggest that AD and VaD share risk factors as well as pathological markers. Both diseases are phenotypically heterogeneous as well as genetically heterogeneous. It is likely there is a smaller subset of individuals with classic disease symptoms, but in older community-dwelling persons it will be clinically difficult to make a clear distinction between the two. These recent findings have implications for clinical practice as well as furthering our understanding of pathophysiological processes underlying the dementias of old age.

ACKNOWLEDGEMENT

This work was funded by the Intramural Research Program of the NIH, National Institute on Aging.

REFERENCES

1. Launer LJ, Andersen K, Dewey ME, et al. Rates and risk factors for dementia and Alzheimer's disease: results from EURODEM pooled analyses. Neurology 1999; 52:78–84.
2. Roman GC, Erkinjuntti T, Wallin A, Pantoni L, Chui HC. Subcortical ischaemic vascular dementia. Lancet Neurol 2002; 1:426–436.
3. American Psychiatric Association. Diagnostic and Statistical Manual of Mental Disorders, 4th edn. Washington DC: American Psychiatric Association 1994.
4. World Health Organization. The ICD-10 Classification of Mental and Behavioural Disorders: Diagnostic Criteria for Research. Geneva: World Health Organization 1993.
5. McKhann G, Drachman D, Folstein M, et al. Clinical diagnosis of Alzheimer's disease: report of the NINCDS-ADRDA Work group under the auspices of the Department of Health and Human Services Task force on Alzheimer's disease. Neurology 1984; 34:939–944.
6. Knopman DS, DeKosky ST, Cummings JL, et. al. Practice parameter: diagnosis of dementia (an evidence-based review). Report of the Quality Standards Subcommittee of the American Academy of Neurology. Neurology 2001; 56:1143–1153.

7. Chui HC, Victoroff JI, Margolin D, et al Criteria for the diagnosis of ischemic vascular dementia proposed by the state of California Alzheimer's Disease Diagnostic and Treatment Centers. Neurology 1992; 42:473–480.
8. Roman GC, Tatemichi TK, Erkinjuntti T, et al. Vascular dementia: diagnostic criteria for research studies. Report of the NINDS-AIREN International Workshop. Neurology 1993; 43:250–260.
9. Farkas E, Luiten PG. Cerebral microvascular pathology in aging and Alzheimer's disease. Prog Neurobiol 2001; 64:575–611.
10. Barber R, Scheltens P, Gholkar A, et al. White matter lesions on magnetic resonance imaging in dementia with Lewy bodies, Alzheimer's disease, vascular dementia, and normal aging. J Neurol Neurosurg Psychiatry 1999; 67:66–72.
11. Backman L, Jones S, Berger AK, Laukka EJ, Small BJ. Cognitive impairment in preclinical Alzheimer's disease: a meta-analysis. Neuropsychology 2005; 19:520–531.
12. Nestor PJ, Scheltens P, Hodges JR. Advances in the early detection of Alzheimer's disease. Nat Med 2004; 10:S34–S41.
13. Jack CR Jr, Petersen RC, Xu Y, et al. Rates of hippocampal atrophy correlate with change in clinical status in aging and AD. Neurology. 2000; 55:484–489.
14. Fein G, Di Sclafani V, Tanabe J, et al. Hippocampal and cortical atrophy predict dementia in subcortical ischemic vascular disease. Neurology 2000; 55:1626–1635.
15. Chui H. Neuropathology lessons in vascular dementia. Alzheimer Dis Assoc Disord 2005; 19:45–52.
16. Mueller SG, Weiner MW, Thal LJ, et al. Ways toward an early diagnosis in Alzheimer's disease: The Alzheimer's Disease Neuroimaging Initiative [ADNI]. Alzheimer's Dem 2005; 1:55–66.
17. Neuropathology Group. Medical Research Council Cognitive Function and Aging Study. Pathological correlates of late-onset dementia in a multicentre, community-based population in England and Wales. Cognitive Function and Ageing Study (MRC CFAS). Lancet 2001; 357:169–175.
18. Petrovitch H, Ross GW, Steinhorn SC, et al. AD lesions and infarcts in demented and non-demented Japanese-American men. Ann Neurol 2005; 57:98–103.
19. Selkoe DJ. Alzheimer disease: mechanistic understanding predicts novel therapies. Ann Intern Med 2004; 140:627–638.
20. De La Torre JC. Vascular basis of Alzheimer's pathogenesis. Ann NY Acad Sci 2002; 977:196–215.
21. Casserly I, Topol E. Convergence of atherosclerosis and Alzheimer's disease: inflammation, cholesterol, and misfolded proteins. Lancet 2004; 363:1139–1146.
22. Markesbery WR. Oxidative stress hypothesis in Alzheimer's disease. Free Radic Biol Med 1997; 23:134–147.
23. Diaz MN, Frei B, Vita JA, Keaney JF Jr. Antioxidants and atherosclerotic heart disease. N Engl J Med 1997; 337:408–416.
24. Rosenfeld ME. Inflammation, lipids, and free radicals: lessons learned from the atherogenic process. Semin Reprod Endocrinol 1998; 16:249–261.
25. McGeer EG, McGeer PL. Brain inflammation in Alzheimer disease and the therapeutic implications. Curr Pharm Des 1999; 5:821–836.
26. Hoyer S. Is sporadic Alzheimr's disease the brain type of non-insulin dependent diabetes mellitus? A challenging hypothesis. J Neural Transm 1998; 105:415–422.
27. Eikelenboom P, van Gool WA. Neuroinflammatory perspectives on the two faces of Alzheimer's disease. J Neural Transm 2004; 111:281–294.

28. Ziegler D. Type 2 diabetes as an inflammatory cardiovascular disorder. Curr Mol Med 2005; 5:309–322.
29. Snowdon DA, Greiner LH, Mortimer JA, et al. Brain infarction and the clinical expression of Alzheimer's disease. The Nun Study. JAMA 1997; 277:813–817.
30. Schneider JA, Wilson RS, Bienias JL, Evans DA, Bennett DA. Cerebral infarctions and the likelihood of dementia from Alzheimer's disease pathology. Neurology 2004; 62:1148–1155.
31. Launer LJ. Demonstrating the case that AD is a vascular disease: epidemiologic evidence. Ageing Res Rev 2002; 1:61–77.
32. Hofman A, Ott A, Breteler MMB, et al. Atherosclerosis, apolipoprotein E, and the prevalence of dementia and Alzheimer's disease in the Rotterdam Study. Lancet 1997; 349:151–154.
33. Skoog I, Lernfelt B, Landahl S, et al. 15-year longitudinal study of blood pressure and dementia. Lancet 1996; 347:1141–1145.
34. Bertram L, Tanzi RE. Alzheimer's disease: one disorder, too many genes? Hum Mol Genet 2004; 13:R135–R141.
35. Farrer L, Cupples LA, Haines JL, et al. Effects of age, sex and ethnicity on the association between apolipoprotein E genotype and Alzheimer's disease. A meta-analysis. JAMA 1997; 278:1349–1356.
36. Daw EW, Payami H, Nemens EJ, et al. The number of trait loci in late-onset Alzheimer's disease. Am J Hum Genet 2000; 66:196–204.
37. Schelleman H, Stricker BH, De Boer A, et al. Drug–gene interactions between genetic polymorphisms and antihypertensive therapy. Drugs 2004; 64:1801–1816.
38. Nicoll JA, Mrak RE, Graham DI, et al. Association of interleukin-1 gene polymorphisms with Alzheimer's disease. Ann Neurol 2000; 47:365–368.
39. Silverman JM, Ciresi G, Smith CJ, Marin DB, Schnaider-Beeri M. Variability of familial risk of Alzheimer disease across the late life span. Arch Gen Psychiatry 2005; 62:565–573.
40. Fratiglioni L, Viitanen M, von Strauss E, et al. Very old women at highest risk of dementia and Alzheimer's disease: incidence data from the Kungsholmen Project, Stockholm. Neurology 1997; 48:132–138.
41. Andersen K, Launer LJ, Dewey ME, et al. for the EURODEM Incidence Research Group. Gender differences in the incidence of AD and vascular dementia: The EURODEM studies. Neurology 1999; 53:1992–1997.
42. Fitzpatrick AL, Kuller LH, Ives DG, et al. Incidence and prevalence of dementia in the Cardiovascular Health Study. J Am Geriatr Soc 2004; 52:195–204.
43. Edland SD, Rocca WA, Petersen RC, Cha RH, Kokmen E. Dementia and Alzheimer disease incidence rates do not vary by sex in Rochester, Minn. Arch Neurol 2002; 59:1589–1593.
44. Di Carlo A, Baldereschi M, Amaducci L, et al. Incidence of dementia, Alzheimer's disease, and vascular dementia in Italy. The ILSA Study. J Am Geriatr Soc 2002; 50:41–48.
45. Barnes L, Wilson RS, Bienias JL, et al. Sex differences and clinical manifestations of Alzheimer's disease. Arch Gen Psychiatr 2005; 62:685–691.
46. Karp A, Kareholt I, Qiu C, et al. Relation of education and occupation-based socioeconomic status to incident Alzheimer's disease. Am J Epidemiol 2004; 159:175–183.
47. Stern Y, Gurland B, Tatamichi TK, et al. Influence of education and occupation on the incidence of Alzheimer's disease. JAMA 1994; 271:1004–1010.
48. Cobb JB, Wolf PA, White R, D'agostino RB. The effect of education on the incidence of dementia and Alzheimer's

disease in the Framingham study. Neurology 1995; 45:1707–1712.

49. Stern Y, Tang MX, Denaro J, Mayeux R. Increased risk of mortality in Alzheimer's disease patients with more advanced educational and occupational attainment. Ann Neurol 1995; 37:590–595.

50. Letenneur L, Launer LJ, Andersen K, et al. for the EURO-DEM Incidence Research Group. Education and the risk for Alzheimer's disease: sex makes a difference. EURODEM pooled analyses. Am J Epidemiol 2000; 151:1064–1071.

51. Lupien SJ, Gaudreau S, Tchiteya, et al. Stress-induced declarative memory impairment in healthy elderly subjects: relationship to cortisol reactivity. J Clin Endocrinol Metab 1997; 82:2070–2075.

52. Sapolsky RM, Uno Hm Robert CS, Finch CE. Hippocampal damage associated with prolonged glucocorticoid exposure in primates. J Neurosci 1990; 10:2897–2902.

53. Stern Y, Alexander GE, Prohovnik I, Mayeux R. Inverse relationship between education and parietotemporal perfusion deficit in Alzheimer's disease. Ann Neurol 1992; 32:371–375.

54. Alexander GE, Furey ML, Grady CL, et al. Association of premorbid intellectual function with cerebral metabolism in Alzheimer's disease: implication for the cognitive reserve hypothesis. Am J Psychiatr 1997; 154:165–172.

55. Verghese J, Lipton RB, Katz MJ, et al. Leisure activities and the risk of dementia in the elderly. N Engl J Med 2003; 348:2508–2516.

56. Diamond MC. Enriching Heredity: The impact of the environment on the anatomy of the brain. New York: Free Press 1988.

57. US Department of Health and Human Services. Reducing the health consequences of smoking: 25 years of progress. Rockville, MD: US Department of Health and Human Services, Public Health Service, Centers for Disease Control, Center for Chronic Disease Prevention and Health Promotion, Office on Smoking and Health (DHHS Publication No. [CDC] 89–8411 1989.

58. Burke A, Fitzgerald GA. Oxidative stress and smoking-induced vascular injury. Prog Cardiovasc Dis 2003; 46:79–90.

59. Traber MG, van der Vliet A, Reznick AZ, Cross CE. Tobacco related diseases: is there a role for antioxidant micronutrient supplementation? Clin Chest Med 2000; 21:173–187.

60. Dallongeville J, Marecaux N, Fruchart J-C, Amouyel P. Cigarette smoking is associated with unhealthy patterns of nutrient intake: a meta analysis. J Nutr 1998; 128:1450–1457.

61. Graves AB, van Duijn CM, Chandra V, et al. Alcohol and tobacco consumption as risk factors for Alzheimer's disease: a collaborative re-analysis of case-control studies. EURO-DEM Risk Factors Research Group. Int J Epidemiol 1991; 20(suppl 2):S48–S57.

62. Newhouse PA, Potter A, Kelton M, Corwin J. Nicotinic treatment of Alzheimer's disease. Neurobiol Aging 2001; 49:268–278.

63. Tyas SL, White LR, Petrovitch H, et al. Mid-life smoking and late-life dementia: The Honolulu-Asia Aging Study. Neurobiol Aging 2003; 24:589–596.

64. Merchant C, Tang M-X, Albert S, et al. The influence of smoking on the risk of Alzheimer's disease. Neurology 1999; 52:1408–1412.

65. Ott A, Slooter AJC, Hofman A, et al. Smoking and risk of dementia and Alzheimer's disease in a population-based cohort study: the Rotterdam Study. Lancet 1998; 351:1840–1843.

66. Humphries SE, Talmud PJ, Hawe E, et al. Apolipoprotein E4 and coronary heart disease in middle-aged men who smoke: a prospective study. Lancet 2001; 358:115–119.

67. Kalmijn S, van Boxtel MP, Verschuren MW, Jolles J, Launer LJ. Cigarette smoking and alcohol consumption in relation to cognitive performance in middle age. Am J Epidemiol 2002; 156:936–944.

68. Cotman CW, Berchtold NC. Exercise: a behavioral intervention to enhance brain health and plasticity. Trends Neurosci 2002; 25:295–301.

69. Pate RR, Pratt M, Blair SN, et al. Physical activity and public health. A recommendation from the Centers for Disease Control and Prevention and the American College of Sports Medicine. JAMA 1995; 273:402–407.

70. Laurin D, Verreault R, Lindsay J, MacPherson K, Rockwood K. Physical activity and risk of cognitive impairment and dementia in elderly persons. Arch Neurol 2001; 58:498–504.

71. Podewils LJ, Guallar E, Kuller LH, et al. Physical activity, APOE genotype, and dementia risk: findings from the Cardiovascular Health Cognition Study. Am J Epidemiol 2005; 161:639–651.

72. Kalmijn S, Launer LJ, Ott A, et al. Dietary fat intake and the risk of incident dementia in the Rotterdam Study. Ann Neurol. 1997; 42:776–782.

73. Kalmijn S. Fatty acid intake and the risk of dementia and cognitive decline: a review of clinical and epidemiological studies. J Nutr Health Aging 2000; 4:202–207.

74. Lucas DL, Brown RA, Wassef M, Giles TD. Alcohol and the cardiovascular system research challenges and opportunities. J Am Coll Cardiol 2005; 45:1916–1924.

75. Seshadri S, Beiser A, Selhub J, et al. Plasma homocysteine as a risk factor for dementia and Alzheimer's disease. N Engl J Med 2002; 346:476–483.

76. Engelhart MJ, Geerlings MI, Ruitenberg A, et al. Dietary intake of antioxidants and risk of Alzheimer disease. JAMA 2002; 287:3223–3229.

77. Commenges D, Scotet V, Renaud S, et al. Intake of flavonoids and risk of dementia. Eur J Epidemiol 2000; 16:357–363.

78. Morris MC, Evans DA, Bienias JL, et al. Dietary intake of antioxidant nutrients and the risk of incident Alzheimer disease in a biracial community study. JAMA 2002; 287:3230–3237.

79. Laurin D, Foley DJ, Masaki KH, White LR, Launer LJ. Vitamin E and C supplements and risk of dementia. JAMA 2002; 288:2266–2268.

80. Luchsinger JA, Tang M-X, Shea S, Mayeux R. Antioxidant vitamin intake and risk of Alzheimer disease. Arch Neurol 2003; 60:203–208.

81. Halliwell B. The antioxidant paradox. Lancet 2000; 355:1179–1180.

82. Launer LJ. Is there epidemiologic evidence that anti-oxidants protect against disorders in cognitive function? J Nutr Hlth Aging 2000; 4:197–201.

83. Laurin D, Masaki KH, Foley DJ, White LR, Launer LJ. Midlife dietary intake of antioxidants and risk of late-life incident dementia. The Honolulu-Asia Aging Study. Am J Epidemiol 2004; 159:959–967.

84. Sano M, Ernesto C, Thomas RG, et al. A controlled trial of selegiline, alpha-tocopherol, or both as treatment for Alzheimer's disease. N Engl J Med 1997; 336:1216–1222.

85. Heart Protection Study Collaborative Group. MRC/BHF Heart Protection Study of antioxidant vitamin supplementation in 20536 high-risk individuals: a randomised placebo-controlled trial. Lancet 2002; 360:23–33.

86. Pullicino PM. Pathogensis of lacunar infarcts and small deep infarcts. In: Pullicino PM, Caplan LR, Hommel M (eds). Advances in Neurology. Raven Press, New York 125–140 1993.

87. Li H, Forstermann U. Nitric oxide in the pathogenesis of vascular disease. J Pathol 2000; 190:244–254.

88. Mattson MP, Zhu H, Yin J, Kindy MS. Presenilin-1 mutation increases neuronal vulnerability to focal ischemia in vivo and to hypoxia and glucose deprivation in cell culture: involvement of perturbed calcium homeostasis. J Neurosci 2000; 20:1358–1364.

89. Bennett SA, Pappas BA, Stevens WD, et al. Cleavage of amyloid precursor protein elicited by chronic cerebral hypoperfusion. Neurobiol Aging 2000; 21:207–214.

90. Alexander RW. Theodore Cooper Memorial Lecture. Hypertension and the pathogenesis of atherosclerosis. Oxidative stress and the mediation of arterial inflammatory response: a new perspective. Hypertension. 1995; 25:155–161.

91. Sugawara T, Kawase M, Lewen A, et al. Effect of hypotension severity on hippocampal CA1 neurons in a rat global ischemia model. Brain Res 2000; 877:281–287.

92. Arendash GW, Su GC, Crawford FC, Bjugstad KB, Mullan M. Intravascular β-amyloid infusion increases blood pressure: implications for a vasoactive role of β-amyloid in the pathogenesis of Alzheimer's disease. Neurosci Lett 1999; 268:17–20.

93. Launer LJ, Masaki K, Petrovitch H, Foley D, Havlik R. The association between midlife blood pressure levels and late-life cognitive function: The Honolulu-Asia Aging Study. JAMA 1995; 274:1846–1851.

94. de Leeuw FE, de Groot JC, Oudkerk M, et al. A follow-up study of blood pressure and cerebral white matter lesions. Ann Neurol 1999; 46:827–833.

95. Tzourio C, Dufouil C, Ducimetiere P, Alperovitch A. Cognitive decline in individuals with high blood pressure: a longitudinal study in the elderly. EVA Study Group. Epidemiology of Vascular Aging. Neurology 1999; 53:1948–1952.

96. Korf ESC, White LR, Scheltens P, Launer LJ. Midlife blood pressure and the risk of hippocampal atrophy. The Honolulu Asia Aging Study. Hypertension 2004; 44:29–34.

97. Launer LJ, Ross GW, Petrovitch H, et al. Midlife blood pressure and dementia: The Honolulu-Asia Aging Study. Neurobiol Aging 2000; 21:49–55.

98. Petrovitch H, White LR, Izmirlian G, et al. Midlife blood pressure and neuritic plaques, neurofibrillary tangles, and brain weight at death: the HAAS. Neurobiol Aging 2000; 21:57–62.

99. Kivipelto M, Helkala EL, Hanninen T, et al. Midlife vascular risk factors and late-life mild cognitive impairment: a population-based study. Neurology 2001; 56:1683–1689.

100. Guo Z, Viitanen M, Fratiglioni L, Winblad B. Low blood pressure and dementia in elderly people. BMJ 1996; 312:805–808.

101. Morris MC, Scherr PA, Hebert LE, et al. Association of incident Alzheimer disease and blood pressure measured from 13 years before to 2 years after diagnosis in a large community study. Arch Neurol 2001; 58:1640–1646.

102. Birns J, Markus H, Kalra L. Blood pressure reduction for vascular risk: is there a price to be paid? Stroke 2005; 36:1308–1313.

103. Guo Z, Fratiglioni L, Zhu L, et al. Occurrence and progression of dementia in a community population aged 75 years and older: relationship of antihypertensive medication use. Arch Neurol 1999; 56:991–996.

104. in't Veld BA, Ruitenberg A, Hofman A, Stricker BH, Breteler MM. Antihypertensive drugs and incidence of dementia: the Rotterdam Study. Neurobiol Aging 2001; 22:407–412.

105. Prince MJ, Bird AS, Blizard RA, Mann AH. Is the cognitive function of older patients affected by antihypertensive treatment? Results from 54 months of the Medical Research Council's trial of hypertension in older adults. BMJ 1996; 312:801–805.

106. Applegate WB, Pressel S, Wittes J, et al. Impact of the treatment of isolated systolic hypertension on behavioral variables. Results from the systolic hypertension in the elderly program. Arch Intern Med 1994; 154:2154–2160.

107. Forette F, Seux ML, Staessen JA, et al. Prevention of dementia in randomized double-blind placebo-controlled Systolic Hypertension in Europe (Syst-Eur) trial. Lancet 1998; 352:1347–1351.

108. Lithell H, Hansson L, Skoog I, et al. The Study on Cognition and Prognosis in the Elderly (SCOPE): principal results of a randomized double-blind intervention trial. J Hypertens 2003; 21:875–886.

109. Bulpitt C, Fletcher A, Beckett N, et al. Hypertension in the Very Elderly Trial (HYVET): protocol for the main trial. Drugs Aging 2001; 18:151–164.

110. de Craen AJ, Gussekloo J, Vrijsen B, Westendorp RG. Meta-analysis of nonsteroidal antiinflammatory drug use and risk of dementia. Am J Epidemiol 2005; 161: 114–120.

111. in t' Veld BA, Ruitenberg A, Hofman A, et al. Nonsteroidal antiinflammatory drugs and the risk of Alzheimer's disease. N Engl J Med 2001; 345:1515–1521.

112. Schmidt R, Schmidt H, Curb JD, et al. Early inflammation and dementia: a 25-year follow-up of the Honolulu-Asia Aging Study. Ann Neurol 2002; 168–174.

113. Engelhart MJ, Geerlings MI, Meijer J, et al. Inflammatory proteins in plasma and the risk of dementia: the Rotterdam Study. Arch Neurol 2004; 61:668–672.

114. Aisen PS, Schafer KA, Grundman M, et al. Effects of rofecoxib or naproxen vs placebo on Alzheimer disease progression: a randomized controlled trial. JAMA 2003; 289:2819–2826.

115. Solomon CG. Reducing cardiovascular risk in type 2 diabetes. N Engl J Med 2003; 348:457–459.

116. Biessels GJ, Bravenboer B, Gispen WH. Glucose, insulin and the brain: modulation of cognition and synaptic plasticity in health and disease: a preface. Eur J Pharmacol 2004; 490:1–4.

117. Dickson DW, Sinicropi S, Yen SA, et al. Glycation and microglial reaction in lesions of Alzheimer's disease. Neurobiol Aging 1996; 17:733–743.

118. Zlokovic B. RAGE mediates amyloid-beta peptide transport across the blood–brain barrier and accumulation in brain. Nat Med 2003; 9:907–913.

119. Yan SD, Chen X, Chen M, et al. RAGE and amyloid-β peptide neurotoxicity in Alzheimer's disease. Nature 1996; 382:685–691.

120. Yaffe K, Blackwell T, Kanaya AM, et al. Diabetes, impaired fasting glucose, and development of cognitive impairment in older women. Neurology 2004; 63:658–663.

121. den Heijer T, Vermeer SE, van Dijk EJ, et al. Type 2 diabetes and atrophy of medial temporal lobe structures on brain MRI. Diabetologia 2003; 46:1604–1610.

122. Schmidt R, Launer LJ, Nilsson LG, et al. Magnetic resonance imaging of the brain in diabetes: The Cardiovascular Determinants of Dementia (CASCADE) Study. Diabetes 2004; 53:687–692.

123. Peila R, Rodriguez BL, Launer LJ. Type 2 diabetes, APOE gene, and the risk for dementia and related pathologies: The Honolulu-Asia Aging Study. Diabetes 2002; 51:1256–1262.
124. Luchsinger JA, Tang MX, Stern Y, Shea S, Mayeux R. Diabetes mellitus and risk of Alzheimer's disease and dementia with stroke in a multiethnic cohort. Am J Epidemiol 2001; 154:635–641.
125. Leibson CL, Rocca WA, Hanson VA, et al. Risk of dementia among persons with diabetes mellitus: a population-based cohort study. Am J Epidemiol 1997; 145:301–308.
126. Ott A, Stolk RP, van Harskamp F, et al. Diabetes mellitus and the risk of dementia: The Rotterdam Study. Neurology 1999; 53;1937–1942.
127. Arvanitakis Z, Wilson RS, Bienias JL, Evans DA, Bennet DA. Diabetes mellitus and risk of Alzheimer disease and decline in cognitive function. Arch Neurol 2004; 61:661–666.
128. Roth CS, Joseph JA, Mason RP. Membrane alterations as causes of impaired signal transduction in Alzheimer's disease and aging. Trends Neurosci 1995; 18:203–206.
129. Howland DS, Trusko SP, Savage MJ, et al. Modulation of secreted beta-amyloid precursor protein and amyloid beta-peptide in brain by cholesterol. J Biol Chem 1998; 273:16576–16582.
130. Bodowitz S, Klein WL. Cholesterol modulates alpha-secretase cleavage of amyloid precursor protein. J Biol Chem 1996; 271:4436–4440.
131. Kivipelto M, Helkala EL, Laakso MP, et al. Apolipoprotein E α4, elevated midlife total cholesterol level, and high systolic blood pressure are independent risk factors for late-life Alzheimer's disease. Ann Intern Med 2002; 137:149–155.
132. Tan ZS, Seshadri S, Beiser A, et al. Plasma total cholesterol level as a risk factor for Alzheimer disease: The Framingham Study. Arch Intern Med 2003; 163:1053–1057.
133. Ettinger WH, Wahl PW, Kuller LH, et al. Lipoprotein lipids in older people. Results from the Cardiovascular Health Study. The CHS Collaborative Research Group. Circulation 1992; 86:858–869.
134. Sparks DL, Sabbagh MN, Connor DJ, et al. Atorvastatin for the treatment of mild to moderate Alzheimer disease: preliminary results. Arch Neurol 2005; 62:753–757.
135. Hong M, Lee VM. Insulin and insulin like growth factor-1 regulate tau phosphorylation in cultured human neurons. J Biol Chem 1997; 272:19547–19553.
136. Craft S, Watson GS. Insulin and neurodegenerative disease: shared and specific mechanisms. Lancet Neurol 2004; 3:169–178.
137. Zhao W, Alkon DL. Role of insulin and insulin receptor in learning and memory. Mol Cell Endocrinol 2001; 177:125–134.
138. Brass BJ, Nonner D, Barrett JN. Differential effects of insulin on choline acetyltransferase and glutamic acid decarboxylase activities in neuron-rich striatal cultures. J Neurochem 1992; 59:415–429.
139. Peila R, Rodriguez BL, White LR, Launer LJ. Fasting insulin and incident dementia in an elderly population of Japanese-American men. Neurology. 2004; 63:228–233.
140. Luchsinger JA, Tang MX, Shea S, Mayeux R. Hyper-insulinemia and risk of Alzheimer disease. Neurology 2004; 63:1187–1192.
141. Kuusisto J, Koivisto K, Mykkanen L, et al. Association between features of the insulin resistance syndrome and Alzheimer's disease independently of apolipoprotein E4 phenotype: cross sectional population based study. BMJ 1997; 315:1045–1049.

II Diagnosis

4

Typical clinical features

Rémi W Bouchard and Martin N Rossor

DEFINITION OF DEMENTIA

Dementia is a 'decline of intellectual function in comparison with the patient's previous level of function'.[1] This decline is usually associated with changes in behaviour and impairment of social and professional activities and is reflected in a decline in basic (BADL) and in instrumental (IADL) activities of daily living. About 5–10 per cent of the population over 65 has some kind of cognitive decline which is considered to be abnormal for this age group. Among these, more than 50 per cent will have a dementia of degenerative aetiology, of which the most common is Alzheimer's disease (AD). However, recent studies have shown that in degenerative dementia it is common to have other pathologies as well, such as AD plus parkinsonian features, AD plus Lewy bodies, and more frequently, AD plus vascular pathology.[2] The diagnosis of dementia is a clinical diagnosis,[3] based on a careful clinical history and examination. Although investigations such as neuroimaging (computerized tomography (CT) and magnetic resonance imaging (MRI)) and laboratory tests are of value to rule out specific aetiologies, they are of no help for the diagnosis of dementia per se and even the aetiology may be suspected on clinical grounds in the majority of cases (see clinical differential features). Most often, the cognitive impairment in dementia is progressive, but a sudden onset does not exclude the diagnosis. The mode of onset and the knowledge of the clinical profile of a dementia syndrome are the basis for the differential diagnosis with respect to the likely aetiology. Although the criteria for the diagnosis of dementia demand multiple domains of cognitive impairment, isolated deficits such as amnesia, dyslexia or dysphasia may be the early manifestations of a dementing process. For example, early language disorder, although unusual in AD, may be the presentation of a particular subtype of AD (see Chapter 5), although other progressive degenerative disorders such as primary progressive aphasia,[4–7] the group of frontotemporal dementias (FTD) and the dementia of vascular aetiology, which may not have a sudden onset, enter the differential diagnosis. For that reason, the standard definition of dementia in the DSM-IV,[8] that requires a memory deficit as the first criterion, should be modifed to include memory and/or any other predominant cognitive domain. In addition, mood and behaviour disturbances should be added as supportive features in the general definition of dementia. In the clinical situations of a progressive focal cognitive deficit, it is preferable to describe the clinical picture as a syndrome until the profile of cognitive impairment permits a more precise diagnosis.

When a patient is consulting a physician for possible dementia, the relatives may have noticed changes in personality or behaviour, some problems with memory, a decreased performance at work or impairment in BADL or IADL. The family often fears a diagnosis of AD – particularly if there is a family history. Alternatively, the relatives may be concerned that the patient has a brain tumour or a decrease of the blood circulation in the brain, or perhaps hope that the problems are related to depression and anxiety from the stress of special events, such as divorce in the family or the death of a close member of the family, or they may even hope it is manipulation. They are rarely concerned about other causes of dementia.

Before looking for the main causes of dementia the clinician has to decide whether the patient has a true dementia or pseudodementia of depression. The main clinical clues are described in Table 4.1. Once the diagnosis of dementia is suspected and pseudodementia unlikely, the clinician may follow the seven steps described below to support the diagnosis and point to specific aetiologies (Table 4.2).

Table 4.1 Some clinical differences between dementia and pseudodementia of depression

Clinical picture	Pseudodementia	Dementia
Mode of onset	Rapid, with change in behaviour	Insidious over a period of months
Mood/behaviour	Stable or apathy, depressed mood	Fluctuating, sometimes apathy, sometimes normal or irritable
Intellectual functions	Many complaints; states being unable to perform tests but results are good on objective tests	Objective deficits on neuropsychological tests but patient minimizes or rationalizes his errors or failures
Self-image	Poor	Normal
Associated symptoms	Anxiety, insomnia, anorexia	Rare: sometimes insomnia
Duration	Variable; symptoms may stop spontaneously or after treatment	Symptoms progress slowly over months and years
Reason for consultation	Self referral; anxious about possible AD; heard about AD	Patient brought to the physician's office by members of the family who notice changes in memory, personality or behaviour
Previous history	Psychiatric history and/or family/personal problems	Familial history of dementia is not uncommon

Table 4.2 The seven steps of the clinical approach for investigating a patient for possible dementia

1. General medical history
2. General neurological history
3. Neurocognitive and behavioural history (for the diagnosis of dementia)
4. Psychiatric history
5. Toxic, nutritional and drug history
6. Familial history
7. Objective examination: physical, neurological and neuropsychological

THE PRACTICAL CLINICAL APPROACH

General medical history

When dementia is secondary to a serious medical illness, it is usually only part of a whole array of symptoms and signs which are often suggestive of the underlying aetiology (e.g. hypothyroidism or neoplasia). The clinician must seek actively these other clues of endocrine disorder, of possible neoplasia (loss of weight, anaemia, asthenia, smoking, etc.), of possible chronic infections, particularly in high-risk patients (syphilis, AIDS), of ischaemic heart disease or valvulopathy (cerebral emboli causing multi-infarct dementia), of connective tissue disorder and deficiency states. It is also important to inquire about arterial hypertension, hyperlipidaemia, diabetes and peripheral arteriosclerosis as risk factors for vascular dementia as well as AD. Even if an AD patient may have other illnesses, in general he does not look sick and most of the questions about his general health lead to negative answers. While taking the history, the physician may observe that the patient exhibits the 'head turning sign' (looking at his caregiver when asked a question), which is a common sign in AD.

General neurological history

The objective of a careful neurological history is to seek specific conditions which could be responsible for the dementia. A previous history of cerebrovascular events is of great importance (transient ischaemic attacks, strokes, previous carotid surgery), as well as head trauma[9] with or without intracranial surgery (brain contusions, subdural haematomas), infections of the central nervous system (encephalitis, meningitis, HIV encephalopathy, opportunistic infections), previous history of epilepsy or recent seizures, history of neurosurgical procedures for brain tumours or hydrocephalus. It is important to enquire about any associated neurological symptoms, such as motor or sensory complaints, gait disorder or impaired co-ordination, loss of control of sphincters or headache at the onset of dementia. These might indicate a structural rather than degenerative cause or associated motor deficits might suggest a subcortical type of dementia (Table 4.3) or at least a mixed pattern.

Neurocognitive functional and behavioural history

The neurocognitive and behavioural history is critical in determining whether the patient has dementia or not. It is important to obtain information and seek examples of different memory problems (short and long term), of problems with temporal and spatial orientation (knowing the dates, orientation in familiar and non-familiar places, car-driving), of language difficulty (fluency, word-finding, conversation), of executive functioning (planning, organizing), of the ability to recognize people, travel, handle money and make decisions. Changes in behaviour or personality, and the degree of interference with BADL and IADL, as well as social or professional activities, must also be identified. This interview has to be done with the caregiver as well as with the patient, since it is common to obtain two different versions, the patient having a tendency to minimize or to rationalize or to be unaware of his cognitive deficits (anosognosia). The examiner must use simple and practical questions related to a specific patient, taking into account the level of education, the profession and the usual interests or activities at home, at work, in hobbies or in social events. The mode of onset, the evolution and the degree of impairment will help in staging the dementia. From taking this history and even before the physical examination, the physician will be able to say whether the profile meets the criteria of the DSM-III-R[10] for dementia, or of the DSM-IV[8] and the NINCDS-

---

Table 4.3 List of the most frequent causes of dementia

Predominantly cortical pattern
- Alzheimer's disease*
- Down's syndrome*
- Fronto-temporal dementias*
- Some cases of corticobasal degeneration*

Predominantly subcortical pattern
- Parkinson's disease*
- Huntington's disease*
- Hydrocephalus
- Progressive supranuclear palsy*
- Multiple system atrophy*
- Subdural haematoma
- Corticobasal degeneration*

Mixed cortical and subcortical pattern
- Prion diseases**
- Multiple sclerosis
- Diffuse Lewy body disease*
- Cerebrovascular diseases
- Frontal lobe degeneration*
- Post-traumatic encephalopathies
- Toxic and anoxic encephalopathies
- Dementia from non-metastatic cancer
- Brain tumours (thalamus, corpus callosum)
- Progressive multifocal leucoencephalopathy
- Frontotemporal dementias with motor neuron disease*
- Deficiency states, endocrine disorders, alcoholism, depression
- Chronic infectious diseases: syphilis, chronic meningitis, AIDS

* Degenerative dementia.

** Kuru, Creutzfeldt–Jakob disease, Gerstmann–Straussler–Scheinker syndrome, fatal familial insomnia.

ADRDA for AD[1], taking into account the updated changes recommended in this chapter for the DSM-IV and the NINCDS-ADRDA criteria.

Psychiatric history

The psychiatric history should establish whether the patient has a pure psychiatric disorder or a dementia in association with psychiatric disease. It will also explore any psychiatric features of a primary dementing illness. It is valuable to focus on previous history of depression and on any depressive symptoms, history of psychosis, personality changes, aggressive behaviour, delusions, hallucinations and paranoid ideation. If psychiatric symptoms are present, it is important to know when in the course of the dementia these symptoms emerged. It is often stated that the psychiatric manifestations in AD occur mainly at the intermediate stage, at least in the selected cohort referred to the neurologist, but there is increasing evidence that subtle psychiatric features may occur earlier.[11,12]

Toxic, nutritional and drug history

Among potential causes of cognitive decline, environmental toxins may play a role (toxic chronic encephalopathies). Aluminium has long been implicated in AD, although studies have given inconsistent results.[13,14] The Canadian Study of Health and Aging showed some increased risk for AD in low educated people who were exposed to glues, pesticides or fertilizers.[14] Although not specifically associated with AD, some nutritional deficiencies may be a risk factor (see below). As far as drugs are concerned, it should be borne in mind that elderly people tend to minimize the significance of chronic use of pills such as benzodiazepines, sleeping pills, herbal medicines and over-the-counter drugs. An elderly person with true but mild cognitive decline may have rapid worsening or delirium induced by drugs and, on the other hand, an unexplained delirium may mask an underlying dementing process. Tricyclic antidepressive medication and anticholinergic drugs in particular can impair cognition and an association between use of neuroleptics and accelerated rate of decline in AD has been reported.[15]

Familial history

The clinician must enquire about possible familial incidence of dementia, mainly in first-degree relatives, of other neurological diseases or of psychiatric illnesses, particularly depression, Parkinson's disease (PD), AD and Down's syndrome.[16–18] Familial history of vascular disease (e.g. arteriosclerosis, strokes, carotid surgery, amyloid angiopathy or, rarely, autosomal dominant arteriopathy (CADASIL)[19]) may give some clues for vascular cognitive impairment in a given patient.

Examination

The general physical examination will focus on the overall physical status, the vital signs and the presence of arteriosclerosis or risk factors for vascular events: fundi, carotid bruits, high blood pressure, peripheral pulses, abdominal aortic aneurism and evidence of heart disease. One should also check for visceromegaly, enlarged lymph nodes and signs of endocrine disorders. In general, the patient who looks unwell is unlikely to have typical AD. A comprehensive neurological examination is necessary in order to answer the following questions: does the patient have signs of raised intracranial pressure? Is there any focal deficit, e.g. gait disturbance, motor or sensory deficit or visual field defect? Are there abnormalities of muscle tone, abnormal movements or primitive reflexes? With the exception of memory, an isolated neurocognitive deficit at the early stage of a dementing syndrome makes the diagnosis of AD less likely. A progressive dysphasia, dyspraxia or frontal syndrome makes a space occupying lesion, vascular lesions or degenerative conditions such as FTD or corticobasal degeneration more likely.

The clinical neuropsychological examination by the physician must include the evaluation of memory (immediate, short term and long term), orientation, language and related literary skills such as calculation and writing, praxis, gnosis, visuospatial and visuoperceptual abilities such as drawing a clock, a cube or superimposed geometric figure; the evaluation of executive functions, judgment and behaviour completes the examination. As a quick screen the Mini-Mental State Examination (MMSE)[20] is widely used. This test, however, has a limited value in some patients and is only a tool within the full clinical neuropsychological examination. Early dementia is suspected with a score below 24 out of 30, but highly educated people with obvious dementia may score 27 or above, and non-demented subjects with modest educational attainment may score as low as 24. A compromise cut-off at 27 is reasonable for most patients, but this test cannot be used as a single tool for diagnosis; it has to be interpreted within the context of the clinical history and examination. A 'within normal' score on the MMSE does not rule out mild cognitive impairment (MCI) or early dementia. The Montreal Cognitive

Assessment (MoCA) has higher sensitivity than the MMSE for screening persons with mild cognitive complaints.[21] Clock drawing has also been found useful for early diagnosis since most AD patients have abnormal drawing even in the early phase, but this test may be impaired for a variety of reasons from perceptual to praxis difficulties.[22] The clock test is a 'live' test to be done by the examiner himself, observing how the patient proceeds. In general any hesitation, if the patient understands the test, is abnormal and a too large space between the 5 and the 6, the 11 and the 12 may be indicating of a true incipient process, even if the final result looks good. Longitudinal follow-up is strongly recommended in those cases. Most patients starting the clock by putting the numbers 12, 3, 6, 9 at the right place will have a normal drawing. Whenever possible, formal neuropsychological assessment to explore and quantitate individual domains of cognitive function should be undertaken as well as functional and behaviour assessment scales. The screening for vascular aetiology using the modified ischaemic scale[23] completes the evaluation of possible dementia in the clinic and provides the initial clues as to the likely aetiology (Table 4.4). This information is in general sufficient to determine whether the patient fulfils the standard criteria for dementia and for AD. From this systematic approach, the clinician should also know whether the early manifestations are predominantly cortical or subcortical, whether the patient has an obvious serious medical illness and whether the cause of the dementia is degenerative or non-degenerative. The laboratory investigations can then be planned accordingly.

Basic laboratory investigations

As a complement to the clinical assessment of dementia, a relatively small number of laboratory tests are recommended for patients with dementia[24–28] (Table 4.5). The authors feel that, contrary to the recommendations of the last consensus conference in Canada,[24] renal function tests and B_{12} are recommended as routine, considering our new knowledge of the vascular risk factors and the fact that B_{12} may be a risk factor for dementia, such as AD, by increasing homocysteine levels.[29] Additional tests would be requested on a case-by-case basis. Neuroimaging and electrophysiological tests are discussed in Chapters 7, 8 and 9.

AETIOLOGY OF COGNITIVE DECLINE

The main causes of cognitive decline can be placed into four categories:

- systemic diseases;
- psychiatric diseases;
- neurological diseases with secondary dementia, e.g. hydrocephalus, brain tumours, subdural haematomas and vascular disease;
- primary degenerative dementias, of which the most common is AD.

It is useful to identify to which category the patient may be assigned, since the first three are most likely to be associated with a treatable cause (Table 4.6). It can be valuable to determine whether the patient has predominantly a cortical, subcortical or mixed pattern (Table 4.7). A cortical dementia will present as impairment of memory, language, praxis, gnosis (the so-called aphaso-apraxo-agnosic syndrome). By contrast, a subcortical dementia is characterized by marked executive-type cognitive slowing and is often associated with personality or behaviour disturbances, speech involvement, and motor deficits such as bradykinesia and gait disorder. Despite controversy regarding this classification, it can be useful as a clue to the underlying aetiology to know when in the course of a dementia such a pattern appears.[30–32] For example, AD is a primary degenerative dementia with predominant cortical features at the onset, whereas progressive supranuclear palsy (PSP) and Huntington's disease are degenerative dementias with predominant early subcortical features. However, the patterns of cortical and subcortical dementia are not confined to

---

Table 4.4 Modified ischaemic score in dementia. Most patients with Alzheimer's disease will score between 0 and 2, the vascular patients more than 4 (oftentimes 7 and more) and the mixed dementia patients between 4 and 7 (modified from Rosen et al[23])

History, symptoms and signs	Yes	No
Sudden onset	2	0
Stepwise course	1	0
Somatic complaints	1	0
Emotional incontinence	1	0
History or presence of hypertension	1	0
History of cerebrovascular accident	2	0
Focal neurological symptoms	2	0
Focal neurological signs	2	0

Table 4.5 Basic laboratory investigations in dementia

	Ref. 24	Ref. 25	Ref. 26	Ref. 27	Ref. 28
Complete blood count (CBC)	All	All	All	All	All
TSH	All	All	All	All	All
T4			All		
Electrolytes	All	All	All	All	All
Blood urea nitrogen (BUN)	*	All	All	All	All
Creatinine	*	All	All	All	All
Calcium	All	All	All	All	All
Glycaemia	All	All	All		All
Alanine aminotransferase (ALT)	*	All	All	All	All
B_{12}	*	All			
Folate		All	All	All	All
Syphilis serology				All	Optional
HIV screen					

TSH: thyroid-stimulating hormone; All: all patients with dementia
*Authors' recommendation now for all subjects under investigation

Table 4.6 Some clinical clues for categorizing patients in the possible degenerative group or in the group of secondary dementia. From the first visit the clinician can classify the patient in one of these categories in order to plan the investigation

Degenerative dementia	Dementia of other aetiology (secondary dementia)
• Patient brought to consultation by a relative • Patient has memory problems or personality changes for at least 6 months • Insidious onset and progressive • Good general health (stable condition) • No history of recent acute medical, neurological or psychiatric event • Unremarkable physical examination • Basic neurological examination within normal limits • Screening neuropsychological tests abnormal	• Rapid onset or course • Significant early motor or gait disturbances • Recent medical or neurological event • Previous history of neurological or psychiatric disease • Recent history of head trauma • General appearance of a sick patient • Patient with known multiple medical problems • Patient taking many medications • Abnormal neurological examination • Alcoholism

the primary degenerative dementias. A subcortical pattern is often found with the secondary dementias such as hydrocephalus and subdural hematomas; many other diseases may have mixed patterns such as vascular diseases, endocrine disorders, deficiency states, chronic infections and psychiatric disease (Table 4.3).

THE STANDARD CRITERIA FOR THE DIAGNOSIS OF AD

The standard criteria widely used for the diagnosis of dementia and of AD are the DSM-IV[8] and the NINCDS-ADRDA.[1] The DSM-IV criteria for AD can be summarized as follows: impairment of memory,

Table 4.7 Summary of common cortical and subcortical clinical features

Impairment	Cortical	Subcortical
Orientation	+++	+
Abstract thinking	+++	+
Short-term memory	+++	+
Long-term memory	++	+
Executive functioning	++	+++
Language	++	±
Speech	±	++
Praxis	++	±
Perceptual problems	++	+
Apathy	+	++
Bradykinesia	+	+++
Behaviour	+	++
Gait	+ (late)	++ (early)

evidence of at least one of the following cognitive impairments: aphasia, apraxia, agnosia or disturbance in executive functioning, gradual onset and progressive decline; the deficits cause significant impairment of social and professional activities, represent a decline from a previous level of functioning, cannot be explained by any other neurological, psychiatric, systemic or substance-induced conditions known to cause cognitive deficits and do not occur only in the context of delirium. Mood and behaviour disturbances, which are common in AD, can be added as supportive features. Although these criteria are acceptable for AD, the requirement of memory impairment as the first criterion does not systematically apply to other dementias such as FTD and vascular dementias and the standard criteria for dementia in general are in the process of being modified in order to include the possibility of impairment of other predominant cognitive domains as the first criterion.

The NINCDS-ADRDA criteria provide three levels of diagnosis:

- probable AD;
- possible AD;
- definite AD.

A 'probable AD' patient has dementia established by clinical examination, documented and confirmed by neuropsychological tests, deficits in two or more areas of cognition, progressive worsening of memory and other cognitive functions, has normal consciousness, had the first symptoms after 40 and below 90 and has no evidence of significant systemic or other brain diseases that could explain the progressive deficit. A 'possible AD' patient is different in that the onset, the clinical presentation (e.g. a single progressive deficit without identifiable cause), or the course, are considered atypical, or there is a second systemic or brain disorder sufficient to produce dementia but which is not considered to be the cause in that particular case. Common secondary diagnoses are low or borderline low B_{12}, hypothyroidism and a vascular lesion on imaging. When a second disease may contribute to the dementia, the clinical profile is usually clearly different from AD. For example, borderline B_{12} deficiency is seen frequently and needs to be evaluated and possibly treated. However, in our experience this is rarely responsible for any significant cognitive decline resembling AD; over a great number of years we have seen patients with AD and borderline B_{12} and none has improved with treatment. These patients follow the usual course of AD when the initial profile was suggestive of AD. By contrast, when B_{12} deficiency is severe to the point of causing dementia, this is usually accompanied by the haematological and the other neurological features of that disease, and the dementia does not have the classical cortical pattern of AD. However, since B_{12} and folate deficiency are common and can contribute to some cognitive decline or may be a risk factor for dementia, including AD (see above), it is recommended to treat patients whose level is under the lower limit of the lab references. This statement also applies to hypothyroidism; when it is severe enough to cause dementia, the clinical picture is not that of AD but rather that of true hypothyroidism. Since this condition is common in elderly people, it is not rare to see patients with the profile of AD who also have hypothyroidism; again in our experience, the treatment of the thyroid dysfunction does not alter the course of the underlying degenerative condition and for these reasons, most 'possible cases' will turn out to be 'probable cases' with time. Definite AD is 'possible' or 'probable' AD with histological confirmation on biopsy or at autopsy. With regard to patients with a single small asymptomatic vascular lesion, particularly a lacune on imaging in AD patients, these were eligible in the past in AD clinical trials. Now with our recent knowledge about the vascular contribution in AD patients, these patients are diagnosed as AD with a possible vascular component and, depending on the size, location and number of lacunes or the degree of white matter involvement, they are considered as mixed dementia patients.

Obviously, some of these criteria might be subject to controversy such as the requirement of memory impairment, not only for dementia in general but also for AD, or of progressive worsening of memory, the evidence of at least one versus two areas of impaired cognition and the arbitrary age range. Thus, some authors have found patients with only one area of cognition impaired and rare cases of AD without significant memory deficit;[33] rarely, AD may commence below the age of 40 years. Although no criteria can be perfect for all cases, they do serve to identify a relatively pure group of AD patients, particularly for research purposes. The criteria provide a high degree of accuracy for clinical diagnosis, in the range of 85–90 per cent, compared with autopsy findings, which is acceptable for clinical trials and other research purposes.[34–36]

TYPICAL CLINICAL PROFILE OF AD

The more we know about AD, the more we find that this disease is heterogeneous in its presentation and course. This has led some to consider that the term AD may encompass more than one disease. Obviously, patients with predominantly language disorder, behaviour disturbances or memory problems at the onset do not have the same involvement in terms of brain structures and neurochemical deficits, and this is substantiated by changes in multiple neurotransmitters in this disease. This apparent heterogeneity has led to the identification of clinical subgroups[37–40] based on the age at onset, the predominant features, the course, the familial incidence, etc. Those atypical presentations of AD may also mean that we are dealing with different diseases such as the group of FTD and the dementias with parkinsonian features, for which the diagnostic criteria are now better defined (Chapter 5)

Despite some controversy regarding heterogeneity,[41] one can identify a common pattern of patient presentation of early AD to the clinician, as described in Vignette 4.1. It is important to state that most patients referred for memory problems which do not cause significant interference with social or professional life or ADL do not have AD. They are more likely to have benign memory problems related to age, or to anxiety, lack of attention, co-existent medical problems or depression. Some will have true mild cognitive deficits without dementia, also called MCI, and some will have symptoms without objective cognitive deficits. Even if some of these patients will later prove to have an insidious onset of dementia, at this stage it is difficult to say that a given patient suffers from early or preclinical AD. Longitudinal studies have been done to identify specific neuropsychological markers at the

---

Vignette 4.1 Usual clinical presentation of early Alzheimer's disease at the physician's office

- The patient usually does not seek medical help on his own. He is brought to the doctor's office by relatives who have noticed impairment in executive functioning and memory, or personality change
- The patient has a tendency to look at his relative when asked any question: the head-turning sign
- The patient has difficulty with recalling the present date
- May have hesitation in language (word finding) and may be anxious
- Has a tendency to minimize and/or to rationalize and may become upset when the relative explains the problems and gives examples
- The patient does not look ill
- On history, memory problems go back to at least 6 months, more for recent events than for long-term memory. Immediate memory is usually spared
- The patient is taking little or no medication
- The spouse says: 'except for his/her memory, health is good'
- No history of recent headache or of seizures
- No history of cerebrovascular accidents
- Medical and neurological examination are unremarkable except for higher cortical functions
- Obvious mild impairment on neuropsychological screening: memory for recent events, some word finding difficulty and constructional apraxia or visuospatial difficulty with clock or geometric figure drawing
- The patient has usually 20–27 on the MMSE and an ischaemic score less than 4 (often 0–2)

early stages and to characterize this important transitional stage between MCI and true dementia.[42] MCI is a very heterogeneous group, some patients having mainly memory complaints, others many cognitive complaints and others complaints of a single cognitive domain (e.g. language) other than memory; only 10–15 per cent will convert to AD per year.[43] One should pay attention to the MCI patients complaining of their memory (called amnestic MCI) since they are more likely to progress to AD.[44] Despite their heterogeneity, these patients are in the group of what could correspond to stage II of the original global deterioration scale (GDS) of Reisberg et al:[45] this scale ranges from I to VII, and the diagnosis of 'possible' AD can be suspected from stage III (see Chapter 15). Another scale, the Clinical Dementia Rating (CDR)[46,47] is a five-step scale ranging from 0 to 3, based on the degree of autonomy of the patient, and includes assessment of impairment in the following domains: memory, orientation, judgment and problem-solving, community affairs, home, hobbies and personal care; the clinical diagnosis can be suspected from stage 0.5. This functional scale has proven useful in research protocols for therapeutic trials by following the scores of each item and the sum of the boxes during the course of a treatment, for example. But the CDR does not include specific assessment of domains such as language, mood and behaviour, praxis, gnosis and motor function (see Chapter 12).

From the clinical point of view, the first stage where the diagnosis of AD is clinically feasible with reasonable accuracy is considered stage I of our 'AD progression scale' (ADPS), compared to the GDS where it is stage III, and the CDR where it is 0.5. Our progression scale for staging AD ranges from I to V, I being the early phase, II and III being the intermediate phases, where most of the deficits become evident, IV and V the late stages where the deficits are severe and associated with motor impairment and behavioural disturbances. Table 4.8 summarizes the common clinical features at each stage with regard to general behaviour, executive functioning, memory, orientation, motor function, mood, abstract thinking, language, praxis and gnosis. Obviously, due to heterogeneity in the symptoms and the course, all the patients do not have all the features at a given stage, but this practical guideline has proven clinically useful for overall staging of the progression of AD in our patients. The patient in Vignette 4.1 shows a classic presentation of early AD, at stage I of the ADPS.

Patients are mainly referred to neurologists for memory or other cognitive problems, especially when these problems have become obvious to the caregiver. However, some personality change may be an early manifestation, but not mentioned unless specifically asked for. When the behaviour component predominates, the patient is usually referred to a psychiatrist; similarly, the elderly patient with many medical problems in addition to dementia is usually referred to a geriatrician (e.g. vascular patients, mixed patterns). These different referral patterns may explain why some authors[11,12] have found that the psychiatric manifestations are quite common and may significantly precede the memory problems. Thus Oppenheim[11] found, in a retrospective analysis, a predominance of psychiatric features in a cohort of patients who were diagnosed as AD according to the classic criteria. At the time of minor changes in personality or behaviour, it would not have been possible to make a diagnosis of AD, since too many other causes could have explained the behavioural disturbance. This implies that a patient with minor changes in personality needs to be carefully followed up for the possible development of dementia, and that in the clinical investigation of patients with early cognitive decline special attention should be paid to changes in personality or behaviour as well as mood changes. Some groups of AD patients may have a rapid evolution,[48–49] but in general the disease progresses over a period of 7–15 years (see Chapter 11). Plateaux are possible. As shown in Table 4.8, most of the deficits become evident in the intermediate stages. As the disease progresses, the patient develops more motor features, such as bradykinesia, increased tone, myoclonus and more disturbing behaviour. When most of the cognitive functions are lost, the patient is usually bedridden with flexion hypertonia. The detailed evolution of the cognitive deficits, functional loss, behaviour and mood disturbances are described in Chapters 13 to 16.

CLINICAL DIFFERENTIAL FEATURES AMONG DEMENTIAS

The basis of the clinical differential diagnosis is:

- the recognition of three main categories of symptoms and signs: the cognitive symptoms, the motor disturbances and the personality/behaviour/mood changes;
- the time in the course of disease when these symptoms or signs occur;
- the mode of onset.[50]

AD, Pick's disease and associated frontotemporal dementias (FTD) are characterized by early cortical features. The FTD occurring on a degenerative basis are most commonly due to Pick's disease, frontal lobe

Table 4.8 Common clinical profile of AD for early, intermediate and late stages; due to heterogeneity, the patients do not have necessarily all the features at a given stage

Stages	Early (mild)	Intermediate (moderate)		Late (severe)	
Features	ADPS I	ADPS II	ADPS III	ADPS IV	ADPS V
General behaviour/ executive functioning	Denial; patient minimizes or rationalizes his problems. *Decreased performance at work.* Social behaviour ± adequate. Can function with some supervision; problems in hobbies; early head-turning sign	Head-turning sign; withdrawal from situations; 'out of work'; needs help for travelling; recognizes relatives; hesitations in clothing; denial of true illness	Decreased interest for toileting and hygiene; may need reminding for shaving, making-up or bathing; apathy, egocentricity; *cannot stay alone*, needs supervision	Social indifference; incontinence, *frontal behaviour*, mannerism; total dependency: needs full care: *institution*	Most functions lost: usually *bedridden*
Memory/orientation	Spatial disorientation for non-familiar places; takes notes for groceries, difficulty recalling recent events, less for remote; forgets what has just read	± Spatial disorientation in familiar places (shopping centre), search for car in car park, forgets things in ADL and IADL, driving problems	Temporo-spatial disorientation; difficulty recalling names of relatives (children) or things such as addresses, phone numbers	Most memories lost; may remember or recognize vaguely familiar voices or faces but ± testable	None and anyway untestable
Motor function	No motor deficit or mild slowing of movement; normal tone	Mild bradykinesia with sometimes slightly increased tone; the patient helps the examiner while being tested; glabellar tap borderline	More extrapyramidal signs (except tremor): slower gait, increased tone, gestural perseverations, myoclonus (mainly hands), early primitive reflexes	Slowness, more parkinsonian features with less expressive face, increased tone; more primitive reflexes, seizures, myoclonus; gait disorder	Flexion hypertonia; cannot walk
Mood/behaviour Abstract thinking	Anxiety, relatively good insight; may have depressed mood; mild personality changes may be early, sometimes before cognitive deficits become evident	Prior personality features accentuated; problems with abstractions and interpretation of proverbs	Early hallucinations and delusions: paranoid ideation, suspiciousness, jealousy; aggressivity, wandering, poor insight, talks about past life; disturbing sexual behaviour	Accusatory, aggressive behaviour, more delusions and hallucinations, loss of insight, agitation, wandering	Patient ± quiet, may scream or grunt

Language and related functions	Word finding difficulty in spontaneous speech; some impairment in following conversation and understanding, but may be normal	Periphrases, circumlocutions, some paraphasias, decreased ideation, difficulty with numbers and decreased verbal comprehension	Semantic verbal paraphasias, echolalia, verbal stereotypy, poor reading and calculation	Semantic jargon progressing to very poor language; hypophonia, pallilalia and sometimes mutism	Mutism or incomprehensible language
Praxis	Normal or slightly impaired visuospatial abilities and constructional apraxia (clock drawing, copy of geometric figures)	Constructional apraxia, imitation apraxia, early possible ideomotor and ideational apraxia	In addition to the other apraxias, may have dressing apraxia; on examination, patient does not know what to do with his hands	Undressing apraxia in addition to the other apraxias but may be difficult to objectivate due to poor comprehension	Too impaired to be testable
Gnosis	Posssible decreased recognition of complex visual forms and decreased sensitivity to contrast	Early autopagnosia, slightly abnormal face–hand test; mild spatial agnosia and early simultagnosia; increased time for stereognostic exploration	Difficulty with bilateral stereognosis, right–left disorientation and possible finger agnosia; abnormal face–hand test misidentifications (TV, mirror)	Whole body autotopagnosia, but difficult to demonstrate due to poor comprehension	Too impaired to be testable

degeneration or the motor neuron disease dementia complex.[51] Prediction of the underlying histopathology is very difficult. The group of degenerative FTD has early cortical features, often with language impairment and behavioural changes, but with relatively preserved event memory early in the illness; this is in striking contrast to AD. By contrast to Pick's disease and AD, most of the other common neurological causes of dementia are associated with early subcortical manifestations,[30–32] and some of the main differential characteristics are described here.

Multi-infarct dementia (MID)[52,53] is easy to recognize, with a history of sudden onset, a stepwise course, multiple specific cognitive deficits, focal neurological signs and, as a rule, well-known risk factors and sometimes previous cerebrovascular events. However, the presence of cerebral infarcts does not exclude the possibility of co-existent AD, which is then referred to as mixed dementia.[54] Binswanger's disease[55] is considered to be of vascular origin and the diagnosis is suggested by a clinical picture of subcortical dementia with gait apraxia, hyperreflexia and personality changes in a patient with risk factors for vascular disease and is supported by periventricular white matter hypodensities on neuroimaging. A pseudobulbar syndrome with dementia in a patient suffering from hypertension would suggest a lacunar state. Cognitive deficits resulting from cerebral infarcts in strategic areas can be recognized by the acute onset of a focal neuropsychological deficit or behavioural change and the finding of a specific ischaemic lesion on neuroimaging. In contrast to MID, vascular dementia secondary to deep white matter disease may have an insidious onset and slow progression.

The difference between AD and Parkinson's disease (PD) is obvious from the motor features at the onset of the latter, but this difference may be more subtle for cognitive deficits, and both diseases may overlap. In general, early neuropsychological features, without dementia, are common in PD and are characterized by apathy, personality changes and articulatory speech disturbances, which is not the case for AD. On the other hand, dementia associated with PD is not rare, and is characterized by classic PD of at least a few years duration before decline appears in many domains, in addition to personality changes, particularly executive functions, memory retrieval, verbal fluency and attention (see Chapter 5).[56] The extrapyramidal syndrome of progressive supra-nuclear palsy (PSP) and the limitation of vertical gaze make it very different from AD. Dementia with Lewy bodies is suspected in patients with a clinical picture of cognitive impairment, fluctuation, hallucinations, early parkinsonian features, delusions, neuroleptic sensitivity and

repeated falls.[57,58] Normal pressure hydrocephalus (NPH) is suggested clinically by the classic syndrome of gait disorder, hyperreflexia and incontinence in a patient with predominant personality or behaviour changes and without the cortical features of AD. By contrast, NPH can be suspected on imaging results. However, caution is recommended in the interpretation of the dilatation of the lateral ventricle in elderly patients (NPH versus subcortical atrophy) if there is no clinical picture suggestive of NPH. In space-occupying lesions, dementia will be preceded by focal neurological signs in the majority of cases, but one has to be aware that subdural haematomas, large meningiomas and tumours of the corpus callosum and of the thalamus may be quite silent in terms of primary deficits at the beginning and that imaging will be of great utility in these conditions. Small asymptomatic meningiomas are commonly found on CT in elderly people, most of the time not associated with any cognitive decline, unless located in very strategic areas. In Huntington's disease, the familial history and the abnormal movements will help in differentiation from AD. A rapidly progressing dementia with extrapyramidal signs and myoclonus would suggest Creutzfeldt–Jakob disease, mainly if supported by the classic periodic pattern on the electroencephalogram, although a new variant has been described in the UK without the typical clinical and electroencephalographical features.[59] The next chapter will review in more detail the differential diagnosis of other dementias.

CONCLUSION

We have described a practical approach for the clinical diagnosis of dementia and its main causes. We stress the fact that the diagnosis of dementia is mainly clinical. Careful history and examination cannot be replaced by laboratory tests or brain imaging. In addition, the accuracy for the diagnosis of dementia and AD is relatively high on clinical grounds and the differential diagnosis of the main neurological causes of dementia is also possible in the majority of the cases.

REFERENCES

1. McKhann G, Drachman D, Folstein M, et al. Clinical diagnosis of Alzheimer's disease: report of the NINCDS-ADRDA Work Group under the auspices of Department of Health and Human Services Task Force on Alzheimer's Disease. Neurology 1984; 34:939–944.
2. Holmes C, Cairns N, Lantos P, et al. Validity of current clinical criteria for Alzheimer's disease, vascular dementia and dementia with Lewy bodies. Br J Psychiatry 1999; 174:45–50.

3. National Institutes of Health: Dementia – Consensus Conference. Differential Diagnosis of Dementing Disease. JAMA 1987; 258:3411–3416.

4. Mesulam MM. Slowly progressive aphasia without generalized dementia. Ann Neurol 1982; 11:592–598.

5. Mesulam MM. Primary progressive aphasia: differentiation from Alzheimer's disease. Ann Neurol 1987; 22:533–534.

6. Karbe H, Kertesz A, Polk M. Profiles of language impairment in primary progressive aphasia. Arch Neurol 1993; 50:193–201.

7. Price BH, Gurvit H, Weintraub S, et al. Neuropsychological patterns and language deficits in 20 consecutive cases of autopsy-confirmed Alzheimer's disease. Arch Neurol 1993; 50:931–937.

8. American Psychiatric Association. Diagnostic and Statistical Manual of Mental Disorders, 4th edn. Washington DC: American Psychiatric Association 1994.

9. Mortimer JA, van Duijn CM, Chandra V, et al. Head trauma as a risk factor for Alzheimer's disease: a collaborative re-analysis of case-control studies. Int J Epidemiol 1991; 20 (suppl 2):S28–S35.

10. American Psychiatric Association, Committee on Nomenclature and Statistics. Diagnostic and Statistical Manual of Mental Disorders, 3rd edn., revised. Washington DC: American Psychiatric Association (1987).

11. Oppenheim G. The earliest signs of Alzheimer's disease. J Geriatr Psychiatry Neurol 1994; 7:116–120.

12. Paquette I. Les manifestations psychiatriques dans la démence: perspective phénoménologique. Rev Can Psychiat 1993; 38:671–677.

13. Doll R. Review: Alzheimer's disease and environmental aluminum. Age Ageing 1993; 22:138–153.

14. Canadian Study of Health and Aging. The Canadian Study of Health and Aging: risk factors for Alzheimer's disease in Canada. Neurology 1994; 44:2073–2080.

15. McShane R, Keene J, Gedling K, et al. Do neuroleptic drugs hasten cognitive decline in dementia? Prospective study with necropsy follow up. BMJ 1997; 314:266–270.

16. Hofman A, Schulte W, Tanja TA, et al. History of dementia and Parkinson's disease in first-degree relatives of patients with Alzheimer's disease. Neurology 1989; 39:1589–1592.

17. Jorm AF, van Duijn CM, Chandra V, et al. Psychiatric history and related exposures as risk factors for Alzheimer's disease: a collaborative re-analysis of case-control studies. Int J Epidemiol 1991; 20(suppl 2):S43–S47.

18. van Duijn CM, Stijnen T, Hofman A. Risk factors for Alzheimer's disease: overview of the EURODEM collaborative re-analysis of case-control studies. Int J Epidemiol 1991; 20(suppl 2):S4–S12.

19. Desmond DW, Moroney JT, Lynch T, et al. The natural history of CADASIL. A pooled analysis of previously published cases. Stroke 1999; 30:1230–1233.

20. Folstein MF, Folstein SE, McHugh PR. 'Mini-mental state': a practical method for grading the cognitive state of patients for the clinician. J Psychiatr Res 1975; 12:189–198.

21. Nasreddine ZS, Philips NA, Bédirian V, et al. The Montreal Cognitive Assessment, MoCA: A Brief Screening Tool For Mild Cognitive Impairment. J Am Geriatr Soc 2005; 53:695–699.

22. Tuokko H, Hadjistavropoulos T, Miller JA, Beattie BL. The Clock Test: a sensitive measure to differentiate normal elderly from those with Alzheimer disease. J Am Geriatr Soc 1992; 40:579–584.

23. Rosen WG, Terry RD, Fould PA, Katzman R, Peck A. Pathological verification of ischemic score in differentiation of dementias. Ann Neurol 1980; 7:486–488.

24. Organizing Committee, Canadian Consensus Conference on the Assessment of Dementia. Assessing dementia: the Canadian consensus. Can Med Assoc J 1991; 144:851–853.

25. Rossor MN. Management of neurological disorders: dementia. J Neurol Neurosurg Psychiatry 1994; 57:1451–1456.

26. Knopman DS, DeKosky ST, Cummings JL, et al. Practice parameter: diagnosis of dementia (an evidence-based review): Report of the Quality Standards Subcommittee of the American Academy of Neurology. Neurology 2001; 56:1143–1153.

27. Corey-Bloom J, Thal LJ, Galasko D, et al. Diagnosis and evaluation of dementia. Neurology 1995; 45:211–218.

28. Geldmacher DS, Whitehouse P. Evaluation of dementia. N Engl J Med 1996; 335:330–336.

29. Wang H-X, Wahlin A, Basun H, et al. Vitamin B12 and folate in relation to the development of Alzheimer's disease. Neurology 2001; 56:1188–1194.

30. Cummings JL. Subcortical dementia: neuropsychology, neuropsychiatry, and pathophysiology. Br J Psychiatry 1986; 149:682–697.

31. Habib M, Donnet A, Ceccaldi M, Poncet M. Syndrome de démence sous-corticale. Presse Méd 1989; 18:719–724.

32. Huber SJ, Shuttleworth EC, Paulson GW, Bellchambers MJG, Clapp LE. Cortical vs subcortical dementia. Arch Neurol 1986; 43:392–394.

33. Huff FJ, Becker JT, Belle SH, et al. Cognitive deficits and clinical diagnosis of Alzheimer's disease. Neurology 1987; 37:1119–1124.

34. Joachim CL, Morris JH, Selkoe DJ. Clinically diagnosed Alzheimer's disease: autopsy results in 150 cases. Ann Neurol 1988; 24:50–56.

35. Morris JC, McKeel DW, Fulling K, Thorack RM, Berg L. Validation of clinical diagnostic criteria for Alzheimer's disease. Ann Neurol 1988; 24:17–22.

36. Sulkava R, Haltia M, Paetau A, Wikström J, Palo J. Accuracy of clinical diagnosis in primary degenerative dementia: correlation with neuropathological findings. J Neurol Neurosurg Psychiatry 1983; 46:9–13.

37. Chui HC, Lee Teng E, Henderson VW, Moy AC. Clinical sub-types of dementia of the Alzheimer's type. Neurology 1985; 35:1544–1550.

38. Mayeux R, Stern Y, Spanton, S. Heterogeneity in dementia of the Alzheimer's type: evidence of sub-groups. Neurology 1985; 35:453–461.

39. Lawlor BA, Ryan TM, Schmeidler J, Mohs RC, Davis KL. Clinical symptoms associated with age of onset in Alzheimer's disease. Am J Psychiatry 1994; 151:1646–1649.

40. Folstein MF. Heterogeneity in Alzheimer's disease. Neurobiol Aging 1989; 10:434–435.

41. Scheltens PH, Vermersch P, Leys D. Hétérogénéité de la maladie d'Alzheimer. Rev Neurol (Paris) 1993; 149:14–25.

42. Feldman HH, Jacova, C. Mild cognitive impairment. Am J Geriatr Psychiatry 2005; 13:645–655.

43. Grundman M, Petersen R.C, Morris JC, et al. Rate of dementia of Alzheimer type (DAT) in subjects with mild cognitive impairment: the Alzheimer's Disease Cooperative Study (Abstract). Neurology 1996; 46:A403.

44. Petersen RC, Doody R, Kurz A, et al. Current concepts in Mild Cognitive Impairment. Arch Neurol 2001; 58: 1985–1992.

45. Reisberg B, Ferris SH, De Leon MJ, Crook T. The Global Deterioration Scale for assessment of primary degenerative dementia. Am J Psychiatry 1982; 139:1136–1139.

46. Hughes CP, Berg L, Danziger WL, Coben LA, Martin RL. A new clinical rating scale for the staging of dementia. Br J Psychiatry 1982; 140:566–572.

47. Berg L. Clinical dementia rating (CDR). Psychopharmacol Bull 1988; 24:637–639.

48. Yesavage JA, Brooks JO, Taylor J, Tinklenberg J. Development of aphasia, apraxia, and agnosia and decline in Alzheimer's disease. Am J Psychiatry 1993; 150:742–747.

49. Chui HC, Lyness SA, Sobel E, Schneider LS. Extrapyramidal signs and psychiatric symptoms predict faster cognitive decline in Alzheimer's disease. Arch Neurol 1994; 51: 676–681.

50. Bouchard R. Maladie d'Alzheimer: éléments neurologiques du diagnostic différentiel. In: Hébert R, ed. Interdisciplinarité en Gérontologie. Édisem: Québec (1990) 153–157.

51. Snowden JS, Neary D, Mann DMA. Fronto-Temporal Lobar Degeneration: Fronto-Temporal Dementia, Progressive Aphasia, Semantic Dementia. Churchill Livingstone: Edinburgh (1996).

52. Hachinski VC, Lassen NA, Marshall J. Multi-infarct dementia. A cause of mental deterioration in the elderly. Lancet 1974; 2:207–210.

53. Hachinski VC. Multi-infarct dementia: a reappraisal. Alzheimer's Dis Assoc Disord 1991; 5:64–68.

54. Hachinski VC. The decline and resurgence of vascular dementia. Can Med Assoc J 1990; 142:107–111.

55. Morris JC, Gado M, Torack RM, Mckeel DW Jr. Binswanger's disease or artefact: a clinical, neuroimaging, and pathological study of periventricular white matter changes in Alzheimer's disease. In: Wurtham RJ, et al. eds, Advances in Neurology, Vol 51: Alzheimer's Disease. Raven Press: New York 1990 47–52.

56. Emre M. Dementia associated with Parkinson's disease. Lancet Neurol 2003; 2:229–237.

57. McKeith IG, Galasko D, Kosoka K, et al. Consensus guidelines for the clinical and pathological diagnosis of dementia with Lewy bodies. *Neurology* 1996; 47:1113–1116.

58. McKeith I, Mintzer J, Aarsland D, et al. Dementia with Lewy bodies. Lancet Neurol 2004; 3:19–28.

59. Will RG, Ironside JW, Zeidler M, et al. A new variant of Creutzfeldt–Jakob disease in the UK. Lancet 1996; 347:921–925.

5

Differentiation from non-Alzheimer dementia

Richard Camicioli

INTRODUCTION

Alzheimer's disease (AD) is the most common dementia, accounting for the majority of cases in the elderly. Differentiation of other dementias from AD is important in order to implement an appropriate treatment plan, including providing prognostic information and counselling to patients and their families. As in AD, diagnosing non-Alzheimer's dementia relies on the consideration of demographics, risk factors, the clinical course, examination features (neuropsychological and neurological) and laboratory findings. The severity of symptoms on presentation might influence the accuracy of diagnosis. Complicating the differential diagnosis of dementia is the fact that neurodegenerative and other age-related disorders (such as ischaemic disease) can be overlapping. In an important minority of cases an accurate diagnosis cannot be made in living patients, highlighting the importance of continued efforts to obtain autopsies in people dying with dementia.

We first discuss diagnostic criteria for the most common dementias other than AD (Figure 5.1, Table 5.1). This is followed by a discussion organized according to features that allow differentiation among

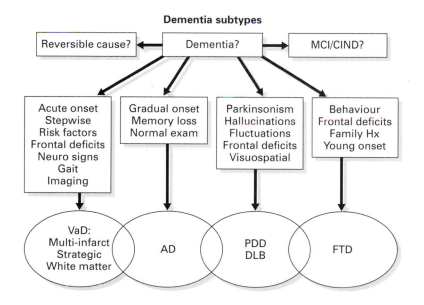

Figure 5.1 Differential diagnostic consideration for common dementias. MCI: mild cognitive impairment; CIND: cognitive impairment not dementia; VaD: vascular dementia; AD: Alzheimer's disease; PDD: Parkinson's disease with dementia; DLB: dementia with Lewy bodies; FTD: frontotemporal dementia

---

Table 5.1 Non-Alzheimer's dementias

- Vascular dementia:
    - Multi-infarct dementia
        - cortical
        - subcortical
    - Subcortical vascular dementia
    - Strategic infarct-related dementia
    - Mixed dementia: Alzheimer/vascular
    - Amyloid angiopathy
    - Hereditary vascular dementias
        - CADASIL
- Dementia with Lewy bodies:
    - Dementia with Lewy bodies (DLB)
        - pure DLB
        - mixed Alzheimer/DLB
    - Parkinson's disease with dementia
- Frontotemporal dementia:
    - Behavioural variant
    - Progressive non-fluent aphasia
    - Semantic dementia
    - Frontotemporal dementia with motor neuron disease
- Other focal neurodegenerative syndromes:
    - Progressive apraxia
        - corticobasal ganglionic degeneration
        - Alzheimer's disease
    - Progressive visuospatial impairment
        - Alzheimer's disease
        - subcortical gliosis
        - Creutzfeld–Jakob disease
- Normal pressure hydrocephalus

- Dementia related to structural pathology:
    - Malignant tumours
    - Benign tumours (depends on location)
    - Abscesses
- Inflammatory disorders:
    - Multiple sclerosis
    - Vasculitis
        - with systemic involvement
        - without systemic involvement
    - Systemic lupus erythematosis
    - Sjögren syndrome
    - Sarcoidosis
    - Bechet's disease
    - Non-vasculitic autoimmune encephalomyelitis (NAIM)
- Infection-related dementias:
    - Creutzfeldt–Jakob disease
    - HIV-related dementia
    - Syphilis
    - Whipple's disease
    - Herpes encephalitis and other viral encephalitides
    - Chronic meningitis
    - Progressive multifocal leukoencephalopathy
    - Subacute sclerosing panencephalitis
- Metabolic-related dementias:
    - B_{12} deficiency
    - Thyroid disease
    - Parathyroid disease
- Toxins:
    - Alcohol
- Hereditary dementias

---

the dementias (Table 5.2). An evolving concept in dementia is the mild cognitive impairment (MCI) that precedes functional impairment required to diagnose dementia. While this prodromal state may occur in many dementias, its relationship to disorders other than AD is not well delineated, and hence we will not specifically consider MCI in this chapter (see Chapter 17).

DEFINITIONS OF COMMON DEMENTIAS

The study of AD has been advanced by the availability of consensus clinical criteria that have been validated against pathological confirmation (see Chapter 1).[1,2]

AD is characterized by an insidious onset of progressive impairment of memory and other areas of cognition, including orientation, language, visuospatial function and praxis. While there is some heterogeneity in the presentation of AD,[3] personality change and marked impairment in attention and executive function raise the possibility of other causes of dementia, such as the frontotemporal dementias (FTD). Marked motor impairment, including abnormal gait, is unusual early in the course of AD and raises the possibility of vascular dementia (VaD) or dementia with Lewy bodies (DLB).[4] Late stage AD patients often have extrapyramidal signs and gait impairment.[5]

Criteria have also been proposed for VaD,[6–8] DLB[9] and FTD.[10,11] Of the common age-associated demen-

---

Table 5.2 Neurological features and selected dementia differential diagnoses

- Cranial nerve findings:
    - Whipple's disease
    - Progressive supranuclear palsy
    - Nieman Pick type C
- Pyramidal signs:
    - Amyotrophic lateral sclerosis
    - Vascular cognitive impairment/dementia
    - Hereditary spastic paraplegia with dementia
        - familial Alzheimer's disease with spastic paraplegia
    - Leukodystrophies
        - adrenoleukodystrophy
        - metachromatic leukodystrophy
        - orthochromatic leukodystrophy
        - Krabbe disease
        - Pelizaeus–Merzbacher disease
- Parkinsonism:
    - Early
    - Parkinson's disease and dementia
    - Dementia with Lewy bodies
    - Progressive supranuclear palsy
    - Late
    - Alzheimer's disease
    - Frontotemporal dementia
- Ataxia:
    - Creutzfeld–Jakob disease
    - Coeliac disease
    - Hashimoto encephalitis
    - Multiple system atrophy
    - Spinocerebellar degeneration
    - Alchohol

- Gait impairment:
    - Vascular cognitive impairment/dementia
    - Normal pressure hydrocephalus
- Neuropathy:
    - HIV
    - Creutzfeld–Jakob disease
    - Paraneoplastic syndromes
    - Vitamin B_{12} deficiency
    - Alcohol
    - Inflammatory disorders
        - sarcoidosis
        - Sjögren syndrome
        - systemic lupus erythematosis
    - Hereditary neuropathy with dementia
        - leukodystrophies
        - mitochondrial disorders
        - hereditary sensory/autonomic neuropathy with dementia
        - polyglucosan body disease
- Apraxia:
    - Corticobasal degeneration
    - Corticobasal ganglionic degeneration
- Seizures/myoclonus:
    - Creutzfeldt–Jakob disease
    - Late Alzheimer's disease
    - Whipple's disease
- Metabolic disorders (with seizure and myoclonus):
    - Mitochondrial encephalopathies
    - Baltic myoclonus (Unverricht Lundborg disease)
    - Lafora disease
    - Ceroid lipofuscinosis
    - Sialidosis
    - GM2 gangliosidosis

---

tias, only Parkinson's disease with dementia (PDD) lacks consensus criteria, so in this case generic dementia criteria are applied.[12] In general, the clinical criteria are not perfect in differentiating dementias from each other. This is partly because of heterogeneity in the clinical presentation of various dementias and because common dementias may have overlapping pathology. In addition, pathological criteria for dementia vary and must be placed in an appropriate clinical context.

Vascular dementia

Vascular dementia, caused by cerebrovascular disease, is generally considered the second most common dementia, accounting for 10–20 per cent of causes of dementia in the elderly. However, pure VaD is relatively uncommon. Cerebrovascular disease is both a risk factor for and can coexist with AD.[13] In fact, mixed AD and cerebrovascular disease is probably more common than VaD.[14] An acute onset, stepwise decline, focal neurological signs, gait impairment and urinary difficulties are suggestive of VaD, especially in the setting of vascular risk factors. Neuroimaging evidence of ischaemic stroke or a haemorrhage temporally associated with, or anatomically consistent with, cognitive deficits is also suggestive of VaD.

It must be kept in mind, however, that VaD is not a uniform entity. Cognitive impairment associated with cerebrovascular disease can be caused by multiple cerebral infarctions, which can be cortical or subcortical, single strategic infarctions or diffuse white matter disease. There are several possible locations of strategic infarctions that would be sufficient to cause dementia: cortical areas include the left angular gyrus, the frontal lobes and the medial temporal lobes, while subcortical areas include the thalamus, genu of the internal capsule and the caudate nucleus.[15,16] Infarction in the anterior cerebral and posterior cerebral territories are particularly likely to be associated with dementia.[17]

The various criteria for VaD are not interchangeable when pathological verification attempts have been made.[18–20] The Hachinski Scale and the National Institute of Neurological Disorders and Stroke Association–Association Internationale pour l'Enseignement en Neurosciences (NINDS-AIREN) criteria are specific in terms of identifying multi-infarct dementia, but sensitivity is low. The California Alzheimer Disease Diagnosis and Treatment Centers (ADDTC) criteria[6,21] and the Mayo Clinic Criteria[22] have improved sensitivity and have reasonable specificity. The more recently proposed criteria incorporate imaging evidence for ischaemic disease, which is critical given that cognitive decline due to cerebrovascular events can be clinically silent.[23]

Many recent studies separate cortical from subcortical vascular dementia and patients who have or have not had clinical strokes versus transient ischaemic events.[24] Neuropsychological assessment – where greater memory deficit is found in AD and where more impairment in executive function is seen in VaD – as well as neuroimaging, can assist in differentiating one disease from the other. In practice, overlapping neuropsychological findings are often found.[21,25,26] A key issue is that of overlapping pathology.

Parkinson's disease with dementia and dementia with Lewy bodies

Pathologically, cortical Lewy bodies can be found in both PDD and DLB. In the former, parkinsonism precedes cognitive changes by one year or longer, whereas in the latter dementia and parkinsonism co-occur within a year of each other. Patients with DLB and PDD also exhibit co-existent AD pathology. The core features of DLB include visual hallucinations, fluctuating cognition and parkinsonism. Two of the three criteria are required for a diagnosis of probable DLB, and one of the three is sufficient for a diagnosis of possible DLB. The clinical picture may be influenced by the degree of co-existent AD and the pattern of regional involvement with Lewy bodies and neurites.[27] Patients with Parkinson's disease (PD) who, by definition, have parkinsonism, are at high risk of developing

dementia, at a rate of up to 10 per cent per year[28] with a prevalence of 20–30 per cent in contemporary cross-sectional studies. When patients with DLB and PDD have been compared with regard to these core features, patients with these two disorders resemble each other, though hallucinations[29] and fluctuations[30] are more common in DLB. Although extrapyramidal signs may be less severe in DLB compared with PDD, response to levodopa may be better in PDD compared with DLB.[31,32] Fluctuations[33] and hallucinations[34] are more common in DLB than in AD, and are also common in PDD. Along with the presence of parkinsonism, these features can assist in differential diagnosis. Rigidity, which suggests an extrapyramidal disorder, such as PD, PDD or DLB, needs to distinguished from paratonia, a non-specific sign in dementia, and spasticity, which suggests pyramidal tract involvement. Sleep disturbance, specifically REM sleep behaviour disorder, is strongly associated with synuclein pathology, including diffuse Lewy bodies,[35] and hence occurs in both DLB and PDD. From a cognitive perspective DLB patients exhibit attention, executive and visuospatial impairment.[36]

Frontotemporal dementias

FTD are distinct degenerative dementias characterized by behavioural and personality changes and circumscribed cognitive deficits predominantly affecting executive function and language. AD can be reliably differentiated from FTD using clinical criteria wherein patients with FTD exhibit a greater degree of behavioural and executive impairment with relative sparing of episodic memory and visuospatial function.[37,38] From a cognitive perspective, VaD, DLB and PDD can sometimes present diagnostic problems since they show greater impairment in executive function and relative sparing of memory, compared to patients with AD, a similar cognitive pattern to FTD. While the clinical history, neurological examination and imaging help in the differentiation of these syndromes, cases of AD with prominent behaviour problems are not uncommon, and FTD can also occur with prominent memory impairment. Behaviour difficulties including decreased insight, decreased attention to personal care, disinhibition, and inappropriate behaviour are prominent in behavioural variant FTD, but also occur in other subtypes of FTD and are important to elicit in establishing the diagnosis.[39–41] Language problems seen in primary progressive aphasia and semantic dementia occasionally lead to diagnostic confusion with AD and VaD if focal presentations of FTD aren't appreciated. AD can present with prominent word finding and language impairment and FTD can be associated with episodic memory impairment. Other 'lobar' degenerative syndromes including progressive apraxia and progressive visuospatial impairment are important to recognize as well.

Pathologically, FTD are histologically varied.[42–44] Findings include non-specific pathology with gliosis and neuronal loss, tau-positive neurons with or without Pick bodies and tau-negative ubiquitin-positive inclusions. The latter pathological changes are often associated with motor neuron disease – familial cases are common. Progressive apraxia is commonly associated with findings consistent with corticobasal ganglionic degeneration,[45] notably ballooned neurons, but can be seen in Pick disease and with AD pathology.[46] Progressive visuospatial impairment is most commonly associated with AD pathology, though Creutzfeldt–Jakob disease (CJD) and non-specific FTD pathology may also be associated with this presentation.[47,48]

Argyrophilic grain disease,[49] neurofilament inclusion disease[50] and late-life hippocampal sclerosis[51–53] are examples of rare entities whose clinical presentation overlaps with FTD and AD. In vivo identification of these entities remains problematic.

DEMOGRAPHICS AND EPIDEMIOLOGY

Early- versus late-onset dementias

Age of onset can help in the differential diagnosis of dementia. A study of the prevalence of dementia in people aged 45–65 years found that Huntington's disease (HD) was the most prevalent at 18 cases/100 000, followed by AD and FTD, which exhibit equal prevalence of 15/100 000.[54] VaD accounted for 8.2 cases and Lewy body dementias accounted for 6.9 cases per 100 000. A second British study found that AD was most prevalent at 41/100 000, followed by VaD at 17.9, FTD at 15.4 and alcohol-related dementia at 13.6 per 100 000.[55] These data can be contrasted with another study examining people aged 65 and older that found the proportion of dementias in the population to be: AD 31.3 per cent; VaD 21.9 per cent; DLB 10.9 per cent; and FLD 7.8 per cent.[56] Another population-based study of people older than 75 years from Finland similarly found 46.7 per cent to have AD, 23.4 per cent VaD, 21.9 per cent Lewy body dementias and 8 per cent other dementias.[57] In the oldest old, aged 85 years and greater, frontal dysfunction was present in 19 per cent, but was accounted for by AD and VaD in the majority of cases, with only 3 per cent having FTD.[58] These data can be helpful when considering the individual dementia patient: early-onset patients are

less likely to have AD and more likely to have dementia related to FTD, HD or alcoholism; later-onset patients are more likely to have AD, VaD and Lewy body related dementia.

Early-onset dementias

Early-onset adult dementias can occur due to typical late-life dementias presenting at an earlier than typical age or to a disorder of childhood onset presenting late.[59,60] For instance, AD can have onset in the twenties. Young-onset AD tends to be familial, accounted for by mutations in genes encoding for presenilin 1 (chromosome 14), presenilin 2 (chromosome 1) and amyloid (chromosome 21). Down's syndrome, with triplication of chromosome 21, is another cause of young-onset dementia associated with AD pathology. VaD and FTD are relatively common in early onset dementia, and can be diagnosed on the basis of clinical findings and neuroimaging features. New variant CJD typically has an early adult onset, with a prolonged clinical course that includes a psychiatric prodrome. Sporadic prion disorders can occur at any age.[61,62] Familial prion disorders such as Gerstmann–Sheinker–Straussler syndrome (GSSS) and familial fatal insomnia typically have an early onset. Multiple sclerosis can lead to considerable cognitive impairment to the degree that patients may have dementia with symptoms and signs that can be quite varied. Neurodegeneration with brain iron accumulation can also present with a young-onset dementia.[63] Subacute sclerosing panencephalitis (SSPE) is an encephalitis associated with prior measles infection that is associated with progressive dementia and myoclonus, generally prior to adulthood.

Metabolic and genetic conditions are associated with early-onset dementia. In general these are rare and are often inherited in an autosomal recessive fashion. These include a number of disorders that are associated with myoclonus and epilepsy, including sialidosis, GM2 gangliosidosis,[64] Lafora disease, ceroid lipofuscinosis and mitochondrial encephalomyopathies.[65] Leukodystrophies associated with dementia, progressive motor impairment and peripheral neuropathy can present in adults. These include adrenoleukodystophy,[66] metachromatic leukodystrophy,[67] orthochromatic leukodystrophy,[68] Krabbe disease,[69] Alexander disease,[70] Pelizaeus–Merzbacher[71] and others.[72,73] Other typically childhood-onset disorders that can present as a dementia in adults include polyglucosan body disease[74] and Nieman Pick type C disease,[75,76] as well as other lipidoses. In general, metabolic conditions should remain in the differential diagnosis of degenerative conditions in adults, especially young adults and in those with unusual clinical features.[77]

Family history

The presence of a family history can provide clues to the aetiology of dementia. While familial AD is well known, a family history of dementia is even more likely in FTD.[78] The most common definable inheritance pattern in FTD is autosomal dominant, occurring in 10–20 per cent or more of cases, depending on the population studied.[79] Family history without a clear inheritance pattern is also common, and can be found in up to 40 per cent of cases.[80,81] A family history is common in AD, but can occur in other late-onset dementias, such as DLB.[82] Although a positive family history may be less common in VaD, this is confounded by shared risk factors between VaD and AD. Familial AD is associated with a number of mutations (see Chapter 27).[83]

HD is common among early-onset dementias associated with an autosomal dominant family history. Dentato-rubralpallidolusyian atrophy (DRPLA) is another autosomal dominant disorder with a movement disorder and dementia.[84] Autosomal dominant VaDs such as CADASIL are a consideration in the appropriate setting.[85]

CLINICAL COURSE

Acute onset

An acute onset may be consistent with vascular causes of dementia, including cerebrovascular disease,[86] vasculitis and amyloid angiopathy (with or without haemorrhage).[87,88] On the other hand, VaD with cognitive impairment is quite heterogeneous and an insidious course is common, especially in subcortical small vessel disease. Complicating matters, a history of vascular risk factors, including past stroke, can place patients at risk for AD.

Causes of delirium should be considered in cognitive impairment of acute onset associated with fluctuations in the level of consciousness, especially in the setting of a possible underlying medical cause.[89] Dramatic fluctuations in the level of consciousness can mimic an acute stroke-like onset and are characteristic of DLB and can be seen in PDD.[30] While delirium can occur in the absence of dementia, they commonly co-occur, dementia being a risk factor for delirium and vice versa.[90]

Rapidly progressive dementias

Creutzfeldt–Jakob disease

A rapidly progressive dementia raises the possibility of CJD, but can be seen in vascular and degenerative dementias, including AD and DLB, as well. CJD is a rapidly progressive dementia that can only be definitively diagnosed by a brain tissue examination showing prion proteins with associated spongiform changes. CJD can be sporadic or familial (associated with mutations in gene coding for the prion protein) or transmissible. Transmissible forms of CJD include iatrogenic and variant CJD. Criteria for probable CJD have been proposed (from http://www.eurocjd.ed.ac.uk/def.htm) and include typical EEG features with at least two of the following clinical features: myoclonus, visual or cerebellar signs, pyramidal/extrapyramidal signs or akinetic mutism. The clinical diagnosis can also be made with a history of a rapidly progressive dementia with duration of less than two years, and at least two of the above clinical features, with a positive 14-3-3 test. The utility of the latter test has come into question because of its variable sensitivity and lack of specificity.[91] Diffusion-weighted magnetic resonance imaging (MRI) may have superior sensitivity compared with EEG, and superior specificity compared to cerebrospinal fluid (CSF) examination.[92] In general, sporadic CJD is inexorably progressive, resulting in death within a year; however, the course of sporadic CJD can be considerably longer.[93] A long duration is common in the autosomal dominant prion disease, GSSS. Variant CJD is a progressive neuropsychiatric disorder ultimately leading to ataxia, dementia and myoclonus (or chorea) without the typical EEG appearance of CJD or the proportion with elevation in the 14-3-3 protein.[94] Young-onset sporadic CJD cases share features of a long neuropsychiatric prodrome with variant CJD.[62]

Findings on MRI that are suggestive of sporadic CJD have been described and include increased signal in the basal ganglia and cortex on diffusion-weighted and FLAIR images.[95,96] Similar changes are found in variant CJD, where they are found in the pulvinar in 70 per cent of cases.[94] It has been proposed that MRI be included among diagnostic criteria given reasonable sensitivity and specificity in some series. Periodic sharp complexes on electroencephalography changes are characteristic, but can occur transiently or late in the course of disease and are thus insensitive.[97] False positives include cases of AD and VaD. While routine cerebrospinal fluid measurements are generally normal in CJD, the 14-3-3 protein detectable using 2-D techniques is elevated in CJD. Test properties probably depend on the specific laboratory where testing is being done and the characteristics of the patient population.

Other rapidly progressive dementias

Rapid progression in symptoms can be seen in AD and DLB.[98,99] Dementia associated with motor neuron disease can also have a rapid course.[100] Syndromes that should be considered in the differential diagnosis of a rapidly progressive dementia include viral encephalitis, paraneoplastic (limbic) encephalitis, central nervous system cancer, Hashimoto's encephalitis, other autoimmune disorders (including antiphospholipid syndrome, systemic lupus erythematosis, sarcoidosis and non-vasculitic autoimmune meningoencephalitis),[101,102] infections and metabolic disorders. Neuroimaging can be helpful in identifying ischaemic changes and other brain lesions.

Infiltrative processes that can lead to a rapidly progressive dementia include intracerebral lymphomatosis,[103] intravascular lymphomatosis[104,105] and miliary metastases.[106] Diencephalic angioencephalopathy is a rare subacutely progressive dementia associated with thalamic symptoms including somnolence.[107]

NEUROLOGICAL EXAM FEATURES

Dementia with motor impairment

Non-specific motor impairments, including generalized slowing, imbalance and gait impairment, are found in the course of all the degenerative dementias, and are even seen in patients with MCI. When prominent, such findings suggest a dementia other than AD.[108] VaD can be diagnosed in the absence of neurological examination findings. However, typical VaD is associated with gait impairment, pyramidal, extrapyramidal or cerebellar signs. Strokes can lead to focal findings based on location and connectivity. Neurological signs and gait impairment are unusual early in the course of AD, and would suggest VaD and DLB among the primary dementia syndromes.[4] Two movement disorders to consider in demented patients with prominent early motor impairment are corticobasal ganglionic degeneration (CBDG), which leads to progressive asymmetric apraxia, and progressive supranuclear palsy (PSP), which is associated with supranuclear gaze palsy and balance impairment.[109–111] Pathological features of CBDG and PSP overlap with those of FTD. Some specific neurological findings that

can be helpful in the differential diagnosis of dementia are considered next.

Abnormal ocular and cranial movements, including oculomasticatory myorhythmic and microsaccadic jerks, are important to seek. The former are seen in Whipple's disease,[112] where dementia, supranuclear gaze palsy and axial parkinsonism are also found. Microsaccadic jerks suggest brainstem pathology and can be seen in patients with PSP, where classically a history of early falls and supranuclear gaze palsy is suggestive of the diagnosis.[113] Abnormal saccadic eye movements are seen in PSP, FTD and HD, reflecting abnormalities in frontostriatal circuitry associated with eye movements. Supranuclear gaze palsy is characteristic of PSP, Nieman Pick type C and Whipple's disease, but can be seen in CBGD[114] and FTD[115] and has been reported in cases of motor neuron disease[116] and familial CJD.[117] The abnormal eye movements of PSP might not be seen early in the course of disease and are not evident in all living patients.

DLB and PDD are characterized by parkinsonism (tremor, bradykinesia, rigidity). Parkinsonism, in addition to other features of dysfunction of the extrapyramidal system, is evident in HD (chorea), PSP (impaired postural reflexes) and CBDG (myoclonus, dystonia). Parkinsonism is present late in the course of FTD.[118] Neuroacanthocytosis is a disorder associated with chorea and peripheral neuropathy, which can be associated with dementia.[119] Acanthocytes can also be seen in pantothenate kinase-associated neurodegeneration, a disorder of brain iron accumulation that generally presents in childhood, but can occur in adults where it can present as a progressive movement disorder with chorea and dementia.[120] Wilson's disease and other disorders of copper metabolism rarely cause dementia, but in the setting of a younger patient with dementia and dystonia or a movement disorder, Wilson's disease should be excluded given the potential for treatment with chelation and diet restriction for copper.

Pyramidal system dysfunction is seen in cerebrovascular disease and associated VaD. Leukodystrophies, in particular adrenoleukodystrophy and metachromatoic leukodystrophy, are associated with cognitive decline and spasticity, which can usually be distinguished from rigidity. Superficial siderosis has been recently recognized as a cause of dementia and progressive neurological deficits.[121] A possibly related problem, central nervous system microbleeds, which can be identified using T2* gradient echo MRI scans, is found in amyloid angiopathy,[122] CADASIL and AD.[123]

Cerebellar ataxia may be seen in these disorders, but is also characteristic of some patients with prion-disease, including GSSS, a hereditary prion disorder. Hereditary ataxia-dementia syndrome includes DRPLA and other spinocerebellar ataxias, such as Machado–Joseph disease.[124] Coeliac disease, vitamin B_{12} deficiency, paraneoplastic syndromes and Hashimoto encephalitis are examples of acquired and potentially treatable ataxia-dementia syndromes. Multiple system atrophy (MSA) and other late-onset ataxias, though not typically associated with frank dementia, are associated with subcortical cognitive deficits, which can be severe.[125] Incontinence, gait ataxia and pyramidal signs in MSA may raise the possibility of normal pressure hydrocephalus (NPH), which can be excluded on the basis of brain imaging. Recently the fragile X pre-mutation has been found to be a relatively common disorder associated with ataxia, tremor, parkinsonism and dementia.[126]

Normal pressure hydrocephalus

NPH is a potentially treatable syndrome defined by dementia associated with gait impairment and urinary urgency or incontinence.[127] NPH patients have hydrocephalus by imaging. If one suspects NPH, causes of obstructive hydrocephalus, MSA (associated with ataxia and incontinence), vascular gait impairment and AD with gait impairment are differential diagnostic considerations. The presence of the clinical triad along with hydrocephalus on imaging is predictive of shunt responders.[128] Clinical features associated with a good response include a shorter duration of illness, lack of prominent cortical cognitive deficits and good response to a removal of cerebrospinal fluid, by external or internal lumbar drainage or by single or repeated lumbar puncture. Neuropsychological and imaging features[129] can be helpful in determining response. For example, anomia on neuropsychological testing or marked hippocampal atrophy might suggest AD and a poorer potential for response to shunting. While longer duration of cognitive impairment is a predictor of poor response, patients may respond despite the presence of negative prognostic indicators.[130] Ancillary tests including intracranial pressure monitoring, measures of CSF compliance and ventricular cysternography have not been consistently helpful in predicting ventricular shunt response.

Seizures and myoclonus

Seizures and myoclonus are relatively rare in dementia patients. Myoclonus is characteristic in CJD, but is also common in AD, especially late in the course of the disorder. Focal myoclonus is also evident in CBGD. A number of young-onset dementias are associated with seizures and myoclonus and are discussed above with young-onset dementia.

NEUROPSYCHOLOGICAL AND BEHAVIOURAL FEATURES

Memory impairment in disorders other than AD

Memory impairment is a defining feature in AD patients who have impaired recall as well as recognition memory. In subcortical dementias, recognition memory is relatively spared. While memory is often impaired in frontotemporal dementia, behavioural difficulties are the most prominent feature. PDD, DLB and VaD exhibit memory deficits associated with response to cueing suggestive of a subcortical dementia.

Subcortical dementias

The term 'subcortical dementias' refers to a dementia where cognitive slowing, apathy, executive dysfunction and pseudobulbar palsy are prominent clinical features in the absence of cortical dementia features,[131] such as aphasia, apraxia and agnosia. While the term might be debated with regard to its relationship to pathological findings, the pattern of cortical versus subcortical cognitive deficits does distinguish between dementias, with subcortical features found prominently in PSP and subcortical VaD. Patients with PDD and DLB present with an intermediate picture.[132] Cortical features are found in AD and in focal cortical degenerative syndromes. Recent studies have compared the pattern of cognitive impairment between subcortical VaD and AD and found that patients with vascular cognitive impairment have relative sparing of memory and worse executive function compared to AD.[25,133,134]

Frontotemporal dementias

FTD have diverse clinical presentations that can be imperfectly matched to a variety of pathologies that are tau-positive (ballooned neurons, Pick bodies) or tau-negative (ubiquitin-positive inclusions or neuronal loss with gliosis).[42,44] More rarely, patients can have AD pathologically. Clinically, the most common variant is associated with prominent personality and behavioural change (FTD-bv). A language disorder represents the next most common presentation. Two variants are recognized: progressive non-fluent aphasia, also known as primary progressive aphasia, and semantic dementia. Progressive asymmetrical apraxia is seen in CBDG, where tau-positive ballooned neurons are the primary pathology. Motor impairment associated with tau pathology is also evident in PSP.

REVERSIBLE DEMENTIAS

While clinical features allow the identification of specific degenerative dementias, it is important to identify potentially reversible dementia syndromes. While completely reversible dementias are rare,[135,136] it is important to keep in mind that common co-morbid conditions may exacerbate symptoms in degenerative dementias (see Chapter 21). Important reversible causes of dementia overlap with causes of delirium (acute systemic or central nervous system infection, metabolic or endocrine derangements, prescription or non-prescription medications). Intracranial pathology – including cerebrovascular disease, tumours and hydrocephalus – are often, but not always, accompanied by associated signs on the general neurological examination, and a progressive course or history. Brain imaging is essential for establishing these diagnoses and provides justification for imaging in patients with dementia. Head trauma in the elderly is often associated with cognitive decline and can often be identified by history. Seizures are associated with fluctuating symptoms (as can be seen in DLB). Depression often co-occurs with dementia and depressive symptoms should be treated regardless of whether or not it is considered the primary cause of cognitive impairment. Among the entities commonly screened for in the evaluation of cognitive impairment, vitamin B_{12} deficiency and thyroid disease can be clinically silent except for cognitive impairment. Alcohol is the most common toxin associated with cognitive impairment. Rarer entities, including autoimmune disorders, can cause dementia syndromes, and can occur in the absence of clues in the history or findings on general examination.

Several infectious diseases may be associated with a progressive dementia. HIV is associated with a subcortical dementia and is an important consideration in individuals with risk factors or those with known infection with HIV, but can sometimes occur in the absence of a history of these predispositions.[137] Though rare, neurosyphilis remains an important cause of dementia to identify because it is potentially treatable.[138] Acute viral encephalitis can leave patients with dementia, and can sometimes present in an indolent fashion. Clues to acute and subacute CNS infection include headache, fever, seizures, systemic complaints, infection of peripheral tissue, rapid progression, focal neurological features (in the setting of abscess with parenchymal involvement) and travel to endemic areas, but may be absent in infections. Immunosuppression predisposes to infections in general, and specific disorders, such as progressive multifocal leukoencephalopathy, are important to consider in this setting. Worldwide tuberculosis and neurocysticercosis are common infections that have a predilection for the central nervous system. Lyme disease is an infection that should be considered in individuals with appropriate symptoms, such as a rash and polyarthritis, from an endemic area. CJD, Whipple's disease and other infections associated with dementia generally offer clues on the clinical examination as noted above. Other infections have abnormalities on CSF examination, including elevated protein, pleiocytosis and evidence of microorganisms on examination or culture. The polymerase chain reaction is useful for amplifying genomic material for specific infections, including herpes simplex and Whipple's disease.

LABORATORY INVESTIGATIONS

Blood tests are generally useful in excluding potential co-morbid conditions noted previously and rarely they can identify metabolic problems that can cause reversible dementia. Guidelines exist for the evaluation of dementia (see Chapter 4).[139,140] In general, it is important to rule out anaemia, renal or hepatic dysfunction, electrolyte abnormalities and abnormal glucose, as these problems can interfere with cognitive function. Most recommendations include checking vitamin B_{12} levels and thyroid function, since these can be associated with insidious cognitive decline. Calcium or phosphate abnormalities raise the concern of parathyroid dysfunction, which is associated with cognitive impairment, parkinsonism and depression.[141]

Neuroimaging in diagnosing non-Alzheimer's dementias

Structural and functional neuroimaging techniques can be helpful in differential diagnosis (see Chapters 7 and 8). Obviously mass lesions and the presence of hydrocephalus will point to specific entities. White matter changes, though not specific, lead to circumscribed diagnostic considerations. Contrast enhancing white matter changes will raise the possibility of infiltrative or inflammatory disorders. AD is associated with progressive atrophy on CT or MRI. While AD is associated with medial temporal atrophy compared to controls, FTD and other dementias can be as well. Asymmetric atrophy or perfusion is evident in CBGD,[142] on MRI scans and positron emission tomography, while PSP patients have midbrain and frontal atrophy.[143,144] Frontal and lateral temporal atrophy is evident in FTD.[145] Single photon emission computerized tomography (SPECT) scans can also be useful in the differential diagnosis of dementia.[146]

Lumbar puncture

Specific tests, including CSF examination, are useful in the appropriate clinical setting (see Chapter 10). Exposure to intravenous drugs or unprotected sex raises the concern of HIV or neurosyphilis, for example. Weight loss or other systemic complaints raises the concern of an underlying neoplasm that might directly (metastasis or carcinomatous meningitis) or indirectly (paraneoplastic) lead to cognitive decline. This should prompt investigations targeted by the clinical picture, including cerebrospinal fluid examination. While elevation in peripheral antibodies may be found in paraneoplastic syndromes, these may be absent; hence a targeted assessment for cancer is a first step in evaluating patients with a suspected paraneoplastic syndrome.[147] Of note, limbic encephalitis can have an autoimmune basis in the absence of a neoplasm.[148,149] Inflammatory disorders of the brain often lead to elevated protein and may lead to elevated cell counts. Multiple sclerosis and other inflammatory disorders can lead to an elevated immunoglobulin index and oligoclonal bands. CSF angiotensin-converting enzyme can be elevated in sarcoidosis.

Peripheral biopsy

Skin and muscle biopsy may be helpful in some dementias and may obviate a brain biopsy if diagnostic. Skin changes may be evident in some dementias such as Sneddon's syndrome.[150] Vasculitis may be evident in skin or muscle biopsy, even in the absence of skin changes. An angiopathy characteristic of CADASIL can be diagnosed on skin biopsy and might be pursued in rapidly progressive dementia with white matter disease.[151] Ceroid lipofuscinosis, also known as Kufs disease in adults, is a progressive myoclonic disorder that is characterized by fingerprint bodies on skin biopsies examined using electron microscopy.[152]

Lafora disease can also be diagnosed by the finding of Lafora bodies on skin biopsies.[153] Polyglucosan body disease is a disorder associated with urinary incontinence, gait impairment and neuropathy, with PAS-positive inclusions on nerve or sweat gland biopsy.[154]

Brain biopsy

Brain biopsy is reserved for cases where there is diagnostic uncertainty and is particularly important in cases where therapeutics may be instituted or altered on the basis of a biopsy.[155] Biopsies may be complicated by seizures, delirium, pneumonia and wound infections. Diagnoses that might lead to specific treatments include inflammatory disorders, including vasculitis, sarcoidosis or non-vasculitic autoimmune meningoencephalitis. Parenchymal or perivascular infiltrative disorders may also be diagnosed definitively via brain biopsy. Whipple's disease and infections by other fastidious organisms can sometimes be diagnosed by biopsy alone. Newer investigative techniques may obviate the need for biopsy. It should be kept in mind that the identification of a non-treatable degenerative syndrome or prion disease can often assist families in decision-making, justifying brain biopsies in some atypical or rapidly progressive cases. It must be kept in mind that biopsies are often non-specific – 43 per cent of the series by Warren et al.[155]

SUMMARY

In summary, a careful clinical approach should allow non-Alzheimer's dementias to be differentiated from typical AD. Given the overlap and the range of dementia presentations, diagnostic uncertainty will remain in a minority of cases. The challenge in such cases is to identify diagnoses for which there are treatments.

ACKNOWLEDGEMENT

The author thanks Thomas Bouchard for assistance with manuscript preparation.

REFERENCES

1. McKhann G, Drachman D, Folstein M, et al. Clinical diagnosis of Alzheimer's disease: report of the NINCDS-ADRDA Work Group under the auspices of Department of Health and Human Services Task Force on Alzheimer's Disease. Neurology 1984; 34:939–944.
2. Newell KL, Hyman BT, Growdon JH, et al. Application of the National Institute on Aging (NIA)–Reagan Institute

criteria for the neuropathological diagnosis of Alzheimer disease. J Neuropathol Exp Neurol 1999; 58:1147–1155.

3. Galton CJ, Patterson K, Xuereb JH, et al. Atypical and typical presentations of Alzheimer's disease: a clinical, neuropsychological, neuroimaging and pathological study of 13 cases. Brain 2000; 123(part 3):484–498.

4. Allan LM, Ballard CG, Burn DJ, et al. Prevalence and severity of gait disorders in Alzheimer's and non-Alzheimer's dementias. J Am Geriatr Soc 2005; 53:1681–1687.

5. Camicioli R, Licis L. Motor impairment predicts falls in specialized Alzheimer care units. Alzheimer Dis Assoc Disord 2004; 18:214–218.

6. Chui HC, Victoroff JI, Margolin D, et al. Criteria for the diagnosis of ischemic vascular dementia proposed by the State of California Alzheimer's Disease Diagnostic and Treatment Centers. Neurology 1992; 42(3 part 1):473–480.

7. Roman GC, Tatemichi TK, Erkinjuntti T, et al. Vascular dementia: diagnostic criteria for research studies. Report of the NINDS-AIREN International Workshop. Neurology 1993; 43:250–260.

8. Wetterling T, Kanitz RD, Borgis KJ. The ICD-10 criteria for vascular dementia. Dementia 1994; 5:185–188.

9. McKeith IG, Galasko D, Kosaka K, et al. Consensus guidelines for the clinical and pathologic diagnosis of dementia with Lewy bodies (DLB): report of the consortium on DLB international workshop. Neurology 1996; 47:1113–1124.

10. Neary D, Snowden JS, Gustafson L, et al. Frontotemporal lobar degeneration: a consensus on clinical diagnostic criteria. Neurology 1998; 51:1546–1554.

11. McKhann GM, Albert MS, Grossman M, et al. Clinical and pathological diagnosis of frontotemporal dementia: report of the Work Group on Frontotemporal Dementia and Pick's Disease. Arch Neurol 2001; 58:1803–1809.

12. Camicioli R, Fisher N. Progress in clinical neurosciences: Parkinson's disease with dementia and dementia with Lewy bodies. Can J Neurol Sci 2004; 31:7–21.

13. Snowdon DA, Greiner LH, Mortimer JA, et al. Brain infarction and the clinical expression of Alzheimer disease. The Nun Study. JAMA 1997; 277:813–817.

14. Langa KM, Foster NL, Larson EB. Mixed dementia: emerging concepts and therapeutic implications. JAMA 2004; 292:2901–2908.

15. Auchus AP, Chen CP, Sodagar SN, et al. Single stroke dementia: insights from 12 cases in Singapore. J Neurol Sci 2002; 203–204:85–89.

16. Szirmai I, Vastagh I, Szombathelyi E, et al. Strategic infarcts of the thalamus in vascular dementia. J Neurol Sci 2002; 203–204:91–97.

17. Tatemichi TK, Desmond DW, Paik M, et al. Clinical determinants of dementia related to stroke. Ann Neurol 1993; 33:568–575.

18. Moroney JT, Bagiella E, Desmond DW, et al. Meta-analysis of the Hachinski Ischemic Score in pathologically verified dementias. Neurology 1997; 49:1096–1105.

19. Pohjasvaara T, Mantyla R, Ylikoski R, et al. Comparison of different clinical criteria (DSM-III, ADDTC, ICD-10, NINDS-AIREN, DSM-IV) for the diagnosis of vascular dementia. National Institute of Neurological Disorders and Stroke–Association Internationale pour la Recherche et l'Enseignement en Neurosciences. Stroke 2000; 31:2952–2957.

20. Gold G, Bouras C, Canuto A, et al. Clinicopathological validation study of four sets of clinical criteria for vascular dementia. Am J Psychiatry 2002; 159:82–87.

21. Lopez OL, Kuller LH, Becker JT, et al. Classification of vascular dementia in the Cardiovascular Health Study Cognition Study. Neurology 2005; 64:1539–1547.

22. Knopman DS, Parisi JE, Boeve BF, et al. Vascular dementia in a population-based autopsy study. Arch Neurol 2003; 60:569–575.

23. Vermeer SE, Prins ND, den Heijer T, et al. Silent brain infarcts and the risk of dementia and cognitive decline. N Engl J Med 2003; 348:1215–1222.

24. Sachdev PS, Brodaty H, Valenzuela MJ, et al. The neuropsychological profile of vascular cognitive impairment in stroke and TIA patients. Neurology 2004; 62:912–919.

25. Tierney MC, Black SE, Szalai JP, et al. Recognition memory and verbal fluency differentiate probable Alzheimer disease from subcortical ischemic vascular dementia. Arch Neurol 2001; 58:1654–1659.

26. Ballard CG, Burton EJ, Barber R, et al. NINDS AIREN neuroimaging criteria do not distinguish stroke patients with and without dementia. Neurology 2004; 63:983–988.

27. McKeith IG, Dickson DW, Lowe J, et al. Diagnosis and management of dementia with Lewy bodies. Third report of the DLB consortium. Neurology 2005; 65:1863–1872.

28. Aarsland D, Andersen K, Larsen JP, et al. Prevalence and characteristics of dementia in Parkinson disease: an 8-year prospective study. Arch Neurol 2003; 60:387–392.

29. Aarsland D, Ballard C, Larsen JP, et al. A comparative study of psychiatric symptoms in dementia with Lewy bodies and Parkinson's disease with and without dementia. Int J Geriatr Psychiatry 2001; 16:528–536.

30. Ballard CG, Aarsland D, McKeith I, et al. Fluctuations in attention: PD dementia vs DLB with parkinsonism. Neurology 2002; 59:1714–1720.

31. Burn DJ, Rowan EN, Minett T, et al. Extrapyramidal features in Parkinson's disease with and without dementia and dementia with Lewy bodies: a cross-sectional comparative study. Mov Disord 2003; 18:884–889.

32. Molloy S, McKeith IG, O'Brien JT, et al. The role of levodopa in the management of dementia with Lewy bodies. J Neurol Neurosurg Psychiatry 2005; 76:1200–1203.

33. Ferman TJ, Smith GE, Boeve BF, et al. DLB fluctuations: specific features that reliably differentiate DLB from AD and normal aging. Neurology 2004; 62:181–187.

34. Ballard C, McKeith I, Harrison R, et al. A detailed phenomenological comparison of complex visual hallucinations in dementia with Lewy bodies and Alzheimer's disease. Int Psychogeriatr 1997; 9:381–388.

35. Boeve BF, Silber MH, Parisi JE, et al. Synucleinopathy pathology and REM sleep behavior disorder plus dementia or parkinsonism. Neurology 2003; 61:40–45.

36. Collerton D, Burn D, McKeith I, et al. Systematic review and meta-analysis show that dementia with Lewy bodies is a visual-perceptual and attentional-executive dementia. Dement Geriatr Cogn Disord 2003; 16:229–237.

37. Rosen HJ, Hartikainen KM, Jagust W, et al. Utility of clinical criteria in differentiating frontotemporal lobar degeneration (FTLD) from AD. Neurology 2002; 58:1608–1615.

38. Knopman DS, Boeve BF, Parisi JE, et al. Antemortem diagnosis of frontotemporal lobar degeneration. Ann Neurol 2005; 57:480–488.

39. Mendez MF, Perryman KM, Miller BL, et al. Behavioral differences between frontotemporal dementia and Alzheimer's disease: a comparison on the BEHAVE-AD rating scale. Int Psychogeriatr 1998; 10:155–162.

40. Kertesz A, Nadkarni N, Davidson W, et al. The Frontal Behavioral Inventory in the differential diagnosis of frontotemporal dementia. J Int Neuropsychol Soc 2000; 6:460–468.

41. Srikanth S, Nagaraja AV, Ratnavalli E. Neuropsychiatric symptoms in dementia–frequency, relationship to dementia

severity and comparison in Alzheimer's disease, vascular dementia and frontotemporal dementia. J Neurol Sci 2005; 236:43–48.

42. Hodges JR, Davies RR, Xuereb JH, et al. Clinicopathological correlates in frontotemporal dementia. Ann Neurol 2004; 56:399–406.

43. Johnson JK, Diehl J, Mendez MF, et al. Frontotemporal lobar degeneration: demographic characteristics of 353 patients. Arch Neurol 2005; 62:925–930.

44. Kertesz A, McMonagle P, Blair M, et al. The evolution and pathology of frontotemporal dementia. Brain 2005; 128(part 9):1996–2005.

45. Graham NL, Bak TH, Hodges JR. Corticobasal degeneration as a cognitive disorder. Mov Disord 2003; 18:1224–1232.

46. Green RC, Goldstein FC, Mirra SS, et al. Slowly progressive apraxia in Alzheimer's disease. J Neurol Neurosurg Psychiatry 1995; 59:312–315.

47. Renner JA, Burns JM, Hou CE, et al. Progressive posterior cortical dysfunction: a clinicopathologic series. Neurology 2004; 63:1175–1180.

48. Tang-Wai DF, Graff-Radford NR, Boeve BF, et al. Clinical, genetic, and neuropathologic characteristics of posterior cortical atrophy. Neurology 2004; 63:1168–1174.

49. Tolnay M, Clavaguera F. Argyrophilic grain disease: a late-onset dementia with distinctive features among tauopathies. Neuropathology 2004; 24:269–283.

50. Cairns NJ, Grossman M, Arnold SE, et al. Clinical and neuropathologic variation in neuronal intermediate filament inclusion disease. Neurology 2004; 63:1376–1384.

51. Blass DM, Hatanpaa KJ, Brandt J, et al. Dementia in hippocampal sclerosis resembles frontotemporal dementia more than Alzheimer disease. Neurology 2004; 63:492–497.

52. Hatanpaa KJ, Blass DM, Pletnikova O, et al. Most cases of dementia with hippocampal sclerosis may represent frontotemporal dementia. Neurology 2004; 63:538–542.

53. Lippa CF, Dickson DW. Hippocampal sclerosis dementia: expanding the phenotypes of frontotemporal dementias? Neurology 2004; 63:414–415.

54. Ratnavalli E, Brayne C, Dawson K, et al. The prevalence of frontotemporal dementia. Neurology 2002; 58:1615–1621.

55. Harvey RJ, Skelton-Robinson M, Rossor MN. The prevalence and causes of dementia in people under the age of 65 years. J Neurol Neurosurg Psychiatry 2003; 74:1206–1209.

56. Stevens T, Livingston G, Kitchen G, et al. Islington study of dementia subtypes in the community. Br J Psychiatry 2002; 180:270–276.

57. Rahkonen T, Eloniemi-Sulkava U, Rissanen S, et al. Dementia with Lewy bodies according to the consensus criteria in a general population aged 75 years or older. J Neurol Neurosurg Psychiatry 2003; 74:720–724.

58. Gislason TB, Sjogren M, Larsson L, et al. The prevalence of frontal variant frontotemporal dementia and the frontal lobe syndrome in a population based sample of 85 year olds. J Neurol Neurosurg Psychiatry 2003; 74:867–871.

59. Coker SB. The diagnosis of childhood neurodegenerative disorders presenting as dementia in adults. Neurology 1991; 41:794–798.

60. Sampson EL, Warren JD, Rossor MN. Young onset dementia. Postgrad Med J 2004; 80:125–139.

61. Martindale J, Geschwind MD, De Armond S, et al. Sporadic Creutzfeldt–Jakob disease mimicking variant Creutzfeldt–Jakob disease. Arch Neurol 2003; 60:767–770.

62. Boesenberg C, Schulz-Schaeffer WJ, Meissner B, et al. Clinical course in young patients with sporadic Creutzfeldt–Jakob disease. Ann Neurol 2005; 58:533–543.

63. Cooper GE, Rizzo M, Jones RD. Adult-onset Hallervorden–Spatz syndrome presenting as cortical dementia. Alzheimer Dis Assoc Disord 2000; 14:120–126.

64. Frey LC, Ringel SP, Filley CM. The natural history of cognitive dysfunction in late-onset GM2 gangliosidosis. Arch Neurol 2005; 62:989–994.

65. Shahwan A, Farrell M, Delanty N. Progressive myoclonic epilepsies: a review of genetic and therapeutic aspects. Lancet Neurol 2005; 4:239–248.

66. Luda E, Barisone MG. Adult-onset adrenoleukodystrophy: a clinical and neuropsychological study. Neurol Sci 2001; 22:21–25.

67. Shapiro EG, Lockman LA, Knopman D, et al. Characteristics of the dementia in late-onset metachromatic leukodystrophy. Neurology 1994; 44:662–665.

68. Letournel F, Etcharry-Bouyx F, Verny C, et al. Two clinicopathological cases of a dominantly inherited, adult onset orthochromatic leucodystrophy. J Neurol Neurosurg Psychiatry 2003; 74:671–673.

69. Jardim LB, Giugliani R, Pires RF, et al. Protracted course of Krabbe disease in an adult patient bearing a novel mutation. Arch Neurol 1999; 56:1014–1017.

70. Namekawa M, Takiyama Y, Aoki Y, et al. Identification of GFAP gene mutation in hereditary adult-onset Alexander's disease. Ann Neurol 2002; 52:779–785.

71. Nance MA, Boyadjiev S, Pratt VM, et al. Adult-onset neurodegenerative disorder due to proteolipid protein gene mutation in the mother of a man with Pelizaeus–Merzbacher disease. Neurology 1996; 47:1333–1335.

72. Simon DK, Rodriguez ML, Frosch MP, et al. A unique familial leukodystrophy with adult onset dementia and abnormal glycolipid storage: a new lysosomal disease? J Neurol Neurosurg Psychiatry 1998; 65:251–254.

73. Jacob J, Robertson NJ, Hilton DA. The clinicopathological spectrum of Rosenthal fibre encephalopathy and Alexander's disease: a case report and review of the literature. J Neurol Neurosurg Psychiatry 2003; 74:807–810.

74. Klein CM, Bosch EP, Dyck PJ. Probable adult polyglucosan body disease. Mayo Clin Proc 2000; 75:1327–1331.

75. Hulette CM, Earl NL, Anthony DC, et al. Adult onset Niemann–Pick disease type C presenting with dementia and absent organomegaly. Clin Neuropathol 1992; 11:293–297.

76. Shulman LM, David NJ, Weiner WJ. Psychosis as the initial manifestation of adult-onset Niemann–Pick disease type C. Neurology 1995; 45:1739–1743.

77. Gray RG, Preece MA, Green SH, et al. Inborn errors of metabolism as a cause of neurological disease in adults: an approach to investigation. J Neurol Neurosurg Psychiatry 2000; 69:5–12.

78. Grasbeck A, Horstmann V, Nilsson K, et al. Dementia in first-degree relatives of patients with frontotemporal dementia. A family history study. Dement Geriatr Cogn Disord 2005; 19:145–153.

79. Chow TW, Miller BL, Hayashi VN, et al. Inheritance of frontotemporal dementia. Arch Neurol 1999; 56:817–822.

80. Rosso SM, Donker Kaat L, Baks T, et al. Frontotemporal dementia in The Netherlands: patient characteristics and prevalence estimates from a population-based study. Brain 2003; 126(part 9):2016–2022.

81. Goldman JS, Farmer JM, Van Deerlin VM, et al. Frontotemporal dementia: genetics and genetic counseling dilemmas. Neurologist 2004; 10:227–234.

82. Harding AJ, Das A, Kril JJ, et al. Identification of families with cortical Lewy body disease. Am J Med Genet B Neuropsychiatr Genet 2004; 128:118–122.

83. Raux G, Guyant-Marechal L, Martin C, et al. Molecular diagnosis of autosomal dominant early onset Alzheimer's disease: an update. J Med Genet 2005; 42:793–795.

84. Vinton A, Fahey MC, O'Brien TJ, et al. Dentatorubral-pallidoluysian atrophy in three generations, with clinical courses from nearly asymptomatic elderly to severe juvenile, in an Australian family of Macedonian descent. Am J Med Genet A 2005; 136:201–204.

85. Dong Y, Hassan A, Zhang Z, et al. Yield of screening for CADASIL mutations in lacunar stroke and leukoaraiosis. Stroke 2003; 34:203–205.

86. Rabinstein AA, Romano JG, Forteza AM, et al. Rapidly progressive dementia due to bilateral internal carotid artery occlusion with infarction of the total length of the corpus callosum. J Neuroimaging 2004; 14:176–179.

87. Greenberg SM, Vonsattel JP, Stakes JW, et al. The clinical spectrum of cerebral amyloid angiopathy: presentations without lobar hemorrhage. Neurology 1993; 43: 2073–2079.

88. Harkness KA, Coles A, Pohl U, et al. Rapidly reversible dementia in cerebral amyloid inflammatory vasculopathy. Eur J Neurol 2004; 11:59–62.

89. American Psychiatric Association. Diagnostic criteria from DSM-IV-TR. Washington DC: American Psychiatric Association 2000.

90. McCusker J, Cole M, Dendukuri N, et al. Delirium in older medical inpatients and subsequent cognitive and functional status: a prospective study. CMAJ 2001; 165:575–583.

91. Geschwind MD, Martindale J, Miller D, et al. Challenging the clinical utility of the 14-3-3 protein for the diagnosis of sporadic Creutzfeldt–Jakob disease. Arch Neurol 2003; 60:813–816.

92. Tschampa HJ, Kallenberg K, Urbach H, et al. MRI in the diagnosis of sporadic Creutzfeldt–Jakob disease: a study on inter-observer agreement. Brain 2005; 128(part 9):2026–2033.

93. Brown P, Rodgers-Johnson P, Cathala F, et al. Creutzfeldt–Jakob disease of long duration: clinicopathological characteristics, transmissibility, and differential diagnosis. Ann Neurol 1984; 16:295–304.

94. Will RG, Zeidler M, Stewart GE, et al. Diagnosis of new variant Creutzfeldt–Jakob disease. Ann Neurol 2000; 47: 575–582.

95. Shiga Y, Miyazawa K, Sato S, et al. Diffusion-weighted MRI abnormalities as an early diagnostic marker for Creutzfeldt–Jakob disease. Neurology 2004; 63:443–449.

96. Young GS, Geschwind MD, Fischbein NJ, et al. Diffusion-weighted and fluid-attenuated inversion recovery imaging in Creutzfeldt–Jakob disease: high sensitivity and specificity for diagnosis. AJNR 2005; 26:1551–1562.

97. Steinhoff BJ, Zerr I, Glatting M, et al. Diagnostic value of periodic complexes in Creutzfeldt–Jakob disease. Ann Neurol 2004; 56:702–708.

98. Tschampa HJ, Neumann M, Zerr I, et al. Patients with Alzheimer's disease and dementia with Lewy bodies mistaken for Creutzfeldt–Jakob disease. J Neurol Neurosurg Psychiatry 2001; 71:33–39.

99. Reinwald S, Westner IM, Niedermaier N. Rapidly progressive Alzheimer's disease mimicking Creutzfeldt–Jakob disease. J Neurol 2004; 251:1020–1022.

100. Catani M, Piccirilli M, Geloso MC, et al. Rapidly progressive aphasic dementia with motor neuron disease: a distinctive clinical entity. Dement Geriatr Cogn Disord 2004; 17:21–28.

101. Caselli RJ, Boeve BF, Scheithauer BW, et al. Nonvasculitic autoimmune inflammatory meningoencephalitis (NAIM): a reversible form of encephalopathy. Neurology 1999; 53:1579–1581.

102. Gomez-Puerta JA, Cervera R, Calvo LM, et al. Dementia associated with the antiphospholipid syndrome: clinical and radiological characteristics of 30 patients. Rheumatology (Oxford) 2005; 44:95–99.

103. Rollins KE, Kleinschmidt-DeMasters BK, Corboy JR, et al. Lymphomatosis cerebri as a cause of white matter dementia. Hum Pathol 2005; 36:282–290.

104. Han JH, Kim JH, Yim H. Intravascular lymphomatosis of the brain. Report of a case using an intraoperative cytologic preparation. Acta Cytol 2004; 48:411–414.

105. Heinrich A, Vogelgesang S, Kirsch M, et al. Intravascular lymphomatosis presenting as rapidly progressive dementia. Eur Neurol 2005; 54:55–58.

106. Rivas E, Sanchez-Herrero J, Alonso M, et al. Miliary brain metastases presenting as rapidly progressive dementia. Neuropathology 2005; 25:153–158.

107. Tihan T, Burger PC, Pomper M, et al. Subacute diencephalic angioencephalopathy: biopsy diagnosis and radiological features of a rare entity. Clin Neurol Neurosurg 2001; 103:160–167.

108. Waite LM, Broe GA, Grayson DA, et al. Motor function and disability in the dementias. Int J Geriatr Psychiatry 2000; 15:897–903.

109. Osaki Y, Ben-Shlomo Y, Lees AJ, et al. Accuracy of clinical diagnosis of progressive supranuclear palsy. Mov Disord 2004; 19:181–189.

110. Soliveri P, Monza D, Paridi D, et al. Cognitive and magnetic resonance imaging aspects of corticobasal degeneration and progressive supranuclear palsy. Neurology 1999; 53: 502–507.

111. Bak TH, Crawford LM, Hearn VC, et al. Subcortical dementia revisited: similarities and differences in cognitive function between progressive supranuclear palsy (PSP), corticobasal degeneration (CBD) and multiple system atrophy (MSA). Neurocase 2005; 11:268–273.

112. Louis ED, Lynch T, Kaufmann P, et al. Diagnostic guidelines in central nervous system Whipple's disease. Ann Neurol 1996; 40:561–568.

113. Litvan I, Bhatia KP, Burn DJ, et al. Movement Disorders Society Scientific Issues Committee report: SIC Task Force appraisal of clinical diagnostic criteria for Parkinsonian disorders. Mov Disord 2003; 18:467–486.

114. Shiozawa M, Fukutani Y, Sasaki K, et al. Corticobasal degeneration: an autopsy case clinically diagnosed as progressive supranuclear palsy. Clin Neuropathol 2000; 19: 192–199.

115. Soliveri P, Rossi G, Monza D, et al. A case of dementia parkinsonism resembling progressive supranuclear palsy due to mutation in the tau protein gene. Arch Neurol 2003; 60:1454–1456.

116. Okuda B, Yamamoto T, Yamasaki M, et al. Motor neuron disease with slow eye movements and vertical gaze palsy. Acta Neurol Scand 1992; 85:71–76.

117. Bertoni JM, Brown P, Goldfarb LG, et al. Familial Creutzfeldt–Jakob disease (codon 200 mutation) with supranuclear palsy. JAMA 1992; 268:2413–2415.

118. Rinne JO, Laine M, Kaasinen V, et al. Striatal dopamine transporter and extrapyramidal symptoms in frontotemporal dementia. Neurology 2002; 58:1489–1493.

119. Rampoldi L, Danek A, Monaco AP. Clinical features and molecular bases of neuroacanthocytosis. J Mol Med 2002; 80:475–491.

120. Verkkoniemi A, Somer M, Rinne JO, et al. Variant Alzheimer's disease with spastic paraparesis: clinical characterization. Neurology 2000; 54:1103–1109.

121. Fearnley JM, Stevens JM, Rudge P. Superficial siderosis of the central nervous system. Brain 1995; 118(part 4): 1051–1066.

122. Remes AM, Finnila S, Mononen H, et al. Hereditary dementia with intracerebral hemorrhages and cerebral amyloid angiopathy. Neurology 2004; 63:234–240.

123. Hanyu H, Tanaka Y, Shimizu S, et al. Cerebral microbleeds in Alzheimer's disease. J Neurol 2003; 250:1496–1497.

124. Ishikawa A, Yamada M, Makino K, et al. Dementia and delirium in 4 patients with Machado–Joseph disease. Arch Neurol 2002; 59:1804–1808.

125. Osaki Y, Wenning GK, Daniel SE, et al. Do published criteria improve clinical diagnostic accuracy in multiple system atrophy? Neurology 2002; 59:1486–1491.

126. Hall DA, Berry-Kravis E, Jacquemont S, et al. Initial diagnoses given to persons with the fragile 3 associated tremor/ataxia syndrome (FXTAS). Neurology 2005; 65: 299–301.

127. Hebb AO, Cusimano MD. Idiopathic normal pressure hydrocephalus: a systematic review of diagnosis and outcome. Neurosurgery 2001; 49:1166–1184; discussion 1184–1186.

128. Vanneste J, Augustijn P, Tan WF, et al. Shunting normal pressure hydrocephalus: the predictive value of combined clinical and CT data. J Neurol Neurosurg Psychiatry 1993; 56:251–256.

129. Golomb J, de Leon MJ, George AE, et al. Hippocampal atrophy correlates with severe cognitive impairment in elderly patients with suspected normal pressure hydrocephalus. J Neurol Neurosurg Psychiatry 1994; 57:590–593.

130. Poca MA, Mataro M, Matarin M, et al. Good outcome in patients with normal-pressure hydrocephalus and factors indicating poor prognosis. J Neurosurg 2005; 103:455–463.

131. Albert ML, Feldman RG, Willis AL. The 'subcortical dementia' of progressive supranuclear palsy. J Neurol Neurosurg Psychiatry 1974; 37:121–130.

132. Aarsland D, Litvan I, Salmon D, et al. Performance on the dementia rating scale in Parkinson's disease with dementia and dementia with Lewy bodies: comparison with progressive supranuclear palsy and Alzheimer's disease. J Neurol Neurosurg Psychiatry 2003; 74:1215–1220.

133. Canning SJ, Leach L, Stuss D, et al. Diagnostic utility of abbreviated fluency measures in Alzheimer disease and vascular dementia. Neurology 2004; 62:556–562.

134. Graham NL, Emery T, Hodges JR. Distinctive cognitive profiles in Alzheimer's disease and subcortical vascular dementia. J Neurol Neurosurg Psychiatry 2004; 75:61–71.

135. Hejl A, Hogh P, Waldemar G. Potentially reversible conditions in 1000 consecutive memory clinic patients. J Neurol Neurosurg Psychiatry 2002; 73:390–394.

136. Clarfield AM. The decreasing prevalence of reversible dementias: an updated meta-analysis. Arch Intern Med 2003; 163:2219–2229.

137. McArthur JC, Brew BJ, Nath A. Neurological complications of HIV infection. Lancet Neurol 2005; 4:543–555.

138. Timmermans M, Carr J. Neurosyphilis in the modern era. J Neurol Neurosurg Psychiatry 2004; 75:1727–1730.

139. Patterson C, Gauthier S, Bergman H, et al. The recognition, assessment and management of dementing disorders: conclusions from the Canadian Consensus Conference on Dementia. Can J Neurol Sci 2001; 28(suppl 1):S3–S16.

140. Petersen RC, Stevens JC, Ganguli M, et al. Practice parameter: early detection of dementia: mild cognitive impairment (an evidence-based review). Report of the Quality Standards Subcommittee of the American Academy of Neurology. Neurology 2001; 56:1133–1142.

141. Benke T, Karner E, Seppi K, et al. Subacute dementia and imaging correlates in a case of Fahr's disease. J Neurol Neurosurg Psychiatry 2004; 75:1163–1165.

142. Taniwaki T, Yamada T, Yoshida T, et al. Heterogeneity of glucose metabolism in corticobasal degeneration. J Neurol Sci 1998; 161:70–76.

143. Cordato NJ, Duggins AJ, Halliday GM, et al. Clinical deficits correlate with regional cerebral atrophy in progressive supranuclear palsy. Brain 2005; 128(part 6):1259–1266.

144. Oba H, Yagishita A, Terada H, et al. New and reliable MRI diagnosis for progressive supranuclear palsy. Neurology 2005; 64:2050–2055.

145. Likeman M, Anderson VM, Stevens JM, et al. Visual assessment of atrophy on magnetic resonance imaging in the diagnosis of pathologically confirmed young-onset dementias. Arch Neurol 2005; 62:1410–1415.

146. Talbot PR, Lloyd JJ, Snowden JS, et al. A clinical role for 99mTc-HMPAO SPECT in the investigation of dementia? J Neurol Neurosurg Psychiatry 1998; 64:306–313.

147. Graus F, Delattre JY, Antoine JC, et al. Recommended diagnostic criteria for paraneoplastic neurological syndromes. J Neurol Neurosurg Psychiatry 2004; 75:1135–1140.

148. Vincent A, Buckley C, Schott JM, et al. Potassium channel antibody-associated encephalopathy: a potentially immunotherapy-responsive form of limbic encephalitis. Brain 2004; 127:701–712.

149. Ances BM, Vitaliani R, Taylor RA, et al. Treatment-responsive limbic encephalitis identified by neuropil antibodies: MRI and PET correlates. Brain 2005; 128: 1764–1777.

150. Adair JC, Digre KB, Swanda RM, et al. Sneddon's syndrome: a cause of cognitive decline in young adults. Neuropsychiatry Neuropsychol Behav Neurol 2001; 14: 197–204.

151. Markus HS, Martin RJ, Simpson MA, et al. Diagnostic strategies in CADASIL. Neurology 2002; 59:1134–1138.

152. Ivan CS, Saint-Hilaire MH, Christensen TG, et al. Adult-onset neuronal ceroid lipofuscinosis type B in an African-American. Mov Disord 2005; 20:752–754.

153. Andrade DM, Ackerley CA, Minett TS, et al. Skin biopsy in Lafora disease: genotype-phenotype correlations and diagnostic pitfalls. Neurology 2003; 61:1611–1614.

154. Bigio EH, Weiner MF, Bonte FJ, et al. Familial dementia due to adult polyglucosan body disease. Clin Neuropathol 1997; 16:227–234.

155. Warren JD, Schott JM, Fox NC, et al. Brain biopsy in dementia. Brain 2005; 128:2016–2025.

6

Neuropsychological assessment

Constant Rainville, Nicole Caza, Sylvie Belleville and Brigitte Gilbert

VIGNETTE

Mrs Jones is a 73-year-old woman who used to be a teacher and lives alone following the death of her husband a year ago. Her daughter accompanies her at a medical appointment. Mrs Jones' score on the Mini-Mental State Examination (MMSE) is 26/30. She can undertake the main activities of daily living independently (bathing and dressing, preparing meals, using the telephone, doing housework and taking medication). During the interview, Mrs Jones is alert, cooperative, answers the questions asked and has no word-finding difficulties on conversation. Although she acknowledges difficulty in recalling new events, orienting herself in unfamiliar places and finding appropriate words, she argues that this is just normal for her age. Her daughter has noticed a gradual decline of her cognitive capacities, including forgetfulness (recent conversations, appointments), occasional writing errors and a tendency to jot down notes. In spite of the fact that the patient has always managed her finances in the past, the daughter now has to oversee her mother's financial transactions. Moreover, she reports that her mother is more disorganized and anxious whenever her routine is disrupted. This was particularly obvious on a recent occasion when her children invited her to a restaurant. She lost track of the conversation, repeated herself and was less aware than before of recent public events, although she reported reading the newspaper on a daily basis. In light of the elements described here, the practitioner requested a neuropsychological assessment.

INTRODUCTION

The case of Mrs Jones is typical of many early Alzheimer's disease (AD) patients. Family often notice progressive changes in daily abilities although the patient himself seems less concerned about them. Difficulties often seem to affect memory and executive functions. As screening exam (MMSE) is above the cut-off score of 24/30, the question remains as to whether these changes can be part of normal ageing. A neuropsychological assessment will help to determine the answer to this question.

The present chapter delineates the neuropsychological assessment issues raised by cognitive impairments in neurodegenerative disease, such as AD. Despite considerable scientific advances, it is not yet possible to diagnose AD based on evidence from brain imaging, neurophysiological assessment or other biological tests. Because there are no definitive markers of AD, the neuropsychological assessment plays a key role in supporting the diagnosis, particularly in the initial stage. The purpose of this chapter is to outline the general principles that should guide the neuropsychological assessment of AD patients and to review the main cognitive domains that should be addressed along with relevant tasks available to assess them, especially in early stages of AD. Notably, this chapter does not provide an exhaustive description of all of the various tests available to the neuropsychologist in order to evaluate cognitive functions in dementia. Several good summaries of these options are available elsewhere.[1–4]

THE ROLE OF THE NEUROPSYCHOLOGICAL ASSESSMENT

The purpose of the neuropsychological assessment may vary according to the context surrounding the evaluation, and consequently this will affect the nature and the number of tests. The main objective of the neuropsychological assessment is to obtain a clear picture of the cognitive profile of a patient suspected of having dementia. In other words, the nature of the cognitive deficits, their severity and their functional consequences need to be addressed. The impact of these deficits on the individual's activities, such as work, leisure and social relationships, is also considered in collaboration with informants and other health professionals. In addition, recording preserved capacities and ways to facilitate learning (e.g. use of cueing) fall under the scope of the evaluation. As requested by the referring physician, the neuropsychologist offers an opinion as to whether the cognitive profile is typical of AD, more characteristic of other dementias (e.g. frontotemporal, subcortical) or part of the spectrum that encompasses normal ageing.

Neuropsychological assessment is also useful for providing information about the progression of cognitive dysfunction and response to treatment, pharmacological or otherwise. Knowledge about changes in the different cognitive functions over time is important for patient management and can be used to provide strategies and guidance to the patient and the caregivers. Notably, many of the neuropsychological tests are vulnerable to practice effects. That is, when a test is used repeatedly, the performance can improve because of increased familiarity with the test material and procedure, rather than as a result of any real change in the underlying cognitive skills. In the context of a progressive disease such as AD, the rate of decline may therefore be underestimated. In order to minimize practice effect, annual assessments with parallel versions should be conducted. However, this would not reduce the effect of increased familarity with the general procedure. Thus, these issues should be considered in the qualitative interpretation of the data.

GENERAL PRINCIPLES IN NEUROPSYCHOLOGICAL ASSESSMENT

Neuropsychological assessment includes a series of steps guided by an hypothesis-testing procedure. Generally, the process begins with the collection of information from clinical records (history, results of neurological evaluation, brain imaging data, etc.) and is guided by the pattern and history of complaints expressed by the patient and/or the informant and by initial clinical observations. By spending time talking to or observing the patient, the clinician can identify deficits in a number of domains. Clinicians must also establish a positive relationship with patients to ensure a good collaboration. This collaboration is crucial as results obtained on tests need to reflect optimal performances. In order to test the hypothesis about the nature of the deficits, a qualitative analysis of the over-

all behaviour is an important part of the assessment. Does the patient complain of cognitive difficulties? Is he or she aware when his performance on a task is impaired? Are depressive symptoms present? Is the patient apathetic? Does he or she have difficulty concentrating on a task? Is the discourse fluent or repetitive? The clinician can also obtain a large amount of information from relatives, caregivers or other people who knew the patient pre-morbidly and can report changes in behaviour. Time should be taken to discuss memory complaints, behaviour and personality changes, and activities of daily living with an informant.

An optimal neuropsychological assessment should employ simple general procedural guidelines. Within a session, demanding tasks should be alternated with less demanding ones and care should be taken to ensure that self-esteem is preserved throughout the interview. Ideally, at least two different sessions should be devoted to the assessment to promote convergent validity in the results. Different factors, such as stress and tiredness, can influence cognitive performance (especially attention and memory functions) and those can be minimized by distributing the testing across different time periods. Obviously, sensory loss, low educational level, cultural differences and linguistic barriers should all be considered when planning the neuropsychological assessment and when interpreting the results. Everyday memory can be assessed by inquiring about the previous testing session.

In the assessment process, test batteries or global scales covering global aspects of cognition may be administered if necessary. The main purpose of these global assessment scales is to detect the presence of cognitive dysfunction and provide quantitative scores that can be used to quantify the severity of dementia. Screening tests include the MMSE[5] and a somewhat longer version, the 3MS,[6] the Blessed Dementia Rating Scale[7] and the Mattis Dementia Rating Scale.[8] These tests share a number of characteristics: they are multidimensional, they allow for a relatively brief examination, they address issues that are of relevance for everyday life and they are often applicable to people with a low level of education.

The ideal assessment would obviously attempt to evaluate all cognitive domains relatively extensively. However, this would be a lengthy process and thus impractical in most clinical settings. A choice must be made on the basis of the expected clinical profile (see Table 6.1). As suggested above, it should be based on a hypothesis-testing procedure and it should incorporate tasks based on more recent cognitive models, although their speculative nature must be recognized. Theoretical approaches are particularly important in ambiguous

Table 6.1 Common (or typical) clinical profile of patients with AD at the early and mild stages of the disease. It should be noted that AD is heterogeneous in its presentation and course. Patients at a given stage do not necessarily present with all of the features described below

	Earlier stage	Mild to moderate stage
General behaviours	Tendency to minimize or rationalize memory problems; impairment in social activities; mild personality changes; apathy may occur; may have depressed mood and anxiety	Denial of impairments; personality features accentuated; withdrawal from complex situations
Memory		
Episodic	Difficulty with learning and retrieving new information, especially after a delay; recognition is better than recall; providing cues generally improves memory; remote events are better preserved than recent ones	Poor recall and recognition of events; disorientation in time and space; memory for remote events is increasingly impaired
Semantic	Some word-finding difficulties in spontaneous speech and picture naming (anomia); knowledge of common objects and concepts is relatively unimpaired	Increasing loss of knowledge, especially for uncommon objects or specific features of an object; difficulty with names of objects and people
Working	Impairment in activities involving online processing such as following a conversation, reasoning and problem solving; impaired word span	Pervasive and severe impairment which has an impact on activities of daily living; impaired word and digit span
Executive function	Difficulty with activities involving planning and organization of behaviours, particularly in novel situations; decreased performance at work, but can function with some supervision	Difficulty in everyday activities such as preparing meals and managing a budget; impairment in open-ended tasks and multistep behaviours; difficulties in understanding complex task instructions; problems may also appear in hobbies
Attention/inhibition	Difficulty coordinating two simultaneous tasks (divided attention)	Difficulty following conversations with numerous people and inhibiting irrelevant actions
Language	Impaired word production; spelling errors, especially with irregular words; tendency to make semantic paraphasias (*tiger* instead of *lion*); word comprehension is relatively unimpaired	Impaired word comprehension; use of circumlocutions; discourse may be empty
Praxis		
Limb	Normal or slightly impaired for some meaningless gestures	Difficulty imitating some gestures
Constructional	Drawing on command is more sensitive than copying; difficulties often reported in a variety of copying tasks (e.g. clock, Rey Complex Figure Test); copies of three-dimensional figures are more impaired (e.g. cube)	Impairment in copying familiar models (e.g. house, bicycle, cube) and unfamiliar models; difficulty drawing superimposed geometric figures
Gnosis	May be a mild agnosia but generally related to an impaired semantic memory system	Possible impairment in recognition of complex forms; difficulties in figure-ground analysis
Space orientation	Spatial disorientation in non-familiar environments (especially in driving conditions); no difficulty navigating familiar territories	Difficulties in spatial orientation may appear in familiar environments

cases, as in the differentiation between early dementia and normal ageing in persons who are quite intelligent and well educated, such as Mrs Jones. Detection of subtle cognitive dysfunction needs a more systematic approach than screening tasks and scales. In addition, theoretical approaches allow for a better description of the cognitive profile, which helps differentiate between different neuro-degenerative diseases. Finally, performance should always be interpreted in light of the clinician's experience and judgment. Neuropsychological assessment goes beyond the boundaries of task administration. Specifically, both clinical observation (behaviour, emotions) and qualitative information obtained from test completion (e.g. type of errors) are important for the interpretation of the results.

THE MAIN COGNITIVE DOMAINS

Working memory and attention

Working memory (WM) is a multicomponent cognitive activity involved in the online processing and maintenance of information.[9] It is increasingly construed as an attentional controller and, for this reason, there is some overlap between the tasks that can be used to measure the more dynamic aspects of WM and some aspects of attention (e.g. divided attention, control of attention) or executive functions (e.g. inhibition). In this chapter, we will attempt to distinguish tasks as a function of the putative components that they likely reflect. However, because clinical tasks are not 'pure' measures of cognitive processes, they inevitably tap only partially on these different yet very similar processes.

There is increasing evidence in favour of a pervasive, severe and early impairment of WM in AD.[10,11] In addition, different attentional systems have been found to be impaired in this population.[12] WM is involved in numerous actions, or activities involving online processing including discourse comprehension, reasoning and problem solving. Attention plays a role in a large range of activities such as driving and way finding. Impairment of these cognitive processes is thought to be responsible for a substantial portion of the difficulties experienced by AD patients in their daily lives, particularly at an early stage of the disease. Thus clinicians have been increasingly attentive to the assessment of attentional control and WM. In the case of Mrs Jones, impairment of WM could account for the difficulties she experienced in completing tasks that were less familiar to her or in following conversations involving numerous persons.

Digit span,[13] the ability to report a short series of digits, has been used as a classical measure of the passive maintenance capacity of WM. Unfortunately, the digit span task has little sensitivity to early AD (see reference 14 for a review). WM tasks that are most detrimental to persons with AD are those that involve a re-organization of the material in memory or concurrent maintenance and processing. A complete assessment of AD should therefore include at least one of these types of WM tasks. Moreover, some tasks are well designed and incorporate appropriate norms for older persons. The clinician can interpret a discrepancy between the score on the digit backward and digit forward scales of the Wechsler Memory Scale III (WMS-III)[13] as reflecting a deficit in manipulating information. Notably, some individuals use a visuospatial approach in the digit backward condition and results on this task should thus be interpreted with caution. Additionally, the letter–number sequencing subtest of the WMS-III can be used in combination with the spatial memory subtest to obtain a WM index. Unfortunately, this index is not sensitive to AD.[13] In contrast, the alpha-span task,[15] which requires reporting a series of words in their alphabetical order, is seriously impeded by AD.[11] In addition, the Brown–Peterson procedure in which participants are asked to report a short series of items (typically three) following a short delay filled by a demanding task is severely reduced in AD.[10,16] This impairment would reflect patients' difficulties in coordinating two simultaneous tasks.

In spite of the importance of including attention in the clinical assessment of AD, there is a scarcity of specific measures of attention available to the clinician. Attention capacities include selective, focused and divided attention. Not all of these aspects are impaired in AD. The dysfunction includes mainly divided attention and some aspects of selective attention such as set inhibition.[12] These are aspects that are also part of the executive functions assessment (see below) but will be reviewed here briefly. Within selective attention, inhibition can be measured with normed tasks such as the Stroop procedure,[17] in which patients are asked to name aloud the ink of colour words that are printed in an incongruent colour (e.g. the word 'red' printed in green ink), or the Hayling test.[18,19] In the Hayling test the clinician provides sentences in which the last word is missing and the patient is asked to complete it with a word that bears no relation with the sentence. Because the word is highly constrained semantically (e.g. he mailed a letter without a __[20]), participants need to inhibit a prepotent response to perform the task adequately. If the clinician feels that focused attention is impaired, the Paced

Auditory Serial Addition Test (PASAT)[21,22] can be used to measure this component. In this task, the patient is asked to add digits to the preceding one in the list. It thus involves both focused attention and some WM capacities (for normative values see references 1, 23, 24). In addition, it is worth pointing out that this is a demanding task, which may be frustrating for more severely impaired patients, and that simplified versions of the task are available.[25] Finally, divided attention can be measured with a paper-and-pencil task developed by Baddeley and collaborators[26,27] that involves repeating short sequences of digits while completing a simple visuomotor task. Because one of the tasks in this paradigm requires memory, it has also been used to measure WM capacities.

Executive functions

Executive functions (EF) refer to a broad range of processes which are involved in activities such as decision making, planning or cognitive flexibility.[28–31] At the most basic level, current consensus regards EF as a process or set of processes whose primary purpose is to facilitate adaptation to novel and/or complex situations.[32–35]. EF enable a person to establish new behaviour patterns and ways of thinking. EF account for the adaptive abilities in situations where established ways of behaving, or routines, are no longer useful or appropriate. EF operate in the majority of mental tasks that are driven by strategies and are not performed automatically. Thus, executive dysfunctions interfere with many other forms of cognition. Executive dysfunctions have a negative effect on daily functioning.[36–38] As is the case for Mrs Jones, one may observe difficulties in everyday activities in terms of planning, preparing meals, managing the budget, selecting clothing appropriate for the weather, etc .[39,40] They are also associated with neuropsychiatric symptoms.[41,42]

Several researchers have suggested that executive dysfunction is common in AD.[12,36,43–46] A number of cross-sectional and longitudinal studies have revealed that EF are the first non-memory domains to be impaired, usually prior to problems with language or visuospatial abilities.[12,41,47,48] Some studies have identified subgroups of AD in which executive impairment is more pronounced, but these tend to become more generalized as the dementia progresses.[40,49]

A variety of tests are available for the assessment of EF impairments. The most commonly used will be considered here. With the Stroop test,[17] some studies have indicated that AD patients are particularly sensitive to interference.[50–54] Many studies[55–60] have also reported impairments in the Trail Making Test (TMT)[61], which may reflect impairment in shifting capacities. Defects in the TMT were also reported[62] in the early clinical stage of AD. Recent studies underlined the interest to consider the qualitative features of performance in AD.[50,55,63,64] An impairment in shifting abilities in AD has also been shown in the Wisconsin Card Sorting Test,[65] which is a measure of cognitive flexibility.[66,67] The verbal fluency test is considered to impose comparable demands upon executive control processes such as effortful retrieval. There are different forms of this test (category, letter, first names and supermarket fluency) which have different degrees of discrimination between patients with AD and normal control subjects in terms of sensitivity and specificity.[68] The verbal fluency test has been said to be a useful screening test.[69–71] For instance, in the Isaacs Set Test of verbal semantic fluency,[72] the performances were abnormally low nine years before the clinical diagnosis.[73] Performance in this test is in relation to the degree of severity of the AD.[70] The Tower of London task, originally developed by Shallice,[74] is now well recognized for measuring EF. Specifically, it is a non-verbal task that evaluates planning abilities, which imply the attainment of a goal through a series of intermediate steps. This test was found to be sensitive to executive dysfunctions in different neurodegenerative diseases.[75,76] In this test, AD patients were impaired in comparison to controls.[77] Qualitative analysis revealed that they made a significantly higher number of rule violations.[77] The examiner must be careful since there are now many versions of this test, with different procedures and data scoring systems.[78–84]

Episodic memory

Episodic memories refer to specific events that occurred at a particular time and place, making them unique and personal.[85,86] This memory system allows one to retrieve personal memories and create new ones. Episodic memory is thought to involve different memory processes (encoding, storage and retrieval), each of which may be affected by brain disease. In AD, a cognitive history from both the patient and an informant typically reveals memory complaints. Indeed, Mrs Jones' difficulty recalling recent conversations and appointments is suggestive of episodic memory impairment. Such a deficit progressively leads to disorientation, both with time and space. This may be illustrated by a difficulty with remembering today's date, or by problems with finding one's way in unfamiliar places, as reported by Mrs Jones.

Although the course of the disease may vary from one individual to another, episodic memory impairment is a cardinal feature of AD and dementia in general.[87] Studies show that the capacity to learn and retrieve new information is severely affected very early during the time course of the disease[88–92] (for a review see reference 89). Patients show poor recall, especially with longer delays, and have a tendency to make intrusions by recalling words that were not on the presented list. However, rates of forgetting appear to be equivalent in AD patients and healthy controls, at least when measured by recognition tasks.[91,92] Episodic memory measures provide the most useful indicator of early AD and, therefore, this type of memory should be thoroughly evaluated in patients.

An amnestic syndrome is typically observed in AD patients, as damage tends to affect medial temporal structures bilaterally.[93–95] An exhaustive evaluation of episodic memory should include both verbal and non-verbal memory. Several verbal memory tests may be used, including the California Verbal Learning Test[96,97] or the Logical Memory subtest from the WMS-III.[13] Although no test provides a pure measure of a memory component, the Free and Cued Selective Reminding Test,[98] a recent version derived from Bushke's Selective Reminding Test,[99–101] allows assessment of the relative contribution of different constituents of memory. It has also been shown to identify persons at risk for future dementia.[102] This test maximizes learning by promoting deep semantic encoding and controlling for attention and other cognitive processing deficits that may also affect memory performance. In the encoding phase of the test, the patient must search for items (e.g. *eagle*) based on semantic cues (e.g. *bird*) given by the examiner; these cues may be used later during retrieval to elicit recall of items not retrieved by free recall. A recognition task is also administered. Patients with mild AD show very little learning over trials with very poor recall – that is only slightly helped with semantic cueing but remains abnormal – and impaired recognition that is characterized by a tendency to make false positive responses.[102] However, as the disease progresses, patients become more impaired and performance on many tests becomes limited by floor effects. Non-verbal memory may be assessed using the immediate and delayed recall of the Rey–Osterreith Complex Figure Test[103] or the Visual Reproduction subtest from the WMS-III.[13] In those tests patients with AD are severely impaired, even with short delays.

Semantic memory

Semantic memory is conceived as the repository for all culturally-shared knowledge, i.e. information that is not related to personal events, as is the case for episodic memory.[85] It comprises general information about people, including one's self, knowledge about objects, concepts and facts, as well as linguistic knowledge, such as words and their meaning (further discussed in the language section).

Numerous studies show that semantic memory is impaired in the majority of AD patients, even in very early AD or pre-dementia stage.[104–109] Impairment of semantic memory typically reflects the hierarchical organization of this memory system; patients at the early stage of the disease are generally more impaired on specific features of an object (e.g. *whether a lion has stripes or not*) while more general semantic categories (e.g. *wild animal*) remain relatively well preserved up until more advanced stages of the disease. A widely accepted view is that semantic memory is organized in a collection of modality-specific subsystems[110,111] (although see reference 112 for an alternative view). In AD, the semantic impairment is generally ubiquitous: it is found for the same object, within and across different modalities (auditory, visual or somatosensory), and independently of the physical characteristic of the stimulus (picture or word[113,114]) Anomia represents one of the most common manifestations of semantic impairment in AD patients, as illustrated by Mrs Jones' occasional word-finding problems.[115] Several tests are sensitive to semantic impairment in early AD. A recent study by Diehl and colleagues[116] revealed that the combined use of the MMSE with some tasks that are dependent on semantic memory allows for differential diagnosis between early AD and other dementias. These tasks include picture naming tasks, such as the Boston Naming Test[117] or the short version.[118] Many studies indicate that patients are impaired on picture naming as well as the naming of famous faces.[109] When the patient fails to provide the name of a particular object in a picture naming task, the clinician should probe the patient's semantic memory by asking more general knowledge questions regarding the item. However, in AD anomia must be distinguished from abnormal visuospatial abilities.[113] Several studies have also found AD patients to be impaired on verbal fluency, in particular for semantic relative to letter categories[88,104,119–121] (see reference 122 for meta-analysis). Although semantic fluency involves executive processes that are known to be impaired in AD patients (see previous section), this task is also considered to measure semantic processing, as performance depends on the accessibility of category members and the integrity of semantic associations. In both the semantic and letter fluency tasks, AD patients give fewer responses than controls. However, only the semantic task enables discrimination between other types of dementia, with the tendency for AD patients to have smaller clusters (i.e. items in a subcategory) and switch less often to another cluster.[123–125] The assessment of associations in semantic memory without verbal input/output may be conducted using a picture matching task, such as the Pyramids and Palm Trees Test[126] or the Associative Match subtest from the Birmingham Object Recognition Battery (BORB).[127] Finally, a more exhaustive neuropsychological assessment of semantic memory in AD should measure the ability to use common objects or make certain gestures (described in the Apraxia section).

Language

Language is a complex activity that operates at many levels (e.g. single word, sentence or discourse). Here, we essentially focus on single word processing, as this level has been extensively studied in AD patients (see references 128 and 129 for narrative aspects of language in AD). The patient's spontaneous discourse during the interview may serve as an indicator of language status and guide assessment of single word processing. For example, the clinician should evaluate whether the patient's discourse is fluent and meaningful, and whether simple commands are easily understood.

Language may be partitioned into two broad categories: production and comprehension. Early AD patients are essentially impaired on word production while comprehension is typically affected at more advanced stages of the disease.[124,130,131] Patients are especially sensitive to the lexical properties of words: selection of items to be tested should take into consideration word characteristics, such as frequency of usage, regularity in the spelling-to-sound correspondence and age of acquisition.[132–134] For example, in picture naming tasks, patients generally perform better with more frequent words and those acquired earlier in childhood.

The assessment of single word production and comprehension should include both verbal and written words. Word production may be evaluated with a picture naming task (as already discussed in the semantic memory section); patients have a tendency to make semantic paraphasias (*tiger* instead of *lion*). Spelling errors are often observed in early AD;[135,136] spelling may be assessed orally or with a dictation that includes both regular (*red*) and irregular (*blood*) words, with varying frequency of usage. Patients are generally more impaired on irregular words relative to regular ones, as the former do not have regular spelling-to-sound correspondence. The same items

should be used to assess reading skills in Alzheimer patients. Word comprehension may also be evaluated by asking the patient to execute a simple and a more complex command with real objects, such as 'touch the pencil and fold the sheet of paper' or those found in the Token Test.[137] However, not all aspects of language are impaired in AD; phonological processing and syntax are generally preserved, at least in the early stage.

Agnosia and limb apraxia

Agnosia refers to a deficit in the recognition of stimuli (e.g. pictures, objects) in a specific modality (visual, tactile) because of an impairment in perceptual processing. In the earlier stage of AD, the presence of agnosia is generally related to an impaired semantic memory system (see above). More basic perceptual abilities are typically preserved in early AD (but see reference 139 for the report of visual agnosia in some variants of AD).

Limb apraxia refers to the inability to perform learned skilled movements and is usually measured by asking participants to perform pantomimes of tool use (e.g. asking the patient to imitate the use of scissors), symbolic gestures (asking the patient to execute a military salute) or to imitate meaningless gestures. This ability may be tested with the CHCN Apraxia Battery.[138] Limb apraxia is usually observed in moderate to severe AD,[140] although some authors report limb apraxia in the early stage, in those patients with early and marked semantic memory deficit.[141]

Spatio-cognition

Impairments in a wide range of the so-called 'visuospatial abilities' have been reported in early AD. Despite the frequency of disturbance in this cognitive domain, there are relatively few studies that assessed it systematically and the amount of material devoted to this subject is generally small. One difficulty in the evaluation of spatio-cognition is that activities qualified as visuospatial are disparate (e.g. space perception, mental rotation, drawing, space orientation). Accordingly, tests evaluating them are varied and involve multiple aspects.

Visuospatial functioning tends to be sensitive to impairment in AD, in particular in the moderate stage.[142–146] In some cases, visuospatial dysfunction can be the initial presenting cognitive deficit in AD,[142–147] but it is a relatively rare occurrence. In AD, the figure-ground analysis is severely affected.[148–150] In the Visual Object and Space Perception Battery,[151] in the early stages, Binetti and colleagues[152] found that visual and spatial perception was not significantly different from a matched control group. The patients were impaired only in the task in which they had to name the stimulus (Silhouettes task), which requires access to semantic and lexical knowledge. Different studies[153,154] showed deficits in the judgment of line orientation evaluated with the Benton Line Orientation Test.[157] Moreover, qualitative analyses indicated that some error types were much more frequent in AD patients.[156] Some authors[157–159] reported a deficit in spatial rotation, measured with the Standardized Road-map Test of Direction Sense of Money et al.[160] For Kurylo et al[161] this test is a robust visuospatial measure which allows for discrimination between people with dementia and normal control subjects. However, significant impairments in this test were not systematically found by others.[162,163]

Impairments in constructional abilities in AD are commonly observed,[59,145,164,165] and they vary in proportion to the overall severity of the dementia.[166–167] AD patients were found to be impaired in a variety of drawing and copying tasks[168–170] of familiar models (e.g. a bicycle, a cube) and unfamiliar models, such as the copying of the Rey–Osterrieth Complex Figure.[103,163,168,171] Tasks that reveal impairment in visuospatial abilities also include the Clock Drawing Test, which is sensitive to the severity of the disease.[172–176] Other authors[165,175] have suggested that drawing on command (spontaneous drawings or drawings from memory) may be more sensitive than reproduction drawings in the early course of the disease. Similarly, AD patients have more difficulties with three-dimensional figures than with two-dimensional ones.[169,177–179] Constructional abilities can be evaluated by some subtests of the WAIS, such as the Block Design, on which mildly demented AD subjects have been shown to be impaired.[59,166,180] It is important to note that, although constructional tasks involve visual and spatial integration, they have a wide range of complexity and, accordingly, are involved at different degrees of EF (e.g. the Rey–Osterrieth Complex Figure).

One major issue of visuospatial deficits in AD concerns space orientation (SO). Indeed, deficits in SO are often rapidly recognized because of the negative effect that they have on daily functioning.[165,177,181–185] As is the case for Mrs Jones, patients in the early stage of the disease are usually able to go from their home to their destination and back without difficulty, while their ability to navigate in less familiar territories is somewhat deteriorated.[158,186,187] Ideally, the assessment of SO should be conducted with regard to a number of factors such as the nature of the environment (e.g. natural/architectural), the complexity of the task (in terms of decision-making) and the level of familiarity of the environment.[188,189] SO performances in AD, in an ecological environment, may be studied in the conceptual framework of EF. That is, to reach a destination, the individual has to make a series of decision and to develop an overall plan.[190] In this approach, AD patients were found to be impaired in both these processes.[191,192]

CONCLUSION

The neuropsychological assessment plays a major role in the evaluation of age-related disorders whenever cognitive dysfunctions are suspected. Evaluation of the patient's cognitive status requires the documentation of cognitive changes as well as behavioural and functional changes (Table 6.2). There are different methods of measuring these changes in the elderly (e.g. psychometric or cognitive), and each of these methods have their advantages and drawbacks. Regardless of which method is used, there is consensus regarding the need for a multidimensional assessment. Moreover, there is a growing belief that it is necessary to base the assessment on theoretical models and, at a more general level, to rely on a hypothesis testing approach. Such an approach goes beyond merely reporting the patterns of deficits and spared functions. This is particularly relevant in cases where the pattern of deficits is not 'prototypical'. For instance, the scores of educated individuals, such as Mrs Jones, may remain within the normal limits proposed by standardized tests. In such cases, it may be difficult to determine whether the actual scores reflect the person's pre-morbid cognitive abilities or a decline from a higher level of functioning. The reduction of the diagnostic error is based on both the clinical judgment, a crucial value, and the selection of the most appropriate of the theoretical approaches in order to make a valuable contribution to the assessment of the individual.

Table 6.2 Summary of the main cognitive components to assess for an efficient and comprehensive evaluation (3–4 hours), characteristics that the test should include and suggestion of tests

Process measured	Test characteristics	Example of test
Memory		
Episodic	Measures both recall and recognition after a delay; maximizes learning; evaluates the effects of cues on memory performance; both verbal and non-verbal material should be tested	Buschke's Selective Reminding Test; recall of the Rey–Osterrieth Complex Figure test
Semantic	Includes items from different semantic categories and with varying frequency of occurrence	Boston Naming Test; verbal fluency (letter and semantic category)
Working memory	Processes involved in the online processing and maintenance of information more than passive storage	Alpha-span task; Brown-Peterson procedure; reading span or calculation span
Executive function	Processes involved in decision-making, planning and cognitive flexibility	Tower of London task
Attention/inhibition	Processes involved in selection of information	Stroop test; trail making test
Language	Should include word production and comprehension, in both verbal and written modalities	Boston Naming Test; Token test; writing to dictation; reading
Praxis		
Limb	Processes involved in the ability to perform skilled movements	CHCN apraxia battery
Constructional	Processes involved in visual and spatial integration	Copy of Rey–Osterrieth Complex Figure or clock drawing test
Gnosis	Processes involved in the recognition of stimuli	Boston Naming Test
Space orientation	Capacity to reach a destination in a familiar or unfamiliar environment	Standardized Road-map Test of Direction Sense of Money; space orientation task in an ecological environment

REFERENCES

1. Spreen O, Strauss E. A Compendium of Neuropsychological Tests: Administration, Norms, and Commentary. New York: Oxford University Press 1998.
2. McCaffrey RJ, Puente AE. Handbook of Neuropsychological Assessment: A Biopsychosocial Perspective. New York: Plenum Press 1992.
3. Gilandas A. Handbook of Neuropsychological Assessment. Toronto: Grune & Stratton 1984.
4. Lezak MD. Neuropsychological Assessment. 4th edn. New York: Oxford University Press 2004.
5. Folstein MF, Folstein SE. 'Mini-Mental State': a practical method for grading the cognitive state of patients for the clinician. J Psychiatr Res 1975; 12:189–198.
6. Teng EL, Chui HC. The Modified Mini-Mental State (3MS) examination. J Clin Psychiatry 1987; 48:314–318.
7. Blessed G, Tomlinson BE, Roth M. The association between quantitative measures of dementia and of senile change in the cerebral grey matter of elderly subjects. Br J Psychiatry 1968; 114:797–811.

8. Mattis S. Dementia Rating Scale Professional Manual. Odessa: Psychological Assessment Resources 1988.

9. Baddeley AD. Working Memory. Oxford: Clarendon Press 1986.

10. Belleville S, Peretz I, Malenfant D. Examination of the working memory components in normal aging and in dementia of the Alzheimer type. Neuropsychologia 1996; 34:195–207.

11. Belleville S, Rouleau N, Van der Linden M, Collette F. Effect of manipulation and irrelevant noise on working memory capacity of patients with Alzheimer's dementia. Neuropsychology 2003; 17:69–81.

12. Perry RJ, Hodges JR. Attention and executive deficits in Alzheimer's disease. A critical review. Brain 1999; 122 (part 3): 383–404.

13. Wechsler D. Wechsler Memory Scale III, 3rd edn. San Antonio: The Psychological Corporation 1997.

14. Belleville S, Crépeau F, Caza N, Rouleau N. La mémoire de travail dans la démence de type Alzheimer. In: Agniel A, Eustache F, eds. Neuropsychologie Clinique des Démences: Evaluations et Prises en Charge. Marseille: Solal 1995.

15. Belleville S, Rouleau N, Caza N. Effect of normal aging on the manipulation of information in working memory. Mem Cognit 1998; 26:572–583.

16. Morris RG. Short-term forgetting in senile dementia of the Alzheimer's type. Cogn Neuropsychol 1986; 3:77–97.

17. Stroop JR. Studies of interference in serial verbal reactions. J Exp Psychol 1935; 18:643–662.

18. Burgess PW, Shallice T. Fractionnement du syndrome frontal. Rev Neuropsychol 1994; 4:345–370.

19. Shallice T, Burgess PW. Deficits in strategy application following frontal lobe damage in man. Brain 1991; 114 (part 2): 727–741.

20. Burgess PW, Shallice T. The Hayling and Brixton Test. Thames Valley Test Company, Bury St Edmunds, Suffolk. 1997.

21. Gronwall DM. Paced auditory serial-addition task: a measure of recovery from concussion. Percept Mot Skills 1977; 44:367–373.

22. Gronwall D, Sampson H. The Psychological Effects of Concussion. Auckland: Auckland University Press 1974.

23. Diehr MC, Heaton RK, Miller W, Grant I. The Paced Auditory Serial Addition Task (PASAT): norms for age, education, and ethnicity. Assessment 1998; 5:375–387.

24. Wiens AN, Fuller KH, Crossen JR. Paced Auditory Serial Addition Test: adult norms and moderator variables. J Clin Exp Neuropsychol 1997; 19:473–483.

25. Zimmermann P, Fimm B. Tests d'évaluation de l'attention (TEA). Würselen: Psytest 1994.

26. Baddeley A, Della Sala S, Papagno C, Spinnler H. Dual-task performance in dysexecutive and nondysexecutive patients with a frontal lesion. Neuropsychology 1997; 11:187–194.

27. Greene JD, Hodges JR, Baddeley AD. Autobiographical memory and executive function in early dementia of Alzheimer type. Neuropsychologia 1995; 33:1647–1670.

28. Fuster JM. Synopsis of function and dysfunction of the frontal lobe. Acta Psychiatr Scand Suppl 1999; 395:51–57.

29. Luria AR. Les Fonctions Corticales Supérieures de l'homme. Paris: Presse Universitaires de France 1966.

30. Luria AR. The Working Brain. New York: Penguin Press 1973.

31. Stuss DT, Benson DF. The Frontal Lobes. New York: Raven Press 1986.

32. Burgess PW. Theory and methodology in executive function research. In: Rabbitt P, ed. Methodology of Frontal and Executive Function. New York: Psychology Press 1997; 81–116.

33. Burgess P. Assessment of executive function. In: Halligan PW, Kischka U, Marshall JC, eds. Handbook of Clinical Neuropsychology. Oxford: Oxford University Press 2003.

34. Karnath HO, Wallesch CW. Inflexibility of mental planning: a characteristic disorder with prefrontal lobe lesions? Neuropsychologia 1992; 30:1011–1016.

35. Rabbitt P. Introduction: methodologies and models in the study of executive function. In: Rabbitt P, ed. Methodology of Frontal and Executive Function. Perth: Psychology Press 1997 1–38.

36. Patterson MB, Mack JL, Gelmacher DS, Whitehouse PJ. Executive functions and Alzheimer's disease: problems and prospects. Eur J Neurol 1996; 3:5–15.

37. Lezak M. Neuropsychological Assessment 3rd edn. Oxford: Oxford University Press 1995.

38. Roman GC, Royall DR. Executive control function: a rational basis for the diagnosis of vascular dementia. Alzheimer Dis Assoc Disord 1999; 13(suppl 3):S69–S80.

39. Willis SL, Allen-Burge R, Dolan MM, et al. Everyday problem solving among individuals with Alzheimer's disease. The Gerontologist 1998; 38:569–577.

40. Ashford JW, Kumar V, Barringer M, et al. Assessing Alzheimer severity with a global clinical scale. Int Psychogeriatr 1992; 4:55–74.

41. Chen ST, Sultzer DL, Hinkin CH, Mahler ME, Cummings JL. Executive dysfunction in Alzheimer's disease: association with neuropsychiatric symptoms and functional impairment. J Neuropsychiatr Clin Neurosci 1998; 10:426–432.

42. Jeste DV, Wragg RE, Salmon DP, Harris MJ, Thal LJ. Cognitive deficits of patients with Alzheimer's disease with and without delusions. Am J Psychiatry 1992; 149: 184–189.

43. Carlesimo GA, Fadda L, Lorusso S, Caltagirone C. Verbal and spatial memory spans in Alzheimer's and multi-infarct dementia. Acta Neurol Scand 1994; 89:132–138.

44. Royall DR. Precis of executive dyscontrol as a cause of problem behavior in dementia. Exp Aging Res 1994; 20: 73–94.

45. Collette F, Van der Linden M, Salmon E. Executive dysfunction in Alzheimer's disease. Cortex 1999; 35:57–72.

46. Sultzer DL. Mental Status Examination. In: Coffey CE, Cummings JL, eds. Textbook of Geriatric Neuropsychiatry. Washington: American Psychiatric Press 1994 111–127.

47. Almkvist O. Neuropsychological features of early Alzheimer's disease: preclinical and clinical stages. Acta Neurol Scand Suppl 1996; 165:63–71.

48. Bhutani GE, Montaldi D, Brooks DN, McCulloch J. A neuropsychological investigation into frontal lobe involvement in dementia of the Alzheimer type. Neuropsychology 1992; 6:211–224.

49. Baddeley A, Della Sala S, Spinnler H. The two-component hypothesis of memory deficit in Alzheimer's disease. J Clin Exp Neuropsychol 1991; 13:372–380.

50. Amieva H, Lafont S, Rouch-Leroyer I, et al. Evidencing inhibitory deficits in Alzheimer's disease through interference effects and shifting disabilities in the Stroop test. Arch Clin Neuropsychol 2004; 19:791–803.

51. Amieva H, Lafont S, Auriacombe S, et al. Inhibitory breakdown and dementia of the Alzheimer type: a general phenomenon? J Clin Exp Neuropsychol 2002; 24:503–516.

52. Fisher LM, Freed DM, Corkin S. Stroop Color-Word Test performance in patients with Alzheimer's disease. J Clin Exp Neuropsychol 1990; 12:745–758.

53. Koss E, Ober BA, Delis DC, Friedland RP. The Stroop color-word test: indicator of dementia severity. Int J Neurosci 1984; 24:53–61.

54. Spieler DH, Balota DA, Faust ME. Stroop performance in healthy younger and older adults and in individuals with dementia of the Alzheimer's type. J Exp Psychol Hum Percept Perform 1996; 22:461–479.

55. Amieva H, Lafont S, Auriacombe S, et al. Analysis of error types in the trial making test evidences an inhibitory deficit in dementia of the Alzheimer type. J Clin Exp Neuropsychol 1998; 20:280–285.

56. Greenlief CL, Margolis RB, Erker GJ. Application of the Trail Making Test in differentiating neuropsychological impairment of elderly persons. Percept Mot Skills 1985; 61:1283–1289.

57. Mitrushina M, Satz P, Van Gorp W. Some putative cognitive precursors in subjects hypothesized to be at-risk for dementia. Arch Clin Neuropsychol 1989; 4:323–333.

58. Laflèche G, Albert M. Executive function deficits in mild Alzheimer's disease. Neuropsychology 1995; 9:313–320.

59. Storandt M, Botwinick J, Danziger W, et al. Psychometric differentiation of mild senile dementia of the Alzheimer type. Arch Neurol 1984; 41:497–499.

60. Chertkow H, Bub D, Bergman H, et al. Increased semantic priming in patients with dementia of the Alzheimer's type. J Clin Exp Neuropsychol 1994; 16:608–622.

61. Reitan RM. Manual for Administration of Neuro-psychological Test Batteries for Adults and Children. Tucson, Arizona: Reitan Neuropsychological Laboratories, Inc. 1979.

62. Herlitz A, Hill RD, Fratiglioni L, Backman L. Episodic memory and visuospatial ability in detecting and staging dementia in a community-based sample of very old adults. J Gerontol A Biol Sci Med Sci 1995; 50:M107–M113.

63. Amieva H, Lafont S, Rainville C, Dartigues J-F, Fabrigoule C. Analysis of inhibitory errors in patients with dementia of the Alzheimer's disease and normal elderly adults in two verbal tasks. Brain Cogn 1998; 37:58–60.

64. Cahn DA, Salmon DP, Bondi MW, et al. A population-based analysis of qualitative features of the neuropsychological test performance of individuals with dementia of the Alzheimer type: implications for individuals with question-able dementia. J Int Neuropsychol Soc 1997; 3: 387–393.

65. Berg EA. A simple objective technique for measuring flexibility of thinking. J Gen Psychol 1948; 39:15–22.

66. Bondi MW, Monsch AU, Butters N, Salmon DP, Paulsen J. Utility of a modified version of the Wisconsin Card Sorting Test in the detection of dementia of the Alzheimer type. Clin Neuropsychol 1993; 7:161–170.

67. Paolo AM, Axelrod BN, Troster AI, Blackwell KT, Koller WC. Utility of a Wisconsin Card Sorting Test short form in persons with Alzheimer's and Parkinson's disease. J Clin Exp Neuropsychol 1996; 18:892–897.

68. Monsch AU, Bondi MW, Butters N, et al. Comparisons of verbal fluency tasks in the detection of dementia of the Alzheimer type. Arch Neurol 1992; 49:1253–1258.

69. Alberca R, Salas D, Perez-Gil JA, Lozano P, Gil-Neciga E. [Verbal fluency and Alzheimer's disease.] Neurologia 1999; 14:344–348.

70. Anterion CT, Honore S, Cougny H, Grosmaitre C, Laurent B. [IContribution of lexical recall in the Set Test in Alzheimer disease screening.] Rev Neurol (Paris) 2001; 157(11 part 1):1377–1382.

71. Dastoor D, Schwartz G, Nair N. Category Retrieval and Verbal Fluency from Semantic Memory in Cognitively Impaired and Healthy Elderly Subjects. Toronto: Roman Research Institute 1993.

72. Isaacs B, Kennie AT. The Set test as an aid to the detection of dementia in old people. Br J Psychiatry 1973; 123:467–470.

73. Amieva H, Jacqmin-Gadda H, Orgogozo JM, et al. The 9 year cognitive decline before dementia of the Alzheimer type: a prospective population-based study. Brain 2005; 128(part 5):1093–1101.

74. Shallice T. Specific impairments of planning. Phil Trans R Soc Lond B Biol Sci 1982; 298:199–209.

75. Carlin D, Bonerba J, Phipps M, et al. Planning impairments in frontal lobe dementia and frontal lobe lesion patients. Neuropsychologia 2000; 38:655–665.

76. Piquard A, Derouesne C, Lacomblez L, Sieroff E. [Planning and activities of daily living in Alzheimer's disease and frontotemporal dementia.] Psychol Neuropsychiatr Vieil 2004; 2:147–156.

77. Rainville C, Amieva H, Lafont S, et al. Executive function deficits in patients with dementia of the Alzheimer's type: a study with a Tower of London task. Arch Clin Neuropsychol 2002; 17:513–530.

78. Anderson V. Assessing executive functions in children: bio-logical, psychological and developmental considerations. Neuropsychol Rehab 1998; 8:319–349.

79. Allamano N, Della Sala S, Laicona M, Pasetti C, Spinnler H. Problem solving ability in aging and dementia: norma-tive data on a non-verbal test. Ital J Neurol Sci 1987; 8:111–120.

80. Culberston WC, Zillmer EA. The Tower of London: a standardized approach to assessing executive functioning in children. Arch Clin Neuropsychol 1998; 13:285–302.

81. Culbertson WC, Moberg PJ, Duda JE, Stern MB, Weintraub D. Assessing the executive function deficits of patients with Parkinson's disease: utility of the Tower of London–Drexel. Assessment 2004; 11:27–39.

82. Krikorian R, Bartok J, Gay N. Tower of London procedure: a standard method and developmental data. J Clin Exp Neuropsychol 1994; 16:840–850.

83. Schnirman GM, Welsh MC, Retzlaff PD. Development of the Tower of London – Revised. Assessment 1998; 5: 355–360.

84. Unterrainer JM, Rahm B, Leonhart R, Ruff CC, Halsband U. The Tower of London: the impact of instructions, cueing, and learning on planning abilities. Brain Res Cogn Brain Res 2003; 17:675–683.

85. Tulving E. Episodic and semantic memory. In: Tulving E, Donaldson W, eds. Organization of Memory. New York: Academic Press 1972; 382–403.

86. Tulving E. Elements of Episodic Memory. New York: Clarendon Press & Oxford University Press 1983.

87. American Psychiatric Association. Diagnostic and Statistical Manual of Mental Disorders. Washington: American Psychiatric Association 1994.

88. Butters N, Granholm E, Salmon DP, Grant I, Wolfe J. Episodic and semantic memory: a comparison of amnesic and demented patients. J Clin Exp Neuropsychol 1987; 9:479–497.

89. Morris RG, Kopelman MD. The memory deficits in Alzheimer-type dementia: a review. Q J Exp Psychol A 1986; 38:575–602.

90. Grady CL, Haxby JV, Horwitz B, et al. Longitudinal study of the early neuropsychological and cerebral metabolic changes in dementia of the Alzheimer type. J Clin Exp Neuropsychol 1988; 10:576–596.

91. Christensen H, Kopelman MD, Stanhope N, Lorentz L, Owen P. Rates of forgetting in Alzheimer dementia. Neuropsychologia 1998; 36:547–557.

92. Kopelman MD. Rates of forgetting in Alzheimer-type dementia and Korsakoff's syndrome. Neuropsychologia 1985; 23:623–638.

93. Braak H, Braak E. Neuropathological stageing of Alzheimer-related changes. Acta Neuropathol (Berl) 1991 82:239–259.

94. Damasio A. The anatomic basis of memory disorders. Semin Neurol 1984; 4:223–225.

95. Hyman BT, Arriagada PV, Van Hoesen GW, Damasio AR. Memory impairment in Alzheimer's disease: an anatomical perspective. In: Parks WR, Zec RF, Wilson RS, eds. Neuropsychology of Alzheimer's Disease and Other Dementias. Oxford: Oxford University Press 1993; 138–150.

96. Delis DC, Kramer JH, Kaplan E, Ober BA. The California Verbal Learning Test. New York: The Psychological Corporation 1987.

97. Delis DC, Massman PJ, Kaplan E, et al. Alternate form of the California Verbal Learning Test: development and reliability. Clin Neuropsychol 1991; 5:154–162.

98. Grober E, Buschke H, Crystal H, Bang S, Dresner R. Screening for dementia by memory testing. Neurology 1988; 38:900–903.

99. Buschke H. Cued recall in amnesia. J Clin Neuropsychol 1984; 6:433–440.

100. Buschke H, Fuld PA. Evaluation of storage, retention, and retrieval in disordered memory and learning. Neurology 1974; 11:1019–1025.

101. Grober E, Buschke H. Genuine memory deficits in dementia. Devel Psychol 1987; 3:13–36.

102. Grober E, Lipton RB, Hall C, Crystal H. Memory impairment on free and cued selective reminding predicts dementia. Neurology 2000; 54:827–832.

103. Osterrieth P. Le test d'une figure complexe. Arch Psychol 1941; 30:206–356.

104. Chertkow H, Bub D. Semantic memory loss in dementia of Alzheimer's type. What do various measures measure? Brain 1990; 113(part 2):397–417.

105. Hodges JR, Patterson K. Is semantic memory consistently impaired early in the course of Alzheimer's disease? Neuroanatomical and diagnostic implications. Neuropsychologia 1995; 33:441–459.

106. Hodges JR, Salmon DP, Butters N. Semantic memory impairment in Alzheimer's disease: failure of access or degraded knowledge? Neuropsychologia 1992; 30:301–314.

107. Martin A. Representation of semantic and spatial knowledge in Alzheimer's patients: implications for models of preserved learning in amnesia. J Clin Exp Neuropsychol 1987; 9:191–224.

108. Martin A. Semantic knowledge in patients with Alzheimer's disease: evidence for degraded representations. In: Bäckman L, ed. Memory Functioning in Dementia. Amsterdam: Elsevier Science 1992; 119–134.

109. Vogel A, Gade A, Stokholm J, Waldemar G. Semantic memory impairment in the earliest phases of Alzheimer's disease. Dem Geriatr Cogn Disord 2005; 19:75–81.

110. Allport DA. Distributed memory, modular subsystems, and dysphasia. In: Newman SK, Epstein R, eds. Current Perspectives in Dysphasia. Edinburgh: Churchill Livingstone 1985.

111. Warrington EK. The selective impairment of semantic memory. Quart J Exp Psychol 1975; 27:635–657.

112. Caramazza A, Hillis AE, Rapp BC, Romani C. The multiple semantics hypothesis: multiple confusions? Cogn Neuropsychol 1990; 7:161–189.

113. Huff FJ, Corkin S, Growdon JH. Semantic impairment and anomia in Alzheimer's disease. Brain Language 1986; 28:235–249.

114. Hodges JR, Patterson K, Oxbury S, Funnell E. Semantic dementia. Progressive fluent aphasia with temporal lobe atrophy. Brain 1992; 115:1783–1806.

115. Hodges JR, Graham N, Patterson K. Charting the progression in semantic dementia: implications for the organisation of semantic memory. Memory 1995; 3:463–495.

116. Diehl J, Monsch AU, Aebi C, et al. Frontotemporal dementia, semantic dementia, and Alzheimer's disease: the contribution of standard neuropsychological tests to differential diagnosis. J Geriatr Psychiatry Neurol 2005; 18:39–44.

117. Kaplan E, Goodglass H, Weintraub S. Boston Naming Test. Philadelphia: Lea & Febiger 1983.

118. Williams BW, Mack W, Henderson VW. Boston Naming Test in Alzheimer's disease. Neuropsychologia 1989; 27:1073–1079.

119. Diaz M, Sailor K, Cheung D, Kuslansky G. Category size effects in semantic and letter fluency in Alzheimer's patients. Brain Language 2004; 89:108–114.

120. Monsch AU, Bondi MW, Butters N, et al. A comparison of category and letter fluency in Alzheimer's disease and Huntington's disease. Neuropsychology 1994; 8:25–30.

121. Monsch AU, Bondi MW, Butters N, et al. Comparisons of verbal fluency tasks in the detection of dementia of the Alzheimer type. Arch Neurol 1992; 49:1253–1258.

122. Henry JD, Crawford JR. A meta-analytic review of verbal fluency performance following focal cortical lesions. Neuropsychology 2004; 18:284–295.

123. Troyer AK, Moscovitch M, Winocur G, Leach L, Freedman M. Clustering and switching on verbal fluency tests in Alzheimer's and Parkinson's disease. J Int Neuropsychol Soc 1998; 4:137–143.

124. Martin A, Fedio P. Word production and comprehension in Alzheimer's disease: the breakdown of semantic knowledge. Brain Language 1983; 19:124–141.

125. Troster AI, Salmon DP, McCullough D, Butters N. A comparison of the category fluency deficits associated with Alzheimer's and Huntington's disease. Brain Language 1989; 37:500–513.

126. Howard D, Patterson K. The Pyramids and Palm Trees Test: A Test of Semantic Access from Pictures to Words. Bury St Edmunds: Thames Valley Test Company 1992.

127. Humphrey G, Riddoch MJ. Birmingham Object Recognition Battery (BORB). Hove, UK: Lawrence Erlbaum Associates 1993.

128. Cardebat D, Démonet JF, Doyon B. Narrative discourse in dementia. In: Brownell G, Joanette Y, eds. Narrative Discourse in Neurologically Impaired and Normal Aging Adults. San Diego: Singular Publishing Group 1993.

129. Croisile B, Ska B, Brabant MJ, et al. Comparative study of oral and written picture description in patients with Alzheimer's disease. Brain Language 1996; 53:1–19.

130. Bayles KA. Language function in senile dementia. Brain Language 1982; 16:265–280.

131. Bayles KA, Tomoeda CK, Trosset MW. Relation of linguistic communication abilities of Alzheimer's patients to stage of disease. Brain Language 1992; 42:454–472.

132. Caza N, Moscovitch M. Effects of cumulative frequency, but not of frequency trajectory, in lexical decision times of older adults and patients with Alzheimer's disease. J Memory Language. 2005; 35:533–545.

133. Balota DA, Ferraro FR. A dissociation of frequency and regularity effects in pronunciation performance across young adults, older adults, and individuals with senile dementia of the Alzheimer type. J Memory Language 1993; 32:573–592.

134. Hughes JC, Graham N, Patterson K, Hodges JR. Dysgraphia in mild dementia of Alzheimer's type. Neuropsychologia 1997; 35:533–545.

135. Platel H, Lambert J, Eustache F, et al. Characteristics and evolution of writing impairment in Alzheimer's disease. Neuropsychologia 1993; 31:1147–1158.

136. Rapcsak SZ, Arthur SA, Bliklen DA, Rubens AB. Lexical agraphia in Alzheimer's disease. Arch Neurol 1989; 46: 65–68.

137. De Renzi E, Vignolo LA. The Token Test: a sensitive test to detect disturbances in aphasics. Brain 1962; 85:665–678.

138. Ska B, Caramelli P, Croisile B, et al. Protocole d'Evaluation de la Production des Gestes. [Gestures Production Assesssment Battery.] Montreal: Centre de Recherche de l'Institut Universitaire de Gériatrie de Montréal 1994.

139. Goethals M, Santens P. Posterior cortical atrophy. Two case reports and a review of the literature. Clin Neurol Neurosurg 2001; 103:115–119.

140. Parakh R, Roy E, Koo E, Black S. Pantomime and imitation of limb gestures in relation to the severity of Alzheimer's disease. Brain Cogn 2004; 55:272–274.

141. Dumont C, Ska B, Joanette Y. Conceptual apraxia and semantic memory deficit in Alzheimer's disease: two sides of the same coin? J Int Neuropsychol Soc 2000; 6:693–703.

142. Martin A, Brouwers P, Lalonde F, et al. Towards a behavioral typology of Alzheimer's patients. J Clin Exp Neuropsychol 1986; 8:594–610.

143. Butter CM, Trobe JD, Foster NL, Berent S. Visual-spatial deficits explain visual symptoms in Alzheimer's disease. Am J Ophthalmol 1996; 122:97–105.

144. Mendez MF, Mendez MA, Martin R, Smyth KA, Whitehouse PJ. Complex visual disturbances in Alzheimer's disease. Neurology 1990; 40:439–443.

145. Cummings JL, Benson DF. Dementia: A Clinical Approach. Boston: Butterworth–Heinemann 1992.

146. Neary D, Snowden JS. Perceptual disorder in Alzheimer's disease. Semin Ophthalmol 1987; 2:151–158.

147. Crystal HA, Horoupian DS, Katzman R, Jotkowitz S. Biopsy-proved Alzheimer disease presenting as a right parietal lobe syndrome. Ann Neurol 1982; 12:186–188.

148. Kurylo DD, Corkin S, Growdon JH. Perceptual organization in Alzheimer's disease. Psychol Aging 1994; 9:562–567.

149. Mendola JD, Cronin-Golomb A, Corkin S, Growdon JH. Prevalence of visual deficits in Alzheimer's disease. Optom Vis Sci 1995; 72:155–167.

150. Trobe JD, Butter CM. A screening test for integrative visual dysfunction in Alzheimer's disease. Arch Ophthalmol 1993; 111:815–818.

151. Warrington EK, James M. The Visual Object and Space Perception Battery. Thames Valley Test Company: Bury St Edmunds, Suffolk, UK. Gaylord MI: National Rehabilitation Services, 1991.

152. Binetti G, Cappa SF, Magni E, et al. Disorders of visual and spatial perception in the early stage of Alzheimer's disease. Ann NY Acad Sci 1996; 777:221–225.

153. Eslinger PJ, Benton AL. Visuoperceptual performances in aging and dementia: clinical and theoretical implications. J Clin Neuropsychol 1983; 5:213–220.

154. Eslinger PJ, Damasio AR, Benton AL, Van Allen M. Neuropsychologic detection of abnormal mental decline in older persons. JAMA 1985; 253:670–674.

155. Benton AL, Varney NR, Hamsher KD. Visuospatial judgment. A clinical test. Arch Neurol 1978; 35:364–367.

156. Ska B, Poissant A, Joanette Y. Line orientation judgment in normal elderly and subjects with dementia of Alzheimer's type. J Clin Exp Neuropsychol 1990; 12:695–702.

157. Armstrong CL, Cloud B. The emergence of spatial rotation deficits in dementia and normal aging. Neuropsychology 1998; 12:208–217.

158. Liu L, Gauthier L, Gauthier S. Spatial disorientation in persons with early senile dementia of the Alzheimer type. Am J Occup Ther 1991; 45:67–74.

159. Rainville C, Marchand N, Passini R. Performances of patients with a dementia of the Alzheimer type in the Standardized Road-map Test of Direction Sense. Neuropsychologia 2002; 40:567–573.

160. Money J, Alexander D, Walker HT. A Standardised Road-map Test of Direction Sense. Baltimore: Johns Hopkins University Press 1976.

161. Kurylo DD, Corkin S, Rizzo JF, Growdon JH. Greater relative impairment of object recognition than of visuospatial abilities in Alzheimer's disease. Neuropsychology 1996; 10:74–81.

162. Flicker C, Ferris SH, Crook T, Reisberg B, Barbus RT. Equivalent spatial-rotation deficits in normal aging and Alzheimer's disease. J Clin Exp Neuropsychol 1988; 10: 387–399.

163. Brouwers P, Cox C, Martin A, Chase T, Fedio P. Differential perceptual-spatial impairment in Huntington's and Alzheimer's dementias. Arch Neurol 1984; 41:1073–1076.

164. Bayles KL, Kaszniak AW, Tomoeda C. Communication and Cognition in Normal Aging and Dementia. Boston: College-Hill 1987.

165. Strub RL, Black FW. Neurobehavioral Disorders: A Clinical Approach. Philadelphia: FA Davis Company 1988.

166. Berg L, Danziger W, Storandt M, et al. Predictive features in mild dementia of the Alzheimer type. Neurology 1984; 34:563–569.

167. Stub RL, Black PM. The clinical diagnosis of Alzheimer's disease: relative sensitivity of various mental status and neurological examination test items. Ann Neurol 1988; 20:129.

168. Ska B. Fonctions visuo-spatiales et praxiques dans la démence de type Alzheimer. In: Habib M, Joanette Y, Puel M, eds. Démences et Syndromes Démentiels: Approche Neuropsychologique. Paris: Masson 1991; 189–201.

169. Moore V, Wyke MA. Drawing disability in patients with senile dementia. Psychol Med 1984; 14:97–105.

170. Ober BA, Jagust WJ, Koss E, Delis DC, Friedland RP. Visuoconstructive performance and regional cerebral glucose metabolism in Alzheimer's disease. J Clin Exp Neuropsychol 1991; 13:752–772.

171. Binetti G, Cappa SF, Magni E, et al. Visual and spatial perception in the early phase of Alzheimer's disease. Neuropsychology 1998; 12:29–33.

172. Dastoor D, Schwartz G, Kurzman D. Clock drawing – an assessment technique in dementia. J Clin Exp Gerontol 1991; 13:69–85.

173. Sunderland T, Hill JL, Mellow AM, et al. Clock drawing in Alzheimer's disease. A novel measure of dementia severity. J Am Geriatr Soc 1989; 37:725–729.

174. Salmon DP, Butters N. Neuropsychologic assessment of dementia in the elderly. In: Katzman R, Rowe JW, eds. Principles of Geriatric Neurology. Philadelphia: FA Davis Company 1992; 144–163.

175. Zec RF. Neuropsychological functioning in Alzheimer's disease. In: Parks RW, Zec RF, Wilson RS, eds. Neuropsychology of Alzheimer's Disease and other Dementias. New York: Oxford University Press 1993; 3–80.

176. Royall DR, Cabello M, Polk MJ. Executive dyscontrol: an important factor affecting the level of care received by older retirees. J Am Geriatr Soc 1998; 46:1519–1524.

177. Henderson VW, Mack W, Williams BW. Spatial disorientation in Alzheimer's disease. Arch Neurol 1989; 46:391–394.

178. Pan GD, Stern RA, Sano M, Mayeux R. Clock-drawing in neurological disorders. Behav Neurol 1989; 2:39–48.

179. Kirk A, Kertesz A. On drawing impairment in Alzheimer's disease. Arch Neurol 1991; 48:73–77.

180. Johanson AM, Gustafson L, Risberg J. Behavioral observations during performance of the WAIS Block Design Test related to abnormalities of regional cerebral blood flow in organic dementia. J Clin Exp Neuropsychol 1986; 8:201–209.

181. Branconnier RJ, DeVitt DR. Early detection of incipient Alzheimer's disease: some methodological considerations on computerized diagnosis. In: Reisberg B, ed. Alzheimer's Disease: The Standard Reference. New York: Academic Press 1983; 214–227.

182. De Leon MJ, Potegal M, Gurland B. Wandering and parietal signs in senile dementia of Alzheimer's type. Neuropsychobiology 1984; 11:155–157.

183. Cogan DG. Visual disturbances with focal progressive dementing disease. Am J Ophthalmol 1985; 100:68–72.

184. Eustache F, Agniel A, Dary M, et al. Sériation chronologique des symptômes comportementaux et instrumentaux dans les démences de type Alzheimer. Rev Neuropsychol 1993:37–61.

185. Ylieff M, Brach B, Ronvaux B. Le traitement des troubles de l'orientation dans l'espace familier dus aux états démen-tiels de la vieillesse. In: Lévesque L, Marat O, eds. Un Défi Simplement Humain. Montréal: Editions du Renouveau Pédagogique 1988.

186. Beatty WW, Bernstein N. Geographical knowledge in patients with Alzheimer's disease. J Geriatr Psychiatry Neurol 1989; 2:76–82.

187. Cherrier MM, Mendez M, Perryman K. Route learning performance in Alzheimer disease patients. Neuropsychiatry Neuropsychol Behav Neurol 2001; 14:159–168.

188. Rainville C, Joanette Y, Passini R. Les troubles de l'orientation dans l'espace dans la démence de type Alzheimer. Rev Neuropsychol 1994; 4:3–45.

189. Rainville C. Les troubles de la représentation anticipatrice et de la représentation spatiale dans la maladie d'Alzheimer. Montréal: Université de Montréal 1992.

190. Rainville C, Passini R. Communication et résolution de problème (spatial) dans la maladie d'Alzheimer. In: Michel B, ed. Monographie de Recherche sur l'Alzheimer. Marseille, France: Salal 2005.

191. Rainville C, Passini R, Marchand N. A multiple case study of wayfinding of the Alzheimer type: decision making. Aging, Neuropsychol Cogn 2001; 8:54–71.

192. Passini R, Rainville C, Marchand N, Joanette Y. Wayfinding in dementia of the Alzheimer type: planning abilities. J Clin Exp Neuropsychol 1995; 17:820–832.

7

Structural brain imaging

António J Bastos Leite, Frederik Barkhof and Philip Scheltens

INTRODUCTION

The number of elderly people is increasing rapidly, and this tendency will continue in the near future. As a consequence of the aged population, an increase in neurological illnesses is expected, such as neurodegenerative dementias, cerebrovascular disease (CVD) and movement disorders.[1]

Since dementia is a growing health problem[2,3] with an enormous impact on society, measures should be taken to restructure the diagnostic algorithms and rehabilitation support.[3] From the diagnostic point of view, structural neuroimaging with either a non-contrast computed tomography (CT) or magnetic resonance (MR) imaging is already recommended for the initial evaluation of patients with dementia,[4] and is increasingly being used to support the clinical diagnosis beyond the traditional exclusionary approach.[5] Additionally, there is an increasing urge for an early and more accurate diagnosis of dementia given the current availability of therapies, such as cholinesterase inhibitors, that for the most frequent dementias[6–9] improve or stabilize cognition, treat behavioural symptoms and delay institutionalization.[10] Moreover, the recognition of conditions that may precede dementia and may be more amenable to intervention[11–14] also raises the importance of an earlier diagnosis.

In the future, the introduction of new therapies, for example the anti-amyloid drugs[15] for Alzheimer's disease (AD), will reinforce the need for a more rigorous and early diagnosis, given the expectation that the earlier a specific therapy can be started, the more effective it will be in preventing or slowing disease progression.

AD is the most common cause of dementia, with prevalence rates higher than 40 per cent at the age of 85 and a total annual cost approaching 70 billion dollars in the United States of America.[16–18] It is pro-jected that the prevalence will nearly quadruple over the next 50 years, by which time approximately 1 in 45 Americans will be affected by this disease.[3]

A large proportion of patients with dementia have a combination of degenerative and vascular pathology in the brain,[19–27] and there are multiple causes of dementia other than AD. Vascular dementia (VaD), dementia with Lewy bodies (DLB) and frontotemporal dementia (FTD) are the most common causes after AD. Parkinson's disease (PD) can also be associated with dementia, as well as some rare atypical parkinsonian syndromes.[28] Argyrophilic grain disease is probably an underestimated cause of dementia in old patients.[29] Huntington's disease is an autosomal dominant inherited condition characterized by chorea, behavioural disturbances and cognitive deterioration,[28] whose genetic defect is already known.[30] One of the main features of prionic diseases, like Creutzfeldt–Jakob disease, is rapidly progressive dementia.[28] Cases of amyotrophic lateral sclerosis and parkinsonism–dementia complex, the so-called Lytico–Bodig disease, are extremely rare and occur almost exclusively in the Chamorran population of southern Guam.[28,31] Other causes of dementia include infections, inflammatory white matter diseases, metabolic disorders, drugs and toxins, heavy metal poisoning, lipophilic substances, renal insufficiency and dialysis, paraneoplastic syndromes, tumours, radiotherapy, cranial trauma, hydrocephalus and idiopathic calcinosis of Fahr.[28]

Although there are established clinical criteria for the diagnosis of diseases causing dementia,[32–35] the definite diagnosis was always believed to be histopathological. Currently, not even neuropathology can be considered a gold standard anymore. There are considerable discrepancies between different post-mortem pathological criteria and clinical information is still needed for a correct classification.[36] For example, Polvikoski et al,[37] in an autopsy-controlled, prospective, population-based study on the prevalence of AD in very old people ($\geq$ 85 years), found that 55 per cent of the individuals with neuropathological criteria for AD were either non-demented during life or classified as having VaD. Conversely, they also found that 35 per cent of those with clinical AD did not fulfil the neuropathological criteria.

CHOICE OF IMAGING MODALITY

CT without contrast is sufficient to rule out almost all surgically manageable causes of dementia,[38] but except in cases where MR is contraindicated, not available or not affordable, there is no reason to prefer CT over MR.[39] When CT is the only alternative, axial thin slices parallel to the long axis of the temporal lobe (using a negative scan angle) should be obtained.[40]

MR without contrast is the preferred imaging modality for dementia, and the protocol should include at least axial T2-weighted images (T2-WI), axial fluid-attenuated inversion recovery (FLAIR) or proton density-weighted images (PD-WI), axial gradient-echo T2*-weighted images (T2*-WI) and coronal high resolution T1-weighted images (T1-WI) perpendicular to the long axis of the temporal lobe. Axial T2-WI, FLAIR and PD-WI are crucial for the detection of cerebrovascular pathology and white matter changes. Axial T1-WI facilitate the distinction between ischaemic lacunae (hypointense on T1-WI) and focal incomplete infarcts (isointense on T1-WI), and are useful for the assessment of global brain atrophy. Coronal high resolution T1-WI are extremely important to evaluate medial temporal lobe atrophy (MTA). Axial gradient-echo T2*-WI are needed to detect microbleeds and calcifications.[28]

Functional imaging techniques have also been applied to the diagnosis of dementia.[39,41–43] Single photon emission computed tomography (SPECT) evaluates brain perfusion but does not yield absolute quantification of blood flow, and positron emission tomography (PET) is currently used almost exclusively to evaluate the brain's glucose metabolism. At present, SPECT and PET are second-line investigations employed when MR is inconclusive (e.g. in early AD and FTD cases). In the future, SPECT and PET may become more important, especially due to the development of radioligands for in vivo detection of AD pathology.[44,45] Currently, PET imaging is already reimbursed in the United States of America for dementia patients who have atypical symptoms that preclude a clinical diagnosis.

ALZHEIMER'S DISEASE

Neuropathological changes underlying AD first occur in the medial temporal lobe.[46] Therefore, structural neuroimaging in AD is focused on detection of Medial Temporal Lobe Atrophy (MTA), particularly of the hippocampus, parahippocampal gyrus (including the entorhinal cortex) and amygdala. MR and CT are indeed sensitive to MTA in AD,[47–49] correlating with AD pathology at postmortem.[50,51] MTA can be assessed using visual rating scales, linear measurements of temporal lobe structures and volumetry of the hippocampus.[40,52–54] Volumetric analyses are time-consuming and therefore not well suited for clinical practice.[55] Moreover, MR studies comparing volumetric and visual assessment of MTA found there is no advantage of volumetry in differentiating AD patients from controls.[55–57] Linear measurements of the temporal horns are reliable, can be used in routine clinical settings and have the advantage of being applicable both to CT and MR.[53,58] The visual rating of MTA[52] is based on subjective evaluation of the choroidal fissure width, the temporal horn width and the hippocampal height (Table 7.1) using coronal high resolution T1-

Table 7.1 Visual rating scale for medial temporal lobe atrophy			
Score	Width of choroidal fissure	Width of temporal horn	Height of hippocampus
0	Normal	Normal	Normal
1	↑	Normal	Normal
2	↑↑	↑	↓
3	↑↑↑	↑↑	↓↓
4	↑↑↑	↑↑↑	↓↓↓

↑ = increased, ↓ = decreased. Reproduced with permission of Scheltens et al[52]

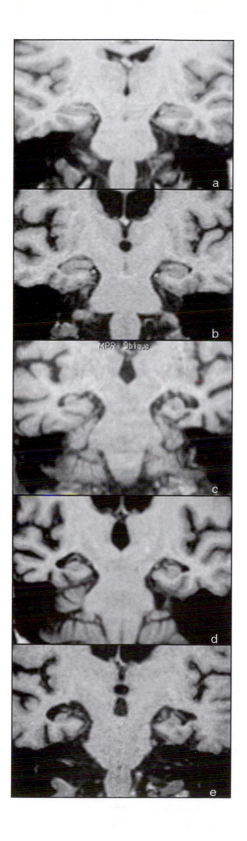

Figure 7.1 Coronal high resolution T1-weighted images perpendicular to the long axis of the temporal lobe showing the different degrees of medial temporal lobe atrophy (MTA), according to the visual rating scale proposed by Scheltens et al:[52] (a) absence of atrophy (MTA = 0), (b) minimal atrophy (MTA = 1), (c) mild atrophy in the right side (MTA = 2), severe atrophy on the left (MTA = 4), (d) moderate atrophy (MTA = 3), and (e) severe atrophy (MTA = 4)

weighted images perpendicular to the long axis of the temporal lobe (Figure 7.1). It is easily applicable in clinical practice, but slightly observer dependent.[59] In a review[5] of studies employing visual rating scales or linear measurements to evaluate MTA, the weighted sensitivity and specificity for detection of patients with AD (versus controls) were, respectively, 85 per cent and 88 per cent.

Because the initial neuropathological changes in AD occur in the entorhinal cortex,[46] some volumetric MR studies compared the discriminative power of measurements in both the entorhinal cortex and hippocampus to identify patients with early stages of AD. Although they found that both regions are affected, they did not find advantage by assessing the entorhinal cortex as an alternative for the hippocampus.[60,61]

Besides the existence of MTA, the most important structural imaging feature of AD is progression of such atrophy. Jack et al[62] found a yearly decline in hippocampal volume approximately 2.5 times greater in patients with AD than in normal aged subjects, and a relationship exists between memory loss and hippocampal damage across the spectrum from normal aging to dementia.[63] However, neuroanatomical changes over time may be too mild, diffuse or topographically complex to be detected by simple visual inspection or even with manually traced measurements of regions of interest. New serial volumetric imaging techniques developed in the past few years represent an added value to identify subtle structural brain abnormalities, which have brought extensive neocortical changes to the fore.[64,65] In addition, voxel based morphometry (VBM), a voxel-wise, fully automated and unbiased technique that enables comparisons of the local brain tissue concentration between groups of subjects,[66] when applied to compare normal elderly controls with AD patients, demonstrates in these patients: MTA, global cortical atrophy (with relative sparing of the sensorimotor cortex, occipital poles and the cerebellum) as well as atrophy of the caudate nuclei and medial thalami.[67] Furthermore, VBM shows that patients with early onset AD have greater neocortical atrophy at the temporoparietal junction, but less hippocampal atrophy, than patients with late onset AD.[68]

MR studies employing thin-section coronal T2-WI have suggested it is possible to demonstrate shrinkage of the substantia innominata, a finding more pronounced in AD patients who respond to cholinesterase inhibitors, but that may also occur in other dementias.[69–71]

MILD COGNITIVE IMPAIRMENT

Identification of patients with mild cognitive impairment (MCI), a transitional stage between normal aging and AD,[12] is an area where modern imaging techniques might yield the greatest added value, since clinical criteria may be poorly specific.[38] Hippocampal atrophy determined by MR volumetry was found to predict conversion to AD,[72] and entorhinal cortex volumetry might even better distinguish MCI from AD.[73] Visual rating of MTA is a good alternative to hippocampal volumetry, although not so accurate.[74] Finally, VBM shows that MCI patients have less grey matter in the medial temporal lobe, insula and thalamus than normal elderly controls, but more grey matter in the parietal association areas and cingulate cortex than AD patients.[75]

Functional neuroimaging studies can also accurately identify converters from MCI to AD, and even from normal aging to MCI.[76–79] Combinations of serial volumetric studies and cognitive or functional imaging assessments may prove to be the best option in the near future.[80–82] Prospective studies on the effect of white matter lesions in conversion from MCI to dementia are also warranted,[83,84] as well as on their impact in transition to disability.[85]

ALZHEIMER'S DISEASE WITH CEREBROVASCULAR DISEASE AND OTHER PATHOLOGIES

The most frequent combination of brain pathologies in dementia is that which results from both degenerative and vascular lesions,[20–22,24–27] but there are also combinations among different types of degenerative pathologies, namely between AD, PD and DLB.[19,24,26]

Additional pathologies in AD can lower the threshold for dementia or increase its severity, and may represent an independent target for treatment. For example, the burden of AD pathology is lower in cases of AD mixed with other pathologies than in cases of pure AD,[21,23,86,87] and patients with brain infarcts fulfilling neuropathological criteria for AD have poorer

cognitive function and higher prevalence of dementia than those without infarcts,[21,22] especially when they have lacunae in the basal ganglia, thalamus or in deep white matter.[21] Dementia may also occur in a considerable proportion of post-stroke patients, particularly in those with MTA.[88,89] Moreover, when there is neuroimaging evidence of mixed pathology (degenerative and vascular), atrophy correlates better with dementia than CVD,[90–93] and may even result from both ischaemic and degenerative injuries.[90]

Neuroimaging is very useful for the diagnosis of cerebrovascular disease (CVD), particularly of small vessel disease which is frequently not suspected clinically[94,95] and more often associated with dementia than large vessel disease.[96] MR signal abnormalities of deep white and grey matter[97] occurring in AD, VaD and usual ageing can be considered as a surrogate marker for small vessel disease.[5,98]

DEMENTIA WITH LEWY BODIES

Formerly considered a variant of AD, DLB is now recognized as a common degenerative dementia characterized by an often rapidly progressive syndrome also including fluctuations in cognitive function and spontaneous parkinsonism,[7,34,99] but the precise nosological relationships between DLB, AD and PD dementia (PDD) are not yet completely clarified.[34,99]

MR studies comparing DLB, AD, VaD and normal controls found that, although MTA was more frequent and severe in all dementia groups than in controls, subjects with DLB had significantly lower MTA scores and larger temporal lobe, hippocampal and amygdala volumes than those with AD. Therefore, in the differentiation of DLB from AD, the absence of MTA may be considered suggestive of DLB.[100,101] Conversely, atrophy of the putamen is a feature of DLB, but not of AD.[102]

Functional studies found occipital hypoperfusion and hypometabolism in DLB[103,104] that do not seem to be associated with occipital atrophy.[105]

DEMENTIA ASSOCIATED WITH PARKINSON'S DISEASE

Contrary to the initial assumption that cognitive function would be spared, it is now recognized that patients with PD may develop dementia, as their age increases.[106] When fully developed, Parkinson's Disease with Dementia (PDD) and DLB overlap both clinically and pathologically. If the previous history is unknown, patients with each of these disorders may be indistinguishable. Currently, an arbitrary rule used for the distinction between these disorders is to consider that in DLB the onset of dementia should occur within 12 months of parkinsonism, and in PDD only after more than 12 months.[99,106]

Whereas PDD was claimed not to be associated with a specific pattern of MR abnormalities,[107] Laakso et al[108] found severe hippocampal atrophy in these patients, which is surprising considering the aforementioned similarity between PDD and DLB. Additionally, functional studies found patterns of brain hypoperfusion and hypometabolism in PDD not very different from those described in AD.[106] One explanation for these findings may be that PDD patients included in the referred studies had coexistent Alzheimer pathology.

FRONTOTEMPORAL LOBAR DEGENERATION

Frontotemporal lobar degeneration (FTLD) accounts for a substantial proportion of primary degenerative dementia cases occurring before the age of 65 years.[35] Recent clinical criteria proposed by Neary et al[35] discern three main prototypic syndromes – frontotemporal dementia (FTD), progressive non-fluent aphasia (PNA) and semantic dementia (SD), also known as progressive fluent aphasia or temporal variant of FTLD. In addition to the sporadic form, there are also familial cases of FTLD, often linked to chromosome 17 abnormalities.

Neuroimaging studies in patients with clinical and pathological diagnosis of FTLD may show a pattern of marked anterior temporal and frontal atrophy resulting in the so-called 'knife edge' appearance and in dilatation (ballooning) of the temporal and frontal horns of the lateral ventricles (Figure 7.2), in some cases associated with predominantly frontal white matter changes.[109,110] Characteristically, FTLD affects more the temporal pole, but relatively spares the posterior part of the hippocampus.[111]

Asymmetric atrophy is also a distinctive feature of FTLD, particularly of SD and PNA. Selective inferolateral and anterior left temporal atrophy is characteristic of SD. In PNA, atrophy appears to be more diffuse and involves the left frontal and perisylvian structures.[112–115] One variant of FTLD affecting the right temporal lobe presents with progressive prosopagnosia.[115]

Studies employing SPECT for the differential diagnosis between FTD and other dementias found hypoperfusion in the same regions where atrophy occurs,[116,117] and since hypoperfusion or hypometabo-

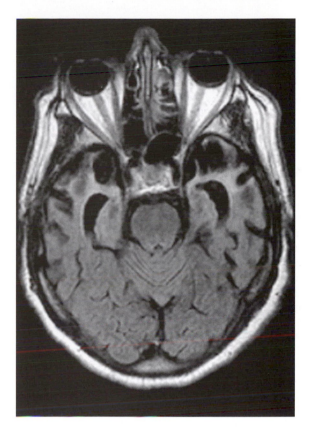

Figure 7.2 Axial fluid-attenuated inversion recovery image of a patient with frontotemporal dementia revealing severe anterior temporal lobe atrophy with 'knife edge' appearance, dilatation of the ventricular temporal horns and subcortical hyperintensity

lism may precede volume loss, functional studies can be useful in early cases.

DEMENTIA AND ATYPICAL PARKINSONIAN SYNDROMES

Characteristic findings on routine MR imaging can contribute to the identification of atypical parkinsonian syndromes[118,119] that may be associated with dementia.[120,121]

Asymmetric atrophy involving the posterior frontal and parietal regions contralateral to the clinically most affected side occurs in the vast majority of patients with corticobasal degeneration (CBD). Mild signal changes on FLAIR and PD-WI in the atrophic cortex have been described in some of these patients.[122] On the other hand, despite the existence of pathological changes in the basal ganglia, MR imaging abnormalities of these structures were almost never reported.[122]

Midbrain atrophy and diffuse hyperintensity on T2-WI in the mesencephalic tegmentum and tectum are characteristic of progressive supranuclear palsy (PSP), and occur due to predominance of pathology in these regions.[123,124] Midbrain atrophy can be simply and accurately assessed measuring the antero-posterior midbrain diameter on axial T2-WI,[119,125] but visual assessment using sagittal T1-WI should also be done, because when there is midbrain atrophy the mesencephalic caudo-cranial dimension is reduced and the third ventricle's floor appears more superiorly concave than normal.[118,122] Besides the infratentorial abnormalities, VBM and serial volumetric studies also show a distinct pattern of mesio-frontal atrophy in PSP.[126,127]

Although asymmetric frontoparietal atrophy in CBD and mesencephalic atrophy in PSP are considered the most useful aids to the clinical diagnosis,[128] other neuroimaging abnormalities have also been described. Asymmetric involvement of the corpus striatum and thalamus in CBD was disclosed by PET in addition to asymmetric cortical hypometabolism.[129] Moreover, patients with PSP and cognitive impairment studied with both MR and PET were found to have predominantly anterior corpus callosum atrophy as well as predominantly frontal cortical hypometabolism.[130]

VASCULAR DEMENTIA

VaD is the second most common type of dementia.[131] The most specific diagnostic criteria for VaD are the National Institute of Neurological Disorders and Stroke (NINDS)–Association Internationale pour la Recherche et l'Enseignement en Neurosciences (AIREN) criteria. These criteria emphasize the heterogeneity of both clinical syndromes and pathological subtypes of VaD, the need to establish a temporal relationship between stroke and the onset of dementia as well as the importance of brain imaging to support clinical findings.[33]

The main clinicopathological subtypes of VaD are large vessel VaD and small vessel VaD. Ischaemic–hypoperfusive VaD and haemorrhagic VaD may also be considered as separate groups. Large vessel VaD can be further subdivided into multi-infarct dementia and strategic infarct dementia (caused by vascular lesions located in strategic regions of the brain, such as the hippocampus, paramedian thalamus and the thalamocortical networks). Small vessel disease may also affect strategic regions. Binswanger's disease, lacunar state (état lacunaire) and cerebral autosomal dominant arteriopathy with subcortical infarcts and leucoencephalopathy (CADASIL) are examples of subcortical ischaemic small vessel VaD. Cerebral amyloid angiopathies (CAA) are considered as a subtype of cortical–subcortical small vessel disease, but they have associated large vessel pathology as well. Both CADASIL and some forms of CAA have a genetic basis.[131–134]

Most patients with the diagnosis of VaD have small vessel rather than large vessel disease.[96,135] Therefore, research criteria were formulated specifically for subcortical ischaemic VaD, now recognized as the most broad and homogeneous subtype.[136]

Given that patients with coexistent AD and CVD (mixed dementia) represent an important and previously underestimated group,[137] the causal relation between vascular lesions alone and dementia is only clear in the following circumstances: when patients are young and it is unlikely they have associated Alzheimer pathology; when cognitive functions are normal before stroke, impaired immediately after and do not worsen over time; when vascular lesions are located in strategic regions and when well-defined vasculopathies known to cause dementia are proven, such as CADASIL or CAA. In other circumstances, it is probable that patients may have a combination of degenerative and vascular pathology.[138,139]

Because the NINDS-AIREN criteria consider structural neuroimaging crucial for the diagnosis of VaD,[33] operational definitions for the radiological part of these criteria were proposed, both in terms of topography and severity of lesions (Table 7.2).[140]

T2-weighted MR sequences are far more sensitive for the detection of CVD than CT,[141] although CT was found to be more specific than MR in predicting subsequent symptomatic CVD.[94] In addition, the sensitivity of T2-WI for detection of thalamic lesions in patients with probable VaD is superior to FLAIR, and given the great clinical importance of these lesions, FLAIR should not be used as the only T2-weighted sequence.[142]

Infarcts may either be complete or incomplete. Complete infarcts correspond to areas of tissue destruction, whereas incomplete infarcts may only represent demyelination and oedema. Hypointensity on T1-WI usually represents tissue destruction, and may thus be considered as a surrogate marker for complete infarcts. Therefore, lesions hyperintense on T2-WI and isointense on T1-WI may just correspond to demyelination.[143,144] FLAIR has the additional advantage of easily identifying cystic lesions,[145] and the combination of FLAIR with T1-WI may be useful to differentiate the more aggressive lesions from those that might have less power to cause cognitive impairment.[144]

Table 7.2 Operational definitions for the imaging guidelines of the National Institute of Neurological Disorders and Stroke (NINDS)–Association Internationale pour la Recherche et l'Enseignement en Neurosciences (AIREN) criteria for vascular dementia

Topography

Large vessel stroke – arterial territorial infarct involving the cortical grey matter

- Anterior cerebral artery (ACA) – only bilateral ACA infarcts are sufficient to meet the NINDS-AIREN criteria
- Posterior cerebral artery (PCA) – infarcts in the PCA territory can only be included when they involve the following regions:
   1. paramedian thalamus
   2. inferior medial temporal lobe
- Association areas – a medial cerebral artery (MCA) infarct needs to involve the following regions:
   1. parietotemporal (e.g., angular gyrus)
   2. temporo-occipital
- Watershed carotid territories – a watershed infarct is defined as an infarct in the watershed area between MCA and ACA or between MCA and PCA, in the following regions:
   1. superior frontal region
   2. parietal region

Small vessel disease

- Ischaemic pathology resulting from occlusion of small perforating arteries may become apparent as white matter lesions or as ischaemic lacunae:
   1. multiple basal ganglia, thalamic and frontal white matter lacunae – the criteria are met when there are at least two lacunae in the basal ganglia, thalamus or internal capsule, and at least two lacunae in the frontal white matter
   2. extensive periventricular white matter lesions
   3. bilateral thalamic lesions

Severity

- Large vessel disease of the dominant hemisphere – if there is a large vessel infarct, the criteria are only met when the infarct is located in the dominant hemisphere. In the absence of clinical information, the left hemisphere is considered dominant
- Bilateral large vessel hemispheric strokes – the infarct located in the non-dominant hemisphere should involve an area listed under topography. The infarct located in the dominant hemisphere does not need to meet the topography criteria
- Leukoencephalopathy involving at least one quarter of the total white matter – extensive white matter lesions are considered to involve at least one quarter of the total white matter when they are confluent – grade 3 in the age-related white matter changes (ARWMC) scale[141] – in at least two regions, and beginning confluent – grade 2 in the ARWMC scale – in two other regions. A lesion is considered confluent when it measures >20 mm or it consists of ≥2 smaller lesions fused by connecting bridges

Fulfilment of radiological criteria for probable VaD

- Large vessel disease – a lesion must be scored in at least one subsection of both topography and severity (both the topography and severity criteria should be met)
- Small vessel disease – for white matter lesions, both the topography and severity criteria should be met; for multiple lacunae and bilateral thalamic lesions, only the topography criterion is sufficient

Modified with permission of van Straaten et al[140]

Complete infarcts of deep small vessels are defined as lacunar infarcts, and some authors consider this definition also dependent on size (from 2–3 to 15–20 mm in diameter).[131,146,147] Misclassification between lacunar infarcts and enlarged perivascular (Virchow–Robin) spaces may occur, but most of the enlarged Virchow–Robin spaces measure <2 mm, and normally surround perforating arteries entering the striatum at the anterior perforated substance.[148,149] Their appearance in large numbers reflects focal brain atrophy around blood vessels and may lead to the so called *état criblé*, especially in the basal ganglia.[148,150,151] Moreover, the association of enlarged Virchow–Robin spaces and white matter lesions with cognitive impairment occurs,[152] and widening of Virchow–Robin spaces can be considered as a measure of focal atrophy.[153]

White matter changes on MR imaging are visible as diffuse hyperintense abnormalities on T2-WI, FLAIR and PD-WI, without prominent hypointensity on T1-WI. On CT, white matter changes appear as mildly hypodense areas. Since their occurrence increases progressively with age, they are usually referred to as age-related white matter changes (ARWMC). ARWMC may be considered as a surrogate marker for small vessel disease.[5,98] Moreover, they are associated with vascular risk factors as well as with other types of CVD.[154–156] Since the original scale of Fazekas et al,[97] several others have been proposed for rating ARWMC. Currently, the most complete is that proposed by Wahlund et al, applicable both to CT and MR imaging.[141] According to the NINDS-AIREN criteria, white matter changes alone may be sufficient to cause dementia when at least one quarter of the white matter is involved.[33] Although this proportion has been defined arbitrarily, it is in accordance with the finding that only severe white matter disease is associated with cognitive dysfunction.[157] Extensive and diffuse white matter changes affecting predominantly deep and periventricular white matter, but relatively sparing the U-fibres, occur in Binswanger's disease.[131]

In patients with CADASIL, diffuse white matter signal changes involving the U-fibres occur mainly in the temporal, temporopolar and frontal regions (Figure 7.3).[158–160] Microbleeds, defined by some authors as hypointense foci (<5 mm) on T2-WI or gradient-echo T2*-WI,[161,162] are present in a considerable proportion of these patients, as well as in patients with CAA.[163,164] However, the most typical feature of CAA is the occurrence of cortical–subcortical (lobar) haemorrhages.[164,165]

Deep venous thrombosis and dural arteriovenous fistulae are vascular abnormalities that may rarely cause venous hypertensive encephalopathy or bilateral thalamic congestion, and lead to dementia. MR or conventional angiography is crucial for their diagnosis.[166–168] Conventional angiography is also very useful for the interventional therapy of these abnormalities.[166,167,169]

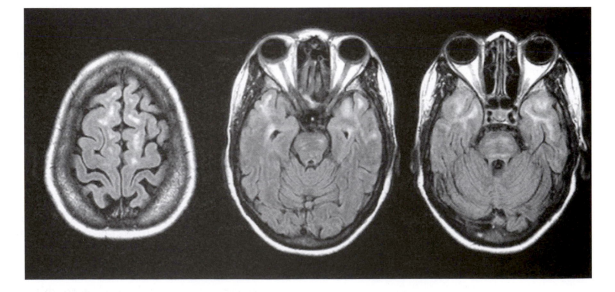

Figure 7.3 Axial fluid-attenuated inversion recovery images revealing diffuse white matter signal changes involving the U-fibres, mainly in the temporal, temporopolar and frontal regions of a patient with cerebral autosomal dominant arteriopathy with subcortical infarcts and leucoencephalopathy (CADASIL)

ROLE OF NEUROIMAGING IN THE DIFFERENTIAL DIAGNOSIS OF DEMENTIA

MR studies performed to investigate the value of MTA for the differential diagnosis of dementia did not find unequivocal results. O'Brien et al[170] carried out a study to determine the specificity of hippocampal atrophy for the differentiation between AD and other conditions associated with cognitive impairment, such as VaD and major depression. They found that ratings of MTA were useful to differentiate AD from other groups. Conversely, Laakso et al[108] found that hippocampal atrophy was not specific to differentiate AD from VaD or PDD, although they couldn't rule out the co-existence of Alzheimer pathology in their VaD or PDD patients. More recently, Barber et al[100,101] found different degrees of hippocampal atrophy occurring in AD, VaD and DLB – the most severe in AD, the less severe in DLB and, although there was also a trend towards less atrophy in DLB compared with VaD, no significant volumetric difference between these two groups was observed. Most likely, these discrepancies reflect studies of different populations, illustrating that the diagnostic accuracy of MTA depends on disease severity.

SPECT and PET studies have also been applied to the differential diagnosis of dementia. Although they are considered useful for the differentiation between AD, VaD and FTD, the discrimination between AD and DLB was found to be difficult based on cerebral metabolism and blood flow.[171,172] In the future, VBM and serial volumetric studies evaluating global brain atrophy may also be useful for the differential diagnosis. However, one should always keep in mind that imaging overlap between different entities may reflect a combination of different pathologies, or even result from differences in pathology distribution.[173,174]

The pattern of white matter signal abnormalities on MR imaging is very important for the differentiation between ischaemic lesions and inflammatory demyelinating lesions. Multiple sclerosis (MS) is the most common inflammatory demyelinating disease and occurs mainly in young people, but it may lead to cognitive dysfunction due to accumulation of white matter lesions, or due to occurrence of cortical and juxtacortical lesions.[28] The most specific MR imaging diagnostic criteria for MS were proposed by Barkhof et al,[175] and currently a modification of them makes part of the guidelines from the International Panel on the diagnosis of MS.[176] MR imaging is also very important for the diagnosis of other disorders that may lead to dementia and primarily affect white matter, such as herpes simplex encephalitis, human immunodeficiency virus encephalitis and progressive multifocal leukoencephalopathy.[28]

Apart from the imaging findings described for the most frequent diseases causing dementia, MR may still show specific imaging patterns of atrophy or signal abnormalities in other disorders. Atrophy of the striatum, most conspicuous on visual inspection in the caudate nucleus, is typical of Huntington's disease,[28] although putaminal atrophy is a better predictor of disease onset in presymptomatic subjects.[177] Rapidly progressive brain atrophy as well as striatal and cortical hyperintensity on FLAIR, PD-WI or T2-WI preceded by signal abnormalities on diffusion-weighted imaging (DWI) occur in patients with Creutzfeldt–Jakob disease.[178–181] Additionally, in the new variant of Creutzfeldt–Jakob disease, bilateral hyperintensity of the pulvinar is a very specific imaging finding.[182]

Normal pressure hydrocephalus (NPH) is a rare disorder that, even more rarely, causes dementia. By definition, it includes the clinical triad of gait disturbance, urinary incontinence and dementia. Gait impairment is the cardinal symptom, while mental deterioration may be subtle or even unrecognized. Initially, NPH was considered to be an idiopathic form of communicating hydrocephalus, but, currently, other forms of communicating hydrocephalus, and even a few non-communicating forms, make part of its spectrum.[183–185] MR is the best imaging modality to evaluate the pulsatile motion of cerebrospinal fluid (CSF) in the cerebral aqueduct, either visually, as a low intensity signal on T2-WI (flow void), or using quantitative phase-contrast measurements. In NPH, both flow void and phase-contrast measurements are increased due to reduced ventricular compliance,[186,187] and it seems that only when they are prominently increased is there prediction of a positive response to shunt therapy.[185,188–190] Given the frequent co-existence of NPH with deep and periventricular white matter ischaemic changes,[191,192] it is a matter of controversy whether NPH alone represents a true disease entity causing dementia.

FUTURE PERSPECTIVES

The big future challenge of neuroimaging techniques in the diagnosis of dementia will be to demonstrate pathological processes occurring at a microscopic level, and therefore help to recognize subjects at risk of developing dementia before the occurrence of atrophy as an indicator of substantial tissue loss. For this purpose, a combination of new structural and functional MR techniques, as well as molecular imaging (by means of PET, SPECT or MR microscopy) may play a major role in the future, either for the early diagnosis of diseases causing dementia or to identify persons at risk of developing cognitive impairment.[193]

CONCLUSIONS

The number of elderly people is increasing rapidly and, therefore, an increase in neurodegenerative and cerebrovascular disorders causing dementia is expected. Alzheimer's disease is the most common cause of dementia. Vascular dementia, dementia with Lewy bodies and frontotemporal dementia are the most frequent causes after AD, but a large proportion of patients have a combination of degenerative and vascular brain pathology. Structural neuroimaging in dementia is focused on detection of brain atrophy, especially in the medial temporal lobe. Therefore, MR coronal high resolution T1-weighted images perpendicular to the long axis of the temporal lobe are extremely important. The MR imaging protocol should also include axial T2-weighted images, axial fluid-attenuated inversion recovery or proton density-weighted images and axial gradient-echo T2*-weighted images, for the detection of cerebrovascular pathology. Finally, new serial volumetric imaging studies to identify subtle brain abnormalities may provide surrogate markers for pathological processes which occur in diseases causing dementia and, in conjunction with clinical evaluation, may enable a more rigorous and early diagnosis.

REFERENCES

1. Drayer BP. Imaging of the aging brain. Part II. Pathologic conditions. Radiology 1988; 166:797–806.
2. The incidence of dementia in Canada. The Canadian Study of Health and Aging Working Group. Neurology 2000; 55:66–73.
3. Brookmeyer R, Gray S, Kawas C. Projections of Alzheimer's disease in the United States and the public health impact of delaying disease onset. Am J Public Health 1998; 88: 1337–1342.
4. Knopman DS, DeKosky ST, Cummings JL, et al. Practice parameter: diagnosis of dementia (an evidence-based review). Report of the Quality Standards Subcommittee of the American Academy of Neurology. Neurology 2001; 56:1143–1153.
5. Scheltens P, Fox N, Barkhof F, De Carli C. Structural magnetic resonance imaging in the practical assessment of dementia: beyond exclusion. Lancet Neurol 2002; 1:13–21.
6. Mayeux R, Sano M. Treatment of Alzheimer's disease. N Engl J Med 1999; 341:1670–1679.
7. McKeith I, del Ser T, Spano P, et al. Efficacy of rivastigmine in dementia with Lewy bodies: a randomised, double-blind, placebo-controlled international study. Lancet 2000; 356: 2031–2036.
8. Kumar V, Anand R, Messina J, Hartman R, Veach J. An efficacy and safety analysis of Exelon in Alzheimer's disease patients with concurrent vascular risk factors. Eur J Neurol 2000; 7:159–169.
9. Erkinjuntti T, Roman G, Gauthier S. Treatment of vascular dementia–evidence from clinical trials with cholinesterase inhibitors. J Neurol Sci 2004; 226:63–66.
10. Winblad B, Wimo A. Assessing the societal impact of acetylcholinesterase inhibitor therapies. Alzheimer Dis Assoc Disord 1999; 13(suppl 2):S9–S19.
11. Graham JE, Rockwood K, Beattie BL, et al. Prevalence and severity of cognitive impairment with and without dementia in an elderly population. Lancet 1997; 349:1793–1796.
12. Petersen RC, Smith GE, Waring SC, et al. Mild cognitive impairment: clinical characterization and outcome. Arch Neurol 1999; 56:303–308.
13. Rockwood K, Wentzel C, Hachinski V, et al. Prevalence and outcomes of vascular cognitive impairment. Vascular Cognitive Impairment Investigators of the Canadian Study of Health and Aging. Neurology 2000; 54:447–451.
14. Petersen RC, Stevens JC, Ganguli M, et al. Practice parameter: early detection of dementia: mild cognitive impairment (an evidence-based review). Report of the Quality Standards Subcommittee of the American Academy of Neurology. Neurology 2001; 56 :1133–1142.
15. Citron M. Strategies for disease modification in Alzheimer's disease. Nat Rev Neurosci 2004; 5:677–685.
16. Evans DA, Funkenstein HH, Albert MS, et al. Prevalence of Alzheimer's disease in a community population of older persons. Higher than previously reported. JAMA 1989; 262: 2551–2556.
17. Carr DB, Goate A, Phil D, Morris JC. Current concepts in the pathogenesis of Alzheimer's disease. Am J Med 1997; 103:3S–10S.
18. Small GW, Rabins PV, Barry PP, et al. Diagnosis and treatment of Alzheimer disease and related disorders. Consensus statement of the American Association for Geriatric Psychiatry, the Alzheimer's Association, and the American Geriatrics Society. JAMA 1997; 278:1363–1371.
19. Ince P, Irving D, MacArthur F, Perry RH. Quantitative neuropathological study of Alzheimer-type pathology in the hippocampus: comparison of senile dementia of Alzheimer type, senile dementia of Lewy body type, Parkinson's disease and non-demented elderly control patients. J Neurol Sci 1991; 106:142–152.
20. Hulette C, Nochlin D, McKeel D, et al. Clinical-neuropathologic findings in multi-infarct dementia: a report of six autopsied cases. Neurology 1997; 48:668–672.
21. Snowdon DA, Greiner LH, Mortimer JA, et al. Brain infarction and the clinical expression of Alzheimer disease. The Nun Study. JAMA 1997; 277:813–817.
22. Heyman A, Fillenbaum GG, Welsh-Bohmer KA, et al. Cerebral infarcts in patients with autopsy-proven Alzheimer's disease: CERAD, part XVIII. Consortium to Establish a Registry for Alzheimer's Disease. Neurology 1998; 51:159–162.
23. Esiri MM, Nagy Z, Smith MZ, Barnetson L, Smith AD. Cerebrovascular disease and threshold for dementia in the early stages of Alzheimer's disease. Lancet 1999; 354:919–920.
24. Holmes C, Cairns N, Lantos P, Mann A. Validity of current clinical criteria for Alzheimer's disease, vascular dementia and dementia with Lewy bodies. Br J Psychiatry 1999; 174: 45–50.
25. Kalaria RN, Ballard C. Overlap between pathology of Alzheimer disease and vascular dementia. Alzheimer Dis Assoc Disord 1999; 13:S115–S123.

26. Lim A, Tsuang D, Kukull W, et al. Clinico-neuropathological correlation of Alzheimer's disease in a community-based case series. J Am Geriatr Soc 1999; 47:564–569.

27. Neuropathology Group of the Medical Research Council Cognitive Function and Ageing Study (MRC CFAS). Pathological correlates of late-onset dementia in a multicentre, community-based population in England and Wales. Lancet 2001; 357:169–175.

28. Valk J, Barkhof F, Scheltens P. Magnetic Resonance in Dementia. Berlin, Heidelberg, New York, Barcelona, Hong Kong, London, Milan, Paris, Tokyo: Springer 2002.

29. Braak H, Braak E. Argyrophilic grain disease: frequency of occurrence in different age categories and neuropathological diagnostic criteria. J Neural Transm 1998; 105:801–819.

30. The Huntington's Disease Collaborative Research Group. A novel gene containing a trinucleotide repeat that is expanded and unstable on Huntington's disease chromosomes. Cell 1993; 72:971–983.

31. McGeer PL, Schwab C, McGeer EG, Haddock RL, Steele JC. Familial nature and continuing morbidity of the amyotrophic lateral sclerosis–parkinsonism dementia complex of Guam. Neurology 1997; 49:400–409.

32. McKhann G, Drachman D, Folstein M, et al. Clinical diagnosis of Alzheimer's disease: report of the NINCDS-ADRDA Work Group under the auspices of Department of Health and Human Services Task Force on Alzheimer's Disease. Neurology 1984; 34:939–944.

33. Roman GC, Tatemichi TK, Erkinjuntti T, et al. Vascular dementia: diagnostic criteria for research studies. Report of the NINDS-AIREN International Workshop. Neurology 1993; 43:250–260.

34. McKeith IG, Galasko D, Kosaka K, et al. Consensus guidelines for the clinical and pathologic diagnosis of dementia with Lewy bodies (DLB): report of the consortium on DLB international workshop. Neurology 1996; 47:1113–1124.

35. Neary D, Snowden JS, Gustafson L, et al. Frontotemporal lobar degeneration: a consensus on clinical diagnostic criteria. Neurology 1998; 51:1546–1554.

36. Nagy Z, Esiri MM, Joachim C, et al. Comparison of pathological diagnostic criteria for Alzheimer disease. Alzheimer Dis Assoc Disord 1998; 12:182–189.

37. Polvikoski T, Sulkava R, Myllykangas L, et al. Prevalence of Alzheimer's disease in very elderly people: a prospective neuropathological study. Neurology 2001; 56:1690–1696.

38. Frisoni GB. Structural imaging in the clinical diagnosis of Alzheimer's disease: problems and tools. J Neurol Neurosurg Psychiatry 2001; 70:711–718.

39. Petrella JR, Coleman RE, Doraiswamy PM. Neuroimaging and early diagnosis of Alzheimer disease: a look to the future. Radiology 2003; 226:315–336.

40. Jobst KA, Smith AD, Szatmari M, et al. Detection in life of confirmed Alzheimer's disease using a simple measurement of medial temporal lobe atrophy by computed tomography. Lancet 1992; 340:1179–1183.

41. Silverman DH, Small GW, Chang CY, et al. Positron emission tomography in evaluation of dementia: regional brain metabolism and long-term outcome. JAMA 2001; 286:2120–2127.

42. Frisoni GB, Scheltens P, Galluzzi S, et al. Neuroimaging tools to rate regional atrophy, subcortical cerebrovascular disease, and regional cerebral blood flow and metabolism: consensus paper of the EADC. J Neurol Neurosurg Psychiatry 2003; 74:1371–1381.

43. Kantarci K, Jack CR Jr. Neuroimaging in Alzheimer disease: an evidence-based review. Neuroimaging Clin N Am 2003; 13:197–209.

44. Nordberg A. PET imaging of amyloid in Alzheimer's disease. Lancet Neurol 2004; 3:519–527.

45. Sair HI, Doraiswamy PM, Petrella JR. In vivo amyloid imaging in Alzheimer's disease. Neuroradiology 2004; 46:93–104.

46. Braak H, Braak E. Neuropathological staging of Alzheimer-related changes. Acta Neuropathol (Berl) 1991; 82:239–259.

47. Seab JP, Jagust WJ, Wong ST, et al. Quantitative NMR measurements of hippocampal atrophy in Alzheimer's disease. Magn Reson Med 1988; 8:200–208.

48. Kido DK, Caine ED, LeMay M, et al. Temporal lobe atrophy in patients with Alzheimer disease: a CT study. AJNR 1989; 10:551–555.

49. de Leon MJ, George AE, Stylopoulos LA, Smith G, Miller DC. Early marker for Alzheimer's disease: the atrophic hippocampus. Lancet 1989; 2:672–673.

50. Davis PC, Gearing M, Gray L, et al. The CERAD experience, Part VIII: Neuroimaging–neuropathology correlates of temporal lobe changes in Alzheimer's disease. Neurology 1995; 45:178–179.

51. Bobinski M, de Leon MJ, Wegiel J, et al. The histological validation of post mortem magnetic resonance imaging-determined hippocampal volume in Alzheimer's disease. Neuroscience 2000; 95:721–725.

52. Scheltens P, Leys D, Barkhof F, et al. Atrophy of medial temporal lobes on MRI in 'probable' Alzheimer's disease and normal ageing: diagnostic value and neuropsychological correlates. J Neurol Neurosurg Psychiatry 1992; 55:967–972.

53. Frisoni GB, Beltramello A, Weiss C, et al. Linear measures of atrophy in mild Alzheimer disease. AJNR 1996; 17:913–923.

54. Jack CR Jr, Petersen RC, O'Brien PC, Tangalos EG. MR-based hippocampal volumetry in the diagnosis of Alzheimer's disease. Neurology 1992; 42:183–188.

55. Wahlund LO, Julin P, Lindqvist J, Scheltens P. Visual assessment of medial temporal lobe atrophy in demented and healthy control subjects: correlation with volumetry. Psychiatry Res 1999; 90:193–199.

56. Desmond PM, O'Brien JT, Tress BM, et al. Volumetric and visual assessment of the mesial temporal structures in Alzheimer's disease. Aust NZ J Med 1994; 24:547–553.

57. Wahlund LO, Julin P, Johansson SE, Scheltens P. Visual rating and volumetry of the medial temporal lobe on magnetic resonance imaging in dementia: a comparative study. J Neurol Neurosurg Psychiatry 2000; 69:630–635.

58. Frisoni GB, Geroldi C, Beltramello A, et al. Radial width of the temporal horn: a sensitive measure in Alzheimer disease. AJNR 2002; 23:35–47.

59. Scheltens P, Launer LJ, Barkhof F, Weinstein HC, van Gool WA. Visual assessment of medial temporal lobe atrophy on magnetic resonance imaging: interobserver reliability. J Neurol 1995; 242:557–560.

60. Juottonen K, Laakso MP, Partanen K, Soininen H. Comparative MR analysis of the entorhinal cortex and hippocampus in diagnosing Alzheimer disease. AJNR 1999; 20:139–144.

61. Xu Y, Jack CR Jr, O'Brien PC, et al. Usefulness of MRI measures of entorhinal cortex versus hippocampus in AD. Neurology 2000; 54:1760–1767.

62. Jack CR Jr, Petersen RC, Xu Y, et al. Rate of medial temporal lobe atrophy in typical aging and Alzheimer's disease. Neurology 1998; 51:993–999.

63. Petersen RC, Jack CR, Jr., Xu YC, et al. Memory and MRI-based hippocampal volumes in aging and AD. Neurology 2000; 54:581–587.

64. Fox NC, Crum WR, Scahill RI, et al. Imaging of onset and progression of Alzheimer's disease with voxel-compression

mapping of serial magnetic resonance images. Lancet 2001; 358:201–205.

65. Ashburner J, Csernansky JG, Davatzikos C, et al. Computer-assisted imaging to assess brain structure in healthy and diseased brains. Lancet Neurol 2003; 2:79–88.

66. Ashburner J, Friston KJ. Voxel-based morphometry–the methods. Neuroimage 2000; 11(6 part 1):805–21.

67. Karas GB, Burton EJ, Rombouts SA, et al. A comprehensive study of gray matter loss in patients with Alzheimer's disease using optimized voxel-based morphometry. Neuroimage 2003; 18:895–907.

68. Frisoni GB, Testa C, Sabattoli F, et al. Structural correlates of early and late onset Alzheimer's disease: voxel based morphometric study. J Neurol Neurosurg Psychiatry 2005; 76: 112–114.

69. Sasaki M, Ehara S, Tamakawa Y, et al. MR anatomy of the substantia innominata and findings in Alzheimer disease: a preliminary report. AJNR 1995; 16:2001–2007.

70. Hanyu H, Tanaka Y, Sakurai H, Takasaki M, Abe K. Atrophy of the substantia innominata on magnetic resonance imaging and response to donepezil treatment in Alzheimer's disease. Neurosci Lett 2002; 319:33–36.

71. Hanyu H, Asano T, Sakurai H, et al. MR analysis of the substantia innominata in normal aging, Alzheimer disease, and other types of dementia. AJNR 2002; 23:27–32.

72. Jack CR, Jr., Petersen RC, Xu YC, et al. Prediction of AD with MRI-based hippocampal volume in mild cognitive impairment. Neurology 1999; 52:1397–1403.

73. Du AT, Schuff N, Amend D, et al. Magnetic resonance imaging of the entorhinal cortex and hippocampus in mild cognitive impairment and Alzheimer's disease. J Neurol Neurosurg Psychiatry 2001; 71:441–447.

74. Visser PJ, Verhey FR, Hofman PA, Scheltens P, Jolles J. Medial temporal lobe atrophy predicts Alzheimer's disease in patients with minor cognitive impairment. J Neurol Neurosurg Psychiatry 2002; 72:491–497.

75. Karas GB, Scheltens P, Rombouts SA, et al. Global and local gray matter loss in mild cognitive impairment and Alzheimer's disease. Neuroimage 2004; 23:708–716.

76. Johnson KA, Jones K, Holman BL, et al. Preclinical prediction of Alzheimer's disease using SPECT. Neurology 1998; 50:1563–1571.

77. de Leon MJ, Convit A, Wolf OT, et al. Prediction of cognitive decline in normal elderly subjects with 2-[(18) F]-fluoro-2-deoxy-D-glucose/positron-emission tomography (FDG/PET). Proc Natl Acad Sci USA 2001; 98:10966–10971.

78. Okamura N, Arai H, Maruyama M, et al. Combined analysis of CSF tau levels and [(123)I]iodoamphetamine SPECT in mild cognitive impairment: implications for a novel predictor of Alzheimer's disease. Am J Psychiatry 2002; 159: 474–476.

79. Chetelat G, Desgranges B, de la Sayette, V, et al. Mild cognitive impairment: can FDG-PET predict who is to rapidly convert to Alzheimer's disease? Neurology 2003; 60: 1374–1377.

80. Kantarci K, Xu Y, Shiung MM, et al. Comparative diagnostic utility of different MR modalities in mild cognitive impairment and Alzheimer's disease. Dement Geriatr Cogn Disord 2002; 14:198–207.

81. Chetelat G, Baron JC. Early diagnosis of Alzheimer's disease: contribution of structural neuroimaging. Neuroimage 2003; 18:525–541.

82. Jack CR Jr, Shiung MM, Gunter JL, et al. Comparison of different MRI brain atrophy rate measures with clinical disease progression in AD. Neurology 2004; 62:591–600.

83. Wolf H, Ecke GM, Bettin S, Dietrich J, Gertz HJ. Do white matter changes contribute to the subsequent development of dementia in patients with mild cognitive impairment? A longitudinal study. Int J Geriatr Psychiatry 2000; 15: 803–812.

84. DeCarli C, Miller BL, Swan GE, et al. Cerebrovascular and brain morphologic correlates of mild cognitive impairment in the National Heart, Lung, and Blood Institute Twin Study. Arch Neurol 2001; 58:643–647.

85. Pantoni L, Basile AM, Pracucci G, et al. Impact of age-related cerebral white matter changes on the transition to disability – the LADIS study: rationale, design and methodology. Neuroepidemiology 2004; 24:51–62.

86. Nagy Z, Esiri MM, Jobst KA, et al. The effects of additional pathology on the cognitive deficit in Alzheimer disease. J Neuropathol Exp Neurol 1997; 56:165–170.

87. Goulding JM, Signorini DF, Chatterjee S, et al. Inverse relation between Braak stage and cerebrovascular pathology in Alzheimer predominant dementia. J Neurol Neurosurg Psychiatry 1999; 67:654–657.

88. Henon H, Pasquier F, Durieu I, et al. Preexisting dementia in stroke patients. Baseline frequency, associated factors, and outcome. Stroke 1997; 28:2429–2436.

89. Henon H, Pasquier F, Durieu I, Pruvo JP, Leys D. Medial temporal lobe atrophy in stroke patients: relation to pre-existing dementia. J Neurol Neurosurg Psychiatry 1998; 65:641–647.

90. Fein G, Di Sclafani, V, Tanabe J, et al. Hippocampal and cortical atrophy predict dementia in subcortical ischemic vascular disease. Neurology 2000; 55:1626–1635.

91. Mungas D, Jagust WJ, Reed BR, et al. MRI predictors of cognition in subcortical ischemic vascular disease and Alzheimer's disease. Neurology 2001; 57:2229–2235.

92. Du AT, Schuff N, Laakso MP, et al. Effects of subcortical ischemic vascular dementia and AD on entorhinal cortex and hippocampus. Neurology 2002; 58:1635–1641.

93. Mungas D, Reed BR, Jagust WJ, et al. Volumetric MRI predicts rate of cognitive decline related to AD and cerebrovascular disease. Neurology 2002; 59:867–873.

94. Lopez OL, Becker JT, Jungreis CA, et al. Computed tomography – but not magnetic resonance imaging – identified periventricular white-matter lesions predict symptomatic cerebrovascular disease in probable Alzheimer's disease. Arch Neurol 1995; 52:659–664.

95. Massoud F, Devi G, Moroney JT, et al. The role of routine laboratory studies and neuroimaging in the diagnosis of dementia: a clinicopathological study. J Am Geriatr Soc 2000; 48:1204–1210.

96. Esiri MM. Which vascular lesions are of importance in vascular dementia? Ann NY Acad Sci 2000; 903: 239–243.

97. Fazekas F, Chawluk JB, Alavi A, Hurtig HI, Zimmerman RA. MR signal abnormalities at 1.5 T in Alzheimer's dementia and normal aging. AJR 1987; 149:351–356.

98. Scheltens P, Barkhof F, Valk J, et al. White matter lesions on magnetic resonance imaging in clinically diagnosed Alzheimer's disease. Evidence for heterogeneity. Brain 1992; 115(part 3):735–748.

99. McKeith I, Mintzer J, Aarsland D, et al. Dementia with Lewy bodies. Lancet Neurol 2004; 3:19–28.

100. Barber R, Gholkar A, Scheltens P, et al. Medial temporal lobe atrophy on MRI in dementia with Lewy bodies. Neurology 1999; 52:1153–1158.

101. Barber R, Ballard C, McKeith IG, Gholkar A, O'Brien JT. MRI volumetric study of dementia with Lewy bodies: a

comparison with AD and vascular dementia. Neurology 2000; 54:1304–1309.

102. Cousins DA, Burton EJ, Burn D, et al. Atrophy of the putamen in dementia with Lewy bodies but not Alzheimer's disease: an MRI study. Neurology 2003; 61:1191–1195.

103. Imamura T, Ishii K, Hirono N, et al. Occipital glucose metabolism in dementia with Lewy bodies with and without parkinsonism: a study using positron emission tomography. Dement Geriatr Cogn Disord 2001; 12: 194–197.

104. Lobotesis K, Fenwick JD, Phipps A, et al. Occipital hypoperfusion on SPECT in dementia with Lewy bodies but not AD. Neurology 2001; 56:643–649.

105. Middelkoop HA, van der Flier WM, Burton EJ, et al. Dementia with Lewy bodies and AD are not associated with occipital lobe atrophy on MRI. Neurology 2001; 57: 2117–2120.

106. Emre M. Dementia associated with Parkinson's disease. Lancet Neurol 2003; 2:229–237.

107. Huber SJ, Shuttleworth EC, Christy JA, et al. Magnetic resonance imaging in dementia of Parkinson's disease. J Neurol Neurosurg Psychiatry 1989; 52:1221–1227.

108. Laakso MP, Partanen K, Riekkinen P, et al. Hippocampal volumes in Alzheimer's disease, Parkinson's disease with and without dementia, and in vascular dementia: an MRI study. Neurology 1996; 46:678–681.

109. Knopman DS, Christensen KJ, Schut LJ, et al. The spectrum of imaging and neuropsychological findings in Pick's disease. Neurology 1989; 39:362–368.

110. Larsson E, Passant U, Sundgren PC, et al. Magnetic resonance imaging and histopathology in dementia, clinically of frontotemporal type. Dement Geriatr Cogn Disord 2000; 11:123–134.

111. Laakso MP, Frisoni GB, Kononen M, et al. Hippocampus and entorhinal cortex in frontotemporal dementia and Alzheimer's disease: a morphometric MRI study. Biol Psychiatry 2000; 47:1056–1063.

112. Hodges JR, Patterson K. Nonfluent progressive aphasia and semantic dementia: a comparative neuropsychological study. J Int Neuropsychol Soc 1996; 2:511–524.

113. Abe K, Ukita H, Yanagihara T. Imaging in primary progressive aphasia. Neuroradiology 1997; 39:556–559.

114. Chan D, Fox NC, Scahill RI, et al. Patterns of temporal lobe atrophy in semantic dementia and Alzheimer's disease. Ann Neurol 2001; 49:433–442.

115. Hodges JR. Frontotemporal dementia (Pick's disease): clinical features and assessment. Neurology 2001; 56(11 suppl 4):S6–S10.

116. Charpentier P, Lavenu I, Defebvre L, et al. Alzheimer's disease and frontotemporal dementia are differentiated by discriminant analysis applied to (99m)Tc HmPAO SPECT data. J Neurol Neurosurg Psychiatry 2000; 69:661–663.

117. Sjogren M, Gustafson L, Wikkelso C, Wallin A. Frontotemporal dementia can be distinguished from Alzheimer's disease and subcortical white matter dementia by an anterior-to-posterior rCBF-SPET ratio. Dement Geriatr Cogn Disord 2000; 11:275–285.

118. Savoiardo M, Strada L, Girotti F, et al. MR imaging in progressive supranuclear palsy and Shy–Drager syndrome. J Comput Assist Tomogr 1989; 13:555–560.

119. Schrag A, Good CD, Miszkiel K, et al. Differentiation of atypical parkinsonian syndromes with routine MRI. Neurology 2000; 54:697–702.

120. Litvan I, Agid Y, Calne D, et al. Clinical research criteria for the diagnosis of progressive supranuclear palsy (Steele–

121. Grimes DA, Lang AE, Bergeron CB. Dementia as the most common presentation of cortical-basal ganglionic degeneration. Neurology 1999; 53:1969–1974.

122. Savoiardo M, Grisoli M, Girotti F. Magnetic resonance imaging in CBD, related atypical parkinsonian disorders, and dementias. In: Litvan I, Goetz CG, Lang AE, eds. Corticobasal Degeneration and Related Disorders. Philadelphia, Baltimore, New York, London, Buenos Aires, Hong Kong, Sydney, Tokyo: Lippincott Williams and Wilkins; 2000; 197–208.

123. Yagishita A, Oda M. Progressive supranuclear palsy: MRI and pathological findings. Neuroradiology 1996; 38: S60–S66.

124. Aiba I, Hashizume Y, Yoshida M, et al. Relationship between brainstem MRI and pathological findings in progressive supranuclear palsy–study in autopsy cases. J Neurol Sci 1997; 152:210–217.

125. Warmuth-Metz M, Naumann M, Csoti I, Solymosi L. Measurement of the midbrain diameter on routine magnetic resonance imaging: a simple and accurate method of differentiating between Parkinson disease and progressive supranuclear palsy. Arch Neurol 2001; 58:1076–1079.

126. Brenneis C, Seppi K, Schocke M, et al. Voxel based morphometry reveals a distinct pattern of frontal atrophy in progressive supranuclear palsy. J Neurol Neurosurg Psychiatry 2004; 75:246–249.

127. Paviour DC, Schott JM, Stevens JM, et al. Pathological substrate for regional distribution of increased atrophy rates in progressive supranuclear palsy. J Neurol Neurosurg Psychiatry 2004; 75:1772–1775.

128. Soliveri P, Monza D, Paridi D, et al. Cognitive and magnetic resonance imaging aspects of corticobasal degeneration and progressive supranuclear palsy. Neurology 1999; 53: 502–507.

129. Nagahama Y, Fukuyama H, Turjanski N, et al. Cerebral glucose metabolism in corticobasal degeneration: comparison with progressive supranuclear palsy and normal controls. Mov Disord 1997; 12:691–696.

130. Yamauchi H, Fukuyama H, Nagahama Y, et al. Atrophy of the corpus callosum, cognitive impairment, and cortical hypometabolism in progressive supranuclear palsy. Ann Neurol 1997; 41:606–614.

131. Roman GC, Erkinjuntti T, Wallin A, Pantoni L, Chui HC. Subcortical ischaemic vascular dementia. Lancet Neurol 2002; 1:426–436.

132. Kurz AF. What is vascular dementia? Int J Clin Pract Suppl 2001; 120:5–8.

133. Jellinger KA. The pathology of ischemic-vascular dementia: an update. J Neurol Sci 2002; 203–204:153–157.

134. Jellinger KA. Vascular-ischemic dementia: an update. J Neural Transm Suppl 2002; 62:1–23.

135. Scheltens P, Kittner B. Preliminary results from an MRI/CT-based database for vascular dementia and Alzheimer's disease. Ann NY Acad Sci 2000; 903: 542–546.

136. Erkinjuntti T, Inzitari D, Pantoni L, et al. Research criteria for subcortical vascular dementia in clinical trials. J Neural Transm Suppl 2000; 59:23–30.

137. Erkinjuntti T. Clinical deficits of Alzheimer's disease with cerebrovascular disease and probable VaD. Int J Clin Pract Suppl 2001; 120:14–23.

138. Pasquier F, Leys D. Why are stroke patients prone to develop dementia? J Neurol 1997; 244:135–142.

Richardson–Olszewski syndrome): report of the NINDS-SPSP international workshop. Neurology 1996; 47:1–9.

139. Leys D, Erkinjuntti T, Desmond DW, et al. Vascular dementia: the role of cerebral infarcts. Alzheimer Dis Assoc Disord 1999; 13(suppl 3):S38–S48.

140. van Straaten EC, Scheltens P, Knol DL, et al. Operational definitions for the NINDS-AIREN criteria for vascular dementia: an interobserver study. Stroke 2003; 34:1907–1912.

141. Wahlund LO, Barkhof F, Fazekas F, et al. A new rating scale for age-related white matter changes applicable to MRI and CT. Stroke 2001; 32:1318–1322.

142. Bastos Leite AJ, van Straaten EC, Scheltens P, Lycklama G, Barkhof F. Thalamic lesions in vascular dementia: low sensitivity of fluid-attenuated inversion recovery (FLAIR) imaging. Stroke 2004; 35:415–419.

143. Fazekas F, Kleinert R, Offenbacher H, et al. The morphologic correlate of incidental punctate white matter hyperintensities on MR images. AJNR 1991; 12:915–921.

144. Udaka F, Sawada H, Kameyama M. White matter lesions and dementia: MRI-pathological correlation. Ann NY Acad Sci 2002; 977:411–415.

145. Barkhof F, Scheltens P. Imaging of white matter lesions. Cerebrovasc Dis 2002; 13(suppl 2):21–30.

146. Fisher CM. Lacunar strokes and infarcts: a review. Neurology 1982; 32:871–876.

147. Loeb C. Dementia due to lacunar infarctions: a misnomer or a clinical entity? Eur Neurol 1995; 35:187–192.

148. Braffman BH, Zimmerman RA, Trojanowski JQ, et al. Brain MR: pathologic correlation with gross and histopathology. 1. Lacunar infarction and Virchow–Robin spaces. AJR 1988; 151:551–558.

149. Bokura H, Kobayashi S, Yamaguchi S. Distinguishing silent lacunar infarction from enlarged Virchow–Robin spaces: a magnetic resonance imaging and pathological study. J Neurol 1998; 245:116–122.

150. Poirier J, Derouesne C. The concept of cerebral lacunae from 1838 to the present. Rev Neurol (Paris) 1985; 141:3–17.

151. Awad IA, Johnson PC, Spetzler RF, Hodak JA. Incidental subcortical lesions identified on magnetic resonance imaging in the elderly. II. Postmortem pathological correlations. Stroke 1986; 17:1090–1097.

152. Maclullich AM, Wardlaw JM, Ferguson KJ, et al. Enlarged perivascular spaces are associated with cognitive function in healthy elderly men. J Neurol Neurosurg Psychiatry 2004; 75:1519–1523.

153. Barkhof F. Enlarged Virchow–Robin spaces: do they matter? J Neurol Neurosurg Psychiatry 2004; 75:1516–1517.

154. Breteler MM, van Swieten JC, Bots ML, et al. Cerebral white matter lesions, vascular risk factors, and cognitive function in a population-based study: the Rotterdam Study. Neurology 1994; 44:1246–1252.

155. Lindgren A, Roijer A, Rudling O, et al. Cerebral lesions on magnetic resonance imaging, heart disease, and vascular risk factors in subjects without stroke. A population-based study. Stroke 1994; 25:929–934.

156. Longstreth WT Jr, Manolio TA, Arnold A, et al. Clinical correlates of white matter findings on cranial magnetic resonance imaging of 3301 elderly people. The Cardiovascular Health Study. Stroke 1996; 27:1274–1282.

157. Boone KB, Miller BL, Lesser IM, et al. Neuropsychological correlates of white-matter lesions in healthy elderly subjects. A threshold effect. Arch Neurol 1992; 49:549–554.

158. Skehan SJ, Hutchinson M, MacErlaine DP. Cerebral autosomal dominant arteriopathy with subcortical infarcts and leukoencephalopathy: MR findings. AJNR 1995; 16:2115–2119.

159. Yousry TA, Seelos K, Mayer M, et al. Characteristic MR lesion pattern and correlation of T1 and T2 lesion volume with neurologic and neuropsychological findings in cerebral autosomal dominant arteriopathy with subcortical infarcts and leukoencephalopathy (CADASIL). AJNR 1999; 20:91–100.

160. Auer DP, Putz B, Gossl C, et al. Differential lesion patterns in CADASIL and sporadic subcortical arteriosclerotic encephalopathy: MR imaging study with statistical parametric group comparison. Radiology 2001; 218:443–451.

161. Offenbacher H, Fazekas F, Schmidt R, et al. MR of cerebral abnormalities concomitant with primary intracerebral hematomas. AJNR 1996; 17:573–578.

162. Fazekas F, Kleinert R, Roob G, et al. Histopathologic analysis of foci of signal loss on gradient-echo T2*-weighted MR images in patients with spontaneous intracerebral hemorrhage: evidence of microangiopathy-related microbleeds. AJNR 1999; 20:637–642.

163. Lesnik Oberstein SA, van den Boom R, van Buchem MA, et al. Cerebral microbleeds in CADASIL. Neurology 2001; 57:1066–1070.

164. Greenberg SM, Finklestein SP, Schaefer PW. Petechial hemorrhages accompanying lobar hemorrhage: detection by gradient-echo MRI. Neurology 1996; 46:1751–1754.

165. Knudsen KA, Rosand J, Karluk D, Greenberg SM. Clinical diagnosis of cerebral amyloid angiopathy: validation of the Boston criteria. Neurology 2001; 56:537–539.

166. Hurst RW, Bagley LJ, Galetta S, et al. Dementia resulting from dural arteriovenous fistulas: the pathologic findings of venous hypertensive encephalopathy. AJNR 1998; 19:1267–1273.

167. Tanaka K, Morooka Y, Nakagawa Y, Shimizu S. Dural arteriovenous malformation manifesting as dementia due to ischemia in bilateral thalami. A case report. Surg Neurol 1999; 51:489–493.

168. Krolak-Salmon P, Montavont A, Hermier M, Milliery M, Vighetto A. Thalamic venous infarction as a cause of subacute dementia. Neurology 2002; 58:1689–1691.

169. Chow K, Gobin YP, Saver J, et al. Endovascular treatment of dural sinus thrombosis with rheolytic thrombectomy and intra-arterial thrombolysis. Stroke 2000; 31:1420–1425.

170. O'Brien JT, Desmond P, Ames D, et al. Temporal lobe magnetic resonance imaging can differentiate Alzheimer's disease from normal ageing, depression, vascular dementia and other causes of cognitive impairment. Psychol Med 1997; 27:1267–1275.

171. Salmon E, Sadzot B, Maquet P, et al. Differential diagnosis of Alzheimer's disease with PET. J Nucl Med 1994; 35:391–398.

172. Talbot PR, Lloyd JJ, Snowden JS, Neary D, Testa HJ. A clinical role for 99mTc-HMPAO SPECT in the investigation of dementia? J Neurol Neurosurg Psychiatry 1998; 64:306–313.

173. Victoroff J, Ross GW, Benson DF, Verity MA, Vinters HV. Posterior cortical atrophy. Neuropathologic correlations. Arch Neurol 1994; 51:269–274.

174. Black SE. Focal cortical atrophy syndromes. Brain Cogn 1996; 31:188–229.

175. Barkhof F, Filippi M, Miller DH, et al. Comparison of MRI criteria at first presentation to predict conversion to clinically definite multiple sclerosis. Brain 1997; 120:2059–2069.

176. McDonald WI, Compston A, Edan G, et al. Recommended diagnostic criteria for multiple sclerosis: guidelines from the International Panel on the diagnosis of multiple sclerosis. Ann Neurol 2001; 50:121–127.

177. Harris GJ, Codori AM, Lewis RF, et al. Reduced basal ganglia blood flow and volume in pre-symptomatic, gene-tested persons at-risk for Huntington's disease. Brain 1999; 122(part 9):1667–1678.

178. Finkenstaedt M, Szudra A, Zerr I, et al. MR imaging of Creutzfeldt–Jakob disease. Radiology 1996; 199:793–798.

179. Demaerel P, Heiner L, Robberecht W, Sciot R, Wilms G. Diffusion-weighted MRI in sporadic Creutzfeldt–Jakob disease. Neurology 1999; 52:205–208.

180. Collie DA, Sellar RJ, Zeidler M, et al. MRI of Creutzfeldt–Jakob disease: imaging features and recommended MRI protocol. Clin Radiol 2001; 56:726–739.

181. Tribl GG, Strasser G, Zeitlhofer J, et al. Sequential MRI in a case of Creutzfeldt–Jakob disease. Neuroradiology 2002; 44:223–226.

182. Zeidler M, Sellar RJ, Collie DA, et al. The pulvinar sign on magnetic resonance imaging in variant Creutzfeldt–Jakob disease. Lancet 2000; 355:1412–1418.

183. Vanneste J, Hyman R. Non-tumoural aqueduct stenosis and normal pressure hydrocephalus in the elderly. J Neurol Neurosurg Psychiatry 1986; 49:529–535.

184. Bradley WG. Normal pressure hydrocephalus: new concepts on etiology and diagnosis. AJNR 2000; 21:1586–1590.

185. Vanneste JA. Diagnosis and management of normal-pressure hydrocephalus. J Neurol 2000; 247:5–14.

186. Bradley WG Jr, Kortman KE, Burgoyne B. Flowing cerebrospinal fluid in normal and hydrocephalic states: appearance on MR images. Radiology 1986; 159:611–616.

187. Barkhof F, Kouwenhoven M, Scheltens P, et al. Phase-contrast cine MR imaging of normal aqueductal CSF flow. Effect of aging and relation to CSF void on modulus MR. Acta Radiol 1994; 35:123–130.

188. Bradley WG Jr, Whittemore AR, Kortman KE, et al. Marked cerebrospinal fluid void: indicator of successful shunt in patients with suspected normal-pressure hydrocephalus. Radiology 1991; 178:459–466.

189. Bradley WG Jr, Scalzo D, Queralt J, et al. Normal-pressure hydrocephalus: evaluation with cerebrospinal fluid flow measurements at MR imaging. Radiology 1996; 198:523–529.

190. Egeler-Peerdeman SM, Barkhof F, Walchenbach R, Valk J. Cine phase-contrast MR imaging in normal pressure hydrocephalus patients: relation to surgical outcome. Acta Neurochir Suppl (Wien) 1998; 71:340–342.

191. Bradley WG Jr, Whittemore AR, Watanabe AS, et al. Association of deep white matter infarction with chronic communicating hydrocephalus: implications regarding the possible origin of normal-pressure hydrocephalus. AJNR 1991; 12:31–39.

192. Bradley WG. Normal pressure hydrocephalus and deep white matter ischemia: which is the chicken, and which is the egg? AJNR 2001; 22:1638–1640.

193. Bastos Leite AJ, Scheltens P, Barkhof F. Pathological aging of the brain: an overview. Top Magn Reson Imaging 2004; 15:369–389.

8

Functional brain imaging

Agneta Nordberg

POSITRON EMISSION TOMOGRAPHY

Positron emission tomography (PET) can assess a broad range of functional parameters such as metabolic activity (e.g. glucose metabolism), cerebral blood flow (CBF), neurotransmitter activities and receptor binding, measured with high accuracy. A quantification and three-dimensional imaging of distinct physiological variables are obtained which make PET a powerful tool for the evaluation of brain function in normal and disease states. In the PET procedure, a positron-emitting compound synthesized by a cyclotron is administered systemically and is then taken up by the brain, where it releases positrons (positively charged electrons) which collide with electrons which are annihilated, releasing two gamma rays at 180° to each other. A ring of radiation detectors surrounding the head is used to measure the location of radioactivity within the brain.

PET has proven to be a suitable method for evaluation of functional changes in brain ageing and dementia.[1–3] PET may help in the early diagnosis of Alzheimer's disease (AD), especially if PET investigations can reveal dysfunctional activity prior to losses of neuronal cells. PET can thereby be considered as a clinical instrument revealing dysfunctional changes earlier in the course of the disease than CT and probably also MRI. A correlation between reduction in glucose metabolism in the brain and loss of neurons and gliosis has been reported in AD.[4,5] Correlation between dementia severity prior to death and various features of postmortem neuropathology is well known. These features reflect terminal stages and these correlations provide limited insight into the early course of the disease, while imaging such as PET can provide additional insight.

Recently new PET tracers have been introduced for in vivo measurement of activated glia[6] and amyloid[7] in brain of AD patients. The development of PET ligands with application to dementia has been an emerging field during recent years (Table 8.1). Oxygen metabolism and CBF have been measured in brain using ^{15}oxygen (^{15}O) and ^{11}C-butanol.[8,9] When using ^{15}O, the radioactive half-life is two minutes (as compared to 25 minutes for ^{11}C compounds); the arterial blood radioactivity is sampled for a scanning period of 60 seconds using an autoradiographical method. The regional cerebral metabolic rate of glucose can be estimated using ^{18}F-fluorodeoxyglucose (^{18}F-FDG, radioactive half-life 110 minutes).[10] The tracer is injected intravenously and arterial plasma radioactivities and

Table 8.1 PET and SPECT ligands used in AD

PET radioligands	Functional activity
^{11}C-Butanol	Cerebral blood flow
^{15}O-H$_2$O	Cerebral blood flow
^{18}F-Fluoro-deoxyglucose	Glucose utilization
^{11}C-Nicotine	Nicotinic receptors
^{11}C-Benztropine	Muscarinic receptors
^{11}C-NMP	Muscarinic receptors
^{18}F-6-L-Dopa	Dopamine receptors
^{18}F-Setoperone	5-HT$_2$ receptors
^{11}C-β-CFT	Dopamine reuptake sites

SPECT radioligands	Functional activity
^{99m}TC-HMPAO	Cerebral blood flow
^{99m}Tc-exametazime	Cerebral blood flow
^{122}I-QNB	Muscarinic receptors
^{122}I-IBZM	Dopamine D$_2$ receptors
^{122}I-FP-CIT	Dopamine transporter
^{122}I-Iodobenzovesamicol	Cholinergic terminal density
^{122}I-Iomazenil	GABA$_A$ receptors
^{122}I-5-I-R91150	5HT$_{2A}$

glucose concentration are followed during a scanning period of 30–60 minutes. Since the ^{18}F-FDG technique does not depend on circulation parameters, it gives images with higher resolution than for CBF and is therefore often used in the diagnostic evaluation of dementia by PET. In order to obtain a deeper understanding of the transmitter deficits in brains of demented patients, receptor ligands for measuring cholinergic (muscarinic and nicotinic), dopaminergic and serotonergic receptors have so far been used in PET studies in AD patients.[2,11–13] Ligands for measuring dopamine re-uptake sites[14] and enzyme activity such as acetylcholinesterase activity[15] have also been introduced for studies in AD patients (Table 8.1). It is expected that new selective radioligands for studying nicotinic receptor subtypes will be available soon.[16,17]

PET provides the clinician not only with a visual image interpretation in colour scales but also, more importantly, with quantitative regional brain data which can be used for objective evaluation of the diagnostic accuracy. Relative metabolic rates (with reference to spared brain regions) are used often instead of expressing absolute metabolic rates, since the latter can often show high variability in normal subjects. Several brain regions including the cerebellum,[18] the sensorimotor cortex,[19] visual cortex[20] and the pons[21] have been used as reference regions. The regions used as reference structures may also be metabolically impaired in severe dementia. A method using a denominator in calculating metabolic ratios was proposed by Herholz and colleagues.[22] This latter method has been successfully used in studies performed between several European PET centres to standardize the PET procedure in AD[22] and in large multicentre European cohort studies.[23] The metabolic ratio discriminates AD from normal subjects with an accuracy of 90 per cent.[23] Automated analysis can help to discriminate between AD and can be used in a clinical setting.[24] Voxel-based analysis using statistical parametric mapping (SPM) increased the understanding of the anatomical basis of the cerebral glucose metabolism deficts in AD brains.[25]

SINGLE PROTON EMISSION COMPUTED TOMOGRAPHY (SPECT) IN DEMENTIA

The high cost of PET and its limitation to centres equipped with cyclotrons have increased the interest in developing the single proton emission computed tomography (SPECT) technique. SPECT might be a valuable instrument in routine clinical work in differentiating AD from normal ageing and other dementias, although the spatial resolution as well as quantitative accuracy of SPECT is inferior to that of PET. It is estimated that PET has a 10–20-fold higher sensitivity than SPECT. Knowledge about the metabolic trapping of the SPECT ligands such as ^{99m}Tc-HMPAO is not yet available. Comparison of SPECT imaging with PET for the measurement of CBF has been performed.[26–28] SPECT studies with ^{99m}Tc-HMPAO seem to reflect roughly CBF measured by PET.[26] A correlation has been observed between CBF and cognitive status (Mini-Mental State Examination).[28] Although the SPECT studies often do not provide the researcher with quantitative data, the activity can be defined in relation to a reference area.[26–30] In addition to radio-tracers measuring CBF, SPECT radioligands for the measurement of neuroreceptors and transmitter uptake sites have been applied in AD (Table 8.1).

FUNCTIONAL MAGNETIC RESONANCE IMAGING

Functional magnetic resonance imaging (fMRI) is a relatively new imaging technique which is used to detect weak signals from the human brain non-invasively. This technique offers the possibility of measuring metabolic changes due to neuronal activity by a blood oxygen dependent technique.[3,31] By imaging the difference in oxygenated and deoxygenated blood, focal brain activity can be studied without the use of radioactive ligands and contrast agents. Magnetic resonance spectroscopy (MRS) offers the possibility of measuring neuron specific substances as N-acetyl aspartate (NAA) and other compounds like choline, myoinositol and different phosphorus metabolites.[32]

PET STUDIES IN ALZHEIMER'S DISEASE

Glucose metabolism

Impairment in cortical CBF and glucose metabolism is a common feature in AD.[1,3,33–35] Changes have been observed by PET in the parietotemporal cortical areas and also in the frontal cortex of the AD brain, with sparing of regions such as the visual cortex and sensorimotor cortex (Figure 8.1). The pattern of impaired glucose metabolism in the individual AD patients might vary and can be symmetric or asymmetric in the hemispheres. Subgroups of AD patients have been characterized with predominant parieto-temporal hypometabolism, paralimbic, left hemisphere neocortical and frontal deficits.[36] These metabolic subgroups were considered to be related more to underlying

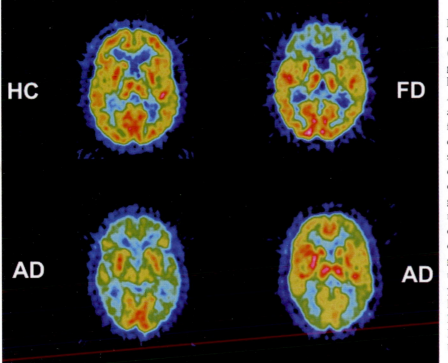

Figure 8.1 Positron emission tomography (PET) scan of cerebral glucose metabolism in an healthy control (HC), two Alzheimer patients (AD) and one patient with frontotemporal lobe dementia (FD). The PET sections are through the cerebral cortex at the level of basal ganglia. The glucose metabolism was measured following a tracer dose of ^{18}F-FDG i.v. The colour indicates regional glucose metabolism umol/min/100g, red high, yellow medium and blue low glucose metabolism. FDG; fluorodeoxyglucose. Photo: Uppsala PET centre, Uppsala.

pathology than dementia as well as the cognitive status measured by clinical and neuropsychological assessments and the degree of hypometabolism found by PET.[1] A difference in regional glucose metabolism has been reported between presenile and senile dementia of AD type.[25,37–40] The presenile form (age of onset 49–65 years) showed more pronounced reduction in glucose metabolism in the right parieto-temporal cortex compared with the senile form (age of onset 66–79).[25,41] These data do not support the left hemispheric vulnerability in presenile forms of AD as suggested by neuropsychological studies.[42] The metabolic impairment in late-onset forms of AD might be more general and less region-specific. In mildly affected patients, a significant correlation has been observed between initial metabolic glucose ratio and subsequent decline in cognition during follow-up.[24]

In the early course of AD the changes probably and mainly represent disturbances in neuronal function, while later in the course of the disease, partial volume artifacts due to cell loss can be prominent.[33] Interestingly, hypometabolic regions in AD have been shown to be activated in response to behavioural tasks,[43] although this activation of brain areas in diseased brains might indicate increased attentional load because of impaired cognitive ability.[44] A shift in metabolic rates to the right hemispheres was observed in

AD patients during cognitive processing, while age-matched controls showed a shift to the left hemisphere.[45] Interestingly, some studies indicate no correlation between glucose metabolism measured in vivo and density of neurofibrillary tangles and senile plaques measured in autopsy brains,[46,47] while other studies suggest that the presence of neurofibrillary tangles is related to the cerebral glucose metabolism.[48]

A crucial question is how early in the course of AD can hypofunction in brain mechanisms be observed by imaging techniques such as PET? According to neuropathological studies,[49] the evolution of AD occurs during many years prior to the emergence of symptoms. Although AD families with chromosomal aberrations are rare, it is important to perform longitudinal PET studies in these families. A similar pattern in deficits in regional glucose metabolism has been observed in AD patients carrying the chromosome-21 codon 717 mutation, the Swedish encoded 670/671 APP double mutation, and the presenilin 1 (PS1) mutation.[50–53] Reduction in cerebral glucose metabolism has been observed in the presymptomatic stage in individuals at risk of familial AD with deficits in glucose metabolism measured in the parieto-temporal cortical regions of the brain with increasing age in carriers of the APP and PS1 encoded mutations, but not in non-carriers.[50–53] Metabolic changes in the brain are revealed by PET in the APP 670/671 mutation carriers earlier than by MRI, EEG, SPECT and neuropsychological testing.[54]

The apolipoprotein E4 (apoE ε4) is generally over-represented in patients with AD. A lower glucose metabolism has been reported particularly in the parietal cortex of cognitive normal apoE ε4 carriers at risk of AD compared to non ε4 allele carrriers.[55–59] ApoE ε4 allele AD carriers do not differ in their regional cortical pattern of deficits in cerebral glucose metabolism compared to ε3 carriers at the same cognitive level.[60] When age-matched, however, the AD patients with ε4 alleles show more pronounced deficits in glucose metabolism compared to ε3 carriers.[61]

Neuroreceptor changes

The cholinergic and serotonergic systems appear to be particularly vulnerable to changes in AD.[62] Losses in nicotinic receptors have been observed in AD brains with ^{11}C-nicotine as ligand[11,17] and the losses in binding of ^{11}C-nicotine correlate significantly with the cognitive status of the AD patients.[11] The dopaminergic system in demented patients has been studied by PET using ^{18}F-labelled 6-L-dopa. While a reduction in tracer uptake has been observed in the putamen of patients with Parkinson's disease, no change in the uptake of ^{18}F-dopa was observed in AD patients, although the latter had shown extrapyramidal signs.[12,63] Losses in $5HT_2$ receptors have been detected in the temporal and frontal cortices of AD patients using ^{18}F-setoperone,[13] which is in accordance with findings in earlier postmortem studies.[64,65]

Amyloid imaging

During the last 10 years great attempts have been made to develop suitable compounds for imaging amyloid in vivo in AD patients using PET, MRI, SPECT and multiphoton microscopy techniques.[7,66,67] The small molecule approach appears to be most promising. Three PET compounds, ^{18}F-FDDNP,[68] ^{11}C-PIB[69] and ^{11}C-SB-13,[70] have so far reached testing in AD patients. ^{18}F-FDDNP is assumed to bind to both amyloid and neurofibrillary tangles,[68] while ^{11}C-PIB binds solely to fibrillar amyloid.[69] ^{11}C-PIB shows a high retention in brain, especially to different cortical regions (Figure 8.2). ^{11}C-PIB shows a robust difference in retention in brain association cortex between mild AD patients and healthy controls.[69] An equal retention is observed in AD patients and controls in brain areas such as white matter, cerebellum and pons, known for their low amyloid deposition in mild AD. The PIB retention in AD patients negatively correlates in the parietal cortex with deficits in cerebral glucose metabolism.[69] Amyloid imaging appears to be a promising diagnostic technique, but further studies need to be performed in different forms of dementia, MCI patients and presymptomatic carriers of genetic forms of AD to further evaluate the potential of the PET ligand. Amyloid imaging holds promise as a surrogate marker for evaluating the efficacy of anti-amyloid therapies including immunization therapy.

Differentiation between dementias

PET is a useful tool to distinguish AD patients from those suffering from other forms of dementia. This

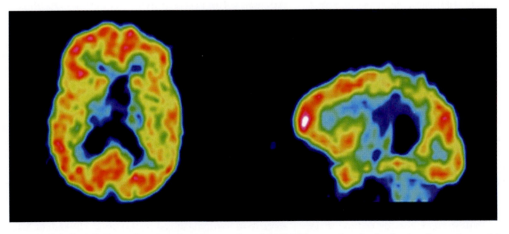

Figure 8.2 Serial plans showing the topography of 11C-PIB retention in the brain of a patient with mild Alzheimer's disease (AD). The scan to the left shows the axial and the scan to the right shows the sagittal standardised uptake values (SUV) of PIB images. Red indicates high, yellow medium and blue low retention. Photo: Uppsala Imanet AB, Uppsala and Karolinska institutet, Karolinska University Hospital Huddinge, Stockholm, Sweden.

might be of special importance in the early course of the disease where the clinical assessment does not indicate unequivocally that the patient might suffer from AD. In frontal lobe dementia, a hypometabolism is observed mainly in the frontal cortex (Figure 8.1); but in the early course of the frontal lobe dementia, the deficits in glucose metabolism might be quite discrete and involve regions such as the anterior temporal cortex, but also the putamen, globus pallidum and thalamus.[71–74] Patients with semantic dementia show a hypometabolism in the left temporal lobe and in the right temporal pole while patients with frontotemporal dementia showed a symmetric hypometabolism in the frontal lobes.[73] The deficits in glucose metabolism seen in frontal lobe dementia differ from the pattern observed in AD patients with bilateral or unilateral parieto-temporal hypometabolism which might also involve frontal regions of the brain (Figure 8.1). Franceschi et al[74] showed that patients with frontotemporal lobe degeneration and apathetic syndrome showed a reduction in frontal glucose metabolism in the dorsolateral and frontal medial cortex, while in patients with disinhibition symptoms, the cerebral glucose metabolism was reduced in the interconnected limbic structures. Furthermore, a reduction was observed in the HT_2 receptors measured by ^{11}C-MDL as the PET ligand.[74] PET studies with pathologically confirmed Pick's disease cases have shown a reduction in glucose metabolism in the frontal and anterior temporal cortex.[75,76]

Dementia with Lewy bodies (DLB) has been recognized as a clinical entity of primary degenerative dementia.[77] Similarly to AD patients, the DLB patients show lower glucose metabolism in the fronto-parieto-temporal cortex, but in addition also show occipital glucose hypometabolism.[78] It has been suggested that reduced glucose metabolism in the medial and lateral occipital cortex of DLB patients can be used to differentiate DLB from AD.[78] PET can confirm the clinical symptoms of the patients by allowing discrimination between the diseases.[77]

In patients with Parkinson's disease, a decrease in glucose metabolism has been observed in the brain, although the changes are mainly considered to be less prominent than in AD. Demented patients with Parkinson's disease have shown parieto-temporal deficits in glucose metabolism, while non-demented patients showed widespread cortical hypometabolism.[79] When comparing the metabolic differences in Parkinson's and AD diseases, a greater reduction in glucose metabolism was observed in the visual cortex, while metabolism was relatively preserved in the medial temporal cortex of patients with Parkinson's disease compared to AD.[80] Hilker et al performed PET studies measuring both dopaminergic (^{18}F-dopa) and cholinergic (^{11}C-MP4A) activity in the brain of Parkinson patients.[81] Demented Parkinson patients showed much more reduced ^{11}C-MP4A binding in the parietal cortex compared to non-demented Parkinson patients, while the striatal ^{18}F-dopa binding was similar in demented and non-demented Parkinson patients.[81]

Patients with multi-infarct dementia might show slight global reduction in glucose metabolism. Scattered focal defects in metabolic activity can be observed by PET throughout the cortex and white matter[82] in patients with larger lesions. A more predominant involvement in the cingulate and superior frontal gyri with respect to changes in cerebral blood flow has been reported for vascular dementia compared to AD.[83]

SPECT STUDIES IN ALZHEIMER'S DISEASE

SPECT can show similar regional changes to PET in AD,[84] although spatial resolution and accuracy might differ. The sensitivity for clinical diagnosis of probable AD has been estimated as 80 per cent with SPECT[85] compared with 92–94 per cent with PET.[86,87] SPECT investigations might allow the clinician to differentiate between AD and vascular dementia (multi-infarct dementia).[88] When Mielke and colleagues[89] compared PET to SPECT they found that the differentiation between AD and vascular dementia was easier and more significant with PET as compared to SPECT. An age-related decrease in CBF and glucose metabolism was observed in brains of AD and vascular dementia patients.[89] Thirty-five different combinations of perfusion deficits in AD brains have been observed by SPECT, supporting the heterogeneity of AD.[90] The sensitivity of the AD diagnosis based on SPECT findings with a selected specificity of 90 per cent is considered to be dependent on the disease stage (mild: 40–70 per cent; severe: 80–90 per cent).[91]

When comparison was made between the spatial normalized PET and SPECT scans in AD, corresponding findings between PET and SPECT was limited to changes in the tempoparietal and posterior cingluate in mild to moderate AD.[92]

A different pattern of CBF change compared with AD was observed in patients with Korsakoff psychosis.[93] Thus, changes in cognitive impairment in Korsakoff patients were found to be linked to CBF changes in the frontal cortex.[93] SPECT studies have shown bilateral hypofrontal perfusion in patients with frontal lobe dementia.[94] Recent studies also suggest that the left frontal lobe might be especially involved in this type of dementia.[95] SPECT has also been used for investigating several other miscellaneous dementia disorders such as normal pressure hydrocephalus, Huntington's disease, Parkinson's disease, AIDS-associated dementia complex, Creutzfeldt–Jakob disease and motor neurone disease.[92,96]

SPECT and PET activation studies

An interesting field for further exploration is the use of SPECT and PET for functional activation studies of patients during memory testing. The SPECT technique has shown some usefulness in brain activation as, for example, in studies during verbal memory tests in AD.[97] While the control subjects increased their cortical CBF, especially in the frontal cortex, during the memory task AD patients failed to improve their CBF in this brain region.[97] A significant correlation was reported between memory performance and CBF in the right lateral frontal region of AD patients.[98] Brain regions associated with episodic retrieval differ between young and old healthy controls as well as AD patients.[99,100] Functional PET studies support the role of the hippocampus and medial cortex as well as the frontal cortex in episodic memory as studied in both healthy subjects and AD patients.[99,100] Different activation patterns are associated with different cognitive performances as reviewed by Cabeza and Nyberg in a review of 275 PET and fMRI studies.[101] Activation studies might be important in the future for detecting early signs for disease (presymptomatic marker?) as well as in the development of new drug treatment strategies.

Receptor changes

Attempts have also been made to use SPECT for tracing receptor changes in AD patients. Muscarinic receptors have been reported in SPECT studies to be decreased in number as well as being relatively preserved in number.[102–104] Wyper and colleagues[104] concluded from their SPECT studies that muscarinic receptors are mainly preserved in the brain of AD patients in mild to moderate forms of the disease, while reductions are seen in the late stages of the disorder. SPECT ligands for visualizing nicotinic receptors in AD patients are under development.[16,17] ^{123}I-Iodobenzovesamicol, an analogue of vesamicol, binds to the presynaptic vesicular acetylcholine transporter and, as a possible marker of presynaptic cholinergic terminal density, has been used in SPECT studies of AD patients.[105] The reduction in binding was more pronounced in AD patients less than 65 years of age compared to older AD patients. A loss of

striatal D2 receptors using ^{123}I-IBZM (iodobenzamide) and SPECT has been reported in AD patients,[106–108] while in patients with Parkinson's disease and without medication mainly normal values were found.[109,110] Cooloby et al[111] used ^{123}I-FP-CIT to visualize loss of dopamine transporter by SPECT. A bilateral reduction in uptake of ^{123}I-FP-CIT was observed in the caudate nucleus of AD patients compared to age-matched controls.[111] Patients with Parkinson's disease and dementia of Lewy bodies showed a bilateral reduction in uptake of ^{123}I-FP-CIT bilaterally in the caudate, anterior and posterior putamen compared to both controls and AD.[111] ^{123}I-Iomazenil, a tracer for $GABA_A$ receptors, has shown a reduced distribution in the temporal and parietal cortical regions in AD patients as a possible sign for synapse losses.[112] $5HT_{2A}$ receptors have been measured by the antagonist [123]I-5–I-R91150 and SPECT.[112] In addition to an age-related decrease in the cortical regions a further reduction in $5HT_{2A}$ binding was observed in several AD patients.[113]

MRS AND fMRI STUDIES IN ALZHEIMER'S DISEASE

NMR – a non-invasive optical technique – detects a frequency dependent signal from individual atomic nuclei and from populations of such nuclei in brain tissue. By using this technique a reduction in N-acetyl aspartate (NAA) has been reported in AD patients compared to age-matched controls.[32,114–116] An increase in the cerebral myoinositol concentration has also been reported in AD patients,[32,115,116] while different phosphorus metabolites were unchanged in the brain of AD patients compared to controls. Kantarci et al[117] have suggested that it might be possible to differentiate between different dementia groups by using MR spectroscopy.[118]

Fallgatter and coworkers[119] used fMRI to measure changes in concentrations of oxy- and deoxyhaemoglobin in the brain of AD patients during verbal fluency tests. In contrast to healthy controls, the AD patients did not show a hemispherical asymmetry in CBF during the verbal fluency test.[119] Hock and colleagues found a reduced concentration of oxygenated haemoglobin in the parietal cortex in AD patients during brain activation (verbal fluency).[120] fMRI studies have shown involvement of the posterior parahippocampal cortex in encoding processes and the more anterior part in retrieval processes.[121] The medial temporal lobe has also been found in fMRI studies to be activated during encoding of visual association in healthy volunteers.[122] It has been suggested that the visual association task may provide a sensitive measure by which to study anterograde amnesia, which is prevalent in AD.[121] Rombouts et al[123] demonstrated a default mode network response in AD compared to controls. AD patients showed no deactivation but rather a sustained activation in brain regions such as the parietal and posterior cingulate cortices.[123]

Mild cognitive impairment

Mild cognitive impairment (MCI) is considered as a clinical entity representing a transitional state between cognitive normal ageing and clinical AD. The cause of MCI may, however, be heterogeneous and can be divided into amnestic, multiple domain or single non-memory domain.[124] There is a wide range in the progression of MCI, varying from 1 to 25 per cent per year.[125] Functional imaging is important in order to predict the likelihood of progression from MCI to AD. Metabolic reduction in the temporoparietal cortex, posterior cingulate gyrus and hippocampus has been reported to be associated with a greater risk of developing AD.[126–129] fMRI studies in MCI patients have shown less activation in the posterior cingulate and right hippocampus compared to controls.[130] MCI patients have shown less deactivation in the anterior frontal, precuneus and posterior cingulate cortex during a visual encoding task compared to control subjects.[131] Functional imaging studies might be used as an early marker for AD pathology. Amyloid imaging[7] in MCI patients with PIB will contribute to further understanding of the underlying pathological mechanism of early AD.

TREATMENT STRATEGIES IN AD STUDIED BY FUNCTIONAL IMAGING

Functional brain imaging studies offer a unique opportunity to study dynamic effects in the brain induced by drug treatment. So far the cholinesterase inhitors in particular have been evaluated by PET, SPECT or functional MRI (Table 8.2 and Figure 8.3). Studies on treatment with anti-amyloid drugs are expected to increase in the near future. The advantage with this type of study is that they can be performed in parallel with the measurement of other functional parameters, including EEG and cognitive tests and the measurement of biological markers in cerebrospinal fluid (CSF) such as β-amyloid, tau and phosphotau proteins. Pharmacokinetic studies may provide valuable information about the penetration of the drug to the CSF and the dosage range for therapeutic efficacy. In comparison to traditional clinical trials, fewer patients are probably needed in imaging studies to obtain a significant result.

CONCLUSIONS

Significant progress has been made in recent years in the development and application of functional brain imaging techniques in neurogeriatrics, an important

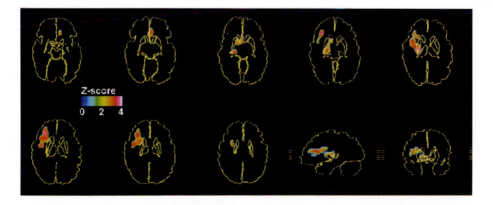

Figure 8.3 Effect of long-term treatment with the cholinesterase inhibitor on cerebral glucose metabolism in Alzheimer (AD) patients. The figure shows cerebral glucose metabolism after 12 months treatment with rivastigmine, minus baseline values in 11 AD patients (statistical z-score map showing only the significant cluster). Reproduced with permission from Springer Verlag.[141]

Table 8.2 Treatment strategies for AD studies by functional imaging

Imaging technique	Ligand	Effect exerted upon
PET		
Piracetam[132]	^{18}F-FDG	Metabolism
Phosphatidylserine[133]	^{18}F-FDG	Metabolism
Physostigmine[134,135]	^{18}F-FDG	Metabolism
	$H_2{}^{15}O$	Blood flow
Tacrine[136,137]	^{18}F-FDG	Metabolism
	^{11}C-Nicotine	Nicotinic receptors
	^{11}C-Benztropine	Muscarinic receptors
Rivastigmine[138,139]	^{18}F-FDG	Metabolism
Donepezil[140]	^{18}F-FDG	Metabolism
Galantamine[141]	^{18}F-FDG	Metabolism
NGF[142,143,144]	^{11}C-Butanol	Blood flow
	^{11}C-Nicotine	Nicotinic receptors
	^{18}F-FDG	Metabolism
SPECT		
Physostigmine[145,146]	^{99m}Tc-HMPAO	Blood flow
Velnacrine[147]	^{99m}Tc-HMPAO	Blood flow
Tacrine[148–151]	^{99m}Tc-HMPAO	Blood flow
Linopiridine[152]	^{99m}Tc-HMPAO	Blood flow
Idazoxan[153]	^{99m}Tc-HMPAO	Blood flow
Donepezil[154]	^{99m}Tc-HMPAO	Blood flow
Rivastigmine[155]	^{99m}Tc-HMPAO	Blood flow
MRI		
Donepezil[156]	fMRI	Brain activation
Galantamine[157]	fMRI	Brain activation
Donepezil[158]	MRI	Brain volume
Abeta immunization[159]	MRI	Brain volume

clinical instrument which allows an early diagnosis of dementia. The various techniques are important tools in the differential diagnosis. So far, PET has been shown to be superior to SPECT in sensitivity, but the high cost of investigations limits availability. Hopefully, SPECT techniques will further develop and allow quantitative measurements. New SPECT ligands may increase the possibility of measuring neuroreceptors and other aspects of neurotransmitter function. In addition, fMRI is a promising technique with several clinical applications. Functional imaging techniques may occupy a unique position in the development of new treatment strategies in dementia. Important information about the mechanism of action of drugs, as well as therapeutic dose ranges, can be obtained. These techniques will undoubtedly play an important role in the clinical pharmacological approach to neurogeriatrics in the future.

REFERENCES

1. Rapoport SI. Positron emission tomography in Alzheimer's disease in relation to disease pathogenesis: a critical review. Cerebrovasc Brain Metab Rev 1991; 3:297–335.
2. Nordberg A. Clinical studies in Alzheimer patients with positron emission tomography. Behav Brain Res 1993; 57: 215–234.
3. Petrella JR, Coleman RE, Doraiswamy PM. Neuroimaging and early diagnosis of Alzheimer disease: a look to the future. Radiology 2003; 226:315–336.
4. McGeer EG, Kamo H, Harrop R, et al. Comparison of PET, MRI and CT with pathology in a proven case of Alzheimer's disease. Neurology 1986; 36:1569–1574.

5. McGeer EG, McGeer PL, Harrop R, et al. Correlations or regional postmortem enzyme activities with premortem local glucose metabolic rate in Alzheimer's disease. J Neurosci Res 1990; 27:612–619.

6. Cagnin A, Brooks DJ, Kennedy AM et al. In-vivo measurement of activated microglia in dementia. Lancet 2001; 358: 461–467.

7. Nordberg A. PET imaging of amyloid in Alzheimer's disease. Lancet Neurol 2004; 3:519–527.

8. Fox PT, Minthun MA, Reiman EM, et al. Enhanced detection of focal brain responses using intersubject averaging and change distribution analysis of subtracted PET images. J Cereb Blood Flow Metab 1988; 8:642–653.

9. Mintun MA, Raichle ME, Martin WRW, et al. Brain oxygen utilization measured with O-15 radiotracers and positron emission tomography. J Nucl Med 1984; 25:177–187.

10. Reivich M, Kuhl D, Wolf A, et al. The 18-F-fluorodeoxyglucose method for the measurement of local cerebral glucose utilization in man. Circ Res 1979; 44:127–137.

11. Nordberg A, Lundqvist H, Hartvig P et al. Kinetic analysis of regional (S)(−)11C-nicotine binding in normal and Alzheimer brains. In vivo assessment using positron emission tomography. Alzheimer Dis Assoc Disord 1995; 9:21–27.

12. Tyrell PJ, Sawle GV, Ibanez V, et al. Clinical and positron emission tomographic studies in the 'extrapyramidal syndrome' of dementia of the Alzheimer type. Arch Neurol 1990; 47:1318–1323.

13. Blin J, Baron JC, Dubois B, et al. Loss of brain 5-HT2 receptors in Alzheimer's disease. Brain 1993; 116:497–510.

14. Rinne JO, Sahlberg N, Routtinine H, et al. Striatal uptake of the dopamine reuptake ligand [^{11}C]-CFT is reduced in Alzheimer's disease assessed by positron emission tomography. Neurology 1998; 50:152–156.

15. Iyo M, Fukushi K, Nagatsuka S, et al. Measurement of acetylcholinesterase by positron emission tomography in the brain of healthy controls and patients with Alzheimer's disease. Lancet 1997; 349:1805–1809.

16. Gallezot J-D, Bottlaender M, Grégoire M-C et al. In vivo imaging of human cerebral nicotinic acetylcholine receptors with 2–^{18}F-fluoro-A-85380 and PET. J Nucl Med 2005; 46:240–247.

17. Nordberg A. Visualization of nicotinic and muscarinic receptors in brain by positron emission tomography. In: Giacobini E, Pepeu G, eds. The Brain Cholinergic System. Oxford: Taylor & Francis 2006.

18. Kuhl DE, Small GW, Riege WH, et al. Cerebral metabolic pattern before the diagnosis of probable Alzheimer's disease. J Cereb Blood Flow Metab 1987; 7(suppl):S406.

19. Haxby JV, Grady CL, Koss E, et al. Heterogenous anterior–posterior metabolic pattern in dementia of Alzheimer type. Arch Neurol 1990; 47:753–760.

20. Duara R, Barker W, Pascal S, et al. The sensitivity and specificity of PET in aging and dementia. J Cereb Blood Flow Metab 1989; 9(suppl 1):S567.

21. Minoshima S, Frey KA, Foster NL, Kuhl DE. Preserved pontine glucose metabolism in Alzheimer disease: a reference region for functional brain image (PET) analysis. J Comput Assist Tomogr 1995; 19:541–547.

22. Herholz K, Perani D, Salmon E, et al. Comparability of FDG PET studies in probable Alzheimer's disease. J Nucl Med 1993; 34:1460–1465.

23. Herholz K, Nordberg A, Salmon E, et al. Impairment of neocortical metabolism predicts progression in Alzheimer's disease. Dement Geriatr Cogn Disord (1999) 10: 494–504.

24. Herholz K, Salmon E, Perani D, et al. Discrimination between Alzheimer dementia and controls by automated

analysis of multicenter FDG PET. NeuroImage 2002; 17: 302–316.

25. Kim EJ, Cho SS, Jeong Y, et al. Glucose metabolism in early onset versus late onset Alzheimer's disease: an SPM analysis of 120 patients. Brain 2005; 128:1790–1801.

26. Gemmell HG, Evans NTS, Bession JAO, et al. Regional cerebral blood flow imaging: a quantitative comparison of technetium-99m-HMPAO SPECT with ^{15}O$_2$ PET. J Nucl Med 1990; 30:1595–1600.

27. Heiss WD, Herholz K, Podreka I, et al. Comparison of [^{99m}TC]HMPAO SPECT with [^{18}F] fluoromethane PET in cerebrovascular disease. J Cereb Blood Flow Metab 1990; 10: 687–697.

28. Messa C, Perani D, Ludignani G, et al. High resolution technetium-99m-HMPAO SPECT in patients with probable Alzheimer's disease: comparison with fluorine-18-FDG PET. J Nucl Med 1994; 35:210–216.

29. Robert Ph, Migneco O, Darcourt J, et al. Correlation between ^{99m}Tc-HMPAO brain uptake and severity of dementia in Alzheimer's disease: assessment using an automatized technique. Dementia 1992; 3:15–20.

30. Perani D, Di Piero V, Vallar G, et al. Technetium-99m HMPAO-SPECT studies of regional cerebral perfusion in early Alzheimer's disease. J Nucl Med 1988; 29:1507–1514.

31. Ogawa S, Lee TM, Nayak AS, Glynn P. Oxygenation-sensitive contrast in magnetic resonance imaging of rodent brain at high fields. Magn Reson Med 1990; 14:68–78.

32. Kantarci K, Petersen RC, Boeve BF, et al. 1H MR spectroscopy in common dementia. Neurology 2004; 63:1393–1398.

33. Ferris SH, De Leon MJ, Wolf AP, et al. Positron emission tomography in the study of aging and senile dementia. Neurobiol Aging 1980; 1:127–131.

34. Frackowiak RSJ, Pozzilli C, Legg NJ, et al. Regional cerebral oxygen supply and utilization in dementia: a clinical and physiological study with O-15 and positron tomography. Brain 1981; 104:753–778.

35. De Leon MJ, Ferris SH, George AE, et al. Computed tomography and positron emission transaxial tomography evaluation of normal aging and Alzheimer's disease. J Cereb Blood Flow Metab 1983; 3:391–394.

36. Grady CL, Haxby JV, Schapiro MB, et al. Subgroups in dementia of the Alzheimer type identified using positron emission tomography. J Neuropsychiatry Clin Neurosci 1990; 2:373–384.

37. Grady CL, Haxby JV, Horvitz B, et al. Neuropsychological and cerebral metabolic function in early vs late dementia of Alzheimer type. Neuropsychologia 1987; 25:807–816.

38. Small GW, Kuhl DE, Riege WH, et al. Cerebral glucose metabolic pattern in Alzheimer's disease. Effect of gender and age in dementia onset. Arch Gen Psychiatry 1989; 46: 527–532.

39. Mielke R, Herholz K, Grond M, et al. Differences of regional cerebral glucose metabolism between presenile and senile dementia of Alzheimer type. Neurobiol Aging 1991; 13:93–98.

40. Salmon P, Colette F, Degueldre C, Franck G. Voxel-based analysis of confounding effects of age and dementia severity on cerebral metabolism in Alzheimer's disease. Hum Brain Mapp 2000; 10:39–48.

41. Ichimiya A, Herholz K, Mielke R, et al. Difference of regional cerebral metabolic pattern between presenile and senile dementia of Alzheimer type: a factor analytic study. J Neurol Sci 1994; 123:11–17.

42. Filly CM, Kelly J, Heaton RK. Neuropsychologic feature of early and late Alzheimer's disease. Arch Neurol 1986; 43: 574–576.

43. Duara R, Barker WW, Chang J, et al. Viability of neocortical function of behavioural activation state PET studies in Alzheimer's disease. J Cereb Blood Flow Metab 1992; 12: 927–934.
44. Grady CL, Haxby JV, Horwitz J, et al. Activation of cerebral blood flow during a visuoperceptual task in patients with Alzheimer-type dementia. Neurobiol Aging 1993; 14:35–44.
45. Miller JD, de Leon MJ, Ferris SH, et al. Abnormal temporal lobe response in Alzheimer's disease during cognitive processing as measured by 11C-2–deoxy-D-glucose and PET. J Cereb Blood Flow Metab 1987; 7:248–251.
46. McGeer PL, Kamo H, Harrop T, et al. Comparison of PET, MRI, CT with pathology in a proven case of Alzheimer's disease. Neurology 1986; 36:1569–1574.
47. Duara R, Barker WW, Pascal S, et al. Lack of correlation of regional neuropathology to the regional PET metabolic deficit in Alzheimer's disease. J Cereb Blood Flow Metab 1991; 11(suppl 2):S19.
48. De Carli C, Attack JR, Ball MJ et al. Postmortem neurofibrillary tangle densities but not senile plaque densities are related to regional metabolic rates for glucose during life in Alzheimer's disease patients. Neurodegeneration 1992; 1: 113–121.
49. Braak H, Braak E. Evolution of the neuropathology of Alzheimer's disease. Acta Neurol Scand 1996; 93(suppl 165): 3–12.
50. Kennedy AM, Newman S, McCaddon A, et al. Familial Alzheimer's disease. Brain 1993; 116:309–324.
51. Nordberg A, Viitanen M, Almkvist O, et al. Longitudinal PET studies in families with chromosomes 14 and 21 encoded Alzheimer's disease. In: Iqbal K, Mortimer J, Winblad B, Wisniewski H (eds). Research Advances in Alzheimer's Disease and Related Disorders. Chichester: John Wiley 1995; 243–250.
52. Kennedy AM, Frackowiak RSJ, Newman SK, et al. Deficits in cerebral glucose metabolism demonstrated by positron emission tomography in individuals at risk of Alzheimer's disease. Neurosci Lett 1995; 186:17–20.
53. Perani D, Grassi F, Sorbi S, et al. PET study in subjects from two Italian FAD families with APP717 Val to Ilue mutation. Eur Neurol 1997; 4:214–220.
54. Wahlund LO, Basun H, Almkvist O, et al. A follow up study of the family with the Swedish APP 670/671 Alzheimer's disease mutation. Dement Geriat Cogn Disord 1999; 10: 526–533.
55. Small GW, Maziotta JC, Collins MT, et al. Apolipoprotein E type 4 allele and cerebral glucose metabolism in relatives at risk for familial Alzheimer disease. JAMA 1995; 273: 942–947.
56. Reiman EM, Caselli RJ, Yun LS, et al. Preclinical evidence of Alzheimer's disease in persons homozygous for the epsilon 4 allele for apolipoprotein E. N Engl Med 1996; 334:752–758.
57. Small GW, Ercoli LM, Silverman DHS, et al. Cerebral metabolic and cognitive decline in persons at genetic risk for Alzheimer's disease. Proc Natl Acad Sci USA 2000; 97: 6037–6042.
58. Reiman EM, Chen K, Alexander GE, et al. Functional abnormalities in young adults at risk for late-onset Alzheimer's dementia. Proc Natl Acad Sci USA 2004; 101: 284–289.
59. Reiman EM, Chen K, Alexander GE, et al. Correlation between apolipoprotein E e4 gene dose and brain-imaging measurements of regional hypometabolism. Proc Natl Acad Sci USA 2005; 102:8299–8302.
60. Corder EH, Jelic V, Basun H, et al. No difference in cerebral glucose metabolism in patients with Alzheimer's disease and differing apolipoprotein E genotype. Arch Neurol 1997; 54: 273–277.
61. Drzezga A, Riemenschneider M, Strassner B, et al. Cerebral glucose metabolism in patients with AD and different APOE genotypes. Neurology 2005; 64:102–107.
62. Nordberg A. Neuroreceptor changes in Alzheimer's disease. Cerebrovasc Brain Metab Rev 1992; 4:303–328.
63. Martin WR, Palmer MR, Patlak CS, et al. Nigrostriatal function in human studied with positron emission tomography. Ann Neurol 1989; 26:535–542.
64. Perry EK, Perry RH, Candy JM, et al. Cortical serotonin-S2 receptor binding abnormalities in patients with Alzheimer's disease: comparison with Parkinson's disease. Neurosci Lett 1984; 51:353–357.
65. Bowen DM, Najlerahim A, Procter AW, et al. Circumscribed changes of the cerebral cortex in neuropsychiatric disorders of later life. Proc Natl Acad Sci USA 1989; 86: 9504–9508.
66. Ebmeier KP, Donaghey C, Dougall NJ. Neuroimaging in dementia. Int Rev Neurobiol 2005; 67:43–72.
67. Wu C, Pike VW, Wang Y. Amyloid imaging: from benchtop to bedside. Curr Topics Develop Biol 2005; 70:171–213.
68. Shogi-Jadid K, Small GW, Agdeppa ED, et al. Localization of neurofibrillary tangles and beta-amyloid plaques in the brain of living patients with Alzheimer disease. Am J Geriatr Psychiatry 2002; 10:24–35.
69. Klunk WE, Engler H, Nordberg A, et al. Imaging brain amyloid in Alzheimer's disease with Pittsburgh Compound B. Ann Neurol 2004; 55:306–319.
70. Verhoeff NP, Wilson AA, Takeshita S, et al. In-vivo imaging of Alzheimer disease beta-amyloid with [11C] SB-13 PET. Am J Geriatr Psychiatry 2004; 12:584–595.
71. Grimmer T, Diehl J, Drzezga A, Forstl H, Kurz A. Region-specific decline of cerebral glucose metabolism in patients with frontotemporal dementia: a prospective 18F-FGD-PET study. Dement Geriatr Cogn Disord 2004; 18:32–36.
72. Jeong Y, Cho SS, Park JM, et al. 18F-FDG PET finding in frontotemporal dementia: an SPM analysis of 29 patients. J Nucl Med 2005; 46:233–239.
73. Diehl J, Grimmer T, Drzezga A, et al. Cerebral metabolic patterns at early stage of frontotemporal dementia and semantic dementia. A PET study. Neurobiol Aging 2004; 25: 1051–1056.
74. Franceschi M, Anchisi D, Pelati O, et al. Glucose metabolism and serotonin receptors in the frontotemporal lobe degeneration. Ann Neurol 2005; 57:216–225.
75. Kamo H, McGeer PL, Herrop R, et al. Positron emission tomography and histopathology in Pick's disease. Neurology 1987; 37:439–445.
76. Salmon E, Franck G. Positron emission tomography study in Alzheimer's disease and Pick's disease. Arch Gerontol Geriatr Suppl 1989; 1:241–247.
77. McKeith IG, Galasko D, Koska K, et al. Consensus guidelines for the clinical and pathological diagnosis of dementia with Lewy bodies (DLB): report of the consortium on DLB international workshop. Neurology 1996; 47:1113–1124.
78. Ishii K, Imamura T, Sasaki M, et al. Regional cerebral glucose metabolism in dementia with Lewy bodies and Alzheimer's disease. Neurology 1998; 51:125–130.
79. Peppard RF, Martin WRW, Carr G, et al. Cerebral glucose metabolism in Parkinson's disease with and without dementia. Arch Neurol 1992; 49:1262–1268.
80. Vander Borght T, Minoshima S, Giordani B, et al. Cerebral metabolic differences in Parkinson's and Alzheimer's diseases matched for dementia severity. J Nucl Med 1997; 38: 797–802.

81. Hilker R, Thomas AV, Klein JC, et al. Dementia in Parkinson disease: functional imaging of cholinergic and dopaminergic pathways. Neurology 2005; 65:1716–1722.

82. Benson DE, Kuhl DE, Hawkins RA, et al. The fluoro-deoxyglucose 18F scan in Alzheimer's disease and multi-infarct dementia. Arch Neurol 1983; 40:711–714.

83. Nagata K, Maruya H, Yuya H, et al. Can PET data differentiate Alzheimer's disease from vascular dementia? Ann NY Acad Sci 2000; 903:252–261.

84. Messa C, Perani D, Lucignani G, et al. High resolution technetium-99m-HMPAO SPECT in patients with probable Alzheimer's disease: comparison with fluorine-18-F-FDG PET. J Nucl Med 1994; 35:210–216.

85. Holman BL, Jonson KA, Gerada B, et al. The scintigraphic appearance of Alzheimer's disease: prospective study using technetium-99m-HMPAO SPECT. J Nucl Med 1992; 8: 978–981.

86. Salmon E, Sadozt B, Maquet P, et al. Differential diagnosis of Alzheimer's disease with PET. J Nucl Med 1994; 35: 391–398.

87. Herholz K. FDG PET and differential diagnosis of dementia. Alzheimer Dis Assoc Disord 1995; 9:6–16.

88. Gemmel HG, Sharp PF, Bession JAO, et al. Differential diagnosis in dementia using the cerebral blood flow agent ^{99m}Tc HMPAO: a SPECT study. J Comput Assist Tomogr 1987; 11:398–402.

89. Mielke R, Pietrzyk U, Jacob A, et al. HMPAO SPECT and FDG PET in Alzheimer's disease and vascular dementia: comparison of perfusion and metabolic pattern. Eur J Nucl Med 1994; 21:1052–1060.

90. Zimmer R, Leucht E, Rädler T, et al. Variability of cerebral blood flow deficits in ^{99m}Tc-HMPAO SPECT in patients with Alzheimer's disease. J Neural Transm 1997; 104: 689–701.

91. Ryding E. SPECT measurements of brain function in dementia: a review. Acta Neurol Scand 1996; 94(suppl 168):54–58.

92. Herholz K, Schopphoff H, Schmidt M, et al. Direct comparison of spatially normalized PET and SPECT scans in Alzheimer patients. J Nucl Med 2002; 43:21–26.

93. Hunter R, McLuskie R, Wyper D, et al. The pattern of function-related regional cerebral blood flow investigated by single photon emission tomography with ^{99m}Tc-HMPAO in patients with presenile Alzheimer's disease and Korsakoff's psychosis. Psychol Med 1989; 19:847–855.

94. Miller BL, Cummings JL, Villaneuva-Meyer J. Frontal lobe degeneration: clinical, neuropsychological and SPECT characteristics. Neurology 1991; 41:1374–1382.

95. Frisoni GB, Pizzolato G, Geroldi C, et al. Dementia of the frontal type: Neuropsychological and ^{99m}Tc-HMPAO SPECT features. J Geriatr Psychiatry Neurol 1995; 8:42–48.

96. Waldemar G. Functional brain imaging with SPECT in normal ageing and dementia. Cerebrovasc Brain Metab Rev 1995 7:89–130.

97. Riddle W, O'Carrol RE, Dougall N, et al. A single photon emission computerized tomography study of regional brain function underlying verbal memory in patients with Alzheimer-type dementia. Br J Psychiatry 1993; 163: 166–172.

98. Cardebat D, Démonet JF, Puel M, et al. Brain correlates of memory processes in patients with dementia of Alzheimer's type: a SPECT activation study. J Cereb Blood Flow Metab 1998; 18:457–462.

99. Bäckman L, Almkvist O, Anderson J, et al. Brain activation of young and older adults during implicit and explicit retrieval. J Cogn Neurosci 1997; 9:378–391.

100. Bäckman L, Andersson JLR, Nyberg L, et al. Brain regions associated with episodic retrieval in normal aging and Alzheimer's disease. Neurology 1999; 52:1861–1870.

101. Cabeza R, Nyberg L. Imaging cognition ll: an empirical review of 275 PET and fMRI studies. J Cogn Neurosci 2000; 12:1–47.

102. Weinberger DR, Gibson R, Coppola R, et al. The distribution of cerebral muscarinic receptors in-vivo in patients with dementia. Arch Neurol 1991; 48:169–176.

103. Weinberger DR, Jones D, Reba RC, et al. A comparison of FDG PET and IQNB SPECT in normal subjects and patients with dementia. J Neuropsychiatry Clin Neurosci 1992; 4:239–249.

104. Wyper DJ, Brown D, Patterson J, et al. Deficits in iodine-labelled 3-quinuclidinyl benzilate binding in relation to cerebral blood flow in patients with Alzheimer's disease. Eur J Nucl Med 1992; 20:379–386.

105. Kuhl DE, Minoshima S, Fessler JA, et al. In vivo mapping of cholinergic terminals in normal aging, Alzheimer's disease and Parkinson's disease. Ann Neurol 1996; 40:399–410.

106. Chabriat H, Levasseur M, Vidailhet M, et al. In vivo SPECT imaging of D2 receptor with iodine-iodosuride: results in supranuclear palsy. J Nucl Med 1992; 33: 1481–1485.

107. Pizzolato G, Chierichetti F, Fabbri M, et al. Reduced striatal dopamine receptors in Alzheimer's disease: single photon emission tomography study with the D2 tracer [1231]-1B2M. Neurology 1996; 47:1065–1068.

108. Van Royen E, Verhoeff NF, Speelman JD, et al. Multiple system atrophy and progressive supranuclear palsy. Diminished striatal D2 dopamine receptor activity demonstrated by 123I-IBZM single proton emission computed tomography. Arch Neurol 1993; 50:513–516.

109. Costa DC, Verhoeff NP, Cullum ID, et al. In vivo characterization of 3-iodo-6-methoxybenzamide ^{123}I in humans. Eur J Nucl Med 1990; 16:813–816.

110. Brucke T, Wegner NP, Asenbaum S, et al. Dopamine D2 receptor imaging and measurement with SPECT. Adv Neurol 1993; 60:494–500.

111. Colloby SJ, O'Brien JT, Fenwick JD, et al. The application of statistical parametric mapping to ^{123}I-FP-CIT SPECT in dementia with Lewy bodies, Alzheimer's disease and Parkinson's disease. NeuroImage 2004; 23:956–966.

112. Soricelli A, Postiglione A, Grivet-Fojala M, et al. Reduced cortical distribution volume of iodine-123 iomazenil in Alzheimer's disease as a measurement of loss of synapses. Eur J Nucl Med 1996; 23:1323–1328.

113. Versijpt J, Van Laere KJ, Dumont F, et al. Imaging of the 5-HT2A system: age-, gender-, and Alzheimer's disease-related findings. Neurobiol Aging 2003; 24:553–561.

114. Miller BL, Moats RA, Shonk T, et al. Alzheimer's disease: depiction of increased cerebral myo-inositol with proton MR spectroscopy. Radiology 1993; 187:433–437.

115. Shiino A, Matsuda M, Morikawa M, et al. Proton magnetic resonance spectroscopy with dementia. Surg Neurol 1993; 39:143–147.

116. Moats RA, Ernst T, Shonk TK, et al. Abnormal cerebral metabolite concentrations in patients with probable Alzheimer disease. Magn Reson Med 1994; 32:110–115.

117. Kantarci K, Petersen RC, Boeve BF, et al. 1H*MR spectroscopy in common dementia. Neurology 2004; 63: 1393–1398.

118. Murphy DG, Bottomley PA, Salerno JA, et al. An in vivo study of phosphorus and glucose metabolism in Alzheimer's disease using magnetic resonance spectroscopy and PET. Arch Gen Psychiatry 1993; 50:341–349.

119. Fallgatter AJ, Roesler M, Sitzmann L, et al. Loss of functional hemispheric asymmetry in Alzheimer's dementia assessed with nearinfrared spectroscopy. Brain Res Cogn Brain Res 1997; 6:67–72.

120. Hock C, Villringer K, Müller-Spahn F, et al. Decrease in parietal cerebral hemoglobin oxygenation during performance of a verbal fluency task in patients with Alzheimer's disease monitored by means of near-infrared spectroscopy (NIRS) – correlation with simultaneous rCBF–PET measurements. Brain Res 1997; 755:293–303.

121. Gabrieli JDE, Brewer JB, Desmond JE, et al. Separate neural bases of two fundamental memory processes in the human medial temporal lobe. Science 1997; 276: 264–266.

122. Rombouts SARB, Machielsen WCM, Witter MP, et al. Visual association encoding activates the medial temporal lobe: a functional magnetic resonance imaging study. Hippocampus 1997; 7:594–601.

123. Rombouts SARB, Barkhof F, Goekoop R, Stam CJ, Schelten P. Altered resting state networks in mild cognitive impairment and mild Alzheimer's disease: An fMRI study. Hum Brain Mapp 2005; 26:231–239.

124. Petersen RC. Mild cognitive impairment as a diagnostic entity. J Intern Med 2004; 256:183–194.

125. Dawe B, Procter A, Philpot M. Concepts of mild memory impairment in the elderly and their relation to dementia – a review. Int Geriatr Psychiatry 1992; 7:473–477.

126. Arnaiz E, Jelic V, Almkvist O, et al. Impaired cerebral glucose metabolism and cognitive functioning predict deterioration in mild cogntive impairment. Neuroreport 2001; 12: 691–696.

127. Drzezgan A, Lautenschlager N, Siebner H, et al. Cerebral metabolic impairment into Alzheimer's disease: a PET follow-up study. Eur J Nucl Med 2003; 30:1104–1113.

128. Mosconi L, Perani D, Sorbi S, et al. MCI conversion to dementia and APOE genotype. A prediction study with FDG-PET. Neurology 2004; 63:2332–2339.

129. Mosconi L, Tsui WH, De Santi S, et al. Reduced hippocampal metabolism in MCI and AD. Neurology 2005; 64:1860–1867.

130. Huang C, Wahlund LO, Almkvist O, et al. Voxel – and VUI-based analysis of SPECT CBF in relation to clinical and psychological heterogeneity of mild cognitive impairment. Neuroimage 2003; 19(3):1137–1144.

131. Johnson SC, Schmitz TW, Moritz CH, et al. Activation of brain regions vulnerable to Alzheimer's disease: the effect of mild cognitive impairment. Neurobiol Aging 2005; [Epub ahead of print].

132. Heiss WD, Hebold I, Klinkhammer P, et al. Effect of piracetam on cerebral glucose metabolism in Alzheimer's disease as measured by positron emission tomography. J Cereb Blood Flow Metab 1988; 8:613–617.

133. Klinkhammer P, Szelies B, Heiss WD. Effect of phosphatidylserine on cerebral glucose metabolism in Alzheimer's disease. Dementia 1990; 1:197–201.

134. Tune L, Brandt J, Frost JJ, et al. Physostigmine in Alzheimer's disease: effects on cognitive functioning, cerebral glucose metabolism analysed by positron emission tomography and cerebral blood flow analysed by single photon emission tomography. Acta Psychiatr Scand Suppl 1991; 366:61–65.

135. Blin J, Ivanoiu A, Coppens A, et al. Cholinergic neurotransmission has different effects on cerebral glucose consumption and blood flow in young normals, aged normals and Alzheimer's disease patients. Neuroimage 1997; 6:335–343.

136. Nordberg A, Lilja A, Lundqvist H, et al. Tacrine restores cholinergic nicotinic receptors and glucose metabolism in Alzheimer patients as visualized by positron emission tomography. Neurobiol Aging 1992; 13:747–758.

137. Nordberg A, Lundqvist H, Hartvig P, et al. Imaging of nicotinic and muscarinic receptors in Alzheimer's disease: effect of tacrine treatment. Dement Geriatr Cogn Disord 1997; 8:78–84.

138. Potkin SG, Anand R, Fleming K, et al. Brain metabolism and clinical effects of rivastigmine in Alzheimer's disease. Int J Neuropsychopharmacol 2001; 4:223–230.

139. Stefanova E, Wall A, Almkvist O, et al. Longitudinal PET evaluation of cerebral metabolism in rivastigmine treated patients with mild Alzheimer's disease. J Neural Transm 2006; 113: 205–218.

140. Tune L, Tiseo PJ, Ieni J, et al. Donepezil HCL (E2020) maintains functional brain activity in patients with Alzheimer disease: results of a 23-week, double-blind, placebo-controlled study. Am J Geriatr Psychiatry 2003; 11:169–177.

141. Mega MS, Dinov ID, Porter V, et al. Metabolic patterns associated with the clinical response to galantamine therapy; a fluorodeoxyglucose F18 positron emission tomographic study. Arch Neurol 2005; 62:721–728.

142. Olson L, Nordberg A, von Holst H, et al. Nerve growth factors affects ^{11}C-nicotine, blood flow, EEG and verbal episodic memory in an Alzheimer patient. J Neural Transm Park Dis Dement Sect 1992; 4:79–95.

143. Erikdotter Jönhagen M, Nordberg A, Amberla K, et al. Intracerebroventricular infusion of nerve growth factor in three patients with Alzheimer's disease. Dement Geriatr Cogn Disord 1998; 9:246–257.

144. Tuszynski MH, Thal L, Pa M, et al. A phase 1 clinical trial of nerve growth factor gene therapy for Alzheimer disease. Nat Med 2005; 11:551–555.

145. Geany DP, Soper NM, Shepstone BG, et al. Effect of central stimulation on regional blood flow in Alzheimer disease. Lancet 1990; 335:1484–1487.

146. Hunter R, Wyper DJ, Patterson J. Cerebral pharmacodynamics of physostigmine in Alzheimer's disease investigations using ^{99m}Tc-HMPAO SPECT imaging. Br J Psychiatry 1991; 158: 351–357.

147. Ebmeier KP, Hunter R, Curran SM, et al. Cholinesterase inhibitor velnacrine on recognition memory and regional cerebral blood flow in Alzheimer's disease. Psychopharmacology 1992; 108:103–109.

148. Cohen MB, Fitten LJ, Lake RR, et al. SPECT brain imaging in Alzheimer's disease with oral tetrahydroaminoacridine and lecithin. Clin Nucl Med 1992; 17:312–315.

149. Minthon L, Gustafson L, Dalfelt G, et al. Oral tetrahydroaminoacridine treatment of Alzheimer's disease evaluated clinically and by regional blood flow and EEG. Dementia 1993; 4:32–42.

150. Minthon L, Nilsson K, Edvinsson L, et al. Long-term effects of tacrine on regional cerebral blood flow changes in Alzheimer's disease. Dementia 1995; 6:245–251.

151. Reikkinen P, Kuikka J, Soininen H, et al. Tetrahydroaminoacridine modulates technetium-99m labelled ethylene dicysteinate retention in Alzheimer's disease measured with single photon emission computed tomography imaging. Neurosci Lett 1995; 195:53–56.

152. Van Dyck CH, Lin CH, Robinson R, et al. The acetylcholine releaser linopirdine increases parietal regional cerebral blood flow in Alzheimer's disease. Psychopharmacology 1997; 13:217–226.

153. Goodwin GM, Conway SC, Peyro-Saint Paul H, et al. Executive function and uptake of ^{99m}Tc-exametazime

shown by single photon emission tomography after oral idazoxan in probable Alzheimer-type dementia. Psychopharmacology 1997; 131:371–378.

154. Nobili F, Koulibaly M, Vitali P, et al. Brain perfusion follow-up in Alzheimer's patients during treatment with acetyl-cholinesterase inhibitors. J Nucl Med 2002; 43:983–990.

155. Vennerica A, Shanks MF, Staff RT, et al. Cerebral blood flow and cognitive responses to rivastigmine treatment in Alzheimer's disease. Neuroreport 2002; 21: 83–87.

156. Kircher TT, Erb M, Grodd W, Leube DT. Cortical activation during cholinesterase-inhibitor treatment in Alzheimer disease: preminary findings from a pharmaco-fMRI study. Am J Geriatr Psychiatry (2005) 13:1006–1013.

157. Goekoop R, Schelten P, Barkhof P, Rombouts SA. Cholinergic challenge in Alzheimer patients and mild cogntive impairment differentially affects hippocampus activation- a pharmacological fMRI study. Brain 2006; 129:141–157.

158. Hashimoto M, Kazui H, Matsumoto K, Nakano Y, Yasuda M, Mori E. Does donepezil treatment slow the progression of hippocampal atrophy in patients with Alzheimer's disease? Am J Psychiatry 2005; 162:676–682.

159. Fox NC, Black RS, Gilman S, et al. Effect of Abeta immunization (AN1792) on MRI measures of cerebral volume in Alzheimer disease. Neurology 2005; 64: 1563–1572.

9

Electrophysiological tests

Cornelis J Stam

INTRODUCTION

Various neurophysiological tests have been investigated over the years to determine their possible usefulness as diagnostic tools in dementia. Abnormalities in evoked potentials and event-related potentials, in particular the P300, in Alzheimer's disease (AD) and related disorders have been known for a long time.[1–3] However, although these studies can provide a better understanding of the neurophysiological processes underlying cognitive dysfunction in AD, they have not been proven to be clinically useful at the level of individual patients. Perhaps a relatively new type of event-related potential, the mismatch negativity, will turn out to be more useful in this respect.[4] Other attempts to apply new neurophysiological techniques to dementia assessment involve transcranial Doppler and transcranial magnetic stimulation (TMS).[5–8] With TMS, changes in cortical excitability have been shown in Alzheimer's disease.[6] This approach might help to differentiate AD from frontotemporal dementias (FTD) and predict response to treatment with cholinesterase inhibitors.[7,8] Transcranial ultrasound has been used recently to differentiate Parkinson's disease from atypical parkinsonian syndromes.[9] However, although many of these new approaches are fascinating and promising, their clinical usefulness remains to be determined.

In the present chapter we will focus upon the EEG, since this is the neurophysiological test that has been studied most extensively and can be considered to have some established clinical value. Even so, the exact role of the EEG in dementia diagnosis remains a topic of discussion. The widely differing opinions on the usefulness of the EEG in dementia are reflected in the way the EEG is dealt with in the various consensus texts on dementia diagnosis. For instance, while a Scandinavian consensus text recommends to record an EEG in all subjects with suspected dementia, the American text does not even mention EEG as a possible laboratory test.[10,11] Given this lack of consensus and the enormous and rapidly growing literature on the topic, the clinician is faced with the difficult question whether the EEG will be of any use in assessing patients who present with cognitive complaints, and what is the optimal way to use the EEG in this category of patients. This chapter is intended to address this question, and to suggest a practical approach to the use of EEG in dementia diagnosis. First, EEG findings in normal ageing and various types of dementia are discussed. Next, a practical approach to EEG diagnosis in dementia is presented. Finally, new developments and future perspectives are briefly addressed.

EEG CHANGES IN NORMAL AGEING AND DEMENTIA

Normal ageing

Dementia is primarily a disorder of the elderly. Therefore, EEG abnormalities in dementia have to be distinguished from physiological EEG changes due to normal ageing.[12] Especially in the very old, this raises the question what should be considered 'normal' or 'healthy ageing'. Normal ageing could be considered a statistical concept, referring to findings and characteristics in the majority of subjects in a certain age category, even when these findings might reflect subtle abnormalities. Healthy, or successful ageing on the other hand, refers to optimal functioning and the absence of disease. These two different notions should be kept in mind when considering age-related EEG changes.

Ageing affects physiological EEG rhythms, most notably the alpha rhythm. The peak frequency of the alpha rhythm decreases with ageing, from the normal value around 10 Hz to 8 Hz. It is unclear whether the 'normal' slowing of the alpha rhythm reflects a physiological change in the elderly or is due to the increasing prevalence of subclinical brain disease, and in particular dementia in this population. In clinical practice, slowing of the alpha rhythm below 8 Hz should always be considered abnormal in adult subjects at any age. Furthermore, the peak frequency in individual subjects is assumed to be fairly constant over time. Slowing of the alpha rhythm in an individual subject by more than 1 Hz is abnormal, even if the frequency is still within the normal range. Also, asymmetries of the alpha peak frequency are not a feature of normal ageing but suggest brain pathology, in particular vascular disease. The reactivity of the alpha rhythm is also slightly diminished with ageing. However, clear absence of reactivity to eye-opening is always abnormal. The amount of alpha activity decreases with ageing, and the alpha rhythm becomes more conspicuous at posterior temporal sites and less pronounced at occipital sites.

Changes in other physiological EEG rhythms with ageing are less outspoken in the elderly. The prevalence of the mu rhythm decreases whereas the amount of low-amplitude beta activity increases in the elderly. Activity in the theta band constitutes a special problem. In children and young subjects some amount of theta activity is normal, roughly up to an age of 25 to 30 years. Interestingly, the disappearance of theta in the EEG of adults coincides with the completion of myelinization of long range association fibres. With ageing the relative amount of theta starts to increase again. Here it is quite difficult to draw the line between normal ageing and early brain pathology. This issue is further complicated by the fact that detection of moderate amounts of low-amplitude theta activity by visual analysis is difficult and unreliable. Spectral analysis of the EEG can be of some help here. As a rule of thumb, a relative theta power of more than 15 per cent at the occipital electrodes in an awake adult should be considered abnormal.[13] Another possible confounding factor that should be taken into account is the influence of the level of arousal during the EEG recording. Drowsiness, which occurs rapidly and frequently during EEG recordings in the elderly and can be recognized by slow eye movements, is associated with an increase in the relative power in the theta band, especially at the central electrodes (Figure 9.1). This should not be confused with pathological theta.

Ageing is not only associated with changes in physiological EEG rhythms, but also with the emergence of new phenomena, which are assumed to have little or no pathological meaning. The most important example of such a phenomenon is the intermittent theta and delta activity in the temporal regions, often more conspicuous on the left side. Over the age of 60 years such activity is found in 36 per cent of EEG records. When the temporal theta activity fulfils certain criteria it is designated as benign temporal theta of the elderly (BTTE) and is assumed to fall within normal limits.[12] Thus, BTTE is a typical example of 'normal ageing' as opposed to 'healthy ageing'. To qualify as BTTE the following eight requirements have to be fulfilled: (1) the subject should be over 60 years of age; (2) the activity should be localized in the anterior temporal areas; (3) the activity is more outspoken on the left side; (4) the background activity should be normal; (5) the amplitude should not exceed 60 μV; (6) the activity should be reactive; (7) the activity should occur as isolated waves and not as long trains; (8) the activity should occur in less than 1 per cent of the EEG record. When temporal theta and delta activity does not fulfil these requirements it should be considered abnormal, and may possibly reflect vascular brain damage.

Another feature that can be seen in the EEG of healthy elderly and that can easily be mistaken for an EEG abnormality is the so-called 'sleep onset FIRDA'. This consists of short bilaterally synchronous bursts of theta en delta which occur at transitions in the level of arousal. In contrast to the usual frontal intermittent rhythmic delta activity (FIRDA) the sleep-onset FIRDA is not considered to reflect brain dysfunction. Finally, runs of sharply formed rhythmical theta activity, with a sudden start and end, can occur in the elderly without pathological significance. These runs are indicated by the acronym SREDA (subclinical rhythmical electrical discharges of adults) and may be associated with drowsiness. SREDA should be differentiated from the rare but clinically important non-convulsive status epilepticus (sometime called 'petit mal status'), which may present as an acute confusional state and which is associated with continuous epileptic seizure activity on the EEG.[14] This is a severe condition which requires treatment with anti-epileptic drugs.

Alzheimer's disease

AD is the most frequent cause of dementia in the Western population. EEG changes in AD have been described in many studies over the years; reviews can be found in Boerman et al,[15] Jonkman[16] and Jeong.[17] The changes can be characterized by the general concept of 'non-specific diffuse slowing': there is a decrease of fast frequencies (beta and alpha band) and an increase in slow frequencies (theta and delta). An example of an EEG record showing diffuse slowing is shown in Figure 9.2. Loss of fast frequencies occurs

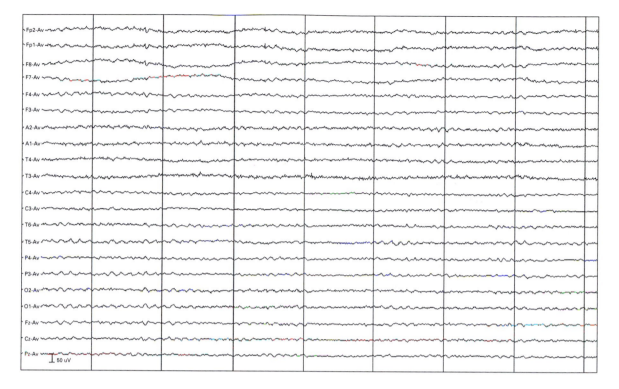

Figure 9.1 EEG showing early signs of drowsiness. The slow, out of phase waves in channels F8 and F7 are due to slow eye movements, which are characteristic for the earliest phase of drowsiness. During drowsiness slowing of the background activity cannot be reliably assessed. (Electrode positions according to the 10–20 system are marked on the left. Av indicates average reference. Vertical bars correspond to seconds. Sensitivity is indicated on the lower left)

relatively early, while the increase in delta is a relatively late phenomenon. The peak frequency of the alpha rhythm decreases, although this is not a very early finding. Increase in relative theta power may be the earliest and, from the point of view of diagnosis, the most sensitive change. Reactivity of the alpha rhythm to eye-opening also decreases, but this is difficult to quantify and almost always occurs in the context of significant slowing of the background activity. Complete absence of reactivity is a rare and late finding. Intermittent slow wave activity in the temporal regions occurs frequently in AD, but not in all patients, and may reflect concurrent vascular pathology rather than intrinsic AD pathology. Focal abnormalities and asymmetries of physiological rhythms or their reactivity are not typical of AD, and may point to vascular pathology. Specific abnormalities such as sharp and triphasic waves or FIRDA occur infrequently in AD, and should always raise suspicion of metabolic or toxic encephalopathy (Figure 9.3).

While slowing is the predominant feature of EEG changes in AD, another characteristic is the loss of synchronization between EEG signals recorded over different brain regions. Synchronization of EEG channels is assumed to reflect functional interactions between the underlying brain regions, and such interactions are probably affected in AD, which has been designated a 'disconnection syndrome'.[18] Functional connectivity is usually assessed by coherence analysis, which is a normalized measure of correlation between EEG channels as a function of frequency.[19] Most authors report a decrease of EEG coherence or related measures in AD, especially in the alpha band, but other bands have also been implicated.[20–31] Loss of interhemispheric coherence in AD correlates with atrophy of the corpus callosum.[32]

What causes the EEG changes in AD is not exactly known, although a few principles can be indicated. First of all it is important to stress that the EEG does not directly reflect neuronal loss or brain atrophy. If a large number of neurons are lost, but the remaining neurons function normally, the EEG will reflect the normal function of these remaining neurons. This notion is captured by the phrase 'dead neurons tell no tales'. Consequently, the EEG abnormalities in AD and other neurodegenerative disorders must reflect

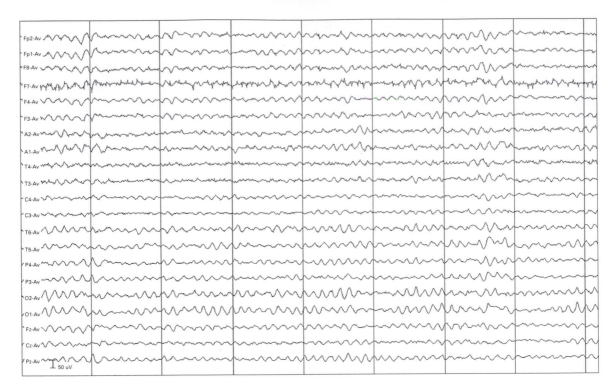

Figure 9.2 EEG with diffuse slowing. The frequency of the background activity is close to 7.5 Hz. The EEG shows little or no anterior to posterior differentiation. This EEG pattern is typical of moderately advanced degenerative dementia, in particular Alzheimer's disease. (Electrode positions according to the 10–20 system are marked on the left. Av indicates average reference. Vertical bars correspond to seconds. Sensitivity is indicated on the lower left)

abnormal functioning of the remaining neurons. There is evidence that a loss of acetylcholine, which is the most important excitatory neuromodulator in the cortex, may be responsible for the slowing of the EEG in AD.[33] Cholinergic projections to the cortex originate in the nucleus basalis of Meynert, which shows a clear loss of neurons in AD.[34] EEG slowing is related to neuron loss in the nucleus of Meynert and cholinergic deficiency in the cortex. In support of this hypothesis, treatment with drugs that activate cortical cholinergic receptors is associated with acceleration of the EEG.[35,36] This phenomenon could be used to identify patients who are more likely to respond to treatment with cholinesterase inhibitors.[37] Animal studies confirm the relation between cholinergic deficiency to nucleus basalis lesions and EEG changes[38] and suggest that loss of cholinergic activity might also be responsible for the reduction of coherence, at least in the higher frequency bands.[39] Disruption of interneuronal synchronization has also been ascribed directly to the amyloid plaques.[40] Some studies have attempted to relate the EEG changes in AD to the APOE genotype. The E4 allele, which is associated with an increased

risk of AD, has been related to more severe EEG slowing[41] and a loss of coherence.[42] Finally, the ubiquitous loss of coherence in AD may also be due to the loss of neurons and axons connecting the involved brain areas.[32]

Many studies have attempted to assess the diagnostic value of the EEG in AD. The reported values for the sensitivity and specificity differ widely, which may be due to differences in the populations examined (stage and severity of dementia; using healthy subjects or subjects with subjective memory complaints as controls) and differences in the various measures used to quantify the EEG abnormalities. Also, many studies involve small groups, and do not provide information on the reproducibility of the results in independent groups. Jonkman has attempted to summarize the available information, taking these limitations into account.[16] In this review, the total accuracy (percentage of correctly classified subjects) varied between 51 and 100 per cent, with a median value of 81 per cent. The best results are reported for slow wave activity in REM sleep, but this is obviously not a very practical approach.[43] On the other hand, the sensitivity of the

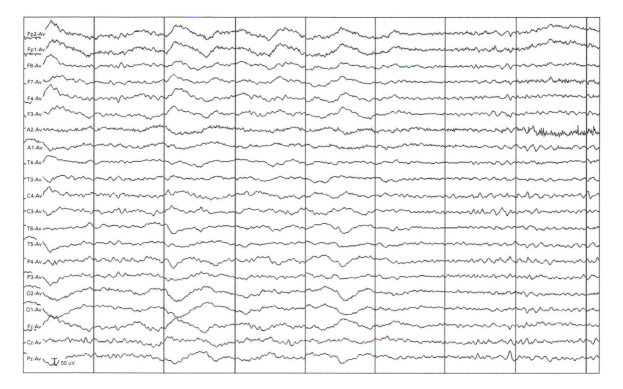

Figure 9.3 EEG showing frontal intermittent rhythmic delta activity (FIRDA). Runs of FIRDA can be seen at the left and in the middle. The delta waves are generalized, but are most pronounced frontally. The waves have a typical 'saw tooth' shape, with a steep rising part and a less steep down going part. FIRDA is seen most frequently in metabolic/toxic encephalopathy, which is often associated with mild delirium. (Electrode positions according to the 10–20 system are marked on the left. Av indicates average reference. Vertical bars correspond to seconds. Sensitivity is indicated on the lower left)

EEG in the early stages of AD can be quite low. Up to 50 per cent of patients with early AD may have normal EEGs,[44] although this may be different for presenile AD where early EEG changes are more likely. So far, various types of quantitative EEG analysis have not been shown to be superior to visual assessment of the EEG in AD.[15,45] Two studies used a simple visual scale, the 'grand total EEG score' or GTE, to assess the value of the EEG in dementia with promising results.[46,47] In the population-based study of Strijers et al the GTE had a sensitivity of and a specificity comparable to MRI assessment of hippocampal atrophy.[46] The study of Claus et al showed that in cases of diagnostic doubt an abnormal EEG makes a diagnosis of AD significantly more likely.[47]

The EEG can also be used in the differential diagnosis of AD and other causes of cognitive dysfunction. Depression can be associated with cognitive complaints but, in contrast to AD, does not give rise to significant EEG abnormalities. According to Jonkman, the total accuracy of the EEG in differentiating

between AD and depression with cognitive complaints is between 69 and 84 per cent.[15] AD and toxic metabolic encephalopathy (with delirium) can both give rise to diffuse EEG abnormalities. However, the EEG abnormalities are usually more severe in toxic metabolic encephalopathy. Features such as triphasic waves, epileptiform abnormalities and FIRDA argue in favour of a metabolic/toxic disorder rather than AD. A simple rule of thumb is the following: 'If the EEG is more affected than the patient, this argues for toxic metabolic encephalopathy; if the patient is more affected than the EEG, this argues for a neurodegenerative disorder such as AD or FTD'. Another frequent clinical problem is the differential diagnosis of AD and vascular dementia (VaD). This differentiation is made more difficult by the fact that AD and vascular problems may occur together. The EEG does not allow an absolute distinction between the two, but some EEG features are considered to be suggestive of vascular pathology: (1) asymmetric frequency and/or reactivity of physiological rhythms, in particular the alpha and the mu rhythm; (2) focal abnormalities, especially in the temporal regions; (3) paroxysmal diffuse abnormalities; (4) sharp waves and epileptiform abnormalities.

The EEG in AD may have prognostic as well as diagnostic significance.[48,49] According to Rodriguez et al,[50] EEG changes predict the occurrence of incontinence, loss of activities of daily life and survival. A loss of beta and, to a lesser extent, alpha is associated with a less favourable prognosis in AD, even after correction for such factors as disease duration, severity, age and such.[51] However, in concluding this section we should remark that the crucial problem when assessing the value of the EEG in dementia diagnosis is not to determine its sensitivity and specificity, or prognosis, but to find out when and how it may aid in clinical decision-making. We will attempt to address this question later in this chapter.

Other degenerative dementias

As is the case with AD, other neurodegenerative disorders that can give rise to dementia may also be associated with normal EEGs in the early stages. This is especially true for FTD, where the EEG can remain normal for quite a long time, although this view has recently been challenged.[52] In an advanced stage mild abnormalities, usually in the form of low voltage, irregular theta, can be found over the frontal and temporal regions, while the alpha rhythm is still preserved. At the group level quantitative analysis can aid in differentiating AD from FTD.[53] In progressive supranuclear palsy the EEG abnormalities are comparable to those in AD. Huntington's disease is often characterized by a so-called 'low voltage' EEG with an amplitude of the background activity lower than 10 µV. According to Markand[54] this EEG pattern is rare in healthy subjects, but can be found in 33 per cent of patients with Huntington's disease.

Parkinson's disease is associated with dementia in 20 to 30 per cent of patients. In non-demented Parkinson patients the EEG is normal. In demented Parkinson patients EEG abnormalities can be found with a pattern comparable to AD.[55] When EEG abnormalities do occur in non-demented Parkinson patients, they may have some predictive value for the later occurrence of dementia.[56] A dementing disorder closely related to both AD and Parkinson's disease is dementia with Lewy bodies (DLB). Some authors have suggested that DLB can be differentiated from AD by the occurrence of more severe EEG abnormalities in DLB.[57] However, in a recent large study no significant EEG differences between AD and DLB could be found.[58] Of interest, in this last study the clinical diagnosis of DLB did not correlate very well with the neuropathological findings. In fact there is some doubt whether DLB can really be differentiated from Parkinson dementia.

Vascular dementia

VaD is a somewhat problematic entity as it involves various types of pathology (vascular white matter changes, lacunar infarcts and multiple cortical infarcts) and their possible relationship with cognitive dysfunction. The basic concept of VaD has three fundamental elements: (1) demonstrated vascular lesions, (2) a dementia syndrome and (3) a causal connection between (1) and (2). In clinical practice it is often difficult to establish this causal connection with certainty. In the case of two or more large cortical infarcts the EEG can be expected to show focal abnormalities (focal flattening, slowing, periodic discharges with or without sharp waves and epileptiform abnormalities); in a more chronic stage these abnormalities tend to diminish. In the case of diffuse vascular white matter changes the EEG can show relatively non-specific slowing as well as intermittent temporal slow waves. As indicated in the section on AD there are some EEG abnormalities that favour vascular pathology over AD: (1) asymmetric frequency and/or reactivity of physiological rhythms, in particular the alpha and the mu rhythm, and asymmetric response on photic stimulation (Farbrot's phenomenon); (2) focal abnormalities, especially in the temporal regions; (3) paroxysmal diffuse abnormalities; (4) sharp waves and epileptiform abnormalities.

Creutzfeldt–Jakob disease

Creutzfeldt–Jakob disease (CJD) is a rare cause of dementia, which is however important in the present discussion because it is associated with characteristic EEG changes which may have diagnostic significance.[59] The EEG changes depend upon the stage of the disease. In the first phase there are predominantly non-specific abnormalities. There may be a disorganization of the background activity with an increase in theta and delta. In the second stage the characteristic periodic discharges can be found. These discharges are usually di- or triphasic, last 200 to 500 mseconds and have amplitudes up to 300 µV. The interval between the periodic discharges may vary between 0.5 and 2 seconds. Often the discharges are associated with myoclonic movements, which sometime have a fixed temporal relation to the discharges. Sometimes the periodic discharges are at first unilateral, and can be classified as PLEDs (periodic lateralized epileptiform discharges). Later in the disease the discharges usually occur in a bilaterally synchronous fashion and should be classified as PSIDDs (periodic short interval diffuse discharges) (Figure 9.4). In the third and final stage of the disease the PSIDDs persist, and the amplitude of the background activity between the discharges decreases until only the periodic discharges remain.

In general it can be stated that absence of periodic discharges after a disease duration of three months or longer makes a diagnosis of CJD unlikely, but does not exclude it. According to Zerr et al,[60] the periodic discharges have a sensitivity of 66 per cent and a specificity of 74 per cent. The 14-3-3 protein in the CSF has a higher sensitivity and specificity, but the EEG is still considered to be important for the diagnosis (see Chapter 5).[60] In a recent study involving 206 autopsy confirmed cases Steinhoff showed that, in subjects with suspected CJD, periodic discharges in the EEG have a sensitivity of 64 per cent and a specificity of 91 per cent.[61]

THE EEG IN DEMENTIA DIAGNOSIS: A PRACTICAL APPROACH

As has become clear in the previous section, the literature on the EEG in dementia, only a fraction of which has been reviewed, is somewhat overwhelming, but it is surprisingly difficult to extract practical guidelines from it. In this section we attempt to give some practical guidelines based on the experience of the Alzheimer Centre of the VU University Medical Center in Amsterdam, The Netherlands. At the Alzheimer Centre new patients with cognitive complaints and suspected dementia undergo a one-day, comprehensive evaluation consisting of a clinical examination, a neuropsychological examination, blood tests, MRI of the brain and an EEG recording. All findings are discussed in a multidisciplinary meeting one and a half weeks later. The multidisciplinary team consists of a neurologist, a psychiatrist, a geriatrician, a nurse, a psychologist and a clinical

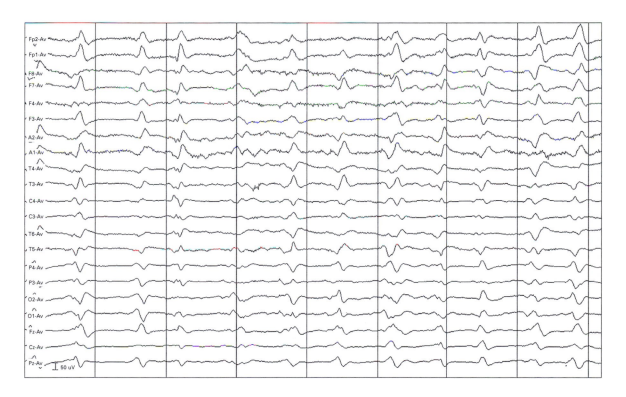

Figure 9.4 EEG showing periodic short interval diffuse discharges (PSIDDs). The discharges occur at more or less regular intervals of slightly less than a second in a generalized way. The discharges have a relatively simple morphology and the background activity between the discharges is almost flat. This EEG pattern is characteristic of advanced Creutzfeldt–Jakob disease, but can also occur in other severe encephalopathies, notably postanoxic encephalopathy. (Electrode positions according to the 10–20 system are marked on the left. Av indicates average reference. Vertical bars correspond to seconds. Sensitivity is indicated on the lower left)

neurophysiologist. The findings of the laboratory tests including the EEG are discussed in relation to the clinical findings and in relation to each other; a final diagnosis is reached by consensus. In case of doubt, the patient is examined again after a half year. This approach, where EEG findings are interpreted in relation to other relevant information and not as absolute facts, has proven quite fruitful. The following guidelines are derived from this experience.

When to record an EEG in suspected dementia?

Two strategies can be followed in determining in whom to record EEGs: a selective and a non-selective approach. In the selective approach, advocated for instance by Walstra et al,[62] EEGs are recorded only when the history and clinical examination suggest the presence of a disorder which requires EEG evaluation. This might be the case in suspected epilepsy, toxic metabolic encephalopathy or CJD. The advantage of this approach is that it makes minimal use of EEG resources, and presumably has a high yield of relevant EEG findings. Alternatively, EEGs can be recorded on a routine basis in all subjects evaluated for dementia. This is the approach followed at the Alzheimer Centre. The disadvantage of this approach is that it implies a considerable demand on facilities for recording EEGs. On the other hand, it turns out that the EEG findings that are most interesting, and that have the most pronounced consequences for clinical decisions, are often unexpected. In other words, the EEG can provide relevant information, even in patients in whom a clear indication for recording an EEG on the basis of the history and clinical examination apparently did not exist.

Two examples of unexpected but relevant EEG findings are (1) unexpected epileptiform abnormalities; (2) frequent apnoeas, suggestive of obstructive sleep apnoea syndrome. Some patients who do not have a clear history of (temporal) epilepsy, and who are not being treated with anti-epileptic drugs, may present with (temporal) epileptiform abnormalities. In our experience this may be the case in about 10 per cent of all patients. This finding has two implications: first, it requires a thorough search for underlying structural abnormalities such as mesio-temporal sclerosis or cortical dysplasia, which may not be obvious on routine MRI; second, even if there are no obvious clinical seizures but only memory complaints, treatment with anti-epileptic drugs should be considered. In some patients such treatment may actually cure the 'dementia'.[63]

Another unexpected but relevant finding is that some patients with cognitive complaints have signifi-

cant (duration longer than 10 seconds) apnoeas during the EEG recording. In such patients there is often a pronounced tendency to fall asleep during the recording, and apnoeas appear usually in non-REM 1. The end of the apnoea is usually characterized by an arousal reaction in the EEG. These patients may suffer from obstructive sleep apnoea syndrome (OSAS), which is known to be associated with cognitive complaints. Also, a relationship between apoE4 and sleep apnoea in AD has been suggested.[64] These patients need to be referred to a specialist sleep centre for further diagnosis (24 hour polysomnographic recordings) and treatment.

Other examples of such unexpected relevant EEG findings can be given, but the main point is clear: they will be missed if the EEG is only recorded in selected cases. Because some of the unexpected findings have clear clinical consequences this argues for recording EEGs in all cases of suspected dementia.

How to record the EEG in dementia?

Recording of the EEG in a patient with cognitive complaints is basically the same procedure as a routine EEG. There are, however, a few points that need to be considered. First, some of the provocation tests used in routine recordings such as hyperventilation and photic stimulation are less relevant for the evaluation of dementia, and can be skipped. On the other hand, it may be useful to include a simple cognitive test during the EEG recording, such as serial subtraction of 7 from 100 or a simple memory task. Such a test may provide information on the reactivity of the EEG during cognitive processing, but its use is still a bit experimental.[65] Another issue to be considered is the level of arousal. As indicated before, even slight drowsiness can be associated with an increase in theta (Figure 9.1). Because relative theta power is one of the earliest and most sensitive indicators of early AD, it is extremely important not to confuse drowsiness related theta with pathological theta. During the EEG recording, care should be taken that the patient is well awake during at least part of the recording. On the other hand, it is also useful to allow the patient to fall asleep during another part of the recording, because this may provoke such abnormalities as epileptiform activity and sleep apnoea.

How to analyse the EEG?

The cornerstone of clinical EEG is still the visual analysis of the EEG record. This is also true when the EEG is used for the evaluation of dementia. There is no evidence that quantitative analysis is superior to visual assessment. However, visual assessment can be made more accurate and reproducible with the use of simple semiquantitative scales such as the GTE.[46,47] EEG evaluation for dementia should take into account subtle abnormalities, such as minor slowing of the alpha frequency, diminished reactivity and an increase in low voltage theta. On the other hand, confusion with normal age-related EEG findings such as BTTE, sleep onset FIRDA and SREDA should be avoided. If quantitative analysis is performed, care should be taken that the epochs used for the analysis are not taken from periods with drowsiness, and the results of quantitative analysis should only be used as an adjunct to visual assessment and not as a replacement. Relying solely on sophisticated quantitative analyses of the EEG is courting disaster.[66] Perhaps the most practical approach is to perform a simple frequency analysis and to determine the alpha peak frequency at O_2 and O_1, and the relative theta power at the same electrodes. This simple analysis can be performed with most modern digital EEG machines.

How to interpret the EEG findings?

EEG interpretation involves two different levels. At the first level, the EEG is described without taking into account any other information than the age and level of arousal of the patient. The EEG should be classified as normal or abnormal for age, and, if abnormal, the nature, distribution and severity of the abnormalities should be indicated, preferably using a semiquantitative scale. At the second level, the EEG findings should be interpreted in the context of the clinical information, but also on the findings of other laboratory tests. At this level it is important to consider whether the EEG supports the clinical diagnosis or suggests alternative possibilities, whether the EEG provides information on prognosis and whether any unexpected EEG findings may be clinically relevant. The second level of interpretation is obviously the more difficult one, because it requires knowledge of both electroencephalography and the clinical aspects of dementia, but it is indispensable to take full advantage of the contribution of the EEG to the diagnostic process. Assessment of the clinical meaning of the EEG findings can be based upon the clinical information provided by the referring clinician on the EEG form, but the most optimal solution is for the clinical neurophysiologist to take part in the multidisciplinary team in which all the findings are discussed. As an aid in the clinical interpretation of EEG findings, a schematic overview of the relation between EEG phenomena and major categories of dementia is given in Table 9.1.

Table 9.1 EEG findings in the major categories of dementia

	SMC	AD	FTD	VD	TME	DLB	CJD
Slowing alpha	− −	+	−	0	+ +	+	+
Diminished reactivity alpha	− −	+	−	0	+	+	+
Asymmetric alpha	− −	−	− −	+	−	−	−
Diff theta	− −	+	−	0	+ +	+	+
Temporal slow waves	0	0	0	+ +	0	+ +	0
Focal abnormalities	− −	−	−	+	−	0	0
Sharp waves	− −	−	− −	+	+	0	0
Periodic discharges	− −	− −	− −	0	+	0	+ +
FIRDA	− −	− −	− −	0	+ +	+	0

SMC: subjective memory complaints; the EEG findings in mild cognitive impairment and depression with cognitive dysfunction resemble this pattern. AD: Alzheimer's disease. Please note that the EEG may be normal in up to 50 per cent with early senile AD, whereas the EEG is often abnormal in presenile AD. FTD: frontotemporal dementia (there may be a slight increase in frontal low voltage theta). VD: vascular dementia. Note that there is often a combination of VD and AD. TME: toxic metabolic encephalopathy, which often manifests clinically as (silent) delirium. DLB: dementia with Lewy bodies (closely related to Parkinson dementia). CJD: Creutzfeldt–Jakob disease. The prevalence of EEG abnormalities in different dementing disorders is indicated as follows: − − almost never; − infrequently; 0 sometimes; + frequently; + + almost always

When to repeat the EEG?

Many patients who are referred to memory clinics these days have only mild complaints. Even after extensive evaluation it is not always possible to make a final diagnosis. Such patients are usually evaluated again after a period of a year or a half year. It is highly recommended to repeat the EEG during such follow-up visits, because this is an objective and sensitive tool to detect slowly progressive brain disease. In particular, slowing of the alpha peak frequency by 1 Hz or more, even when the peak frequency is still within normal limits, is indicative of a progressive encephalopathy. Also, when there is doubt about the relative contribution of a toxic metabolic encephalopathy and a degenerative dementia to the condition of a patient, it may be useful to repeat the EEG, because improvement over time argues against a degenerative dementia.

EEG AND MEG IN DEMENTIA: NEW DEVELOPMENTS AND FUTURE PROSPECTS

The daily practice of EEG in the evaluation of dementia still depends to a large extent upon a straightforward visual analysis of the record, with only minimal support from quantitative analysis. However, there are some interesting developments which may change the way the EEG is used in the evaluation of dementia in the near future. These developments fall into two categories: (1) development of new sophisticated tools to analyse the EEG; (2) using magneto encephalography (MEG) instead of EEG to record the magnetic fields of the brain.

Today quantitative analysis of the EEG is still almost synonymous with the use of so-called linear methods such as frequency analysis and coherence analysis. These methods are based upon the assumption that the EEG is essentially a kind of filtered noise. Since the early 1990s a different approach has been explored. This approach, which is inspired by the theory of non-linear dynamic systems (also called 'chaos theory'), assumes that the brain is a complex, self organizing network of interacting non-linear dynamic systems.[67] The EEG record reflects the dynamics of these underlying networks, and can be analysed with new measures such as the correlation dimension,[68] Lyapunov exponents,[69] Kolmogorov or approximate entropy[69,70] or non-linear measures of synchronization.[71,72] Non-linear analysis of the EEG has suggested that brain dynamics in dementia may be characterized by a loss of complexity and abnormal functional interactions between brain regions.[73,74] There are some indications that combining linear and non-linear EEG analysis may improve the diagnostic accuracy of the EEG in dementia.[75,76] However, although this approach holds promise for the future, at this stage it should be considered still experimental.

Another promising new development is the use of MEG instead of EEG to investigate brain function in Alzheimer's disease. MEG has several theoretical advantages over EEG: (1) it is hardly disturbed by the conductive properties of the intervening tissues such as the skull; (2) with modern whole head systems it is relatively easy to record very large numbers (151 or more) of channels simultaneously; (3) MEG does not require the use of a reference, which is an advantage in studies of functional connectivity. In a pilot study, Berendse et al showed that the MEG in AD is characterized by significant slowing and loss of coherence, not only in the alpha band but essentially in all frequency bands.[77] Temporo-parietal slowing of MEG in AD was also demonstrated by Maestu et al,[78] Fernandez et al,[79] and more recently by Osipova et al.[80] This slowing was found to correlate with hippocampal atrophy.[81,82] Combining non-linear analysis with MEG further extends the scope of functional studies in AD. Using two different measures of brain complexity, van Cappellen et al showed that complexity loss in AD depends upon the frequency bands analysed.[83] Synchronization likelihood analysis of MEG in early AD patients showed a loss of synchronization in the upper alpha, the beta and the gamma band.[84] In this study, non-linear analysis proved to be more sensitive than coherence analysis. MEG may also be useful in discriminating subjects with mild cognitive impairment, which can be an early stage of Alzheimer's disease, from healthy controls.[85] In conclusion, the use of MEG in the evaluation of dementia holds great promise. However, future clinical application will depend upon replication of the results from pilot studies and a wider availability of whole head MEG recording systems in clinical settings.

REFERENCES

1. Moore NC. Visual evoked responses in Alzheimer's disease: a review. Clin Electroencephalogr 1997; 28:137–142.
2. Katada E, Sato K, Ojika K, Ueda R. Cognitive event-related potentials: useful clinical information in Alzheimer's disease. Curr Alzheimer Res 2004; 1:63–69.
3. Olichney JM, Hillert DG. Clinical applications of cognitive event-related potentials in Alzheimer's disease. Phys Med Rehabil Clin N Am 2004; 15:205–233.
4. Pekkonen E. Mismatch negativity in aging and in Alzheimer's disease. Audiol Neurootol 2000; 5:216–224.
5. Asil T, Uzuner N. Differentiation of vascular dementia and Alzheimer's disease: a functional transcranial Doppler ultrasonographic study. J Ultrasound Med 2005; 24:1065–1070.

6. Di Lazzaro V, Oliviero A, Piloto F, et al. Motor cortex hyperexcitability to transcranial magnetic stimulation in Alzheimer's disease. J Neurol Neurosurg Psychiatry 2004; 75:555–559.

7. Pierrantozzi M, Panella M, Palmieri MG, et al. Different TMS patterns of intracortical inhibition in early onset Alzheimer dementia and frontotemporal dementia. Clin Neurophysiol 2004; 115:2410–2418.

8. Di Lazzaro V, Oliviero A, Piloto F, et al. Neurophysiological predictors of long term response to AchE inhibitors in AD patients. J Neurol Neurosurg Psychiatry 2005; 76:1064–1069.

9. Behnke S, Berg D, Naumann M, Becker G. Differentiation of Parkinson's disease and atypical parkinsonian syndromes by transcranial ultrasound. J Neurol Neurosurg Psychiatry 2005; 76:423–425.

10. Wallin A, Brun A, Gustafson L. Swedish consensus on dementia disease. Acta Neurol Scand 1994; 157(suppl):3–31.

11. Knopman DS, DeKosky ST, Cummings JL, et al. Practice parameter: diagnosis of dementia (an evidence-based review). Report of the Quality standards subcommittee of the American Academy of Neurology. Neurology 2001; 56:1143–1153.

12. Klass DW, Brenner RP. Electroencephalography of the elderly. J Clin Neurophysiol 1995; 12:116–131.

13. Soininen H, Partanen J, Laulumaa V, et al. Longitudinal EEG spectral analysis in early stage of Alzheimer's disease. Electroenceph Clin Neurophysiol 1989; 72:290–297.

14. Brenner RP. EEG in convulsive and nonconvulsive status epilepticus. J Clin Neurophysiol 2004; 21:319–333.

15. Boerman RH, Scheltens P, Weinstein HC. Clinical neurophysiology in the diagnosis of Alzheimer's disease. Clin Neurol Neurosurg 1994; 96:111–118.

16. Jonkman EJ. The role of the electroencephalogram in the diagnosis of dementia of the Alzheimer type: an attempt at technology assessment. Neurophysiol Clin 1997; 27:211–219.

17. Jeong J. EEG dynamics in patients with Alzheimer's disease. Clin Neurophysiol 2004; 115:1490–1505.

18. Delbeuck X, Van der Linder M, Colette F. Alzheimer's disease as a disconnection syndrome? Neuropsychol Rev 2003; 13:79–92.

19. Nunez PL, Srinivasan R, Westdorp AF, et al. EEG coherency I: statistics, reference electrode, volume conduction, Laplacians, cortical imaging, and interpretation at multiple scales. Electroenceph Clin Neurophysiol 1997; 103:499–515.

20. Leuchter AF, Newton TF, Cook AA, Walter DO. Changes in brain functional connectivity in Alzheimer-type and multi-infarct dementia. Brain 1992; 115:1543–1561.

21. Besthorn C, Forstl H, Geiger-Kabisch C, et al. EEG coherence in Alzheimer disease. Electroenceph Clin Neurophysiol 1994; 90:242–245.

22. Dunkin JJ, Leuchter AF, Newton TF, Cook IA. Reduced EEG coherence in dementia: state or trait marker? Biol Psychiatry 1994; 35:870–879.

23. Jelic V, Shigeta M, Julin P, et al. Quantitative electro-encephalography power and coherence in Alzheimer's disease and mild cognitive impairment. Dementia 1996; 7:314–323.

24. Locatelli T, Cursi M, Liberati D, Franceschi M, Comi G. EEG coherence in Alzheimer's disease. Electroenceph Clin Neurophysiol 1998; 106:229–237.

25. Knott V, Mohr E, Mahoney C, Ilivitsky V. Electro-encephalographic coherence in Alzheimer's disease: comparisons with a control group and population norms. J Geriatr Psychiatry Neurol 2000; 13:1–8.

26. Stevens A, Kircher T, Nickola M, et al. Dynamic regulation of EEG power and coherence is lost early and globally in

27. Adler G, Brassen S, Jajcevic A. EEG coherence in Alzheimer's dementia. J Neural Transm 2003; 110:1051–1058.

28. Hogan MJ, Swanwick GRJ, Kaiser J, Rowan M, Lawlor B. Memory-related EEG power and coherence reductions in mild Alzheimer's disease. Int J Psychophysiol 2003; 49:147–163.

29. Babiloni C, Miniussi C, Moretti DV, et al. Cortical networks generating movement-related EEG rhythms in Alzheimer's disease: an EEG coherence study. Behav Neurosci 2004; 118:698–706.

30. Koenig T, Prichep L, Dierks T, et al. Decreased EEG synchronization in Alzheimer's disease and mild cognitive impairment. Neurobiol Aging 2005; 26:165–171.

31. Jiang ZY. Abnormal cortical functional connections in Alzheimer's disease: analysis of inter- and intra-hemispheric EEG coherence. J Zheniang Univ Sci B. 2005; 6:259–264.

32. Pogarell O, Teipel SJ, Juckel G, et al. EEG coherence reflects regional corpus callosum area in Alzheimer's disease. J Neurol Neurosurg Psychiatry 2005; 76:109–111.

33. Riekkinen P, Buzsaki G, Riekkinen P Jr, Soininen H, Partanen J. The cholinergic system and EEG slow waves. Electroenceph Clin Neurophysiol 1991; 78:89–96.

34. Francis PT, Palmer AM, Snape M, Wilcock GK. The cholinergic hypothesis of Alzheimer's disease: a review of the progress. J Neurol Neurosurg Psychiatry 1999; 66:137–147.

35. Shigeta M, Persson A, Viitanen M, Winblad B, Nordberg A. EEG regional changes during long-term treatment with tetrahydroaminoacridine (THA) in Alzheimer's disease. Acta Neurol Scand 1993; 149(suppl):58–61.

36. Adler G, Brassen S. Short-term rivastigmine treatment reduces EEG slow-wave power in Alzheimer patients. Neuropsychobiology 2001; 43:273–276.

37. Adler G, Brassen S, Chwalek K, Dieter B, Teufel M. Prediction of treatment response to rivastigmine in Alzheimer's dementia. J Neurol Neurosurg Psychiatry 2004; 75:292–294.

38. Ricceri L, Minghetti L, Moles A, et al. Cognitive and neurological deficits induced by early and prolonged basal forebrain cholinergic hypofunction in rats. Exp Neurol 2004; 189:162–172.

39. Villa AEP, Tetko IV, Dutoit P, Vantini G. Non-linear cortico-cortical interactions modulated by cholinergic afferences from the rat basal forebrain. BioSystems 2000; 58:219–228.

40. Stern EA, Bacskai BJ, Hickey GA, et al. Cortical synaptic integration in vivo is disrupted by amyloid-plaques. J Neurosci 2004; 24:4535–4540.

41. Lehtovirta M, Partanen J, Kononen M, et al. Spectral analysis of EEG in Alzheimer's disease: relation to apolipoprotein E polymorphism. Neurobiol Aging 1996; 4:523–526.

42. Jelic V, Julin P, Shigeta M, et al. Apolipoprotein E ε4 allele decreases functional connectivity in Alzheimer's disease as measured by EEG coherence. J Neurol Neurosurg Psychiatry 1997; 63:59–65.

43. Prinz PN, Larsen LH, Moe KE, Vitiello MV. EEG markers of early Alzheimer's disease in computer selected tonic REM sleep. Electroenceph Clin Neurophysiol 1992; 83:36–43.

44. Soininen H, Riekkinen PJ. EEG in diagnostics and follow up of Alzheimer's disease. Acta Neurol Scand 1992; 139(suppl):36–39.

45. Brenner R, Reynolds ChF III, Ulrich RF. Diagnostic efficacy of computerized spectral versus visual EEG analysis in elderly normal, demented and depressed subjects. Electroenceph Clin Neurophysiol 1988; 69:110–117.

probable DAT. Eur Arch Psychiatry Clin Neurosci 2001; 251:199–204.

46. Strijers RLM, Scheltens Ph, Jonkman EJ, et al. Diagnosing Alzheimer's disease in community-dwelling elderly: a comparison of EEG and MRI. Dement Geriatr Cogn Disord 1997; 8:198–202.

47. Claus JJ, Strijers RLM, Jonkman EJ, et al. The diagnostic value of electroencephalography in mild senile Alzheimer's disease. Clin Neurophysiol 1999; 110:825–832.

48. Helkala EL, Laulumaa V, Soininen H, Partanen J, Riekkinen PJ. Different patterns of cognitive decline related to normal or deteriorating EEG in a 3-year follow-up study of patients with Alzheimer's disease. Neurology 1991; 41: 528–532.

49. Lopez OL, Brenner RP, Becker JT, et al. EEG spectral abnormalities and psychosis as predictors of cognitive and functional decline in probable Alzheimer's disease. Neurology 1997; 48:1521–1525.

50. Rodriguez G, Nobili F, Arrigo A, et al. Prognostic significance of quantitative electroencephalography in Alzheimer patients: preliminary observations. Electroenceph Clin Neurophysiol 1996; 99:123–128.

51. Claus JJ, Ongerboer de Visser BW, Walstra GJM, et al. Quantitative spectral electroencephalography in predicting survival in patients with early Alzheimer disease. Arch Neurol 1998; 55:1105–1111.

52. Chan D, Walters RJ, Sampson EL, et al. EEG abnormalities in frontotemporal lobar degeneration. Neurology 2004; 62: 1628–1630.

53. Yener GG, Leuchter AF, Jenden D, et al. Quantitative EEG in frontotemporal dementia. Clin Electroencephalogr 1996; 27: 61–68.

54. Markand ON. Organic brain syndromes and dementias. In: Daly DD, Pedley TA, eds, Current Practice of Clinical Electroencephalography, 2nd edn. New York: Raven Press 1990.

55. Neufeld MY, Inzelberg R, Korczyn AD. EEG in demented and non-demented Parkinsonian patients. Acta Neurol Scand 1988, 78:1–5.

56. de Weerd AW, Perquin WVM, Jonkman EJ. Role of the EEG in the prediction of dementia in Parkinson's disease. Dementia 1990; 1:115–118.

57. Briel RCG, McKeith IG, Barker WA, et al. EEG findings in dementia with Lewy bodies and Alzheimer's disease. J Neurol Neurosurg Psychiatry 1999; 66:401–403.

58. Londos E, Passant U, Brun A, et al. Regional cerebral blood flow and EEG in clinically diagnosed dementia with Lewy bodies and Alzheimer's disease. Arch Gerontol Geriatr 2003; 36:231–245.

59. Steinhoff BJ, Racker S, Herrendorf G, et al. Accuracy and reliability of periodic sharp wave complexes in Creutzfeldt–Jakob disease. Arch Neurol 1996; 53:162–166.

60. Zerr I, Pocchiari M, Collins S, et al. Analysis of EEG and CSF 14-3-3 proteins as aids to the diagnosis of Creutzfeldt–Jakob disease. Neurology 2000; 55:811–815.

61. Steinhoff BJ, Zerr I, Glatting M, et al. Diagnostic value of periodic complexes in Creutzfeldt–Jakob disease. Ann Neurol 2004; 56:702–708.

62. Walstra GJ, Teunisse S, van Gool WA, van Crevel H. Reversible dementia in elderly patients referred to a memory clinic. J Neurol 1997; 244:17–22.

63. Hogh P, Smith SJ, Scahill RI, et al. Epilepsy presenting as AD: neuroimaging, electrical features, and response to treatment. Neurology 2002; 58:298–301.

64. Bliwise DL. Sleep apnea, APOE4 and Alzheimer's disease. 20 years and counting? J Psychosom Res 2002; 53:539–546.

65. Pijnenburg YAL, van de Made Y, van Cappellen van Walsum AM, et al. EEG synchronization likelihood in mild cognitive impairment and Alzheimer's disease during a working memory task. Clin Neurophysiol 2004; 115:1332–1339.

66. Nuwer MR, Nauser HM. Erroneous diagnosis using EEG discriminant analysis. Neurology 1994; 44:1998–2000.

67. Stam CJ. Chaos, continuous EEG, and cognitive mechanisms: a future for clinical neurophysiology. Am J END Technol 2003 43:1–7.

68. Pritchard WS, Duke DW, Coburn KL. Altered EEG dynamical responsivity associated with normal aging and probable Alzheimer's disease. Dementia 1991; 2:102–105.

69. Stam CJ, Jelles B, Achtereekte HAM, et al. Investigation of EEG non-linearity in dementia and Parkinson's disease. Electroenceph Clin Neurophysiol 1995; 95:309–317.

70. Abasolo D, Hernero R, Espino P, et al. Analysis of regularity in the EEG background activity of Alzheimer's disease patients with Approximate Entropy. Clin Neurophysiol 2005; 116:1826–1834.

71. Jeong J, Gore JC, Peterson BS. Mutual information analysis of the EEG in patients with Alzheimer's disease. Clin Neurophysiol 2001; 112:827–835.

72. Stam CJ, van der Made Y, Pijnenburg YAL, Scheltens Ph. EEG synchronization in mild cognitive impairment and Alzheimer's disease. Acta Neurol Scand 2003; 108:90–96.

73. Jeong J. Nonlinear dynamics of EEG in Alzheimer's disease. Drug Develop Res 2002; 56:57–66.

74. Stam CJ, Montez T, Jones BF, et al. Disturbed fluctuations of resting state EEG synchronization in Alzheimer's disease. Clin Neurophysiol 2005; 116:708–715.

75. Pritchard WS, Duke DW, Coburn KL, et al. EEG-based, neural-net predictive classification of Alzheimer's disease versus control subjects is augmented by non-linear EEG measures. Electroenceph Clin Neurophysiol 1994, 91: 118–130.

76. Stam CJ, Jelles B, Achtereekte HAM, van Birgelen JH, Slaets JPJ. Diagnostic usefulness of linear and nonlinear quantitative EEG analysis in Alzheimer's disease. Clin Electroencephalogr 1996; 27:69–77.

77. Berendse HW, Verbunt JPA, Scheltens Ph, van Dijk BW, Jonkman EJ. Magnetoencephalographic analysis of cortical activity in Alzheimer's disease. A pilot study. Clin Neurophysiol 2000; 111:604–612.

78. Maestu F, Fernandez A, Simos PG, et al. Spatio-temporal patterns of brain magnetic activity during a memory task in Alzheimer's disease. Neuroreport 2001; 12:3917–3922.

79. Fernandez A, Maestu F, Amo C, et al. Focal temporoparietal slow activity in Alzheimer's disease revealed by magnetoencephalography. Biol Psychiatry 2002; 52:764–770.

80. Osipova D, Ahveninen J, Jensen O, Ylikoski A, Pekkonen E. Altered generation of spontaneous oscillations in Alzheimer's disease. Neuroimage 2005; 27:835–841.

81. Fernandez A, Arazzola J, Maestu F, et al. Correlations of hippocampal atrophy and focal low-frequency magnetic activity in Alzheimer disease: volumetric MR imaging – magnetoencephalographic study. Am J Neuroradiol 2003; 24:481–487.

82. Maestu F, Arrazola J, Fernandez A, et al. Do cognitive patterns of brain magnetic activity correlate with hippocampal atrophy in Alzheimer's disease? J Neurol Neurosurg Psychiatry 2003; 74:208–212.

83. van Cappellen van Walsum AM, Pijnenburg YAL, Berendse HW, et al. A neural complexity measure applied to MEG data in Alzheimer's disease. Clin Neurophysiology 2003; 114:1034–1040.

84. Stam CJ, van Cappellen van Walsum AM, Pijnenburg YAL, et al. Generalized synchronization of MEG recordings in Alzheimer's disease: evidence for involvement of the gamma band. J Clin Neurophysiol 2002; 19:562–574.

85. Puregger E, Walla P, Deecke L, Dal-Bianco P. Magneto-encephalographic-features related to mild cognitive impairment. Neuroimage 2003; 20:2235–2244.

10

Biological markers

Douglas Galasko

INTRODUCTION

Biomarkers are laboratory-derived measurements that relate to a disease process. Many markers are being investigated for Alzheimer's disease (AD), including biochemical tests in cerebrospinal fluid (CSF) or plasma, and a variety of indices of brain function, structure or biochemistry obtained by neuroimaging. This chapter will focus on biochemical markers measured in body fluids.

Biomarkers in AD (Table 10.1) can be used as aids to either diagnosis or to treatment. An expert Working Group in 1998 listed several applications to diagnosis, including screening for disease, helping to establish the diagnosis of AD, including very early AD, differential diagnosis of AD from other types of dementias or brain disorders, preclinical diagnosis and characterizing the risk of developing disease.[1] Biomarkers may also be used to follow disease progression, which has implications for treatment as well as clinical use.

Criteria for biomarkers in AD were proposed by the Working Group. An ideal biomarker for AD should detect a fundamental feature of AD pathology and be validated against autopsy proven AD cases. It should diagnose AD precisely, with high enough sensitivity to allow early detection and adequate specificity for differential diagnosis from other causes of dementia. Finally, the ideal biomarker should be reliable, non-invasive, simple to perform and inexpensive. These requirements can be weighted according to the intended use of the biomarker. For example, if a biomarker is used for screening, then high sensitivity, ease of acquisition and low cost are priorities, while specificity for AD can be relatively lower. When a biomarker is used as part of a diagnostic evaluation, both sensitivity and specificity must be high (in excess of 80 per cent). If a biomarker is used as an outcome measure of the response to treatment of AD, then it should show a strong relationship to the clinical progression of dementia.

Table 10.1 Potential uses for biomarkers in Alzheimer's disease (AD)	
Use of marker	**Example of a biomarker in this setting**
Diagnosis	
Predicting AD or stratifying risk	Homocysteine
Screening for AD	Serum panel of proteomic-based markers
Supporting clinical diagnosis of AD, including very early diagnosis at mild cognitive impairment stage	CSF total tau and Aβ42
Differential diagnosis of AD vs other types of dementia	CSF P-tau
Following progression of disease	Progressive atrophy measured by volumetric MRI. No CSF or blood biomarker reliably tracks with AD progression
Following response to disease-modifying treatment	CSF tau, P-tau and F2-isoprostanes; possibly CSF Aβ42

Mild cognitive impairment (MCI) has been described as a possible prodromal stage of AD, identified by symptoms of cognitive decline and mild impairment of cognition on objective testing.[2,3] Amnestic MCI, in which the key area of cognitive impairment was episodic memory,[2] was shown to have a high predictive value for progression to AD. Recently, broader formulations have subdivided MCI into amnestic and non-amnestic varieties according to the areas of mild cognitive deficits. Predicting which patients with MCI have underlying AD pathology and have the highest risk of progressing to overt dementia is important, especially as treatment is initiated early in the course of symptoms. Biomarkers may clarify the extent of risk, and could provide evidence that AD pathological changes may be the substrate of MCI.

APPROACHES TO BIOMARKER DISCOVERY IN ALZHEIMER'S DISEASE

The CSF bathes the brain and is an obvious place to search for altered levels of proteins, lipids or other constituents as evidence of AD pathology or neuro-degeneration. Because lumbar puncture samples CSF that has flowed some distance away from the brain, putative biomarkers should be examined for concentration gradients within the lumbar CSF. Events that are purely intracellular may not be reflected in the CSF, and proteins or other substances released into CSF may fall below the threshold of detectability. Lumbar puncture is a routine neurodiagnostic test, associated with discomfort during the procedure and uncommonly with sequelae such as post-lumbar puncture headache. The risk of post-lumbar puncture headache can be reduced to well below 4 per cent by experienced practitioners and by the use of atraumatic small calibre needles.[4]

Because of the inconvenience of lumbar puncture, a biomarker in the periphery, measurable in blood or urine, would be far easier to use. However, AD pathology is restricted to the brain, and proteins or other substances released into CSF from the brain are greatly diluted when they transit to the bloodstream. Thus it may be unrealistic to find changes in brain-specific proteins in the blood. Biomarker studies on blood or urine assume either that there are systemic changes in AD or that some brain proteins remain detectable in the periphery even after dilution. Predictive biomarkers for AD may be studied in the blood, as indices of inflammation (e.g. cytokines), vascular damage (e.g. homocysteine) or of immune responses to AD pathology (e.g. antibodies against amyloid-beta protein (Aβ)).

Biomarkers for AD have largely been sought using a candidate approach, by measuring proteins or other substances related to lesions of AD or biological processes implicated in the brain. More recently, unbiased searches for biomarkers have been conducted, using methods that separate and measure large numbers of proteins (proteomics), lipids (lipidomics) or small substrates of metabolism (metabolomics). Patterns or profiles of markers (signatures) can be used to identify a disease. Some interesting preliminary findings have been published, in which patients with AD can be discriminated from controls by panels of markers, even using serum.[5] Because of the large numbers of markers that are screened, studies need to be carefully designed to rule out spurious associations, and require confirmation in independent sets of samples. There are many technical challenges in developing methods to assay panels of biomarkers simultaneously, to bring findings from broad-based searches for markers into the clinic.

Candidate markers will be the focus of much of this chapter (Table 10.2). The neuropathology of AD raises many possibilities, because pathological changes include the obligatory senile plaques and neurofibrillary tangles (NFTs), as well as neuronal death, synaptic loss, astroglial and microglial activation, inflammation and oxidative damage.[6] Vascular risk factors also contribute to dementia. Processes such as inflammation or astroglial activation occur in other degenerative disorders and after stroke and may be less specific for AD. Although less specific, biomarkers related to these pathways could be used as part of a panel of biomarkers to aid in diagnosis or to follow treatment. The most obvious candidate biomarkers derive from the biochemistry of the key lesions of AD. Plaques begin as diffuse deposits of amyloid, consisting of aggregates of Aβ which coalesce to form a compact core and over time become surrounded by neuritic changes, activated microglia and reactive astrocytes. Neurons develop cytoskeletal abnormalities consisting of paired helical filaments and NFTs, comprised of aggregates of the microtubule-associated protein tau. Amyloid deposition and other degenerative changes in the brain in AD probably start many years before the clinical onset of the disease and can be detected in the brains of cognitively unimpaired individuals who die at advanced age. The preclinical phase of AD is characterized by an increase in the burden of plaques and tangles, and once this reaches a threshold, symptoms of memory loss and dementia become more likely. It is unlikely that a biomarker will be unique to AD and undetectable in cognitively normal elderly individuals.

Table 10.2 Biomarkers for AD

Biochemical marker	Relevance to AD pathology	Measurable in body fluids	Findings in CSF in AD
AD lesions			
Total Aβ	Deposited in plaques	C, P	Unchanged
Aβ40	More prominent in vascular amyloid deposits	C, P	Unchanged
Aβ42	Major species found in plaques. Increased production in early-onset FAD	C, P	Decreased in CSF
Aβ oligomers	Can cause synaptic damage in vitro	C	? increased in AD
Total tau	Found in NFT in AD brain; released after neuronal damage	C	Increased
Phospho-tau	Main component of paired helical filaments	C	Increased
Oxidative Stress			
F2-isoprostanes	Stable oxidation product, markedly increased in AD brain	C, P, U	Increased
8-hydrodeoxyguanine	Results form DNA damage and elevated in AD brain	U	?
4-Hydroxynonenal	Oxidative damage marker	U	Increased (postmortem)
Inflammation			
Interleukins	Proinflammatory cytokines overexpressed in AD brain	C, P	
TNF-α	Proinflammatory cytokine	C	Sl increase
GM-CSF	Important cytokine for microglial activation and inflammation	C, P	? Sl increase
TGF-β	Multiple roles in inflammatory pathways	C, P	? Sl increase
S-100b	Neurotrophic signalling molecule, made by astrocytes. ? Role in plaque maturation		? Sl increase
α₁-ACT	Non-specific inflammatory marker; Found in plaques in AD		Sl increase
Others			
NTP	Associated with NFT, but not well understood	C, U	Increased
Platelet APP ratio	Uncertain	P	

Aβ: amyloid beta protein; AD: Alzheimer's disease; APP: amyloid precursor protein; FAD: familial AD; GM-CSF: granulocyte-macrophage colony stimulating factor; NFT: neurofibrillary tangles; P: plasma; TGF-β: transforming growth factor-β; TNF-α: tumour necrosis factor-α; α₁-ACT: alpha-1-antichymotrypsin; NTP: neuronal thread protein; C: cerebrospinal fluid; U: urine; Sl: slightly.

DIAGNOSTIC BIOMARKERS IN CSF

Tau and phospho-tau

CSF total tau and phosphorylated tau (P-tau) are the most widely studied and perhaps most promising of all candidate AD biomarkers. Tau is a microtubule-associated protein, specific to neurons, that binds to microtubules in axons and helps to regulate their assembly and transport. Alternate splicing of the tau gene results in six isoforms of the tau protein. Tau protein undergoes complex regulation, controlled in part by phosphorylation by kinase enzymes. Insoluble tau protein is the major component of NFTs in AD, and is highly phosphorylated at amino acids at specific sites in the tau sequence.[7]

Sensitive ELISA assays for tau were developed in the early 1990s and measure all forms of tau (total tau), regardless of phosphorylation state.[8] CSF levels of total tau are consistently increased in patients with AD compared to controls.[9–14] A recent meta-analysis compiled over 30 studies of total tau in AD versus controls and found high sensitivity, in excess of 80 per cent.[15] CSF total tau does not correlate with dementia severity or ApoE genotype. In AD patients, CSF total tau remains stably increased over 3 to 24 months.[12] This suggests that CSF tau levels reflect active or ongoing neurodegeneration. This is further supported by a study of serial CSF after acute stroke, in which total tau levels peaked at 1–2 weeks, and were correlated with the size of infarcts on CT or MRI.[16] Total CSF tau is elevated in many conditions besides AD, limiting its utility in differential diagnosis. Increased levels occur in non-dementing disorders such as traumatic brain injury, acute stroke, encephalitis, ALS and Guillain–Barre syndrome.[8] This suggests that tau is non-specifically released into CSF when axons and neurons are damaged or destroyed. CSF tau levels are extremely high in Creutzfeld–Jakob disease, in which there is typically rapid progression of dementia.[17] In disorders where restricted regions of the brain undergo degeneration, such as Parkinson's disease, CSF total tau is not increased.

To identify markers more specific for AD, ELISAs were developed to measure forms of P-tau, using antibodies that labelled epitopes of phospho-serine or phospho-threonine and stained tau inclusions in neurons. Assays for P-tau phosphorylated at serine199, threonine181,[18] threonine231,[19,20] and serine235[19] have all shown increased levels of P-tau in CSF in AD compared to controls. In general, CSF P-tau and total tau levels show similarly high sensitivity for distinguishing AD from controls, but CSF P-tau has higher specificity for AD than total tau. This has been best established

for P-tau181 and P-tau231.[21] Levels of P-tau181 are not elevated following an acute stroke.[16] Levels of P-tau181 and P-tau231 are infrequently increased in patients with dementia with Lewy bodies, Parkinson's disease and vascular dementia. In some studies, P-tau levels are increased in a percentage of patients with frontotemporal dementia and in tauopathies such as progressive supranuclear palsy (PSP) and corticobasal degeneration (CBD). P-tau levels do not appear to be associated with the severity of AD or with ApoE genotype. Several studies have investigated CSF total tau and P-tau levels in mild cognitive impairment and found increased levels relative to non-demented controls.[22,23] However, studies to date have been relatively small and have not examined how much additive diagnostic value CSF biomarkers provide when used together with sensitive cognitive measures, other clinical methods or imaging.

Amyloid-beta protein (Aβ)

Senile plaques begin as diffuse deposits of amyloid peptide, followed by growth and maturation, when they develop a dense core of aggregated Aβ peptide, less dense surrounding deposits and are surrounded by dystrophic neurites, reactive astrocytes and microglia. Aβ is a 4–5 kDa peptide derived by endoproteolysis of amyloid precursor protein (APP), a single transmembrane protein. This cleavage is carried out by enzymes termed alpha, beta and gamma secretases (reviewed in reference 24). Alpha secretase cleaves APP in the middle of the Aβ sequence, which precludes formation of full length Aβ. Beta secretase cleaves the N-terminal end of the Aβ sequence, releasing a large portion of APP and leaving a C-terminal fragment. The C-terminal fragment is then cleaved by the gamma secretase complex, releasing various species of Aβ. Although Aβ is made by neurons, and non-neuronal cells such as astrocytes, microglial cells and even from platelets, the highest Aβ levels are produced by neurons.

Over 70 per cent of total Aβ ends at amino acid 40, termed Aβ40. The remainder consists of other species, and about 10–15 per cent is Aβ42. Aβ42 forms aggregates or fibrils more readily than shorter forms of Aβ and has greater cellular toxicity in tissue culture models. In early onset familial AD due to mutations in the genes for presenilin or APP, a shift of APP processing occurs, resulting in an increased production of Aβ42.[25] In sporadic AD, there is no evidence of overproduction of Aβ, and it is likely that increased aggregation or decreased clearance from the brain is more important. In brain tissue from patients with AD, Aβ42 is the predominant species found in plaques. Different forms of Aβ may contribute to neurotoxicity, for example oligomers are toxic to synapses and fibrils also show toxicity.[26]

Several forms of Aβ can be measured in CSF, using sensitive assays such as ELISAs. CSF levels of Aβ38 or 40 do not differ in AD patients relative to controls,[27] but Aβ42 is selectively decreased in AD. Aβ42 levels decrease in a dose dependent manner according to the number of ApoE ε4 alleles.[12,28] Many studies have replicated the finding of low Aβ42 in AD[9,12,13,29] and a recent meta-analysis found that the sensitivity of CSF Aβ42 for distinguishing AD from controls exceeded 80 per cent.[15] Studies that included non-AD dementias have found that specificity is lower, varying from 45 to 85 per cent. Low CSF Aβ42 in AD may occur because deposits of Aβ42 may act as a sink and bind normally soluble Aβ42, impairing its diffusion into CSF. Other explanations include decreased clearance of Aβ42 from the brain or possibly decreased production due to compromised neuronal function as AD progresses. Postmortem CSF levels of Aβ42 correlate with the severity of plaque counts, supporting the sink hypothesis.[30] Levels of Aβ42 decrease slightly in moderate to severe AD compared to mild AD. Studies of serial CSF have shown that levels of CSF Aβ42 remain stably decreased for at least 12 months in AD.[28]

Aβ in CSF may be bound to lipid particles or proteins. This pool is not measured by ELISA, which assesses free Aβ. A sensitive electrophoresis method that can strip bound Aβ from carriers has been used to examine CSF Aβ species. This method revealed at least five species of Aβ in CSF, and confirmed the selective decrease in Aβ42 in AD.[31] Levels of Aβ associated with lipid particles purified from CSF were measured in a preliminary study and helped to distinguish mild AD and controls.[32] Recent studies have looked at other specific forms of Aβ in CSF. The N-terminus of Aβ shows variability, perhaps due to differential processing by β-secretase under different physiological conditions. N-terminal truncated forms of Aβ are abundant in postmortem brain tissue,[33] and in one recent study, increased levels of forms of Aβ42 beginning at amino acids other than Aβ1 were increased in MCI.[34] Aβ oligomers have been sought in CSF, but are difficult to measure. A recent study used a highly sensitive nanoparticle assay to detect femtomolar levels of Aβ oligomers in CSF, with the promising findings of increased levels in AD compared to a small number of controls.[35]

Combinations of tau and Aβ

Many studies have simultaneously measured CSF total tau or P-tau and Aβ42. In various combinations, these markers often increase diagnostic accuracy compared

to each marker separately.[12,13] Similarly, CSF tau and Aβ42 have been evaluated in MCI, as recently reviewed.[36] Although studies assessed relatively small numbers of patients, and used inconsistent diagnostic criteria, the general findings were that levels of tau and P-tau are increased and those of Aβ42 decreased in CSF in patients with MCI relative to controls. In some studies, those patients with MCI who showed progressive cognitive decline or progressed to develop clinical AD had high tau and low Aβ42, while those who remained stable did not. As newer markers are developed, it will be interesting to analyse their utility as part of a panel that includes tau and Aβ.[37]

Biomarkers related to oxidative damage

There is evidence of extensive oxidative damage to proteins, lipids (including membranes), DNA and RNA in the brain in AD. Unfortunately, many biomarkers of oxidative damage are unstable and have been difficult to detect in CSF. Isoprostanes are oxidized forms of prostaglandins which are stable and result from lipid peroxidation. A particular group of isoprostanes, denoted F2, appears to be formed primarily during neuronal metabolism and has been measured in CSF. Levels of total F-2 isoprostanes,[38] or of a specific F-2 isoprostane named 8,12-iso-iPF2α-VI,[39] are increased in AD relative to non-demented individuals. Total F-2 isoprostanes are also increased in disorders such as ALS and Huntington's disease. The combination of F-2-isoprostanes and other biomarker measurements may increase sensitivity for AD.[40] Recent studies have found that CSF levels of 8,12-iso-iPF2α-VI were increased in MCI and mild to moderate AD, but not in frontotemporal dementia.[41] This raises the possibility that certain types of oxidative damage may be associated with AD, or the overall degree of lipid peroxidation may be higher in AD than in other degenerative disorders. Unfortunately, sensitive assays for isoprostanes require specialized laboratory methodology, which has limited the more widespread assessment of these interesting markers.

Biomarkers related to lipid metabolism

Lipid levels show marked changes in the brain in AD. A recent study screened many types of lipid molecules in the brain and CSF and found that levels of sulphatides in CSF were decreased in AD and in MCI, relative to non-demented controls.[42] This interesting finding needs to be confirmed. Cholesterol may have important links to AD through several mechanisms. In animal studies, diets rich in cholesterol can increase

Aβ deposits. Levels of cholesterol in the brain and especially in areas of membranes called rafts influence the activity of secretase enzymes responsible for producing Aβ. Serum cholesterol and associated lipoproteins are not altered in patients with AD relative to controls and cholesterol levels in CSF appear to be normal. However, markers more specifically tied to the brain's use of cholesterol may be of interest. 24S-hydroxy cholesterol is a marker of cholesterol efflux from the brain, an index of overall brain utilization of cholesterol. A few studies have reported a slight increase in levels of this marker in AD versus controls, in plasma and CSF, but there is too much overlap for diagnostic utility.[43]

Inflammation

Inflammatory markers are abundant in the brain in AD, including acute phase reactant molecules such as α_1-antichymotrypsin, elements of the complement pathway and cells such as activated microglia and reactive astrocytes, as well as molecules associated with them such as cytokines and chemokines.[44] However, it has not been easy to identify a signature of inflammation in AD. For example, α_1-ACT, an attractive candidate biomarker because it can bind to Aβ and enhance its deposition in the brain, is minimally increased in CSF in AD, with a marked overlap with control values, and is slightly increased in serum only in severe stages of AD.[45] Levels of S-100b, a protein secreted by astrocytes, are slightly increased on average in AD versus controls.[46] However, there is too much overlap for diagnostic utility, and S-100b is increased in a variety of other conditions associated with neuronal damage or inflammation. Although cytokines can be measured by sensitive ELISAs, and are present in the brain in AD, many are undetectable in CSF. A few reports have documented very slight elevations of tumour necrosis factor alpha (TNFα)[47] or transforming growth factor beta (TFGβ) in AD and vascular dementia relative to controls,[48] and one recent study found increased levels of IP-10 in AD.[49] These preliminary findings require more widespread confirmation. In addition to providing diagnostic utility, biomarkers of inflammation could be useful to monitor the effects of anti-inflammatory treatment, which has been widely considered as a means of slowing progression or delaying the onset of AD.

Other CSF biomarkers

A number of other proteins show alterations in CSF in AD. Neuronal thread protein (NTP) was identified over a decade ago based on an antibody which stained plaques. Its role in normal neuronal function and its relation to pathological mechanisms in AD are unclear. CSF levels of NTP are increased in AD, and rise in association with increasing dementia severity.[50] Published studies of NTP have involved small numbers of patients and controls, and its sensitivity and specificity for AD have not been adequately determined. Neurofilament proteins are highly abundant constituents of axonal processes, and axonal damage or degeneration can lead to their release into CSF. Although increased levels of neurofilaments have been reported in CSF in AD and vascular dementia,[51] levels are also increased in a variety of conditions, including multiple sclerosis and head trauma,[52] and even in sciatica.

PERIPHERAL BIOMARKERS: BLOOD, SERUM AND CELLS

Diagnostic markers

Blood draw is much easier than lumbar puncture, therefore a peripheral biomarker would simplify biomarker measurement. Because the pathology of AD is restricted to the brain, and the blood compartment is considerably larger than the CSF space, a biomarker related to the pathology of AD is likely to be highly diluted and difficult to detect after passage from CSF to blood or urine. Some substances cross the blood–brain barrier in reverse, and can be measured in plasma. For example, over 95 per cent of the plasma content of 24S-h-cholesterol, a byproduct of sterol metabolism, originates from the brain. Plasma levels of this marker were minimally increased in AD in one study, but substantially overlapped with control levels. Tau is not detectable in the blood.

Levels of Aβ can be detected in plasma. It is unclear how much of the plasma pool of Aβ originates from clearance from CSF or from production by blood elements such as platelets or lymphocytes or by systemic cells. Studies of transgenic mouse models that progressively deposit Aβ in the brain suggest that plasma and CSF Aβ levels both decrease as more Aβ is deposited in the brain.[53] However, in humans there is no correlation between levels of Aβ40 or 42 in plasma and those in CSF.[54] Although mutations in the APP or presenilin genes lead to increased levels of plasma Aβ or selective increases in Aβ42, in CSF they are associated with decreased Aβ42, even presymptomatically in carriers of PS mutations.[55] Studies of plasma Aβ in AD have been inconsistent. In cross-sectional comparisons, levels of plasma Aβ40 and Aβ42 do not differ significantly between patients with AD or MCI or controls.[56] Levels increase with age[57] and with worsening renal function. In a population-based study of elderly individuals, those with baseline plasma Aβ42 levels in the highest quartile had a 4-fold increased risk of developing AD in the following two years, suggesting that plasma Aβ42 may be a predictor of late onset AD.[58] Levels of plasma Aβ42 are elevated in non-demented first degree relatives and extended family members of patients with AD, with heritability estimated as over 50 per cent, and plasma Aβ42 levels are being used as a quantitative trait in genetic linkage analyses.[58] Although plasma levels of Aβ are of unclear significance in diagnosis of AD, they can be used in treatment studies of secretase inhibitors. A recent study of a gamma secretase inhibitor found that there were dose-dependent decreases in plasma Aβ42 in patients with AD, but CSF Aβ42 did not change in response to treatment.[59]

A wide range of inflammatory markers can be measured in serum. As mentioned above, markers of inflammation such as α_1-ACT show a very slight increase in serum in AD, mainly in patients with advanced dementia. One research group has reported that the specific F2-isoprostane that was increased in CSF can be detected in plasma and urine, and is elevated in AD.[39]

Platelets contain high levels of APP, as well as the secretases needed to process Aβ. Altered ratios of forms of APP found in platelet membranes have been reported in Alzheimer's disease.[60,61] The APP ratios appear to distinguish very mild AD and MCI from controls and are correlated with dementia severity. It is unclear how platelets, which are short-lived and constantly renewed, show changes once AD begins in the brain, and further studies are needed to explain how the APP bands relate to APP and Aβ metabolism.

Predictive biomarkers

As noted above, plasma Aβ may indicate an increased risk of developing AD. Predictive markers are more difficult to study than diagnostic markers, because they require large-scale studies, with longitudinal follow-up and re-evaluation of participants who start out with normal cognition. A combination of risk factors, genetic profiles and biomarkers could provide a signature for individuals who are at higher risk of developing AD. This will facilitate earlier intervention, and could help to guide preventive treatments. Limited progress has been made to date in identifying biomarkers of risk, and some candidates have not stood up consistently to replication.

Homocysteine has received attention as a risk factor for atherosclerosis and vascular disease. An autopsy-based study reported that patients with AD had slightly higher plasma homocysteine levels during life than non-demented controls.[62] In the Framingham study, people with plasma homocysteine levels in the highest quartile had an over 2-fold increased risk of developing dementia when followed for up to eight years.[63] In a study that used MRI to distinguish patients with mild vascular changes from atrophy consistent with AD, increased homocysteine was associated with cerebrovascular disease but not with AD.[64] Homocysteine may need to be interpreted together with levels of B group vitamin.[65] In the Rotterdam study, serum levels of several cytokines were associated with increased risk of incident dementia.[66]

BIOMARKERS AND TREATMENT OF ALZHEIMER'S DISEASE

Biomarkers could be utilized at several stages of drug development for AD.[67] During early stages of drug development, biomarkers can indicate whether the drug hits relevant targets in the brain, and the relationship between drug doses and biological effects. Biomarkers have appeal as outcome measures in clinical trials, because there is less variability in their measurement than in standard clinical or psychometric measures. For a biomarker to be a valid surrogate marker for AD, it should be a substitute for a clinically meaningful endpoint that directly assesses a patient's abilities. To validate a biomarker in this way, a clinical trial will need to demonstrate efficacy of a treatment both on standard clinical measures and on biomarkers. Longitudinal studies of biomarkers in relation to the progression of AD provide data that could be used to interpret change in a treatment trial. For example, the extent of atrophy on volumetric measures of the brain in AD progresses to an extent that can be reliably and accurately measured over 12 months. CSF tau remains stably elevated over at least 12 months in AD. A treatment that achieves neuroprotection would be likely to lead to decreased CSF levels of tau over time, relative to a placebo.

FUTURE DIRECTIONS

As technical methods for analysis of proteins and other small molecules improve, there is great appeal to the strategy of analysing combinations of markers that may yield a signature for the diagnosis of AD, and can allow a variety of cellular processes to be tracked simultaneously. The utility of combining psychometric tests, imaging and biomarkers for diagnosis, very early diagnosis or prediction is receiving attention. Biomarkers are increasingly being used in treatment studies of novel agents in AD. As disease-modifying treatment evolves, early or predictive diagnosis and accurate ways to follow patients over time will gain importance, and are likely to bring biomarkers more clearly into the clinical arena.

ACKNOWLEDGEMENTS

This work was supported by a Merit Grant from the VA and by NIA grant AGO 5131.

REFERENCES

1. Consensus report of the Working Group on: 'Molecular and Biochemical Markers of Alzheimer's Disease'. The Ronald and Nancy Reagan Research Institute of the Alzheimer's Association and the National Institute on Aging Working Group. Neurobiol Aging. 1998; 19:109–116.

2. Petersen RC, Smith GE, Waring SC, et al. Mild cognitive impairment: clinical characterization and outcome. Arch Neurol 1999; 56:303–308.

3. DeCarli C. MIld cognitive imipairment: prevalence, prognosis, aetiology, and treatment. Lancet Neurol 2003; 2: 15–21.

4. Knopman DS, DeKosky ST, Cummings JL, et al. Practice parameter: diagnosis of dementia (an evidence-based review). Report on the Quality Standards Subcommittee of the American Academy of Neurology. Neurology 2001; 56: 1143–1153.

5. Lopez MF, Mikulskis A, Kuzdzal S, et al. High-resolution serum proteomic profiling of Alzheimer's disease samples reveals disease-specific, carrier-protein-bound mass signatures. Clin Chem 2005; 51:1946–1954.

6. Dickson DW. Neuropathology of Alzheimer's disease and other dementias. Clin Geriatr Med 2001; 17:209–228.

7. Lee VM, Goedert M, Trojanowski JQ. Neurodegenerative tauopathies. Ann Rev Neurosci 2001; 24:1121–1159.

8. Vandermeeren M, Mercken M, Vanmechelen E, et al. Detection of tau proteins in normal and Alzheimer's disease cerebrospinal fluid with a sensitive sandwich enzyme-linked immunosorbent assay. J Neurochem 1993; 61:1828–1834.

9. Motter R, Vigo-Pelfrey C, Kholodenko D, et al. Reduction of β-amyloid peptide42 in the cerebrospinal fluid of patients with Alzheimer's disease. Ann Neurol. 1995; 38:643–648.

10. Arai H, Terajima M, Miura M, et al. Tau in cerebrospinal fluid: a potential diagnostic marker in Alzheimer's disease. Ann Neurol. 1995; 38:649–652.

11. Andreasen N, Vanmechelen E, Van de Voorde A, et al. Cerebrospinal fluid tau protein as a biochemical marker for Alzheimer's disease: a community based follow up study. J Neurol Neurosurg Psychiatry 1998; 64:298–305.

12. Galasko D, Chang L, Motter R, et al. High cerebrospinal fluid tau and low amyloid beta42 levels in the clinical diagnosis of Alzheimer disease and relation to apolipoprotein E genotype. Arch Neurol 1998; 55:937–945.

13. Hulstaert F, Blennow K, Ivanoiu A, et al. Improved discrimination of AD patients using beta-amyloid (Aβ 1–42) and tau levels in CSF. Neurology 1999; 52:1555–1562.

14. Shoji M, Matsubara E, Murakami T, et al. Cerebrospinal fluid tau in dementia disorders: a large scale multicenter study by a Japanese study group. Neurobiol Aging 2002; 23:363–370.

15. Sunderland T, Linker G, Mirza M, et al. Decreased β-amyloid1-42 and increased tau levels in cerebrospinal fluid of patients with Alzheimer's disease. JAMA 2003; 289: 2094–2103.

16. Hesse C, Rosengren L, Andreasen N, et al. Transient increase in total tau but not phospho-tau in human cerebrospinal fluid after acute stroke. Neurosci Lett 2001; 297:187–190.

17. Otto M, Wiltfang J, Cepek L, et al. Tau protein and 14-3-3 protein in the differential diagnosis of Creutzfeldt–Jakob disease. Neurology 2002; 58:192–197.

18. Vanmechelen E, Vanderstichele H, Davidsson P, et al. Quantification of tau phosphorylated at threonine 181 in human cerebrospinal fluid: a sandwich ELISA with a synthetic phosphopeptide for standardization. Neurosci Lett 2000; 285:49–52.

19. Ishiguro K, Ohno H, Arai H, et al. Phosphorylated tau in human cerebrospinal fluid is a diagnostic marker for Alzheimer's disease. Neurosci Lett 1999; 270:91–94.

20. Kohnken R, Buerger K, Zinkowski R, et al. Detection of tau phosphorylated at threonine 231 in cerebrospinal fluid of Alzheimer's disease patients. Neurosci Lett 2000; 287: 187–190.

21. Hampel H, Buerger K, Zinkowski R, et al. Measurement of phosphorylated tau epitopes in the differential diagnosis of Alzheimer's Disease: a comparative cerebrospinal fluid study. Arch Gen Psychiatry 2004; 61:95–102.

22. Buerger K, Teipel SJ, Zinkowski Z, et al. CSF tau protein phosphorylated at threonine 231 correlates with cognitive decline in MCI subjects. Neurology 2002; 59:627–629.

23. Blennow K, Hampel H. CSF markers for incipient Alzheimer's disease. Lancet Neurol 2003; 2:605–613.

24. Vassar R, Citron M. Abeta-generating enzymes: recent advances in beta- and gamma-secretase research. Neuron 2000; 27:419–422.

25. Scheuner D, Eckman C, Jensen M, et al. Secreted amyloid beta-protein similar to that in the senile plaques of Alzheimer's disease is increased in vivo by the presenilin 1 and 2 and APP mutations linked to familial Alzheimer's disease. Nat Med 1996; 2:864–870.

26. Walsh DM, Klyubin I, Fadeeva JV, et al. Amyloid-beta oligomers: their production, toxicity and therapeutic inhibition. Biochem Soc Trans 2002; 30:552–557.

27. Schoonenboom NS, Mulder C, Van Kamp GJ. Amyloid beta 38, 40, and 42 species in cerebrospinal fluid: More of the same? Ann Neurol 2005; 58:139–142.

28. Prince JA, Zetterberg H, Andreasen N, et al. APOE epsilon4 allele is associated with reduced cerebrospinal fluid levels of Abeta42. Neurology 2004; 62:2116–2118.

29. Andreasen N, Hesse C, Davidsson P, et al. Cerebrospinal fluid beta-amyloid(1–42) in Alzheimer disease: differences between early- and late-onset Alzheimer disease and stability during the course of disease. Arch Neurol 1999; 56: 673–680.

30. Strozyk D, Blennow K, White LR, Launer LJ. CSF Abeta 42 levels correlate with amyloid-neuropathology in a population-based autopsy study. Neurology 2003; 60: 652–656.

31. Wiltfang J, Esselmann H, Bibl M, et al. Highly conserved and disease-specific patterns of carboxyterminally truncated abeta peptides 1–37/38/39 in addition to 1–40/42

in Alzheimer's disease and in patients with chronic neuroinflammation. J Neurochem 2002; 81:481–496.

32. Fagan AM, Younkin LH, Morris JC, et al. Differences in the Abeta 40/Abeta 42 ratio associated with cerebrospinal fluid lipoproteins as a function of apolipoprotein E genotype. Ann Neurol 2000; 48:201–210.

33. Roher AE, Palmer KC, Yurewicz EC, et al. Morphological and biochemical analyses of amyloid plaque core proteins purified from Alzheimer disease brain tissue. J Neurochem 1993; 61:1916–1926.

34. Vanderstichele H, De Meyer G. Amino-truncated beta-amyloid 42 peptides in cerebrospinal fluid and prediction of progression of mild cognitive impairment. Clin Chem 2005; 51:1650–1660.

35. Georganopoulou DG, Chang L, Nam JM, et al. Nanoparticle-based detection in cerebral spinal fluid of a pathogenic biomarker for Alzheimer's Disease. Proc Natl Acad Sci USA 2005; 102:2273–2276.

36. Andreasen N, Blennow K. CSF biomarkers for mild cognitive impairment and early Alzheimer's Disease. Clin Neurol Neurosurg 2005; 107:165–173.

37. Olsson A, Vanderstichele H, Andreasen N, et al. Simultaneous measurement of beta-amyloid(1–42), total tau, and phosphorylated tau (Thr181) in cerebrospinal fluid by the xMAP technology. Clin Chem 2005; 51:336–345.

38. Montine TJ, Markesbery WR, Morrow JD, Roberts LJ 2nd. Cerebrospinal fluid F2-isoprostane levels are increased in Alzheimer's disease. Ann Neurol 1998; 44:410–413.

39. Pratico D, Clark CM, Lee VM, et al. Increased 8,12-iso-iPF2alpha-VI in Alzheimer's disease: correlation of a noninvasive index of lipid peroxidation with disease severity. Ann Neurol 2000; 48:809–812.

40. Montine TJ, Kaye JA, Montine KS, et al. Cerebrospinal fluid Abeta42, tau, and f2-isoprostane concentrations in patients with Alzheimer disease, other dementias, and in age-matched controls. Arch Pathol Lab Med 2001; 125: 510–512.

41. Grossman M, Farmer J, Leight S, et al. Cerebrospinal fluid profile in frontotemporal dementia and Alzheimer's disease. Ann Neurol 2005; 57:721–729.

42. Han X, Fagan AM, Cheng H, et al. Cerebrospinal fluid sulfatide is decreased in subjects with incipient dementia. Ann Neurol 2003; 54:115–119.

43. Lutjohann D, Papassotiroplous A, Bjrokhem I, et al. Plasma 24S-hydroxycholesterol (cerebrosterol) is increased in Alzheimer and vascular demented patients. J Lipid Res 2000; 41:195–198.

44. Akiyama H, Barger S, Barnum S, et al. Inflammation and Alzheimer's disease. Neurobiol Aging 2000; 21:383–421.

45. DeKosky ST, M.D. I, Wang X, et al. Plasma and cerebrospinal fluid alpha1-antichymotrypsin levels in Alzheimer's disease: correlation with cognitive impairment. Ann Neurol 2003; 53:81–90.

46. Peskind ER, Griffin WS, Akama KT, et al. Cerebrospinal fluid S100B is elevated in the earlier stages of Alzheimer's disease. Neurochem Int 2001; 39:409–413.

47. Tarkowski E, Liljeroth AM, Nilsson A, et al. TNF gene polymorphism and its relation to intracerebral production of TNFalpha and TNFbeta in AD. Neurology 2000; 54:2077–2081.

48. Zetterberg H, Andreasen N, Blennow K. Increased cerebrospinal fluid levels of transforming growth factor-beta1 in Alzheimer's disease. Neurosci Lett 2004; 367:194–196.

49. Galimberti D, Schoonenboom NS, Scarpini E, et al. Chemokines in serum and cerebrospinal fluid of Alzheimer's Disease patients. Ann Neurol 2003; 53:547–548.

50. Kahle PJ, Jakowec M, Teipel SJ, et al. Combined assessment of tau and neuronal thread protein in Alzheimer's disease CSF. Neurology 2000; 54:1498–1504.

51. Rosengren LE, Karlsson JE, Karlsson JO, et al. Patients with amyotrophic lateral sclerosis and other neurodegenerative diseases have increased levels of neurofilament protein in CSF. J Neurochem 1996; 67:2013–2018.

52. Sjogren M, Blomberg M, Jonsson M, et al. Neurofilament protein in cerebrospinal fluid: a marker of white matter changes. J Neurosci Res 2001; 66:510–516.

53. Kawarabayashi T, Younkin LH, Saido TC, et al. Age-dependent changes in brain, CSF, and plasma amyloid beta protein in the Tg2576 transgenic mouse model of Alzheimer's disease. J Neurosci 2001; 21:372–381.

54. Mehta PD, Pirttila T, Patrick BA, et al. Amyloid beta protein 1–40 and 1–42 levels in matched cerebrospinal fluid and plasma from patients with Alzheimer disease. Neurosci Lett 2001; 304:102–106.

55. Moonis M, Swearer JM, Dayaw MP, et al. Familial Alzheimer disease: decreases in CSF Abeta42 levels precede cognitive decline. Neurology 2005; 65:323–325.

56. Fukumoto H, Tennis M, Locascio JJ, et al. Age but not diagnosis is the main predictor of plasma amyloid beta-protein levels. Arch Neurol 2003; 60:958–964.

57. Mayeux R, Tang MX, Jacobs DM, et al. Plasma amyloid beta-peptide 1–42 and incipient Alzheimer's disease. Ann Neurol 1999; 46:412–416.

58. Ertekin-Taner N, Graff-Radford N, Younkin LH, et al. Heritability of plasma amyloid beta in typical late-onset Alzheimer's disease pedigrees. Genet Epidemiol 2001; 21: 19–30.

59. Siemers E, Skinner M, Dean RA, et al. Safety, tolerability, and changes in amyloid beta concentrations after administration of a gamma-secretase inhibitor in volunteers. Clin Neuropharmacol 2005; 28:126–132.

60. Rosenberg RN, Baskin F, Fosmire JA, et al. Altered amyloid protein processing in platelets of patients with Alzheimer disease. Arch Neurol 1997; 54:139–144.

61. Padovani A, Pastorino L, Borroni B, et al. Amyloid precursor protein in platelets: a peripheral marker for the diagnosis of sporadic AD. Neurology 2001; 57:2243–2248.

62. Clarke R, Smith AD, Jobst KA, et al. Folate, vitamin B12, and serum total homocysteine levels in confirmed Alzheimer disease. Arch Neurol 1998; 55:1449–1455.

63. Seshadri S, Beiser A, Selhub J, et al. Plasma homocysteine as a risk factor for dementia and Alzheimer's disease. N Engl J Med 2002; 346:476–483.

64. Miller JW, Green R, Mungas DM, et al. Homocysteine, vitamin B6 and vascular disease in AD patients. Neurology 2002; 58:1471–1475.

65. Kado DM, Karlamangla AS, Huang MH, et al. Homocysteine versus the vitamins folate, B6 and B12 as predictors of cognitive function and decline in older high-functioning adults: MacArthur studies of successful aging. Am J Med 2005; 118:161–167.

66. Engelhart MJ, Geerlings MI, Meijer J, et al. Inflammatory proteins in plasma and the risk of dementia: The Rotterdam study. Arch Neurol 2004; 61:668–672.

67. Frank R, Hargreaves R. Clinical biomarkers in drug discovery and development. Nature Drug Disc 2003; 2:566–580.

III   Natural evolution

11

Natural decline and prognostic factors

Marie Sarazin, Nikki Horne and Bruno Dubois

Alzheimer's disease (AD) progresses at a variable rate, making it difficult to predict the length of delay for a patient to reach clinical milestones, such as the loss of autonomy, institutionalization or even death. The inherent interpatient variability in the disease course also reduces the accuracy with which one can predict the therapeutic response of a given patient. A better knowledge of the natural history of the disease may have important implications for patient care, for the development of interventions and for public health. We will review the current knowledge concerning the main factors that influence cognitive and functional decline in the major degenerative dementias: AD, dementia with Lewy bodies (DLB) and frontotemporal dementia (FTD).

ALZHEIMER'S DISEASE: COGNITIVE DECLINE AND RELATED FACTORS

Cognitive decline in AD

The most prominent feature of AD is the decline in cognitive functions. As AD pathology mainly affects cortical areas involved in memory and cognition (i.e. mesial temporal structures and neocortical associative areas), it is not surprising that cognitive changes can be considered as a marker of disease progression and severity.

Longitudinal studies have shown that the mean annual rate of progression of cognitive impairment is approximately 2–4 points when assessed with the Mini-Mental State Examination (MMSE),[1] 12 points with the Cambridge Cognitive Battery (CAMCOG)[2] and 8 points with the Alzheimer's Disease Assessment Scale–cognitive (ADAS-cog).[3] In clinical trials, patients with mild to moderate AD treated with placebo deteriorated by approximately 5–6 points on the ADAS-cog after one year.[4] Using the modified

MMSE,[5] Stern et al[3] found a mean rate of decline of 3.3 points per 6-month interval that gradually increased as scores dropped from the maximum score of 57 to 20, suggesting that the rate of deterioration is dependent upon baseline cognitive status. Indeed, both the ADAS-cog and the MMSE are less sensitive to change during the early and late stages of AD.[6] As a result, the rate of cognitive decline, as measured with these tests, is not distinctly linear over the entire disease course.[7] This does not signify that the disease progresses in a non-linear way, but rather indicates that current tests do not permit a linear assessment of cognitive domains and that a need exists for tests sensitive to the more severe stages of the disease.

Analysing the annual rate of change in a cohort of patients with AD, Galasko et al[8] found that the MMSE was less sensitive than the Mattis Dementia Rating Scale (Mattis DRS).[9] Performance on the MMSE showed a moderate floor effect and a slight ceiling effect, depending on initial MMSE score, whereas these effects were less prominent for the Mattis DRS. The pattern of MMSE decline was curvilinear. Interestingly, among patients who underwent brain examination, neuropathology of Lewy bodies plus AD (Lewy body variant) was associated with significantly faster cognitive decline.

Little is known about the rate of decline of specific cognitive domains or about their influence on disease severity. It is well recognized that a deficit in episodic memory is the earliest and most predominant cognitive manifestation in AD, a disease thus considered as a progressive amnesic dementia.[10] This is consistent with the precocious involvement of mesial temporal structures, as shown both by new neuro-imaging techniques[11] and by postmortem evidence.[12] Tounsi et al[13] used an episodic memory test with controlled encoding and selective reminding to establish the pattern of long-term episodic memory changes in AD. The authors described the memory pattern of AD as: (1) a very poor delayed free recall, (2) an incomplete improvement by cueing and (3) a high number of intrusions and false recognitions. This pattern, the so-called 'amnesic syndrome of the hippocampal type',[13] is highly suggestive of AD and markedly differs from that of other dementing illnesses.[14] Galasko et al[8] found that delayed recall scores of the MMSE and the Mattis DRS had a very early floor effect in longitudinal studies, indicating that this pattern of episodic memory deficit is observed early in the disease course. Semantic memory impairment is an early feature of AD,[15] possibly arising even before impairment in attentional processing.[16] Aside from memory, aspects of attention and executive function showed the greatest deficit in a longitudinal study.[17] Attentional deficits became apparent after episodic memory impairment and before deficits in visuoperceptual function.[16–18] As the disease progresses, patients demonstrate marked impairments in expressive and receptive language, in the ability to plan and organize activities and in virtually all aspects of cognition.[19]

The follow-up of autosomal dominantly inherited familial AD provides an opportunity to improve our knowledge of the evolution of cognitive deficits from early diagnosis. Godbolt et al[20] followed 19 familial AD patients over a 10-year period (mean duration 5 years). Initial symptoms began very insidiously, sometimes several years before the subjects met accepted criteria for the diagnosis of AD, and were characterized by an impairment of verbal and visual episodic memory. Only formal neuropsychological assessment was able to detect these early memory changes. Additional deficits in other cognitive domains occurred significantly later with a decrease in the MMS score, followed by difficulties for calculation, visuoperceptual and visuospatial skills, naming and then for spelling.

Cognitive performance may predict disease severity in AD. Previous studies have suggested that linguistic deficits, particularly lexical and semantic impairment, are associated with a negative prognosis, thus predicting a rapid illness course and faster cognitive decline.[21–24] More recently, it has been proposed that the relative performance on verbal versus visuoconstructive tasks may predict the rate of decline in AD patients,[25] with lower scores in non-verbal neuropsychological tests predicting a faster progression of functional decline.[25,26] In the early stages of the disease, verbal memory tests, mental control abilities and attention-demanding tasks may help to identify fast decliners as defined by MMSE score decline.[27] Impaired cognitive functions are also correlated with the appearance or exacerbation of behavioural disturbances. For example, impaired fluency, attentional deficits and a low score of construction have been associated with the manifestation of psychotic symptoms.[28–30]

Influence of age

Although debated,[25,26] a young age at onset is generally correlated with faster rates of decline.[22,31,32] More specifically, AD patients with an early onset (before age 65) seem to have a more rapid rate of cognitive decline on the mMMSE when compared to patients with a later disease onset,[33] even after controlling for baseline mMMSE scores. It should be noted that age at onset of the disease might have an additional influence on the pattern of cognitive dysfunction. Jacobs et al[33] found early-onset AD patients to have a distinct cognitive profile characterized by a predominant impairment of attentional skills, whereas late-onset patients scored significantly lower on memory and naming tests.

Influence of motor symptoms

Some motor symptoms can be observed in the course of AD. These symptoms consist of changes in muscular tonus (hypertonia, paratonia or gegenhalten), cogwheel phenomenon, postural instability and gait disorders, slowed speech, myoclonus, etc. Although gathered under the name of 'extrapyramidal signs,' these motor symptoms never comprise a true parkinsonian syndrome, which typically consists of unilateral onset, akineto-rigid syndrome and resting tremor with a good response to levodopa. In addition, extrapyramidal signs rarely respond to levodopa in AD, and their relation to the basal ganglia is far from being demonstrated. Little is known about the progression of these signs. In a cohort study spanning 4 years,[34] extrapyramidal signs progressed rapidly during follow-up, but the rate of progression of these signs, such as bradykinesia, rigidity, gait disorder/postural reflex impairment and tremor, was highly variable across individuals and was not strongly related to the use of neuroleptic medications. Rate of annual change was 4.5 per cent for bradykinesia, 6 per cent for rigidity and 8.9 per cent for gait disorder/postural reflex impairment, and these symptoms were positively correlated. In contrast, tremor was minimal and was confined to postural tremor. Older age was correlated with higher baseline levels of each symptom except tremor, but age was not related to the rate of change. These data were confirmed in a second cohort of early AD followed semi-annually for up to 13.1 years (mean 3.6 years), in which not all motor signs behaved similarly during the course of illness.[35] Resting tremor was less frequent. Motor signs were relatively uncommon at the initial evaluation, but their prevalence increased as the disease progressed (from 3–6 per cent at the first visit to 22–29 per cent at the last visit).

Some longitudinal studies have found the presence of extrapyramidal signs to be indicative of a higher relative risk of reaching moderate cognitive severity.[5,36–39] In all these studies, patients with extrapyramidal signs tend to have a more rapid decline. In a prospective cohort study over a 4-year period,[40] higher levels of parkinsonism at baseline evaluation were reliably associated with lower levels of cognitive function and with faster cognitive decline, without differences in cognitive measures such as repetition, naming, visuoconstruction and memory. A much stronger correlation, however, was found between rates of change in parkinsonism and cognitive function. In fact, the presence of motor signs during the course of AD is associated with a higher risk of important outcomes such as cognitive decline, functional decline, institutionalization and death, even after control for additional covariates, including comorbid disease.[41] This is not surprising because the presence of motor signs testifies for a more diffuse process that invades the neural network involved in motor control, which is normally only marginally impaired in AD, at least until the late stages. Myoclonus alone has been shown to be a significant predictor of a more rapid disease course and of severe cognitive impairment,[5,38,42] although some longitudinal studies did not find the same relationships.[25,43]

Influence of behavioural and psychotic symptoms

Behavioural and psychological symptoms of dementia (BPSD) include depression, apathy, agitation, aggressivity and sleep disruption, as well as psychotic symptoms such as delusions and hallucinations. The prevalence of psychosis and behavioural disturbance increases with disease progression and may herald a poor prognosis.[36,44] In a longitudinal study, Paulsen et al[28] showed that the cumulative incidence of hallucinations and delusions was 20.1 per cent at 1 year, 36.1 per cent at 2 years, 49.5 per cent at 3 years and 51.3 per cent at 4 years. Half of the patients manifested hallucinations or delusions within the 4-year follow-up. Moreover, the severity of cognitive impairment, the rate of cognitive decline and the emergence of gait disorders were predictive of psychotic symptoms. In another longitudinal study, agitation occurred in up to

half of the patients with AD, whereas physical aggression was less common.[45–46] Misidentification delusions doubled in frequency during the 3-year follow-up.[46] Hallucinations are more often visual than auditory. Rarely an early manifestation of the disease, such hallucinations are more common in severe dementia.[46]

Estimates of the prevalence of psychotic symptoms in AD vary widely, from 10 per cent[47] to 73 per cent.[48] This heterogeneity may be due to the fact that BPSD have no regular progression during the course of the illness, but rather periods of exacerbation and remission of the symptoms.[7] The levels of BPSD, especially those of psychosis, depression and agitation, tend to fluctuate over time, resulting in distinct individual differences.[49] Physical aggression, however, may show greater persistence in more advanced stages.[45,46] In a longitudinal study following 60 patients over a period of 2 years, Devanand et al[46] reported that BPSD, specifically misidentification, wandering/agitation and physical aggression, increased during follow-up, and both the frequency and the persistence of symptoms varied. Behavioural disturbances, particularly agitation, were common and persistent during follow-up. Psychotic symptoms were less common and showed moderate persistence over time. In summary, agitation was present in every patient within this period, depression and agitation were both the most common and the most persistent symptoms, anxiety and aggressivity were less persistent and delusions or hallucinations occurred temporarily. In this study, the use of psychotropic medications did not significantly increase the likelihood of symptom persistence.

Depression has a different rate of progression and prevalence than psychosis. Between 10 and 30 per cent of patients with AD meet the diagnostic criteria for major depression, but depression does not seem to be characteristic of any particular stage of the illness.[46,50,51] In a longitudinal study of depression in AD, the prevalence of depressed mood did not change during the 3-year follow-up.[46] In a 1-year prospective study, depression tended to have a duration of 1–5 months, while patients with psychotic symptoms experienced resolution of their symptoms that lasted less than 3 months.[52] Starkstein et al[53] studied the longitudinal course of depression in AD over a period of 2 years. Dysthymia, based on DSM-III-R criteria, was a brief emotional disorder, while the majority of AD patients with major depression (58 per cent) experienced a longer-lasting mood change that persisted over the mean follow-up of 16 months.

Evidence exists that BPSD influence the rate of disease progression. The presence of psychotic symptoms at baseline is strongly and independently predictive of a more rapid decline in mMMSE score and is correlated with an exacerbation of cognitive impairment greater than that of patients without psychotic symptoms.[45,54–56] Among behavioural changes, psychosis and aggressivity are associated with a more rapid rate of cognitive progression.[25,31,57,58] For example, mMMSE scores declined 1.15 points more per 6-month interval among patients with psychosis.[38] Although correlations have been found between BPSD and a more rapid decline,[38,42,45,54–56] McShane et al[59] reported that the association of cognitive decline with psychotic symptoms might be secondary to neuroleptic treatment. Moreover, the frequency and severity of BPS are not strongly correlated with the severity of cognitive and functional impairment.[46,60]

In another way, Hotzler et al[61] examined the course and prevalence of psychopathological features in relation to cognitive status in a cohort study with a 5 year follow-up, and concluded there is a strong association between cognitive dysfunction and the presence of wandering/agitation, psychotic symptoms and physical aggression. Wandering/agitation increased as a function of time and decrement in cognitive function. With time, physical aggression tended to be less frequent and persisted only in the more severely impaired patients. Delusions were maximal with intermediate decline, but remained persistent regardless of cognitive status. Hallucinations were moderately persistent.

Influence of the apolipoprotein ε4 allele (apoε4)

Some studies have failed to show a relationship between apoε4 and cognitive changes, although potential limitations came from the use of the MMSE and the relatively small sample sizes.[62] In other studies, apoε4 was associated with a less aggressive form of AD: the rate of decline on the MMSE was slower.[38] In the late-onset form of the disease, progression, as assessed by changes in global rating scales, was slower in apoεγ homozygotes than heterozygotes, and heterozygotes progressed more slowly than patients with other genotypes.[63] In contrast, in a cohort of over 200 patients followed for an average of 2.4 years, patients with two ε4 alleles declined fastest.[8]

ALZHEIMER'S DISEASE: FUNCTIONAL DETERIORATION AND RELATED FACTORS

Functional decline and nursing home entry

Functional impairment increases with disease progression.[7] In clinical trials, the Disability Assessment for Dementia (DAD) was used to assess the instrumental and basic Activities of Daily Living (ADL) of placebo-treated patients, who deteriorated 2.4–3.5 points from baseline during 5 months of follow-up.[64] Over 12 months on placebo, the decrease in DAD score in mild to moderate AD was 11–13 points.[4] Using the Blessed Dementia Rating Scale (BPRS),[38,65] the mean change in functional decline was 1.20 points per 6-month interval. The IADL and the BDRS assess more demanding cognitive activities than the basic ADL. These scales are thus more sensitive to functional impairment in the early stages of AD,[6] and may be more useful than the basic ADL in longitudinal studies.[7] Indeed, longitudinal data showed that patients could be severely impaired before they exhibit substantial deficits in their basic activities, as measured by the basic ADL activities described in the Physical and Self-Maintenance Scale.[66,67]

There is an increased risk of mortality of 40 per cent in the elderly population with AD, especially in women, as shown by Ganguli et al[68] in a 15-year followed-up and prospective study in Pennsylvania. The mean survival was 5.9 years (SD = 3.7 years), but it was mainly related to age at onset. Others studies have shown shorter survival times.[69]

Despite numerous advances in the knowledge of AD, researchers remain unable to predict the length of time from disease onset to nursing home entry or death. A prospective community-based cohort reported a median time of 5.6 years from the estimated onset of the disease to placement,[70] whereas in a retrospective study the median time was only 2.67 years.[71] In a community-based dementia cohort, Smith et al[72] reported that 40 per cent of the patients were placed in a nursing home during follow-up. Median time from diagnosis to placement was 5.3 years. Placement rates of approximately 10 per cent per year in the 4 to 6 years following initial diagnosis can be expected. Clinical parameters, such as cognition, behaviour, demographic factors and motor symptoms, may influence the rate of functional decline.

Influence of cognition

Functional decline is highly correlated with the severity of cognitive impairment, though this depends on the scales used and on the stage of disease.[7] The rate of functional decline has been shown to be slower for mildly and severely demented patients than for patients with moderate dementia.[73,74] Initial global cognitive status is a significant baseline predictor of time to institutionalization. Level of cognitive impairment, assessed by MMSE, mMMSE or Clinical Dementia Rating (CDR), was a significant risk factor for nursing home placement across all studies that assessed this variable.[22,31,70–72,75] For example, higher mMMSE scores were associated with a reduced risk of placement.[31] In addition, level of functional assistance need[22,76,77] and change in level of assistance[70,71] were significant risk factors for placement.

In a cohort study, the influence of cognitive predictors on loss of autonomy in everyday life was studied in 252 patients with probable AD.[78,79] All patients were seen at 6-month intervals. Cognitive functions were assessed with the mMMSE, which included several additional subtests for a maximum score of 57. The subitems were grouped to cover specific cognitive domains: long-term memory (total score of 8), short-term memory (total score of 20), temporo-spatial memory (total score of 10), language (total score of 17) and construction (total score of 2). Functional capacity was rated with the BDRS[80] and the patient's need for care with the Dependency Scale and the Equivalent Institutional Care. Level of dependency was assessed by the Dependency Scale, which rates the patient's need for care. It is based on interview data and summarises the interviewer's impression of the care the patient received and required, regardless of location. Maximum score is 5. The Equivalent Institutional Care was established from the second section of the Dependency Scale. Categories include limited home care, adult home (a supervised setting with regular assistance in most activities), and health-related facility. Maximal score is 3. Previous studies have demonstrated the robust validity of these scales.[3] Using Cox analyses, global cognitive efficiency, as measured by the total mMMSE[5] score, was associated with an elevated risk of partial or complete loss of autonomy. The analysis of specific neuropsychological domains revealed that temporo-spatial orientation and short-term memory were significantly associated with a greater relative risk of moderate or severe dependency, whereas long-term memory and language were not correlated with the risk of reaching this end point or equivalent institution care. The visuoconstructive score predicted the development of severe dependency. Therefore, the performances in the different cognitive domains assessed with a common scale such as the mMMSE have different weights in terms of predictive power.

Influence of behaviour

As discussed earlier, behavioural symptoms, specifically psychosis and aggressivity, are associated with a faster rate of functional disease progression.[25,31,36,56,57] Furthermore, behavioural symptoms are also correlated with an increased incidence of institutionalization. In a prospective cohort study, the relative risk of need for care equivalent to nursing home placement was increased in patients who had psychotic symptoms at the initial visit.[31,81] Though the presentation of BPSD contributes to premature institutionalization,[31,82,83] quantitative measures of disruptive behaviour assessed by the hallucinations/delusions, aggressions and total scores of the Neuropsychiatric Inventory were not significant risk factors. The ability of caregivers to tolerate disruptive behaviours reduces the likelihood of nursing home placement.[72]

Influence of demographic factors

When compared with a later onset of the disease, early-onset AD was associated with a faster functional decline on the BDRS scale, even after controlling for baseline score.[33] Demographic factors included marital status,[70] age, education, being widowed[71] and gender.[72] In some studies, men have a reduced risk for placement when compared to women, whereas other studies showed that male gender is a positive predictor of nursing home admission and death.[75,84] In a prospective cohort study, the relative risk of the need for care equivalent to nursing home placement was higher for early-onset AD patients.[31] Moreover, survival with early-onset AD increased for patients with at least one E4 allele when compared to patients with other alleles,[85] while time from onset to death was not strongly related to E4 gene dose.[86]

Influence of motor symptoms

Extrapyramidal signs in AD appear to be related to morbidity and mortality.[3,31] In a longitudinal study, Stern et al[3] demonstrated that the presence of extrapyramidal signs was associated with a more rapid increase in BDRS scores. At each 6-month interval, BDRS scores increased an additional 0.59 points in patients with motor symptoms compared to those without. The presence of motor symptoms at the first visit was correlated with a higher relative risk of reaching nursing home entry or death.[3,31] Comorbidity, as rated at initial evaluation, is not a reliable predictor of time to placement,[72] whereas change in medical comorbidity index is considered a significant risk factor.[71] Myoclonus is also a significant predictor of functional impairment, as determined by scoring 15 or more on the BDRS,[3] and it is ultimately a predictor of disease course and death.[31]

DEMENTIA WITH LEWY BODIES

DLB is the second most common neurodegenerative dementia, accounting for 10 to 20 per cent of dementia cases.[87] Typically, patients with DLB have progressive dementia, characterized by fluctuating cognitive states that include periods of worsening confusion and persistent visual hallucinations. According to a review by Lennox[88] and a meta-analysis by Cercy and Bylsma,[89] the mean duration of survival in patients with pure DLB (without concomitant AD pathology at autopsy) is approximately 6 years after the onset of symptoms. In a review of the literature, Walker et al[90] reported that the mean age at disease onset varied between 59 and 79 years and that the disease duration ranged from 1.8 to 9.5 years. Past studies suggested that the mean duration of illness was shorter in DLB patients than in AD patients,[87,91–93] although more recently no difference has been found.[94–96] This might be due to a greater awareness in recent years of the negative side effects of neuroleptics in patients with DLB, thus contributing to a decrease in their prescription and to an increase in survival.[97]

Little is known about the rate of progression of cognitive impairment in DLB or about the factors associated with an accelerated decline. Only five prospective clinical studies have analysed the rate of cognitive decline in DLB.[1,2,98–100] Some of these studies suggested that patients with DLB might decline more rapidly than patients with AD.[2,100] Ballard et al[2] found that patients with DLB experienced a mean decline of 27 points on the CAMCOG in 1 year, compared with a mean decline of 13 points in patients with AD. Moreover, patients with DLB had a significantly greater decline of verbal fluency than the AD group. This difference in rate of cognitive decline, however, may also be related to the finding that DLB patients experience severe neuroleptic reactions, which include rapid cognitive decline.[91] Most recent studies suggest that AD and DLB have similar rates of cognitive decline. In a 3-year follow-up of a cohort of patients with dementia, no evidence indicated that the prognosis of clinically diagnosed DLB patients was worse than that of patients with AD.[90] There was no difference between groups in age at onset, age at death or survival. In a prospective study, Ballard et al[1] reported a similar rate of cognitive decline over 1 year in AD, DLB and vascular dementia. The annual decline for the three dementias was 4–5 points on the MMMS and 12–14 points on the CAMCOG. This study, however, only reported follow-up during 1 year and cannot be extrapolated to longer periods of time. The presence of an apolipoprotein E4 allele appears to be a risk factor for accelerated decline in DLB, influencing the mean annual decline by >3 points on the CAMCOG.[1]

The modified Unified Parkinson's Disease Rating Scale was used to evaluate the progression of parkinsonism over 1 year of follow-up in a prospective cohort of patients suffering from DLB or AD.[101] As expected, parkinsonism was significantly more common in DLB patients (71 per cent) than among patients with AD (7 per cent). In the DLB group, parkinsonism had an annual increase in severity of 9 per cent. The speed of progression was much more rapid in patients who presented with parkinsonism early in the disease course. Parkinsonism was frequent at all severities in DLB patients, but usually present in AD patients when MMSE <10. These results indicate that there may be a difference between early-onset DLB, marked by a rapid decline and parkinsonism, and the more commonly occurring later-onset disease, which is characterized by frequent concomitant Alzheimer's type pathology.[92]

Few data are available regarding the natural course of psychotic symptoms in DLB. Longitudinal studies have suggested that visual hallucinations are significantly more likely to be persistent in dementia with DLB.[102–105] In one study,[105] 77 per cent of 82 DLB patients and 26 per cent of 132 AD patients continued to experience visual hallucinations 1 year after the initial evaluation. In addition, DLB patients were more likely to develop new auditory hallucinations during the follow-up period. Differences in the frequency of delusions between DLB and AD may diminish over the course of the illness.[104] Psychosis does not appear to predict accelerated decline in DLB patients.[105]

FRONTOTEMPORAL DEMENTIA

Several studies have characterized the clinical features that distinguish FTD and AD patients. The core diagnostic features of FTD include early and severe behavioural disorders, speech reduction, frontal dysfunction at neuropsychological testing with preservation of spatial orientation and praxis, normal EEG and predominant frontal or anterior temporal abnormality on imaging.

Few studies have examined the rate of clinical and cognitive decline in FTD. Rascovsky et al[106] reported a faster rate of cognitive decline in patients with FTD as compared to those with AD when measured with the Mattis DRS during 1 year. Mean annual decline was 34 points for FTD and 16.9 points for AD. The difference was particularly pronounced for the conceptualization subscale of the test. In contrast, there were no differential rates of decline on the MMSE. In fact, these discrepancies are not surprising because the Mattis DRS mainly assesses executive functions whereas the MMSE investigates retro-rolandic functions.

In a cohort study with a follow-up of 2–6 years, FTD manifested early behavioural changes with relatively stable global cognition.[107] Behavioural disorders evolved with time, but restlessness and hyperorality were long lasting. Verbal disinhibition decreased with the reduction of speech. However, neither global cognitive scales nor so-called frontal tests were pertinent tools to assess the rate of progression of the disease. The mean MMSE and Mattis DRS scores decreased after 2 years, by 2.3 points and 2.6 points respectively, with important individual variations. Loss of autonomy, related to behavioural changes, appears early in the disease course and remains stable until the late stages. It is therefore not a good item to use to follow the rate of progression in FTD patients. Gregory[108] used the Comprehensive Psychopathological Rating Scale (CPRS) to assess five FTD patients over 3 years.

These patients exhibited a variety of symptom patterns, which did not progress over time. Fronto-temporal dementia covers both the temporal variant of FTD and the frontal variant of FTD. There are no follow-up data regarding this distinction.

In a cohort of 552 patients, Pasquier et al[109] showed that the mean duration of FTD was 2 years longer than AD, but the risk of death after adjustment for age and sex was similar. FTD patients had a longer delay between first symptoms and first visit than AD patients. The mean annual MMSE score decline was 0.9 point.

CONCLUSIONS

Interest in factors that predict and influence rates of cognitive and functional decline in patients with AD has increased. Demographic data such as young age of onset as well as early presence of clinical signs such as extrapyramidal features, behavioural symptoms and global cognitive deficits, are predictors of more rapid decline in AD (Table 11.1). Few data are available in other types of dementia. In future research it would be beneficial to better understand the combined effects of all predictors described in AD in order to better inform and help patients and families to prepare for care.

Table 11.1 Prognostic factors in Alzheimer's disease on the rate of cognitive and functional decline

	Measures of severity	
	Cognitive decline	Functional decline
Prognostic factors		
Young age	Heyman et al 1987[22]	Stern et al 1997[31]
	Rasmusson et al 1996[32]	
	Jacobs et al 1994[33]	
Motor symptoms		
Extrapyramidal signs	Mayeux et al 1985[5]	Stern et al 1994[3]
	Stern et al 1987[36]	Stern et al 1997[31]
	Soininen et al 1992[37]	Scarmeas et al 2005[41]
	Stern et al 1994[38]	
	Richards et al 1995[39]	
	Wilson et al 2000[40]	
Myoclonus	Mayeux et al 1985[5]	Mayeux et al 1985[5]
	Stern et al 1994[38]	Stern et al 1994[3]
	Chui et al 1994[42]	Stern et al 1997[31]
		Stern et al 1994[38]
		Chui et al 1994[42]
Behavioural and psychotic symptoms		
Psychotic symptoms	Stern et al 1994[38]	Mortimer et al 1992[25]
	Chui et al 1994[42]	Stern et al 1997[31]
	Devanand et al 1992[45]	Stern et al 1987[36]
	Jeste et al 1992[54]	Levy et al 1996[56]
	Gilley et al 1991[55]	Mega et al 1996[57]
	Levy et al 1996[56]	Steele et al 1990[81]
	Mortimer et al 1992[25]	
	Stern et al 1997[31]	
	Mega et al 1996[57]	
	Lopez et al 1999[58]	
Aggressivity	Mortimer et al 1992[25]	Mortimer et al 1992[25]
	Stern et al 1997[31]	Stern et al 1997[31]
	Mega et al 1996[57]	Stern et al 1987[36]
	Lopez et al 1999[58]	Levy et al 1996[56]
	Holtzer et al 2003[61]	Mega et al 1996[57]
Neuropsychological factors		
Initial global cognitive impairment		Heyman et al 1987[22]
		Holtzer et al 2003[61]
		Severson et al 1994[70]
		Smith et al 2000[71]
		Smith et al 2001[72]
		Heyman et al 1997[75]
Short term memory, temporospatial disorientation, visuo-constructive score		Sarazin et al 2005[79]

REFERENCES

1. Ballard C, O'Brien JT, Morris CM, et al. The progression of cognitive impairment in dementia with Lewy bodies, vascular dementia and AD. Int Psychogeriatr 2001; 16: 499–503.
2. Ballard C, Patel A, Oyebode F, Wilcock G. Cognitive decline in patients with Alzheimer's disease, vascular dementia and senile dementia of Lewy body type. Age Ageing 1996; 25: 209–13.
3. Stern Y, Albert M, Brandt J, et al. Utility of extrapyramidal signs and psychosis as predictors of cognitive and functional decline, nursing home admission, and death in Alzheimer's disease: prospective analyses from the Predictors Study. Neurology 1994; 44:2300–2307.
4. Torfs K, Feldman H on behalf of the Sabeluzole Study Groups. 12-month decline in cognitive and daily function in patients with mild to moderate Alzheimer's disease: two randomized, placebo-controlled studies. Presented at World Alzheimer Congress Washington, DC, USA, 9–13 July, 2000.
5. Mayeux R, Stern Y, Spanton S. Heterogeneity in dementia of the AD type: evidence of subgroups. Neurology 1985; 35: 53–61.
6. Tariot PN. Maintaining cognitive function in Alzheimer disease: how effective are current treatments? Alzheimer Dis Assoc Disord 2001; 15:S26–S33.
7. Mohs RC, Schmeidler J, Aryan M. Longitudinal studies of cognitive, functional and behavioral change in patients with Alzheimer's disease. Stat Med 2000; 19:1401–1409.
8. Galasko DR, Gould RL, Abramson IS, Salmon DP. Measuring cognitive change in a cohort of patients with Alzheimer's disease. Stat Med 2000; 19:1421–1432.
9. Mattis S. Dementia rating scale. Odessa, Florida. Psychological Assessment Resources 1986.
10. Weintraub S, Mesulam MM. Four neuropsychological profiles in dementia. In: Bohen F, Grafman J, eds. Handbook of Neuropsychology. Amsterdam: Elsevier 1993 253–282.
11. Fox NC, Warrington EK, Rossor MN. Serial magnetic resonance imaging of cerebral atrophy in preclinical Alzheimer's disease. Lancet 1999; 353:2125.
12. Braak H, Del Tredici K, Schultz C, Braak E. Vulnerability of select neuronal types to Alzheimer's disease. Ann NY Acad Sci 2000; 924:53–61.
13. Tounsi H, Deweer B, Ergis AM, et al. Sensitivity to semantic cuing: an index of episodic memory dysfunction in early Alzheimer disease. Alzheimer Dis Assoc Disord 1999; 13: 38–46.
14. Pillon B, Dubois B, Agid Y. Cognitive deficits in non-Alzheimer's degenerative diseases. J Neural Transm 1996; 47:61–71.
15. Hodges JR, Patterson K. Is semantic memory consistently impaired early in the course of Alzheimer's disease? Neuroanatomical and diagnostic implications. Neuropsychologia 1995; 33:441–459.
16. Perry RJ, Hodges JR. Fate of patients with questionable (very mild) Alzheimer's disease: longitudinal profiles of individual subjects' decline. Dement Geriatr Cogn Disord 2000; 11:342–349.
17. Reid W, Broe G, Creasey H, et al. Age at onset and pattern of neuropsychological impairment in mild early-stage Alzheimer disease. A study of a community-based population. Arch Neurol 1996; 53:1056–1061.
18. Grady CL, Haxby JV, Horwitz B, et al. Longitudinal study of the early neuropsychological and cerebral metabolic changes in dementia of the Alzheimer type. J Clin Exp Neuropsychol 1988; 10:576–596.
19. Welsh KA, Butters N, Hughes JP, Mohs RC, Heyman A. Detection and staging of dementia in Alzheimer's disease. Use of the neuropsychological measures developed for the Consortium to Establish a Registry for Alzheimer's Disease. Arch Neurol 1992; 49:448–452.
20. Godbolt AK, Cipolotti L, Watt H, et al. The natural history of Alzheimer disease: a longitudinal presymptomatic and symptomatic study of a familial cohort. Arch Neurol 2004; 61:1743–1748.
21. Boller F, Becker JT, Holland AL, et al. Predictors of decline in AD. Cortex 1991; 27:9–17.
22. Heyman A, Wilkinson WE, Hurwitz BJ, et al. Early onset AD: clinical predictors of institutionalization and death. Neurology 1987; 37:980–984.
23. Huff J, Growdon JH, Corkin S, Rosen TJ. Age at onset and rate of progression of AD. J Am Geriatr Soc 1987; 35:27–30.
24. Knesewich JW, LaBarge E, Edwards D. Predictive value of the Boston Naming Test in mild senile dementia of the AD type. Psychiatry Res 1986; 19:155–161.
25. Mortimer JA, Ebbitt B, Jun SP, Finch MD. Predictors of cognitive and functional progression in patients with probable Alzheimer's disease. Neurology 1992; 42:1689–1696.
26. Drachman DA, O'Donnel B, Lew RA, Swearer JM. The prognosis of AD: how far and how fast best predicts the course. Arch Neurol 1990; 43:851–856.
27. Marra C, Silverini MC, Gainotti G. Predictors of cognitive decline in the early probable Alzheimer's disease. Dement Geriatr Cogn Disord 2000; 11:212–218.
28. Paulsen JS, Salmon DP, Thal LJ. Incidence of and risk factors for hallucinations and delusions in patients with probable AD. Neurology 2000; 54:1965–1971.
29. Lopez OL, Becker JT, Brenner RP, et al. Alzheimer's disease with delusions and hallucinations: neuropsychological and electroencephalographic correlates. Neurology 1991; 41: 906–912.
30. Bylsma F, Folstein M, Devanand D, et al. Delusions and patterns of cognitive impairment in Alzheimer's disease. Neuropsychiatry Neuropsychol Behav Neurol 1994; 7:98–103.
31. Stern Y, Tang MX, Albert MS, et al. Predicting time to nursing home care and death in individuals with Alzheimer disease. JAMA 1997; 277:806–812.
32. Rasmusson DX, Carson KA, Brookmeyer R, Kawas C, Brandt J. Predicting rate of cognitive decline in probable Alzheimer's disease. Brain Cogn 1996; 31:133–147.
33. Jacobs D, Sano M, Marder K, et al. Age at onset of Alzheimer's disease: relation to pattern of cognitive dysfunction and rate of decline. Neurology 1994; 44:1215–1220.
34. Wilson RS, Bennet DA, Gilley DW, et al. Progression of parkinsonian signs in AD. Neurology 2000; 54:1284–1289.
35. Scarmeas N, Hadjigeorgiou GM, Papadimitriou A, et al. Motor signs during the course of Alzheimer disease. Neurology 2004; 63:975–982.
36. Stern Y, Mayeux R, Sano M, Hauser WA, Bush T. Predictors of disease course in patients with probable Alzheimer's disease. Neurology 1987; 37:1649–1653.
37. Soininen H, Helkala EL, Laulumaa V, et al. Cognitive profile of Alzheimer patients with extrapyramidal signs: a longitudinal study. J Neural Transm Park Dis Dement 1992; 4: 241–254.
38. Stern RG, Mohs RC, Davidson M, et al. A longitudinal study of Alzheimer's disease: measurement, rate, and predictors of cognitive deterioration. Am J Psychiatry 1994; 151:390–396.
39. Richards M, McLoughlin D, Levy R. The relationship between extrapyramidal signs and cognitive function in patients with moderate to severe AD. Int J Geriatr Psychiary 1995; 10:395–399.

40. Wilson RS, Bennet DA, Gilley DW, et al. Progression of parkinsonism and loss of cognitive function in AD. Arch Neurol 2000; 57:855–860.

41. Scarmeas N, Albert M, Brandt J, et al. Motor signs predict poor outcomes in Alzheimer disease. Neurology 2005; 64: 1696–1703.

42. Chui HC, Lyness SA, Sobel E, Schneider LS. Extrapyramidal signs and psychiatric symptoms predict faster cognitive decline in Alzheimer's disease. Arch Neurol 1994; 51: 676–681.

43. Lopez O, Wisniewski S, Becker J, Boller F, Dekosky S. Extrapyramidal signs in patients with probable AD. Arch Neurol 1997; 54:969–975.

44. Rosen RC. Sleep and sexual function in the elderly male. Biol Psychiatry 1991; 30:1–3.

45. Devanand DP, Miller L, Richards M, et al. The Columbia University Scale for Psychopathology in Alzheimer's disease. Arch Neurol 1992; 49:371–376.

46. Devanand DP, Jacobs DM, Tang MX, et al. The course of psychopathologic features in mild to moderate Alzheimer's disease. Arch Gen Psychiatry 1997; 54:257–263.

47. Birkett DP. The psychiatric differentiation of senility and arteriosclerosis. Br J Psychiatry 1972; 120:321–325.

48. Leuchter AF, Spar JE. The late-onset psychoses. Clinical and diagnostic features, J Nerv Ment Dis 1985; 173:488–494.

49. Marin DB, Green CR, Schmeidler J, et al. Noncognitive disturbances in Alzheimer's disease: frequency, longitudinal course, and relationship to cognitive symptoms. J Am Geriatr Soc 1997; 45:1331–1338.

50. Ballard CG, Cassidy G, Bannister C, Mohan RN. Prevalence, symptom profile, and aetiology of depression in dementia sufferers. J Affect Disord 1993; 29:1–6.

51. Forsell Y, Jorm AF, Fratiglioni L, Grut M, Winblad B. Application of DSM-III-R criteria for major depressive episode to elderly subjects with and without dementia. Am J Psychiatry 1993; 150:1199–1202.

52. Ballard CG, Patel A, Solis M, Lowe K, Wilcock G. A one-year follow-up study of depression in dementia sufferers. Br J Psychiatry 1996; 168:287–291.

53. Starkstein SE, Chemerinski E, Sabe L, et al. Prospective longitudinal study of depression and anosognosia in Alzheimer's disease. Br J Psychiatry 1997; 171:47–52.

54. Jeste DV, Wragg RE, Salmon DP, Harris MJ, Thal LJ. Cognitive deficits of patients with Alzheimer's disease with and without delusions. Am J Psychiatry 1992; 149:184–189.

55. Gilley DW, Wilson RS, Bennett DA, Bernard BA, Fox JH. Predictors of behavioral disturbance in Alzheimer's disease. J Gerontol 1991; 46:P362–P371.

56. Levy ML, Cummings JL, Fairbanks LA, et al. Longitudinal assessment of symptoms of depression, agitation, and psychosis in 181 patients with Alzheimer's disease. Am J Psychiatry 1996; 153:1438–1443.

57. Mega MS, Cummings JL, Fiorello T, Gornbein J. The spectrum of behavioral changes in AD. Neurology 1996; 46:130–135.

58. Lopez O, Wisniewski S, Becker J, et al. Psychiatric medication and abnormal behavior as predictors of progression in probable AD. Arch Neurol 1999; 56:1266–1272.

59. McShane R, Keene J, Gedling K, et al. Do neuroleptic drugs hasten cognitive decline in dementia? Prospective study with necropsy follow up. BMJ 1997; 314:266–270.

60. Patterson MB, Mack JL, Mackell JA, et al. A longitudinal study of behavioral pathology across five levels of dementia severity in Alzheimer's disease: the CERAD Behavior Rating Scale for Dementia. The Alzheimer's Disease Cooperative Study. Alzheimer Dis Assoc Disord 1997; 11: S40–S44.

61. Holtzer R, Tang MX, Devanand DP, et al. Psychopathological features in Alzheimer's disease: course and relationship with cognitive status. J Am Geriatr Soc 2003; 51:953–960.

62. Growdon JH, Locascio JJ, Corkin S, Gomez-Isla T, Hyman BT. Apolipoprotein E genotype does not influence rates of cognitive decline in Alzheimer's disease. Neurology 1996; 47: 444–448.

63. Frisoni GB, Govoni S, Geroldi C, et al. Gene dose of the epsilon 4 allele of apolipoprotein E and disease progression in sporadic late-onset Alzheimer's disease. Ann Neurol 1995; 37:596–604.

64. Winblad B. Maintaining functional and behavioral abilities in AD. Alzheimer Dis Assoc Disord 2001; 15:S34–S40.

65. Stern Y, Liu X, Albert MS, et al. Modeling the influence of extrapyramidal signs on the progression of Alzheimer's disease. Arch Neurol 1996; 53:1121–1126.

66. Lawton MP, Brody EM. Assessment of older people: self-maintaining and instrumental activities of daily living. Gerontologist 1969; 9:179–186.

67. Green CR, Mohs RC, Schmeidler J, Aryan M, Davis KL. Functional decline in Alzheimer's disease: a longitudinal study. J Am Geriatr Soc 1993; 41:654–661.

68. Ganguli M, Dodge HH, Shen C, Pandav RS, DeKosky ST. Alzheimer disease and mortality: a 15-year epidemiological study. Arch Neurol 2005; 62:779–784.

69. Tschanz JT, Corcoran C, Skoog I, et al and the Cache County Study Group. Dementia: the leading predictor of death in a defined elderly population: the Cache County Study. Neurology 2004; 62:1156–1162.

70. Severson MA, Smith GE, Tangalos EG, et al. Patterns and predictors of institutionalization in community-based dementia patients. J Am Geriatr Soc 1994; 42:181–185.

71. Smith GE, Kokmen E, O'Brien PC. Risk factors for nursing home placement in a population-based dementia cohort. J Am Geriatr Soc 2000; 48:519–525.

72. Smith GE, O'Brien PC, Ivnik RJ, Kokmen E, Tangalos EG, Prospective analysis of risk factors for nursing home placement of dementia patients. Neurology 2001; 57:1467–1473.

73. Galasko D, Bennett D, Sano M, et al. An inventory to assess activities of daily living for clinical trials in Alzheimer's disease. The Alzheimer's Disease Cooperative Study. Alzheimer Dis Assoc Disord 1997; 11:S33–S39.

74. Schmeidler J, Mohs RC, Aryan M. Relationship of disease severity to decline on specific cognitive and functional measures in Alzheimer disease. Alzheimer Dis Assoc Disord 1998; 12:146–151.

75. Heyman A, Peterson B, Fillenbaum G, Pieper C. Predictors of time to institutionalization of patients with AD: the CERAD experience, part XVII. Neurology 1997; 48: 1304–1309.

76. Wolinsky FD, Callahan CM, Fitzgerald JF, Johnson RJ. The risk of nursing home placement and subsequent death among older adults. J Gerontol 1992; 47:S173–S182.

77. Wolinsky FD, Callahan CM, Fitzgerald JF, Johnson RJ. Changes in functional status and the risks of subsequent nursing home placement and death. J Gerontol 1993; 48:S94–S101.

78. Sarazin M, Berr C, Stern Y, et al. Peut-on prédire la gravité de la maladie d'Alzheimer. Rev Neurol (Paris) 2001; 10:A31.

79. Sarazin M, Stern Y, Berr C, et al. Neuropsychological predictors of dependency in patients with Alzheimer disease. Neurology 2005; 64:1027–1031.

80. Blessed G, Tomlinson BE, Roth M. The association between quantitative measures of dementia and of senile changes in the cerebral gray matter of elderly subjects. Br J Psychiatry 1968; 225:797–811.

81. Steele C, Rovner B, Chase GA, Folstein M. Psychiatric symptoms and nursing home placement of patients with Alzheimer's disease. Am J Psychiatry 1990; 147:1049–1051.

82. O'Donnell BF, Drachman DA, Barnes HJ, et al. Incontinence and troublesome behaviors predict institutionalization in dementia. J Geriatr Psychiatry Neurol 1992; 5:45–52.

83. Knopman DS, Berg JD, Thomas R, et al. Nursing home placement is related to dementia progression: experience from a clinical trial, Alzheimer's Disease Cooperative Study. Neurology 1999; 52:714–718.

84. Heyman A, Peterson B, Fillenbaum G, Pieper C. The consortium to establish a registry for Alzheimer's disease (CERAD). Part XIV: Demographic and clinical predictors of survival in patients with Alzheimer's disease. Neurology 1996; 46:656–660.

85. Van Duijn CM, De Knijff P, Wehnert A, et al. The apolipoprotein E2 allele is associated with an increased risk of early-onset Alzheimer's disease and a reduced survival. Ann Neurol 1995; 37:605–610.

86. Corder EH, Saunders AM, Strittmatter WJ, et al. Apolipoprotein E, survival in Alzheimer's disease patients, and the competing risks of death and Alzheimer's disease. Neurology 1995; 45:1323–1328.

87. Perry R, Irving D, Blessed G, Fairbairn A, Perry E. Senile dementia of Lewy body type: a clinically and neuropathologically distinct form of Lewy body dementia in the elderly. J Neurol Sci 1990; 95:119–139.

88. Lennox G. Lewy body dementia. In: Rossor MN, ed. Unusual Dementias. London: Bailliere Tindall 1992.

89. Cercy SP, Bylsma FW. Lewy bodies and progressive dementia: a critical review and metaanalysis. J Int Neuropsychol Soc 1997; 3:179–194.

90. Walker Z, Allen R, Shergill S, Mullan E, Katona C. Three years survival in patients with a clinical diagnosis of dementia with Lewy bodies. Int J Geriatr Psychiatry 2000; 15:267–273.

91. McKeith IG, Fairbairn A, Perry R, Thompson P, Perry E. Neuroleptic sensitivity in patients with senile dementia of Lewy body type. BMJ 1992; 205:673–678.

92. McKeith IG. Cortical Lewy body disease: the view from Newcastle. In: R Levy, R Howards, eds. Developments in Dementia and Functional Disorders in the Elderly. Petersfield: Wrightson Biomedical Publishing 1994.

93. Lippa CF, Smith TW, Swearer JM. Alzheimer's disease and Lewy body disease: a comparative clinicopathology study. Ann Neurol 1994; 35:81–88.

94. Drach LM, Steinmetz HE, Wach S, Bohl J. High proportion of dementia with Lewy bodies in the postmortems of a mental hospital in Germany. Int J Geriatr Psychiatry 1997; 12:301–306.

95. Klatka LA, Louis ED, Schiffer RB. Psychiatric features in diffuse Lewy body disease: a clinicopathologic study using Alzheimer's disease and Parkinson's disease comparison groups. Neurology 1996; 47:1148–1152.

96. Weiner MF, Risser RC, Cullum CM, et al. Alzheimer's disease and its Lewy body variant: a clinical analysis of postmortem verified cases. Am J Psychiatry 1996; 153:1269–1273.

97. McShane R, Gedling D, Reasing M, et al. A prospective study of psychotic symptoms in dementia sufferers: psychosis in dementia. Int Psychogeriatr 1997; 9:57–64.

98. Ballard CG, O'Brien J, Lowery K, et al. A prospective study of dementia with Lewy bodies. Age Ageing 1998; 27:631–636.

99. Olichney JM, Galasko D, Salmon D, et al. Cognitive decline is faster in Lewy bodies variant than in AD. Neurology 1998; 51:351–357.

100. Schoos B, Correy-Bloom J, Sabbagh MN, et al. Plaque only AD; with and without Lewy bodies: what do Lewy bodies add to dementia? Neurology 1998; 50:A281.

101. Ballard C, O'Brien J, Swann A, et al. One year follow-up of parkinsonism in dementia with Lewy bodies. Dement Geriatr Cogn Disord 2000; 11:219–222.

102. Ballard C, McKeith I, Harrison R, et al. A detailed phenomenological comparison of complex visual hallucinations in dementia with Lewy bodies and Alzheimer's disease. Int Psychogeriatr 1997; 9:381–388.

103. McShane R, Gedling K, Reading M, et al. Prospective study of relations between cortical Lewy bodies, poor eyesight, and hallucinations in Alzheimer's disease. J Neurol Neurosurg Psychiatry 1995; 59:185–188.

104. Ballard C, O'Brien JT, Coope B, Wilcok G. Psychotic symptoms in dementia and the rate of cognitive decline. J Am Geriatr Soc 1998; 45:1031–1032.

105. Ballard C, O'Brien J, Swann A, et al. The natural history of psychosis and depression in dementia with Lewy bodies and AD: persistence and new case over 1 year of follow-up. J Clin Psychiatry 2001; 62:46–49.

106. Rascovsky K, Salmon DP, Gilbert J, et al. Rate of cognitive decline differs in AD and frontotemporal dementia. Neurology 2001; 56:S18.005.

107. Pasquier F, Lebert F, Lavenu I, Guillaume B. The clinical picture of frontotemporal dementia: a diagnosis and follow-up. Dement Geriatr Cogn Disord 1999; 10:10–14.

108. Gregory CA. Frontal variant of frontotemporal dementia: a cross-sectional and longitudinal study of neuropsychiatric features. Psychol Med 1999; 29:1205–1217.

109. Pasquier F, Richard F, Lebert F. Natural history of frontotemporal dementia: comparison with Alzheimer's disease. Dement Geriatr Cogn Disord. 2004; 17:253–257.

12

Global assessment measures

Kenneth Rockwood and John C Morris

INTRODUCTION

The diagnosis of dementia is a clinical one, requiring the identification of not just cognitive impairment, but that it is sufficiently severe to interfere with social or occupational functioning. No single cut-point on a given test discriminates dementia from other causes of cognitive impairment. Even neuropathological hallmarks of dementing diseases – the traditional 'gold standard' in dementia diagnosis – do not reliably discriminate between those who would be diagnosed with dementia from those without cognitive impairment.[1] Given that clinical judgment is essential in dementia, it is not surprising that clinical global assessment scales are used routinely both to diagnose and stage dementia, and in research settings, including drug trials where they can be outcome measures.[2] Clinical global scales characterize dementia through multidimensional assessments of cognitive, functional and behavioural aspects of the disorder.[3] Here we critically review some commonly used clinical scales, emphasizing the ones which are judgment based. We note that any comprehensive dementia evaluation will also include cognitive tests that operate relatively independently of clinical judgment, such as the Mini-Mental State Examination (MMSE)[4] and the Alzheimer's disease Assessment Scale cognitive section (ADAS-cog),[5] but such psychometric tests will not be the focus of this chapter.

As opposed to dementia evaluation by cognitive testing alone, global clinical scales employ a semistructured interview to assess changes in behavioural and everyday functioning brought about by intellectual decline. Critically, such information is judged in the context of an individual's past performance. Such contextualization allows consideration of confounding factors, such as education, age, culture and prac-

tice effects, that affect standardized cognitive and neuropsychological testing.[6–8] Moreover, individualization enables more meaningful clinical responses to be looked for in antidementia drug trials. When assessing the full range of dementia severity, global measures are less affected by 'floor' and 'ceiling' effects than longitudinal psychometric testing. Clearly, clinical global measures are characterized by requiring clinical judgment, and this fact is variously perceived as either an advantage or a disadvantage, depending on one's philosophical stance. Scientifically, cases can be made for either approach.[2,3] Given the fact of the memory problems of the patient, global clinical measures are done best when an informant is present who can provide good information about the subject's cognitive functioning, autonomy and behaviour. They can also be time-consuming although, like psychometric tests, this is not inherent.

A recent PET study compared four rating scales, including the Clinical Dementia Rating (CDR),[9] the MMSE, measures of function and caregiver's assessment of cognition. All four identified similar profiles, and a factor analysis found that each was associated with decreased cerebral activity in the parietal and temporal cortices, precuneus and left middle frontal gyrus bilaterally.[10] These data support the underlying validity of the general approach of global scales, particularly for measurement of change. In practice, not all measures are equally responsive,[11] something of critical importance in clinical trials.

In general, global scales can be categorized into three groups, based on their objectives: (1) those that enable a clinical diagnosis of dementia to be made; (2) those that stage the severity of dementia and (3) those that quantify a clinical change in dementia status (Table 12.1).

Table 12.1 Selected global assessment measures.

Measures of diagnosis

Clinical Dementia Rating

Informant Questionnaire on Cognitive Decline in the Elderly

Cambridge Mental Disorders on the Elderly Examination

Dementia Questionnaire[12]

Functional Rating Scale

Brief Cognitive Rating Scale

Measures of severity

Clinical Dementia Rating

Global Deterioration Scale

Functional Rating Scale

Measures of change

Clinical Dementia Rating/CDR sum-of-boxes

Alzheimer Disease Cooperative

Study Group Clinical Dementia Rating Clinical Global Impression of Change

Clinician's Interview-Based Impression of Change-plus

Alzheimer's Disease Cooperative Study Unit Interview-based Impression of Change

Gottfries–Brane–Steen Scale

Goal Attainment Scaling

GLOBAL MEASURES FOR USE IN DIAGNOSIS

The Clinical Dementia Rating (CDR) and the Functional Rating Scale (FRS)

The CDR was developed at the Washington University School of Medicine[9] and last revised in 1993.[13] A new version for clinical trials has been developed by the Alzheimer's Disease Cooperative Study group,[14] and another for use in chronic care facilities.[15] The CDR employs a semi-structured clinical interview with both the patient and an informant to rate performance in six domains: memory, orientation, judgment and problem solving, community affairs, home and hobbies and personal care. The ordinal scale is scored from 0 (no impairment) to 3 (severe dementia). A 'questionable' or very mild impairment category is scaled as 0.5; mild, moderate, and severe impairment are scored as 1, 2 and 3, respectively.

Because the CDR also defines non-demented ageing (CDR = 0), in addition to dementia severity, in practice it additionally has the diagnostic capability of discriminating 'no dementia' from 'dementia' even in its mildest stages (i.e. CDR = 0.5). The reliability of the CDR has been shown to be very good both for physicians and for non-physicians in individual centres and in multicentre trials.[16–19] Its validity has also been demonstrated by clinical progression of Alzheimer's disease (AD) and by autopsy confirmation of AD, even for the earliest symptomatic stages detected by the CDR.[20,21] Substantial longitudinal data for its ability to characterize the course of AD are available.[22,23] The CDR also can serve as a sensitive and specific screening instrument for the detection of dementia in the community.[24]

More recently, the CDR has been used to contribute to the understanding of mild cognitive impairment (MCI), which has been operationally defined as a CDR level of 0.5 by some authors. In its original conceptualization, MCI was understood largely as an amnestic disorder, but as the concept has evolved, it is clear that often many aspects of cognition are involved.[25] At the same time, some CDR-based studies have called important assumptions about MCI into question, by identifying subgroups with varying prognosis within this category.[26] Even so, the CDR has been shown to distinguish usefully between MCI and AD in clinical trials.[27] The CDR has also been analysed as if consisting of two subscales – a cognitive one and one for function. Some support was found for this view, although at present the finding must be considered preliminary.[28]

The Functional Rating Scale[29] (FRS) builds on the CDR by adding domains in social and behavioural aspects of the assessment. It is widely used in Canada, and has formed the basis of clinical assessments in ongoing dementia cohort studies in that country.[30,31] The FRS has also been used in clinical trials.[32]

The Informant Questionnaire on Cognitive Decline in the Elderly (IQCODE)

The IQCODE section is a 26-item, informant-based questionnaire regarding changes in a patient's cognitive performance over the previous 10 years.[33] Each item in the questionnaire is scored in an ordinal fashion from 1 ('very much better now') to 5 ('very much worse now'). Based on the total score, which is compared against community norms, a diagnosis of dementia can be made. A shorter, 16-item version has also been developed.[34] The IQCODE only looks for the presence of a dementia syndrome; it does not attempt to delineate the specific aetiology, such as AD.

This instrument has high test–retest reliability,[34] and it has also performed similarly to the MMSE as a screening test for dementia.[35] Validation studies have demonstrated correlations with the MMSE ranging from 0.37 to 0.78, and more modest correlations with neuropsychological tests. Its diagnostic accuracy, however, has not been validated against autopsy and nor is there information about its ability to detect early dementia. The IQCODE appears not to be influenced by pre-morbid abilities,[35] which also makes it an attractive candidate to understand dementia in people with varying levels of cognitive reserve. Given its ability to supplement test findings with information about a person's cognitive history, the IQCODE has been used in conjunction with cognitive screening tests to increase the efficacy of detecting dementia in community studies.[36]

The Cambridge Mental Disorders of the Elderly Examination (CAMDEX)

The CAMDEX is a standardized clinical instrument developed for use by an expert interviewer.[37,38] Its different sections include a patient interview, cognitive examination, interviewer observations of behaviour and, especially important, a structured interview with a caregiver concerning the patient's present state, past history and family history. Based on these sections, a diagnosis of one of three entities is made: a neurodegenerative disorder, multi-infarct dementia or depression. Information from the caregiver can be scored reliably and the three diagnostic scales of the CAMDEX have been shown to have good discriminating abilities.[39] Progression of the disease has also been described, giving confidence to the description of the early stages of AD.[40]

The Brief Cognitive Rating Scale (BCRS) and Global Deterioration Scale (GDS)

The BCRS[41] assesses the degree of cognitive decline, using defined criteria, across 11 axes. The GDS can be estimated based on the first five axes (concentration, recent memory, past memory, orientation and function/self-care). Each axis is scored on the basis of a semi-structured interview with a caregiver, and follows a hierarchy such that 1 is consistent with no impairment, 4 with mild dementia, and so on to 7, consistent with very severe dementia. Like the CDR, in a typical case of AD, the BCRS shows concordance between the individual scores on its 11 axes. BCRS ratings have been shown to have good inter-rater and test–retest reliabilities. Correlations with selected psychometric

and mental status tests ranged from 0.48 to 0.84, and follow-up data are also available.[42,43] Inter-rater reliability of the individual BCRS axes has been shown to be between 0.76 and 0.97.[44] The GDS and axis 5 of the BCRS (the Functional Assessment Staging Tool – FAST) have been shown to correlate with disease duration,[45] with hippocampal atrophy[46] and with neurofibrillary changes in the hippocampal formation.[47] In addition to its use in clinical practice and prospective studies, the BCRS has been used retrospectively by expert physicians interviewing knowledgeable informants. In that context, it was shown to be useful in retrospective clinical diagnosis as validated by autopsy material.[48]

The GDS appears to be used in Europe on a par with the CDR[49] and is a standard staging measure in Canadian studies.[31,32,50] The BCRS and GDS have also been used to describe patterns of decline in Parkinson's disease.[51]

Critique of measures of diagnosis

Global measures of diagnosis evaluate changes in patient performance in many domains including cognitive abilities and performance on usual activities. In consequence, they aim to be less susceptible to day to day fluctuations that can affect cognitive test performance. This stability, however, requires informants who can provide reliable information about the course of the illness and its effect on that individual's functioning. Global instruments address items that are of relevance to everyday life, and thus can be used in subjects from many different cultures. Moreover, they are applicable to people with limited education. These scales enable a direct assessment of cognitive change that is impossible with a single session of cognitive testing. Furthermore, they have the potential advantage of detecting mild dementia in a patient who is already experiencing functional changes but whose cognitive performance is still within the 'normal range'. On the other hand, global assessment scales, compared with cognitive tests, depend on the availability of an informant, who might not always be present or sufficiently knowledgeable. Finally, the results can be affected by the quality of the relationship between the patient and the informant as well as the emotional state of the latter.

The clinical measures that can specifically detect AD have had an important role in the fall of the two earlier dogmas that dementia is often 'reversible' and that AD is a diagnosis of exclusion. Recognition of the clinical heterogeneity of AD (e.g. different rates of deterioration in different domains) has aided the appreciation of this disorder as the most frequent dementing illness. Previously, it was held that as many as 20 per cent of patients with acquired, progressive cognitive impairment had reversible causes of dementia. While 'reversible' conditions do occur, they are now recognized to be uncommon as the sole cause of dementia,[52] but more often are superimposed on AD.

Experience gained with the global assessment of AD has also helped to refute the notion that the disorder is diagnosed by excluding other causes. While there are cultural differences in the approach to the differential diagnosis of dementia,[53] the existence of a recognizable clinical syndrome means that it is no longer necessary to conduct extensive investigations in all cases to 'rule out' a long list of implausible causes before AD can be diagnosed clinically with confidence.

Clinical global measures have had an important role in improving our understanding of the differential diagnosis of the dementia syndrome. For example, by making atypical patterns clear they assist in the diagnosis of non-AD dementia. This is because the various dementing illnesses are most different in their clinical features when comparisons are made at the earlier stages of dementia; as the condition advances, the clinical characteristics of the various illnesses become more uniform. For example, hallucinations are common in severe AD, but uncommon in the early stages. Clinical global measures readily illustrate that a symptom or sign is occurring 'out of order', i.e. is not congruent with other symptoms and signs for a given stage. Thus, to continue the example, a person who scored 3 or 4 on several domains of the Brief Cognitive Rating Scale (consistent with mild dementia), but who scored 6 on the behavioural axis (due to hallucinations), could readily be seen to have non-congruent symptoms. Thus diagnosis other than AD (e.g. dementia with Lewy bodies – DLB) or in addition to it (e.g. delirium, non-dominate parietal stroke) could be considered.

GLOBAL MEASURES OF SEVERITY

The Clinical Dementia Rating and the Functional Rating Scale as severity measures

The CDR and the FRS can be used to stage the severity of dementia, and their hierarchical construction serves this purpose well. By hierarchy is meant that a score of 3 means a worse severity than a score of 2, and that more than 1, and so on across all patients. This is not necessarily the case, for example, in MMSE scores between patients, where raw MMSE scores are affected by factors such as the subject's past educa-

tional attainment[54] and therefore must be interpreted in a clinical context. The CDR, on the other hand, includes this clinical interpretation in its score. Judgment serves to provide context that is reflected in the score.

The CDR also has the property of concordance in the scores of its six domains, allowing for recognition of the typical stages of AD, and likewise for the FRS. For example, in a typical case of mild AD, not all domains are required or are likely to be of the same severity level, but most would have scores of 0.5 or 1. The presence of widely divergent (i.e. non-concordant) scores between domains (e.g. a mix of 0s, 2s and 3s) would suggest that a non-Alzheimer cause of dementia is present. In this way, it provides a way to understand the heterogeneity of dementia, and how much heterogeneity is tolerable within a given diagnosis.

In addition to the global CDR score, another measure of the severity of cognitive decline can be obtained by the sum-of-boxes score. This summates the ratings of impairment for each of the six categories in the CDR and ranges from 0 (6 categories × level of impairment in each category) to 18 (6 × 3). The CDR sum-of-boxes more quantitatively describes progression of dementia severity.[13]

The Global Deterioration Scale and the Brief Cognitive Rating Scale as severity measures

The GDS[55] rates seven clinically identifiable stages of 'no cognitive decline; subjective complaints without an objective deficit; subjective complaints with some objective deficits which do not meet dementia criteria; mild dementia; moderate dementia; severe dementia; and terminal dementia'. It does not require a structured interview; the assessment is made by a clinician who has access to all sources of information, including an informant. As noted above, however, the GDS can be calculated for the first five axes of the BCRS. It has good reliability and it correlates well with other scales.[41] On the other hand, not all patients with AD follow a dementia trajectory as precisely as is described by the GDS.[56]

GLOBAL MEASURES OF CHANGE

Global measures have been particularly useful in the pretreatment era by making clear which symptoms are usually seen together in AD. As dementia treatment becomes more common, and as more causes of dementia are recognized, the notion of stage congruence becomes more problematic. Two remedies seem reasonable; one is the development of dementia-specific staging measures. For example, typical CDR, FRS or BCRS-like pattern of DLB could be defined, or an entirely new measure to stage DLB could be developed. Second, typical patterns of changes of symptoms under treatment also need to be elaborated.

Another challenge remains in the elucidation of the nature of deficits observed in people with MCI. As noted, the diagnosis and description of MCI is controversial. A better description of the precise nature of the deficits present in people with MCI would help identify patterns of risk of progression to AD and other dementias. Much of the controversy revolves around when MCI is seen as a transient state, a pre-dementia state or early dementia. Global staging measures could help illuminate this important clinical and public policy issue.

The Clinician's Interview-Based Impression of Change-plus (CIBIC-plus)

Guidelines issued by the Food and Drug Administration (FDA) in 1990 endorsed the use of global assessments as a primary outcome measure in clinical trials as the 'ultimate test of the clinical utility of a drug's anti-dementia effects'.[57] It soon became apparent that several global measures of change were being used in different ways across drug trials, prompting the FDA to specify further the requirements of the global improvement scales. The CIBIC-plus evolved as a response to these developments: it assesses the global clinical status of the patient relative to baseline, based on information from semi- structured interviews with the patient and responsible caregiver, without any reference to cognitive test performance from any source. (The term CIBIC by itself involves the same content as CIBIC-plus, except that the clinician interviews only the patient, without any input from caregivers.) It is scored in the absence of specific guidelines for disease progression or treatment effects on a scale of 1–7 (1 = very much improved, 4 = no change, 7 = very much worse).

The rationale of this approach is that if an experienced clinician can perceive clinical change on the basis of an interview, then such changes are likely to be clinically meaningful. The term CIBIC was generic in the FDA's recommendation and no specific instrument was stated as an example. As a result, other constructions have also been used[58,59] for drug trials, although the result in most studies is that 'no change' is the most common designation of patients in both active treatment and placebo groups.[60] This reflects less that no clinically detectable change is occurring than that

clinicians trade off improvement in some areas for decline in others, thus obscuring patterns of treatment.[61,62] An important criticism of the CIBIC-plus is that clinicians appear to find it easier to recognize decline than to recognize improvement.[63] It is probably easier to recognize deterioration than improvement because we have a better idea of what deterioration looks like, given our understanding of dementia progression without treatment. In short, the model of deterioration that clinicians carry in their head is better specified than the model of improvement.[64]

The Alzheimer's Disease Cooperative Study Unit Clinician's Global Impression of Change (ADCS-CGIC)

The ADCS-CGIC is another interview-based global measure of change that involves both patient and caregiver.[58] Compared to the CIBIC-plus, the ADCS-CGIC is more specified with 15 areas incorporating the domains of cognition, behaviour and social and daily functioning, assessed so as to enable the clinician to quantify the degree of change that may have occurred in the patient from the baseline. The rater is instructed not to refer to other study instruments, not to ask about side effects from treatment and not to discuss the subject's functioning with other staff. The change rating is again made on a 7-point scale. Of the various global clinicians' interview-based change scales that currently exist, the ADCS-CGIC has been the most commonly used and has shown good reliability and validity.[56] One of the first worldwide uses of the ADCS-CGIC was a donepezil clinical trial.[65]

The Clinical Dementia Rating as a measure of change

The CDR has been adopted as a primary outcome measure in multicentre antidementia drug trials, and investigators have participated in training protocols for standardization and reliability.[18] The CDR sum-of-boxes performed better than psychometric measures in a longitudinal model of outcomes for intervention studies in AD.[66]

Gottfries–Brane–Steen Scale (GBS)

Published in 1982, the GBS[67] is a structured global instrument encompassing questions related to 'motoric functions' (N = 6), 'intellectual function' (N = 11), 'emotional functions' (N = 3) and 'other symptoms common in dementia' (N = 6). Each question is rated from 0 to 6 using descriptors, with higher scores indicating deterioration (range 0–156). This instrument has been well validated in generic populations with Alzheimer's and vascular dementias. The GBS has been used in AD and vascular dementia trials, where it has been found to be responsive to clinically important changes.[68]

Goal Attainment Scaling (GAS)

GAS is a measure for tracking clinical changes. It was developed in the 1960s for use in community mental health[69] but has been adapted for use in dementia drug studies.[70–72] Importantly, it is patient-centred and individualized. The process is described in detail elsewhere,[73] but boils down to this. First, patients and caregivers describe areas in which they seek to see improvement. Typically they can be grouped in domains such as function, cognition, behaviour, social interaction and leisure activities. On their own, patients and caregivers much more commonly choose the last two than do clinicians.[71] Next, specific problems are identified, using, as much as possible, the words of the patient or caregiver. For example a caregiver might say 'Dad used to want to go out a lot, even after Mom died. But now, he is just content to sit all day long. He won't even go to the lodge unless Uncle Bill comes for him'. After this, a goal is set, e.g. 'I'd like to see Dad want to go out at least once a week and shopping, if only to go to the corner store'. So now we have a patient-centred problem definition (Dad goes out less) and a quantifiable goal (Dad will go out at least once a week). After this, better and worse outcomes can be defined. For example, better would be everything in the goal, plus 'will go to see his friends, and will initiate his own shopping, even if he needs help bringing things home'. A worse outcome would be if he refuses to go to those events. More finely graded levels are also allowed and, for scoring purposes, scoring can be 'on the line' between two levels. At the set 5 points, the extent of attainment can be measured, using a formula that accounts for varying numbers of goals, the weights assigned to them and inter-correlation between goal areas.

GAS has been criticized for being too time-consuming, judgment-based (subjective) and prone to setting goals that are too easy to achieve. Proponents argue that the time is well spent, that what extra time is spent setting goals is compensated for by making follow-up interviews more efficient and that, in a research setting, a controlled design readily overcomes any bias that arises from setting goals that are too 'easy', as this would be the same in treatment and comparison groups. In a clinical setting, 'easy' goals are also easily detected by routine clinical audit, where patterns can readily be discerned.

Critique of measures of change

Since the 1990 FDA guidelines outlining the need for a global assessment instrument that can measure a meaningful clinical change in patients undergoing antidementia drug trials, this topic has received much attention and the field is rapidly evolving. The advantages of the global improvement scales are fairly evident. In drug trials, it is important to document efficacy over and beyond any improvement noted in cognitive or psychometric scores, which are often mild in drug trials and are difficult to interpret in realistic terms. Moreover, many cognitive and psychometric instruments suffer from floor and ceiling effects, especially at the late and early stages of the dementing illness, rendering changes produced by the medication difficult to observe.

The use of global measures of cognitive change has also been defended on the grounds that there is as yet insufficient understanding of the precise treatment effect to be expected in dementia drug trials.[74] Global scales, being more unspecified, can be appropriate instruments to detect whatever changes occur within treatment. However, to capture clinically meaningful changes, the global assessment measure should consider a range of domains that will be important to a patient's quality of life. Using the terminology of Lawton, this would include self-perceived quality of life, psychological well-being and the broad category of 'behavioural competence', which would include, for example, performance in instrumental and personal activities of daily living, behaviour and time use.[75]

The responsiveness of the global clinical measures (either the CIBIC-plus or a Clinical Global Impression of Change) seems best established in mild-moderate AD treated with a cholinesterase inhibitor,[76] a result that seems to carry over as well to the severe stage.[77] The effects with different compounds and diseases, however, have been more variable. Early treatment with linopirdine[78] and with ginkgo biloba[79] showed that these global measures were less sensitive to change than the ADAS-cog. Similarly, another clinical global impression of change measure showed more variable responsiveness in a recent study of atorvastatin in AD, in which the effects of the ADAS-cog were more consistent.[80] The strategy of using global measures in addition to cognitive tests has been endorsed for clinical trials of drugs to treat vascular dementia.[81] Subsequent experience, however, has been variable, with inconsistent effects, for example, of both the CIBIC-plus, an unstructured global outcome measure, and the CDR, a structured measure, at different doses of donepezil.[82] By further contrast, the Clinical Global Impression was more sensitive than standard measures of cognition and behaviour in a recent trial of donepezil in Parkinson's disease dementia.[83] From these variable results it appears that the greater the familiarity with the model of treatment, the more sensitive the measure will be: it appears that clinicians learn what to look for, and then look for it. It is of some interest that while the CIBIC-plus and the ADAS-cog have similar responsiveness, there are few studies which compare whether they identify the same people as benefitting – or not – from treatment.

CONCLUSIONS

Clinical global measures that are judgment based are particularly important in dementia, the diagnosis of which rests on clinical judgment. Clinical measures are used to aid diagnosis, to stage dementia and to judge the effects of dementia treatment. The use of global measures has contributed to improved patient care and better research studies in many ways, not the least of which is by helping to sharpen clinical judgment.

REFERENCES

1. Neuropathology Group. Medical Research Council Cognitive Function and Aging Study. Pathological correlates of late-onset dementia in a multicentre, community-based population in England and Wales. Neuropathology Group of the Medical Research Council Cognitive Function and Ageing Study (MRC CFAS). Lancet. 2001; 357:169–175.
2. Rockwood K. Global assessment measures for dementia drug trials. In: Rockwood K, Gauthier S, eds. Trial Designs and Outcomes in Dementia Therapeutic Research. London: Taylor and Francis 2005; 167–174.
3. Reisburg B, Schneider I, Doody R, et al. Clinical global measures of dementia. Position paper from the International Working Group on Harmonization of Dementia Drug Guidelines. Alzheimer Dis Assoc Disord 1997; 11(suppl 3): S8–S18.
4. Folstein MF, Folstein SE, McHugh PR. Mini-mental state: a practical method for grading the cognitive status of patients by the clinician. J Psychiatry Res 1975; 12:89–198.
5. Rosen WG, Mohs RC, Davis KL. A new rating scale for Alzheimer's disease. Am J Psychiatry 1984; 141:1356–1364.
6. Wiederholt WC, Cahn D, Butters NM, et al. Effects of age, gender and education on selected neuropsychological tests in an elderly community cohort. J Am Geriatric Soc 1993; 41: 639–647.
7. Escobar JI, Burnam A, Karno M, et al. Use of the Mini-Mental State Examination (MMSE) in a community population of mixed ethnicity. J Nerv Ment Dis 1986; 174: 607–614.
8. Galasko D, Abramson I, Corey-Bloom J, et al. Repeated exposure to the Mini-Mental State Examination and the Information – Memory–Concentration tests results in prac-

9. tice effect in Alzheimer's disease. Neurology 1993; 43: 1559–1563.
9. Hughes CP, Berg L. Danziger WL, et al. A new clinical scale for the staging of dementia. Br J Psychiatry 1982; 140: 566–572.
10. Salmon E, Lespagnard S, Marique P, et al. Cerebral metabolic correlates of four dementia scales in Alzheimer's disease. J Neurol 2005; 252:283–290.
11. Rockwood K, Stolee P. Responsiveness of outcome measures in an anti-dementia drug trial. Alzheimer Dis Assoc Disord 2000; 14:182–185.
12. Kawas C, Segal J, Stewart WF, et al. A validation study of the Dementia Questionnaire. Arch Neurol 1994; 51:901–906.
13. Morris JC. The Clinical Dementia Rating (CDR): current version and scoring rules. Neurology 1993; 43:2412–2414.
14. Schafer KA, Tractenberg RE, Sano MK, et al. Reliability of monitoring the clinical dementia rating in multicenter clinical trials. Alzheimer Dis Assoc Disord 2004; 18:219–222.
15. Marin DB, Flynn S, Mare M, et al. Reliability and validity of a chronic care facility adaptation of the Clinical Dementia Rating scale. Int J Geriatr Psychiatry 2001; 16:745–750.
16. Burke WJ, Miller P, Rubin FH, et al. Reliability of the Washington University Clinical Dementia Rating. Arch Neurol 1988; 54:31–32.
17. McCulla M, Coats M, Van Fleet N, et al. Reliability of clinical nurse specialists in the staging of dementia. Arch Neurol 1989; 46:1210–1211.
18. Morris JC, Ernesto C, Schafer K, et al. Clinical Dementia Rating training and reliability in multi-center studies: the Alzheimer's Disease Cooperative Study experience. Neurology 1997; 48:1508–1510.
19. Rockwood K, Strang D, MacKnight C, et al. Inter-rater reliability of the Clinical Dementia Rating in a multi-center trial. J Am Gerontr Soc 2000; 48:588–589.
20. Morris JC, McKeel DW, Fulling K, et al. Validation of clinical diagnostic criteria for Alzheimer's disease. Ann Neurol 1988; 24:17–22.
21. Berg I, McKeel DW, Miller JP, et al. Clinicopathologic studies in cognitively healthy aging and Alzheimer's disease. Arch Neurol 1998; 55:326–335.
22. Berg L, Danziger WL, Storandt M, et al. Predictive features in mild senile dementia of the Alzheimer type. Neurology 1984; 34:563–569.
23. Rubin EH, Storandt M, Miller JP, et al. A prospective study of cognitive function and onset of dementia in cognitively healthy elders. Arch Neurol 1998; 55:395–401.
24. Galasko D, Edland SD, Morris JC, et al. The Consortium to establish a registry for Alzheimer's disease (CERAD). Part XI. Clinical milestones in patients with Alzheimer's disease followed over three years. Neurology 1992; 31:242–249.
25. Winblad B, Palmer K, Kivipelto M. Mild cognitive impairment—beyond controversies, towards a consensus: report of the International Working Group on Mild Cognitive Impairment. J Intern Med 2004; 256:240–246.
26. Morris JC, Storandt M, Miller JP. Mild cognitive impairment represents early-stage Alzheimer disease. Arch Neurol 2001; 58:397–405.
27. Grundman M, Petersen RC, Ferris SH, et al. Mild cognitive impairment can be distinguished from Alzheimer disease and normal aging for clinical trials. Arch Neuro 2004; 61: 59–66.
28. Tractenburg RE, Weiner MF, Cummings JL, et al. Independence of changes in behavior from cognition and function in community-dwelling persons with Alzheimer's disease: a factor analytic approach. J Neuropsychiatry Clin Neurosci 2005; 17:51–60.

29. Feldman H, Schulzer M, Wang S, et al. The Functional Rating Scale (FRS) in Alzheimer's disease: a longitudinal study. In: Iqbal K, Mortimer J, Winbald B, Wisiewski, eds. Research Advantages in Alzheimer's Disease and Related Disorders. London: J Wiley & Sons Ltd 1995; 235–241.

30. Feldman H, Levy AR, Hsiung GY, et al. A Canadian cohort study of cognitive impairment and related dementias (ACCORD): study methods and baseline results. Neuroepidemiology 2003; 22:265–274.

31. Rockwood K, Davis H, MacKnight C, et al. The Consortium to Investigate Vascular Impairment of Cognition: methods and first findings. Can J Neurol Sci 2003; 30:237–243.

32. Feldman H, Gauthier S, Hecker J, et al. A 24-week, randomized, double-blind study of donepezil in moderate to severe Alzheimer's disease. Neurology 2001; 57:613–620. Erratum in: Neurology 2001; 57:2153.

33. Jorm AF, Scott R, Jacomb PA. Assessment of cognitive decline in dementia by informant questionnaire. Int J Geriatric Psychiatry 1989; 4:35–39.

34. Jorm AF. A short form of the Informant Questionnaire on Cognitive Decline in the Elderly (IQCODE): development and cross-validation. Psychol Med 1994; 24:365–374.

35. Jorm AF, Jacomb PA. The informant Questionnaire on Cognitive Decline in the Elderly (IQCODE): socio-demographic correlates, reliability, validity and some norms. Psychol Med 1989; 19:1015–1022.

36. Jorm AF. The Informant Questionnaire on cognitive decline in the elderly (IQCODE): a review. Int Psychogeriatr 2004; 16:275–293.

37. Roth M, Tym E, Mountjoy CQ, et al. CAMDEX: a standardized instrument for the diagnosis of mental disorder in the elderly. Br J Psychiatry 1986; 149:698–709.

38. Hendrie HC, Hall KS, Brittain HM, et al. The CAMDEX: a standardized instrument for the diagnosis of mental disorder in the elderly: a replication with a US sample. J Am Geriatr Soc 1998; 36:402–408.

39. O'Connor DW, Pollitt PA, Hyde JB, et al. A follow-up study of dementia diagnosed in the community using the Cambridge Mental Disorders of the Elderly Examination. Acta Psychiatr Scand 1990; 81:78–82.

40. O'Connor DW, Pollitt PA, Hyde JB, et al. The progression of mild idiopathic dementia in a community population. J Am Geriatr Soc 1991; 39:246–251.

41. Reisberg B, Ferris SH. Brief Cognitive Rating Scale (BCRS). Psychopharmacol Bull 1998; 24:629–636.

42. Flicker C, Ferris SH, Reisberg B. Mild cognitve impairment in the elderly: predictors of dementia. Neurology 1991; 41:1006–1009.

43. Flicker C, Ferris SH, Resiberg B. A longitudinal study of cognitive function in elderly persons with subjective memory complaints. J Am Geriatr Soc 1993; 41:1029–1032.

44. Foster JR, Sclan S, Welkowitz J, Boksay I, Seeland I. Psychiatric assessment in medical long term care facilities: reliability of commonly used rating scales. Int J Geriatr Psychiatry 1998; 3:229–233.

45. Reisberg B, Ferris SH, Franssen E, et al. Mortality and temporal course of probable Alzheimer's disease: a 5-year prospective study. Int Psychogeriatr 1996; 8:291–311.

46. Bobinski M, Weigiel J, Winiewski HM, et al. Atrophy of hippocampal formation subdivisions correlates with stage and duration of Alzheimer disease. Dementia 1996; 6:205–210.

47. Bobinski M, Wegiel J, Tarnawski M, et al. Relationships between regional neuronal loss and neurofibrillary changes in the hippocampal formation and duration and severity of Alzheimer Disease. J Neuropathol Exp Neurol 1997; 56: 414–420.

48. Rockwood K, Howard K, Thomas VS, et al. Retrospective diagnosis of dementia using an informant interview based on the Brief Cognitive Rating Scale. Int Psychogeriatr 1998; 10:53–60.

49. Paulino Ramirez Diaz S, Gil Gregorio P, Manuel Ribera Casado J, et al. The need for a consensus in the use of assessment tools for Alzheimer's disease: the Feasibility Study (assessment tools for dementia in Alzheimer Centres across Europe), a European Alzheimer's Disease Consortium's (EADC) survey. Int J Geriatr Psychiatry 2005; 20:744–748.

50. Sambrook R, Herrmann N, Hebert R, et al. Canadian Outcomes Study in Dementia: study methods and patient characteristics. Can J Psychiatry 2004; 49:417–427.

51. Sabbagh MN, Silverberg N, Birçea S, et al. Is the functional decline of Parkinson's disease similar to the functional decline of Alzheimer's disease? Parkinsonism Relat Disord 2005; 11:311–315.

52. Clarfield AM. The reversible dementias: do they reverse? Am Intern Med 1998; 109:476–486.

53. Clarfield AM, Foley JM. The American and Canadian Consensus Conferences on Dementia: is there consequence? J Am Geriatr Soc 1993; 41:883–886.

54. Tombaugh TN, McIntyre NJ. The Mini-Mental State Examination: a comprehensive review. J Am Geriatr Soc 1992; 40:922–935.

55. Reisberg B, Ferris SH, DeLeon MJ, et al. The global deterioration scale for assessment of primary degenerative dementia. Am J Psychiatry 1982; 139:1136–1139.

56. Eisdorfer C, Cohen D, Paveza GJ, et al. An empirical evaluation of the Global Deterioration Scale for staging Alzheimer's disease. Am J Psychiatry 1992; 149:190–194 [correction, 1129].

57. Leber P. Guidelines for the Clinical Evaluation of Antidementia Drugs. Washington DC: Food & Drug Administration 1990.

58. Schneider LS, Olin JT, Doody RS, et al. Validity and reliability and the Alzheimer's Disease Cooperative Study – Clinical Global Impressions of Change. Alzheimer Dis Assoc Disord 1997; 11(suppl 2):S22–S32.

59. Knopman DS, Knapp MJ, Gracon SI, Davis CS. The Clinician Interview-Based Impression (CIBI): a clinician's global change rating scale in Alzheimer's disease. Neurology 1994; 44:2315–2321.

60. Rockwood K, Joffres K. On behalf of the Halifax Consensus Conference. Improving clinical descriptions to understand the effects of dementia treatment: consensus recommendations. Int J Geriatr Psychiatry 2002; 17: 1006–1011.

61. Joffres C, Graham J, Rockwood K. A qualitative analysis of the Clinician Interview-Based Impression of Change (plus): methodological issues and implications for clinical research. Int Psychogeriatr 2000; 12:403–413.

62. Joffres C, Bucks RS, Haworth J, Wilcock GK, Rockwood K. Patterns of clinically detectable treatment effects with galantamine: a qualitative analysis. Dement Geriatr Cogn Disord 2003; 15:26–33.

63. Quinn J, Moore M, Benson D, et al. A videotaped CIBIC for dementia patients: validity and reliability in a simulated clinical trial. Neurology 2002; 58:433–437.

64. Rockwood K, Wallack M, Tallis R. Alzheimer's disease: understanding treatment success short of a cure. Lancet Neurol 2003; 2:630–633.

65. Rogers SL, Farlow MR, Doody RS, et al. A 24-week, double-blind, placebo-controlled trial of donepezil in patients with Alzheimer's disease. Neurology 1998; 50:136–145.

66. Berg L, Miller JP, Baty J, et al. Mild senile dementia and the Alzheimer type. 4. Evaluation of intervention. Ann Neurol 1992; 31:242–249.

67. Gottfries CG, Brane G, Gullberg B, et al. A new rating scale for dementia syndromes. Arch Gerontol Geriatr 1982; 1:311–330.

68. Brane G, Gottfries CG, Winblad B. The Gottfries–Brane–Steen scale: validity, reliability and application in anti-dementia drug trials. Dement Geriatr Cogn Disord 2001; 12:1–14.

69. Kiresuk T, Sherman, R. Goal attainment scaling: a general method for evaluating community mental health programs. Commun Ment Health J 1968; 4:443–453.

70. Rockwood K, Stolee P, Howard K, Mallery L. Use of Goal Attainment Scaling in a randomized placebo-controlled trial of an anti-dementia drug. Neuroepidemiology 1996; 15:330–338.

71. Rockwood K, Graham JE, Fay S. Goal setting and attainment in Alzheimer's disease patients treated with donepezil. J Neurol Neurosurg Psychiatry 2002; 73:500–507.

72. Rockwood K, Fay S, Song X, et al. Attainment of treatment goals by people with Alzheimer's disease receiving galantamine. CMHJ 2006; 174:1099–1105.

73. Kiresuk TJ, Smith A, Cardillo JE, eds. Goal Attainment Scaling: Applications, Theory, and Measurement. Hillsdale, NJ: Lawrence Erlbaum Associates 1994.

74. Rockwood K. Use of global assessment measures in dementia drug trials. J Clin Epidemiol 1994; 47:101–103.

75. Lawton MP. A multidimensional view of quality of life in frail elderly, In: Birren JE, Lubben JE, Rowe JC, Deutchman DE, eds. The Concept and Measurement of Quality of Life in the Frail Elderly. San Diego: Academic Press Inc 1991; 3–27.

76. Rockwood K. The size of the treatment effect on cognition of cholinesterase inhibition in Alzheimer's disease. J Neurol, Neurosurg Psychiatry 2004; 75:677–685.

77. Feldman H, Gauthier S, Hecker J, et al. Efficacy and safety of donepezil in patients with more severe Alzheimer's disease: a subgroup analysis from a randomized, placebo-controlled trial. Int J Geriatr Psychiatry 2005; 20:559–569.

78. Rockwood K, Beattie L, Eastwood MR, et al. A randomized, controlled trial of linopirdine in the treatment of Alzheimer's disease. Can J Neurol Sci 1997; 24:140–145.

79. LeBars PL, Katz MM, Berman N, et al. A placebo-controlled, double-blind, randomized trial of an extract of Ginkgo biloba for dementia. JAMA 1997; 278:1327–1332.

80. Sparks DL, Sabbagh MN, Connor MJ, et al. Atorvastatin for the treatment of mild to moderate Alzheimer disease: preliminary results. Arch Neurol 2005; 62:753–757.

81. Oliva A, Mani R, Katz R. Regulatory aspects of vascular dementia in the United States. Int Psychogeriatr 2003; 15(suppl 1):293–295.

82. Roman GC, Wilkinson DG, Doody RS, et al. Donepezil in vascular dementia: combined analysis of two large-scale clinical trials. Dement Geriatr Cogn Disord 2005; 20:338–344.

83. Ravina B, Putt M, Siderowf A, et al. Donepezil for dementia in Parkinson's disease: a randomised, double blind, placebo controlled, crossover study. J Neurol Neurosurg Psychiatry 2005; 76:934–939.

13

Depressive syndrome in Alzheimer's disease

Lilian Thorpe

INTRODUCTION

Mood symptoms are very commonly associated with Alzheimer's disease (AD) and related disorders, and can range from subtle and mild to severe symptoms that are the major focus of treatment. Some of the mood symptoms seen in dementia are reactive to difficult life situations, such as the loss of independence (driving, for example). Early symptoms in AD are related to executive deficits, such as impairment in initiation and planning, which may appear as an apathy syndrome, often difficult to differentiate from the decrease in interest and pleasure of depression. Increasing difficulties with cognitive processing, deficits in the development of coping strategies and decreased tolerance to frustration may also give rise to increased mood lability.

Mood symptoms may also be due to a relapsing mood disorder. Although this mood disorder has commonly first presented long before the identification of dementia, an onset after the diagnosis of dementia is not uncommon. Mood disorders in the cognitively impaired elderly might not fulfil formal diagnostic criteria, but they may yet be highly significant to the well-being of the affected person. As is the case in the general elderly, subsyndromal depressions appear to be the most common mood disorders,[1] and, although treatment guidelines for these depressions are less well established, clinical treatment is often necessary.

Mood symptoms in dementia have been associated with additional comorbidity such as decreased functional abilities,[2] increased nursing home placements,[3] increased caregiver stress[4] and increased mortality.[5] The careful assessment and management of mood symptoms in AD is therefore very important.

DIAGNOSTIC CHALLENGES: SYMPTOM OVERLAP BETWEEN DEMENTIA AND DEPRESSION

There is a lot of overlap between symptoms of mood disorders and core symptoms of dementia, such as apathy, sleep disturbance, weight loss and emotional dyscontrol. This makes diagnosis a challenge, and may lead to potential over- and under-diagnosis of mood disorders. Whereas the under-treatment of mood disorders has been well described, along with lost opportunities for improvement of the quality of life and functional abilities, the use of antidepressants in the frail elderly is not free of adverse effects, so it is also important not to overtreat. The rate of psychotropic medication use in general has been increasing over time, including among the elderly with cognitive impairment, so the addition of an antidepressant has the potential for an additional hazard to this frail population. This is the case even with the newer antidepressants, such as the serotonin selective reuptake inhibitors (SSRIs), which have not so much fewer side effects than the tricyclic antidepressants, but different side effects, which may also cause considerable morbidity.

Table 13.1 summarizes symptoms seen in dementia and depression. In general, people with dementia are less concerned about their symptoms, and may even deny these. Those with depression, however, tend to magnify their symptoms and are more likely to bring them to a caregiver as a focus of concern.

Sleep disturbance is a characteristic symptom in both depression and dementia. In dementia, there is a characteristic loss of diurnal sleep variation, resulting in the fragmentation of sleep throughout a 24-hour day. This fragmentation tends to develop over months

Table 13.1 Comparison of symptoms in dementia compared to depression

Symptom	Dementia	Depression
General symptom approach	Frequent unconcern about symptoms or even denial of symptoms	Magnification and elaboration of symptoms
Sleep disturbance	Gradual loss of diurnal sleep variation over months to years (due to brain changes of Alzheimer's disease)	Subacute changes in sleep over weeks to months (increase or decrease)
Change in eating behaviour and weight loss	Gradual loss of weight over months to years. Large increases in weight may sometimes take place secondary to decreased activity, medications and hyperorality in those with very frontal behavioural presentations	Subacute changes of appetite, over weeks to months. Weight may increase or decrease
Depressed mood	None stated or mild, reactive to circumstances and fluctuating	Pervasive, most of the day and nearly every day
Mood dyscontrol (or mood lability)	Gradual increase in the frequency of episodic mood dyscontrol (crying, laughing inappropriately) in the absence of sustained sadness	Subacute increase in crying or other expressions of distress, congruent with sad mood and affect, and more consistent than in dementia. Inappropriate laughing is uncommon
Lack of interest and initiative and poor energy	Gradual loss of interest and initiative (apathy) not accompanied by statements of sadness, tearfulness or other distress	Subacute onset over weeks to months, frequently accompanied by sad mood and affect, as well as statements of hopelessness
Psychomotor agitation	Generally worse during the later part of the day (sundowning)	Often present persistently throughout the day
Guilt or worthlessness	Uncommon	More common
Suicidal thoughts and actions	Uncommon	Common
Decreased concentration	Gradually occurring problem only in the later stages of dementia and often not accompanied by statements of concern	Develops subacutely in depressed patients, who are often very concerned about this

to years and is probably due to biological deficits of the dementing brain.[6] Sleep changes in depression tend to be more subacute, developing over weeks to months. In both depression and dementia total sleep time can be increased as well as decreased.

Weight loss has long been known to be a key symptom of depression, but is now also known to be strongly associated with dementia, even prior to the diagnosis in some studies.[7] Although the reasons for this are not fully understood, it seems plausible that the development of dementia gradually results in the loss of executive abilities necessary to organize appropriate dietary intake and maintain focus on eating behaviour. This may result in a gradual loss of weight over months to years, and eventually necessitates increased environmental support.

Although in many situations weight loss is the outcome of advancing dementia, in some situations dementia may result in considerable increases, rather than decreases in weight. This can occur because of decreased physical activity, as well as from medications that increase weight such as the atypical antipsychotics, particularly olanzapine.[8] Increased orality with excessive and sometimes inappropriate eating might be seen in those with very frontal behavioural presentations.

In depression, changes in eating behaviour are more subacute, occurring over weeks to months, and, similar to the case in dementia, might also include weight gain as well as weight loss.

In the early stages of dementia there may be mild, reactive depressive mood symptoms secondary to the awareness of the illness. This may be particularly so in those who have cared for their own elderly and demented relatives, and who are well aware of the expected evolution of the illness for themselves. Severely and consistently depressed mood is uncommon, however, in the absence of a true mood disorder. In depression, depressed mood is pervasive, present most of the day and present nearly every day. Its severity is frequently greater.

Mood dyscontrol, or mood liability, is different from depressed mood as it tends to be more episodic. It may present without any other symptoms of sadness or other distress and is seen in a variety of brain disorders including dementia.[9] Episodic crying episodes, as well as episodic inappropriate laughter, may at times be very frequent and socially disabling. Mood dyscontrol may be reactive to a stressor that has overwhelmed the person's coping abilities, but if it is very frequent, it is probably secondary to ongoing, biological brain changes. Of course, mood dyscontrol may also be seen in depression, but in this case crying episodes tend to be more frequent and consistent and are congruent with other symptoms of sadness and distress. Inappropriate laughing is rarely seen in depression.

Lack of interest and initiative (apathy) is a typical finding in the course of AD (and other dementias) as the frontal lobes are affected. However, this apathetic presentation develops gradually over months to years, and is generally not associated with expressions of sadness, hopelessness and self harm. In depression there is a subacute decrease of interest and initiative that is somewhat similar to apathy, but this usually develops over weeks to months and is accompanied by other mood symptoms such as sadness and hopelessness. Apathy is thought to be a symptom independent of depression[10] with its own independent aetiology and, unless apathy is secondary to a true depressive disorder, antidepressant medications are generally not useful. Probably first line now in the treatment of apathy in dementia are medications such as the cholinesterase inhibitors.[11] Also of potential use are stimulant medications such as methylphenidate, although these can cause increased agitation and irritability. Dopaminergic drugs may also decrease apathy, yet secondary psychotic symptoms from these limit their usefulness.

Psychomotor agitation becomes more common in the mid to late stages of dementia, particularly in the later part of the day. It is frequently accompanied by wandering, pacing and vocalizations. Psychomotor agitation may be quite difficult to differentiate from a depressive symptom in an older person with an agitated depression, although, in depression, the agitation will probably have developed over a shorter period of time, and will tend to occur throughout the day.

Guilt, worthlessness and hopelessness are not common in dementia, although they are seen commonly in severe depression. Similarly, serious suicidal thoughts and actions are uncommon overall in dementia (although a recent publication has suggested that severe Alzheimer's pathology might be a risk factor for suicide,[12] whereas suicidal thoughts and actions are common in depressive disorder).

DIAGNOSTIC CHALLENGES: SECONDARY DEPRESSIVE SYMPTOMS

Various medical disorders (such as hypothyroidism, stroke and cancers), pain, nutritional deficiency and certain medications may cause significant mood symptoms in the demented elderly. In the presence of significant dementia, communication deficits impair the recognition of these disorders and these underlying conditions may be missed (see Chapter 21). For this reason, the consensus statement on improving the quality of mental health care in United States nursing homes[13] has recommended that residents with new onset or worsening of depressive symptoms, should have a pain assessment, assessment of the nutritional status, assessment of underlying medical conditions and assessment of medications that have the potential to alter cognition and mood. The recommendations also suggest performing a laboratory examination that includes haemoglobin, thyroid function, electrolytes, vitamin B_{12}, relevant serum drug levels and a complete blood cell count.

MAJOR DEPRESSIVE DISORDER AND ALZHEIMER'S DISEASE

Prevalence

Major depressive disorders in AD are less common than depressive symptoms, although most studies have described increased rates compared to the general population. Published prevalence rates have a very large range, presumably because of sampling issues (clinical, convenience and population samples) as well as differing diagnostic schema. Because of this lack of consistency in the information about depression in dementia, an international meeting was held to draft diagnostic criteria. These have now been published by Olin et al.[14] Although the authors of this article cautioned that their criteria were developed on the basis of a consensus process, and further research was needed to confirm their validity, the new criteria seem to represent an improved approach to diagnosis in this difficult clinical area. They might well help clinicians make more consistent diagnoses of mood disorders in AD, and possibly also contribute to more homogeneous prevalence data.

Aetiology

Reasons for the increased prevalence of depressive disorders in AD are not entirely clear. Although there has been some exploration of the potential role insight and awareness of deficits might play in the development of depressive symptoms, it is not generally felt that this is a major factor in the aetiology of major depressive disorders. A more favoured explanation is that neurotransmitter and possibly other structural changes related to the degenerative process of dementia are directly responsible for causing the mood disorder. The face validity of this is bolstered by a body of literature including that associating localized vascular damage to the later development of mood disorders. However, some longitudinal studies have shown an association between mood symptoms and the subsequent development of dementia.[15] This might suggest that the mood disorder itself might have a causal role to play in dementia, possibly through stress-mediated hippocampal damage, although there is much debate about this issue (for a detailed review of this complex topic, see Swab et al[16]). Because mood disorders tend to be relapsing illnesses, this mechanism would ensure a high comorbidity of dementia and mood disorders in later years. A third possibility is that depression is a prodrome of dementia, so that depression does not play a causal role in causing dementia, nor does dementia play a causal role in causing depression, but both might be different dimensions of the same disorder, presenting at different times.

Treatment

There are only a few double-blind placebo-controlled treatment studies of mood disorders in dementia. These include studies with imipramine, citalopram, clomipramine, moclobamide, maprotiline, fluoxetine and sertraline. Possibly because of difficulties with comorbidities and a high level of response to non-pharmacological research conditions, these few studies have not been able to establish strong and unequivocal evidence on the efficacy of antidepressants in depression and dementia, as is summarized in a Cochrane database review.[17] Even less published evidence is available for other treatments in dementia, such as electroconvulsive therapy, and all of these somatic treatments carry with them risks of adverse effects. Fortunately, although it is very difficult to obtain objective evidence on the efficacy of non-pharmacological therapies, some evidence is now available for the successful use of these, which include behavioural, environmental and caregiver approaches.[18,19]

However, even in the absence of a large, consistent research literature, the severity of adverse outcomes caused by comorbid serious depression and dementia often necessitates somatic treatment. Professional consensus suggests that depressive disorder in this clinical situation should be treated in a manner consistent with best practices for other frail elderly people. Fairly specific guidelines for this clinical population have been published by various authors.[20,21] In general, the efficacies of the various groups of antidepressants are thought to be fairly similar.

Adverse effects, drug interactions and pharmacokinetics, however, differ among the groups. Particularly important are anticholinergic properties (common in the tricyclics), as these further worsen cognition as well as cause the usual peripheral symptoms such as constipation. The cardiotoxicity of tricyclic antidepressants also limits their use, especially in patients with cardiac disease, for whom the newer generation of antidepressants is more appropriate.[22] The severity of symptoms of overdose is also more serious for the tricyclics. Significant orthostatic hypotension (such as that caused by the tricyclic antidepressants) can worsen the likelihood of falls. However, it is now clear that the SSRIs also increase (possibly more so) the risk of falls in the elderly, and the mechanism for this is not entirely clear.[23] Other side effects of the SSRIs include gastrointestinal side effects, headache, restlessness and occasional insomnia, hyponatraemia[24] and an adverse impact on sexual function. Of the SSRIs, fluoxetine and its active metabolite have a very long half-life and therefore are not often used in the frail elderly. Citalopram and possibly sertraline may be particularly advantageous because of low levels of drug–drug interactions.

Of the newer antidepressants, bupropion is more likely to cause restlessness, anxiety and insomnia, as well as (rarely) a lowering of the seizure threshold. Venlafaxine is generally well tolerated and has side effects similar to those of the SSRIs. However, it can occasionally cause an increase in diastolic blood pressure. Although trazodone is useful for its sedating effects, its tendency to cause postural hypotension limits its use in frail patients. Mirtazapine has had little formal study in the frail elderly, but may be useful because of its sedating properties and effects on weight gain.

Beneficial effects of antidepressants on pain are of particular interest in the elderly, who commonly suffer from both pain and depression. Dual action antidepressants, i.e. those inhibiting both serotonin and noradrenaline, are more likely to help chronic pain

than the SSRIs.[25] Of these, tricyclics are the best-known and most commonly used group, but their use is limited by side effects, especially as the dosage increases. It is encouraging, therefore, that some of the newer antidepressants such as venlafaxine and duloxetine (and possibly mirtazapine) have also been shown to have pain effects in preliminary research studies.

Table 13.2 presents a summary of selected medications for patients with depression and dementia. Within the different groups of antidepressants, choices of particular usefulness in the elderly are noted with an asterisk.

Electroconvulsive therapy (ECT) may also be useful in older patients with severe depression.[26] It has a very fast onset of action and is extremely useful where there is a serious suicide risk or more severe medical compromise. ECT delirium can be minimized by good anaesthetic technique, including oxygenation and unilateral electrode placement.

Treatment for a significant depressive disorder should continue for at least two years at an adequate dosage for most elderly patients, but this recommendation is less clear in those with dementia. Patients who do not respond to an adequate trial on the first antidepressants may be tried on a different class of

Table 13.2 Antidepressant treatment of patients with depression and dementia

Antidepressant	Comments on use
Tricyclic antidepressants	
*Nortriptyline	Effective antidepressants and additional benefits on pain control, but anticholinergic effects, postural hypotension and cardiotoxicity. Nortriptyline is more sedating than desipramine
Desipramine	
Selective serotonin reuptake inhibitors (SSRIs)	
*Citalopram	Gastrointestinal side effects, headache, insomnia, tremor, sexual dysfunction, SIADH. Citalopram is of particular interest because of low risk of drug–drug interactions
Sertraline	
*Escitalopram	
Other antidepressants	
*Venlafaxine	Gastrointestinal side effects, headache, SIADH. Possibly faster onset of action and beneficial pain effects
*Mirtazapine	Sedation, weight gain, possible pain control. May need to start at 7.5 mg to minimize sedation. Rapid dissolving wafer available helpful in patients with dysphagia
Moclobemide	Nausea, headache and insomnia
Bupropion	Possible excess stimulation, possible lowering of seizure threshold

* Particularly useful choice

antidepressant, or be tried on a lithium augmentation trial. Another possibility is methylphenidate, or a combination of antidepressants, although this increases the risk of adverse medication effects.

CONCLUSION

Mood symptoms are common in AD and related disorders, and may be severe enough to require a variety of interventions. Although the evidence for the efficacy of treatment of depression is not as strong as in older persons without dementia, active treatment is still often indicated to preserve the quality of life of the older person and his or her social network.

REFERENCES

1. Judd LL, Akiskal HS. The clinical and public health relevance of current research on subthreshold depressive symptoms to elderly patients. Am J Geriatr Psychiatry 2002; 10: 233–238.
2. De Ronchi D, Bellini F, Berardi D, et al. Cognitive status, depressive symptoms, and health status as predictors of functional disability among elderly persons with low-to-moderate education: The Faenza Community Aging Study. Am J Geriatr Psychiatry 2005; 13:672–685.
3. Gilley DW, Bienias JL, Wilson RS, et al. Influence of behavioral symptoms on rates of institutionalization for persons with Alzheimer's disease. Psychol Med 2004; 34:1129–1135.
4. Donaldson C, Tarrier N, Burns A. Determinants of carer stress in Alzheimer's disease. Int J Geriatr Psychiatry 1998; 13:248–256.
5. Draper B, Brodaty H, Low LF, Richards V. Prediction of mortality in nursing home residents: impact of passive self-harm behaviors. Int Psychogeriatr 2003; 15:187–196.
6. Wu YH, Swaab DF. The human pineal gland and melatonin in aging and Alzheimer's disease. J Pineal Res 2005; 38: 145–152.
7. Stewart R, Masaki K, Xue QL, et al. A 32-year prospective study of change in body weight and incident dementia: the Honolulu-Asia Aging Study. Arch Neurol 2005; 62: 55–60.
8. Deberdt WG, Dysken MW, Rappaport SA, et al. Comparison of olanzapine and risperidone in the treatment of psychosis and associated behavioral disturbances in patients with dementia. Am J Geriatr Psychiatry 2005; 13: 722–730.
9. Arciniegas DB, Topkoff J. The neuropsychiatry of pathologic affect: an approach to evaluation and treatment. Semin Clin Neuropsychiatry 2000; 5:290–306.
10. Levy ML, Cummings JL, Fairbanks LA, et al. Apathy is not depression. J Neuropsychiatry Clin Neurosci 1998; 10: 314–319.
11. Boyle PA, Malloy PF. Treating apathy in Alzheimer's disease. Dement Geriatr Cogn Disord 2004; 17:91–99. Epub 15 Oct 2003.
12. Rubio A, Vestner AL, Stewart JM, et al. Suicide and Alzheimer's pathology in the elderly: a case-control study. Biol Psychiatry 2001; 49:137–145.
13. American Geriatrics Society; American Association for Geriatric Psychiatry. Consensus statement on improving the quality of mental health care in U.S. nursing homes: management of depression and behavioral symptoms associated with dementia. J Am Geriatr Soc 2003; 51:1287–1298.
14. Olin JT, Schneider LS, Katz IR, et al. Provisional diagnostic criteria for depression of Alzheimer disease. Am J Geriatr Psychiatry 2002; 10:125–128.
15. Dal Forno G, Palermo MT, Donohue JE, et al. Depressive symptoms, sex, and risk for Alzheimer's disease. Ann Neurol 2005; 57:381–387.
16. Swaab DF, Bao AM, Lucassen PJ. The stress system in the human brain in depression and neurodegeneration. Ageing Res Rev 2005; 4:141–194.
17. Bains J, Birks JS, Dening TR. The efficacy of antidepressants in the treatment of depression in dementia. Cochrane Database Syst Rev 2002; (4):CD003944.
18. Teri L, Gibbons LE, McCurry SM, et al. Exercise plus behavioral management in patients with Alzheimer disease: a randomized controlled trial. JAMA 2003; 290:2015–2022.
19. Teri L, Logsdon RG, Uomoto J, McCurry SM. Behavioral treatment of depression in dementia patients: a controlled clinical trial. J Gerontol B Psychol Sci Soc Sci 1997; 52: P159–P166.
20. Baldwin RC, Anderson D, Black S, et al. Guideline for the management of late-life depression in primary care. Int J Geriatr Psychiatry 2003; 18:829–838.
21. Alexopoulos GS, Katz IR, Reynolds CF III, et al. The Expert Consensus Guideline Series: Pharmacotherapy of Depressive Disorders in Older Patients. Postgrad Med Special Report 2001; October:1–86.
22. Roose SP. Considerations for the use of antidepressants in patients with cardiovascular disease. Am Heart J 2000; 140(4 suppl):84–88.
23. Liu B, Anderson G, Mittmann N, et al. Use of selective serotonin-reuptake inhibitors of tricyclic antidepressants and risk of hip fractures in elderly people. Lancet 1998; 351: 1303–1307.
24. Kirby D, Ames D. Hyponatraemia and selective serotonin re-uptake inhibitors in elderly patients. Int J Geriatr Psychiatry 2001; 16:484–493.
25. Briley M. Clinical experience with dual action antidepressants in different chronic pain syndromes. Hum Psychopharmacol 2004; 19(suppl 1):S21–S25.
26. Van der Wurff FB, Stek ML, Hoogendijk WJ, Beekman AT. The efficacy and safety of ECT in depressed older adults: a literature review. Int J Geriatr Psychiatry 2003; 18:894–904.

14

Cognition

Sven Joubert, Steve Joncas, Emmanuel Barbeau, Yves Joanette and Bernadette Ska

INTRODUCTION

Alzheimer's disease (AD) is characterized by the insidious onset of cognitive deficits that progress over the course of several years. The nature of the cognitive impairments and their severity vary greatly throughout the various stages of the disease, some symptoms emerging early in the disease and others occurring in later stages. This chapter will review the main domains of cognition that can be impaired in AD over the course of the disease, including memory, language, executive functions, visuospatial skills and praxis, as well as the evolution of cognitive impairments over the course of the disease. Finally, a short section of this chapter will briefly review atypical presentations of AD, their main presenting cognitive features and their evolution.

Risk factors

The rate of progression and relative severity of cognitive impairments in AD vary from one patient to another. There are a number of risk factors for AD, the most important one being age. For instance, the prevalence of AD is approximately 1 out of 100 Canadians between the ages of 65 and 74, 1 out of 14 between the ages of 75 and 84 and 1 out of 4 after the age of 85.[1] However, there are suggestions that other risk factors might be linked to AD. For example, AD has been found to be more common in women and in individuals with a lower socioeconomic status.[2] AD patients also tend to have less education than healthy individuals matched for age.[3] The reason for this is not well understood, but it may be that more educated people have greater cognitive and intellectual reserves, are able to achieve more during their lifetime and are better able to compensate for their deficits for a longer period of time. Finally, the fact that early onset AD is more frequent in some families and in people with

Down's syndrome reflects genetic risk factors. The role of genetic risk factors decreases with increasing onset age of patients with AD, while the role of environmental risk factors in AD likely increases with onset age (see Chapters 2 and 3).[4]

Heterogeneity in Alzheimer's disease

As it is the case in normal ageing,[5] the neuropsychological profile in AD is not strictly similar from one individual to the other. Heterogeneity in the manifestations of cognitive impairments in AD was first recorded through case reports (e.g. Crystal and collaborators[6]) as well as through multiple case studies realizing double dissociations.[7] Reports have shown that such double dissociations can be found between (e.g. memory vs language) as well as within (e.g. phonological vs semantic abilities) cognitive domains. Numerous group studies have tried to define cognition-based subgroups in AD.[8,9] However, none of these attempts yielded robust conclusions. One reason for such negative results may be that the possible subgroups in AD may be more definable through a longitudinal rather than transverse approach.[10] Indeed, there appears to be considerable heterogeneity in the evolution with time of the pattern of cognitive impairment. The presence of this heterogeneity has to be taken into consideration when examining cognitive abilities in AD. Among other things, evaluation procedures that do not cover all domains and components of cognition could largely be flawed by the presence of such heterogeneity of patterns of cognitive impairments in AD.

MEMORY

Memory is the domain of cognition that is usually affected foremost and that remains impaired most severely during the course of AD. All the different memory processes are affected in the disease (except procedural memory, which is preserved until the last stage), including immediate and working memory, recent memory and remote memory. The extent to which the different components of memory are affected, the order and progression of impairment are usually quite characteristic and are helpful in carrying out a differential diagnosis with other degenerative (e.g. frontotemporal lobar degeneration) and non-degenerative neurological conditions, depression and anxiety. Typically, the ability to retain newly-acquired and recent information is affected first in AD, as well as the ability to remember common and proper names. In the earliest stages, these memory problems and word finding difficulties can be difficult to distinguish from those that healthy elderly individuals sometimes experience. As recent memory becomes more impaired, general knowledge about the world (semantic memory) also slowly fades away, and individuals with AD will start forgetting more distant memories of their own past.

Short-term and working memory

An important component of memory is the ability to record new information and manipulate it during several seconds (usually up to 30 seconds) after it has been registered. This component of memory is commonly referred to as short-term memory. Working memory refers to information that is stored temporarily while it is manipulated simultaneously with other information. Short-term and working memory can apply to both the retention of verbal (e.g. a phonological loop) and visual information (e.g. a visuospatial sketchpad).[11] Short-term and working memory can be assessed by using forward and backward digit span tests, immediate recall of words (such as recalling the three words in the Mini-Mental Sate Examination (MMSE)[12]) and the Brown–Peterson paradigm in which trigrams are repeated successively over a period of 15 to 30 seconds, during which the subject is instructed to simultaneously count backward.[13,14] Short-term and working memory are usually disrupted in the early stages of AD.[15] In terms of working memory processes, it is thought that individuals with AD may experience a phonological loop impairment as well as a disruption of another of its components, namely the central executive system.[16] Several studies have also shown a reduced span for words, digits, letters and spatial locations.[17,18] The 'closing-in phenomenon' observed in figure copying tasks in AD patients has also been attributed to visuospatial working memory deficits.[19] In everyday life, some examples of working

memory defects translate in the patient not remembering what he/she wanted to pull out of the fridge while opening the fridge door or not being able to rehearse a phone number while dialling that number.

Recent memory (anterograde memory)

This aspect of memory refers to information that is consolidated so that it will be retained for a period lasting from 30 seconds to several days or longer. Recent memory allows us to recall the names of persons we have recently met or to recall what we did the day before. However, memory consolidation can occur over longer periods (sometimes weeks and months), and hence the boundary between recent memory and remote memory remains sometimes arbitrary. Recent memory, or what we commonly refer to as anterograde memory, is impaired in the earliest stages of AD, before any other cognitive impairment occurs. This component of memory is believed to be impaired even in the preclinical phase of the disease, several years before diagnosis can be firmly established.[20,21] In the early stage, AD patients are unable to recall what they did the day before, what they had for breakfast the same morning or to remember the content of a movie they saw a few days before. Patients forget the names of people and forget their appointments, lose their personal belongings such as their keys and their clothes, forget to pay their bills, have difficulty learning new information and become spatially and temporally disoriented. Such insidious difficulties are the first sign of the disease and progress more or less rapidly, followed by impairment in other cognitive domains. In neuropsychological practice, recent memory impairments can be evidenced using tests that require remembering word lists, figures and faces over a period of time ranging from several minutes to one week. Some examples of tests commonly used in clinical practice include the Buschke Selective Reminding Test,[22,23] the Logical Memory, Visual Reproduction and Facial Memory subtests of the WMS-III,[24] the California Verbal Learning Test,[25] as well as the Warrington Recognition Memory Test.[26] These tests are helpful to the early diagnosis of AD, particularly when they are used in combination.[27] Delayed recall is generally considered to be one of the best predictors of future dementia.[28,29] On anterograde verbal memory tests, mild AD patients are more impaired on free recall tasks[20] but their performance improves with cueing (cueing only helps in the early phase of AD, however, and is not effective for all individuals). AD patients benefit less from repetition over trials (flatter learning curve than healthy controls). As the disease progresses, patients benefit less from cueing, and total free and cued recall performance decreases. In the late stage, free and cued recall performance is at floor level and patients eventually cannot remember anything after a few minutes. Such tests are also useful in discriminating AD from other degenerative brain diseases, reflecting different patterns of memory impairment and different regions of brain damage. In frontotemporal dementia (FTD), for instance, free recall performance is similar to AD, but FTD patients benefit much more from cueing and the forgetting rate is not as important as in AD.[30]

Remote memory (retrograde memory)

This component of memory refers to memory that lasts from a few days to many years. Remote memory is generally expressed in years and overlaps with what is often designated as long-term memory. This aspect of memory concerns our ability to remember specific episodes of our lives over a period of several decades, including early childhood memories. Remote memory also includes the cultural knowledge that we have acquired during our lifetime (semantic memory). Although they both form declarative memory, semantic memory and episodic memory are considered by many to be functionally distinct and probably partly anatomically distinct components of remote memory.[31]

Autobiographical memory

Autobiographical memory refers to the events that a person has personally experienced, which are anchored in a specific spatial and temporal context. Autobiographical memory is impaired in AD, although specific aspects of autobiographical memory are impaired differently and in different stages of the disease. Because patients develop an anterograde memory disorder in the early stages of the disease, they have difficulties remembering much information that has occurred after the onset of the disease. Consequently, memory of recent years is generally very poor in AD. In contrast, distant events such as childhood memories are generally well preserved in the early stage of the disease and become affected only in the late stage. The destruction of memory follows a temporal gradient in AD (such as in other amnesic syndromes), sparing distant memories and interfering with recent ones along a somewhat linear continuum. This temporally graded memory loss found in antero-grade amnesia was recognized two centuries ago by Ribot[32] and was hence termed Ribot's law. This pattern of autobiographical memory impairment found in AD is distinct from that found in other degenerative dementias affecting memory such as semantic demen-

tia and FTD.[33–35] In semantic dementia, for instance, a reverse temporal gradient is found. Recent memory is generally intact, at least in the early stages of the disease, while more distant memories are lost. There is no clear temporal gradient in FTD.[34] These differences in patterns of retrograde amnesia likely reflect the nature of the memory components that are affected in each disease, as well as differences in the profiles of cortical atrophy associated with each condition. In semantic dementia, for instance, sparing of recent memory has been attributed to the relative preservation of the hippocampal formation (at least in the early stages), which holds a key role in the retention and consolidation of recently-acquired information. In contrast, severely damaged semantic memory in semantic dementia is believed to be caused by early damage to the temporal neocortex, a structure believed to be involved in the permanent storage of long-term memories.[36,37] Memory tests tapping autobiographical memories and semantic knowledge over periods of several decades are particularly useful in differentiating AD from other progressive disorders affecting memory. Memory tests assessing different periods of life include the Autobiographical Memory Interview[38] and the Crovitz Test of Autobiographical Memory.[39]

Semantic memory

The distinction between semantic and episodic memory was first made by Tulving.[31] Semantic memory relates to general knowledge shared by the individuals of the same cultural group and includes language, concepts and factual knowledge acquired over a lifetime. Neuropsychological tests evaluating our knowledge of objects, famous public persons and famous public events over a period of several decades contribute to evaluate the integrity of semantic memory. These tests are usually developed locally because they are sensitive to culture. Semantic memory is usually impaired early in AD and deficits progress slowly until reaching a severe and general semantic breakdown (a 'semantic desert'). Semantic memory impairments in AD can be demonstrated in tasks that require naming pictures or line-drawings of common objects and animals such as with the Snodgrass and Vanderwart battery,[40] in tasks that require to identify objects from their names, in verbal fluency tests (e.g. animals), in visual-verbal semantic matching tasks and in tests that tap general semantic knowledge.

Picture naming errors in AD consist primarily of semantic errors, but also of non-responses and visual errors. They are usually interpreted as reflecting a semantic memory loss concerning the items that are not named correctly rather than reflecting visuoperceptual defects.[41] Verbal fluency tasks (generating semantic category lists) are also impaired early in AD, to a greater extent than letter fluency tasks, the latter exerting greater demands on lexical retrieval abilities than on semantic knowledge.[42,43] General superordinate knowledge is generally better preserved than subordinate knowledge.[41,44] In naming tasks, category-specific effects are often observed in AD (particularly in the later stages), generally affecting natural categories (e.g. animals, fruits and vegetables) to a greater extent than man-made categories (e.g. tools and household objects).[45] This dissociation can sometimes be quite striking in clinical practice, particularly when using comprehensive picture naming tests such as the Snodgrass and Vanderwart battery[40] and when using real objects. Although there is considerable debate as to the putative nature of this dissociation, one theory explains this preference for artifacts over natural kinds in terms of the sensory/functional attributes of these entities and the differential underlying neuroanatomical distribution of these attributes within inferior temporal and frontoparietal regions of the brain.[46,47] Garrard et al[48] have shown the reverse pattern of impairment in a minority of patients (i.e. an advantage for living things), although most patients presented with the classical dissociation. This occasional occurrence of advantage for natural kinds in AD was attributed to variations in the location of cortical atrophy among patients. Patients with early biparietal atrophy were assumed to be disproportionately impaired for man-made objects due to the predominant role of the dorsal stream in functional knowledge of objects.[48] Gonnerman et al[49] suggested that the progression of category specific effects followed a specific course. In the early stage, there appears to be a short period of mild difficulty with artifacts, with no difficulty with biological kinds. Later on, selective and important impairment to biological kinds occurs, while impairment to artifacts remains stable. In the late stages, both biological kinds and artifacts are significantly impaired such that no clear category-specific effects arise.

Some authors have suggested that person-specific semantic knowledge (e.g. famous people) and general knowledge (e.g. objects and animals) may be affected differently in AD.[50,51] There is still debate as to whether they represent distinct semantic domains, but double dissociations have been reported.[52] Several studies have found that AD patients are particularly affected on tests of famous people knowledge (political figures, musicians, singers, athletes). Greene and Hodges[50] demonstrated that AD patients were impaired on all aspects of their Famous Faces and Names Test, including recognition, identification and

naming of celebrities upon presentation of their photographs and their names. Impaired processing of both famous names and faces indicates a multidomain impairment, which is a clear indicator of semantic breakdown. In another study, access to information about famous people was also compromised in AD when compared to normal age-matched controls, both for faces and names.[53] By studying AD patients longitudinally, Greene and Hodges[54] demonstrated that semantic knowledge concerning famous people deteriorated more rapidly than autobiographical knowledge, thus supporting the notion of a fractionation of remote memory. Recently, Estévez-Gonzalez et al[55] showed that mild cognitive impairment (MCI) patients who were diagnosed two years later with AD were significantly impaired in recognizing photographs of famous people in the preclinical phase, more than MCI patients who had not developed dementia. These results suggest that semantic knowledge of famous people may be impaired very early in the course of the disease and may be useful in the early diagnosis of AD. Finally, person-based semantic knowledge would be affected earlier and to a greater extent than general semantic knowledge in early and questionable AD.[51,55] It is commonly accepted that anterograde memory is first impaired in AD, followed by semantic and attentional deficits, and by linguistic and visuospatial impairments later on.[56,57] Some studies suggest, however, that semantic deficits may appear in the earliest phases of the disease.[27,55,58,59]

In summary, the main difficulty found in individuals with AD concerns the acquisition, consolidation and retention of novel information. This memory impairment is followed by a slow and progressive dissolution of the memories accumulated over a lifetime, affecting both the cultural and autobiographical dimensions of these memories. More recent memories are touched first, but with time distant memories also start fading. Then comes a time when the personal history and identity of the individual collapses: first grandchildren are not recognized, followed by children-in-law and eventually the individual's own children. Leaps in generations occur such that the grandchildren will be mistaken for the children, and individuals with AD will be convinced they are currently living periods of their lives that had occurred several decades before. This progressive destruction of an individual's history naturally leads to the collapse of his/her own identity.

ATTENTION AND EXECUTIVE FUNCTIONS

Deficits in attention and executive functions are an important part of the neuropsychological dysfunction of AD and have deleterious impacts on daily living activities,[60,61] such as planning the course of the day and organizing the various activities to be carried out. Royal et al[62] found that a measure of executive functioning was better correlated with functional status than MMSE scores.

Attentional deficits are common in Alzheimer's patients, but the various components of attention appear to be differentially affected in the disease process. Selective attention is typically impaired.[63–66] Most studies showed selective attention deficits in mildly to moderately demented patients, but Perry et al[57] suggested that selective attention could also be altered in minimally demented patients (MMSE > 24). In their review, Perry and Hodges[61] concluded that, in AD patients, the focusing of attention seems to be relatively spared but the ability to disengage and shift their attention is predominantly affected. Divided attention is also impaired early in the disease process.[61,63] There is controversy, however, over the stage at which individuals with AD show impairment in dual task paradigm. Although the performance of mild patients is typically impaired, minimally demented patients do not appear to experience divided attention impairments.[57] The complexity of the task is also an important variable in the patients' performances as they perform relatively well in automatized vs effortful tasks.[65,67] Impairment in divided attention can have practical implications in the patient's daily living. For instance, Camicioli et al[68] concluded that a mental task can interfere with deambulation in AD patients and possibly increase their risk of falling. Sustained attention has not been as extensively studied in AD. It appears to be relatively preserved in minimally demented patients, but altered in mild Alzheimer's patients.[57,65] Alertness is unaffected, at least in mildly to moderately demented patients.[69] Reaction times seem to be longer in mild patients compared to controls, even in some 'very mild' patients in some types of tasks.[70] It is unclear, however, whether it is cognitive processing that is slowed or the response selection and executive element of the tasks.

Executive dysfunction is an early manifestation of AD.[71] Although there are various definitions and models of executive functions, they are generally defined as complex abilities that allow response in an adaptive manner to novel situation.[72] Inhibition, a major component of executive functioning, appears to be impaired early in the course of the disease[16] and may also account for disrupted performance in certain neuropsychological tests.[73] Patients have difficulty inhibiting an automated response in tasks, but also in suppressing a previously relevant rule in order

to learn a new one.[73] Deficits in mental flexibility and set-shifting are also reported in mild to moderate Alzheimer's patients.[74–76] AD patients also tend to make more perseverative errors,[77,78] and planning difficulties have been demonstrated in mild to moderate Alzheimer's patient.[79] As Perry and Hodges[61] point out in their review, it is unclear whether all functions are equally affected in the disease or if there are dissociations in performance between specific aspects of executive functions. Self-awareness is another important aspect of executive functions that is impaired in mild to moderate stages[72] and may occur more frequently in AD than in other types of dementias.[80] In a recent study comparing subjects' self-estimation of objective performance, Barrett et al[81] demonstrated anosognosia in mild to moderate patients relative to controls. It is also common in clinical practice to witness patients being confronted with their difficulties in a testing environment, but nevertheless having difficulties estimating the impact of their illness in their daily life or the burden of their condition on their family.

LANGUAGE

Language disturbances appear early in AD and constitute an important element of the diagnosis, although they are usually overshadowed by impairment of memory and executive functions. Anomia is one of the earliest and most easily recognizable symptoms in AD.[82] Difficulties finding the right word and hesitations become exacerbated as the disease progresses. Word-finding difficulties are particularly evident during confrontation naming tasks such as the Boston Naming Test.[83] In contrast, speech is fluent (although sometimes incoherent), articulation, syntax, morphology and reading abilities are preserved. Many empty words (e.g. *thing*, *do*, *it*) are used as substitutions for missing words, which sometimes makes it difficult to follow what patients are saying. A high proportion of utterances that convey little or no meaning is used. Anomia in AD likely results from a combination of lexical-retrieval difficulties and semantic memory impairments. In the early stage, word-finding problems are more likely due to lexical-retrieval difficulties, but semantic impairments increasingly account for the difficulties as the disease progresses (i.e. lost or degraded meaning of words and concepts; see section on semantic memory). Empty speech, reduction of informative content and overuse of pronouns are also characteristic features of AD. These problems also reflect a semantic defect at the level of individual lexical entries, affecting either the meaning of a word or the meaning of a string of words in the case of a sentence. Semantic memory breakdown is thus probably one of the central causes of language disturbances in AD, accounting for word-finding difficulties,[84] the emptiness of AD patients' discourse,[85] the reduction of information content[85] and the overuse of pronouns without clear referents.[86]

Discourse abilities – or the ability to organize the communicative content by reference to a given type of discourse (e.g. narrative, conversation, descriptions) – is relatively spared in the early stage, although the desire to communicate may be reduced. AD patients often do not complete their sentences and tend to lose track of the conversation, probably at least in part due to working memory impairments. Nevertheless, speech is clearly articulated and sentences are grammatically correct. Discourse requires the integration of basic linguistic abilities, such as naming, but also non-linguistic cognitive abilities, such as selection, organization, and planning.[87,88] Because all of these abilities can be impaired to various degrees in AD, they can lead to somewhat heterogeneous patterns of discourse impairments. In terms of discourse comprehension, AD patients demonstrate better comprehension for central ideas than for details, and better comprehension for literal information than for implied information.[89,90] AD patients are thus able to retain a mental representation of the structure of narratives, at least in the early stage of the disease. They have difficulties, however, with information that is not stated explicitly, which requires in other words the construction of an inference.[90] The difficulties of AD patients with such implicit information can be explained by working memory deficits and/or attentional resource allocation problems.

In the moderate stage, the syntactic complexity of AD patients' speech output diminishes.[91–94] Speech may become paragrammatic (e.g. improper use of syntactic structures or function words). AD patients also have increased problems with the comprehension of syntactically complex sentences. For example, patients show difficulties in processing reversible or passive sentences (e.g. *John loves Mary* and *Mary is loved by John*).[95,96] This ability to process sentences using syntactic information, however, only appears to be lost in the moderate to severe stage of the disease. Memory problems may contribute to the presence of sentence comprehension problems.[82] Paraphasias (e.g. the use of a word for another), and particularly semantic paraphasias and neologisms, become more frequent due to the aggravation of the semantic defect. Perseverations of words and syllables occur more frequently and the speech content is often repetitive. Reading is very disturbed and writing becomes severely disorganized, confirming an already existing pattern of surface dysorthographia and dyslexia. Writing and reading deficits are characterized by the incorrect spelling and reading of irregular words despite normal use of grapheme-to-phoneme transcription rules. During the progression of the disease, the component of language that appears to be the most preserved is phonology. Repetition of words and spontaneous language indicate that the phonological aspects of language production in AD patients remain preserved even in the severe stage of the disease.[97–99] Finally, the late stage of the disease is marked by pallilalia (repetition of their own words), echolalia (repetition of others), reduced fluency and severely reduced speech output evolving toward complete mutism.

PRAXIC ABILITIES

The two main types of apraxia found in AD are visuo-constructional apraxia and limb apraxia. The main features of visuoconstructional apraxia appear in the early stage of the disease.[100–102] Typically, patients have difficulties when they are asked to copy drawings of two-dimensional and three-dimensional figures such as drawing a clock, a cube or the Rey–Osterrieth figure. Visuoconstructional errors are very subtle in the early stage and become more important as the disease progresses (see Figure 14.1). When they are asked to draw, AD patients do not use the space of the page properly. The drawing is not centred and the dimensions of the drawing are reduced.[103] Drawing impairment worsens as the disease progresses.[100] Fewer angles, impaired perspective and fewer spatial relations were also found in drawings of AD patients.[104] Frequent errors consist of omissions, simplifications, perseverations as well as errors in spatial orientation and organization.[105,106] Constructional apraxia is generally viewed as a visuospatial deficit. The 'closing-in phenomenon' observed in AD patients is perhaps one of the best examples of visuospatial dysfunction, where patients tend to copy a figure near the target or overlap the figure with the target in order to compensate for their deficit.[19]

Limb apraxia, or apraxia of voluntary movements, is also present in AD but the nature and the degree of the impairment and the stage at which apraxia appears are quite heterogeneous.[107] Classically, AD patients present signs of ideomotor apraxia in the early stage of the disease, although several studies have shown that early-stage AD patients do not necessarily show problems during the evaluation of limb praxis.[108,109] Therefore, contrary to what has long been

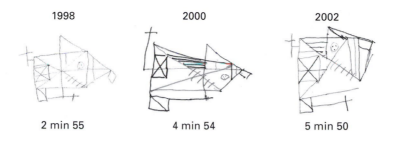

1998   2000   2002

2 min 55   4 min 54   5 min 50

Figure 14.1 Performance of an Alzheimer's patient on the Rey–Osterrieth Complex Figure Test (copy) several years apart

thought, apraxia is not a necessary presenting feature of AD.[110] Ochipa et al[111] suggested that AD patients have an impaired ability to understand the meaning of certain gestures and movements (conceptual apraxia), while their ability to produce gestures remains intact much longer. They demonstrated that AD patients could be impaired at the various levels of conceptual knowledge underlying the execution of actions. Another distinctive feature of apraxia in AD is that individuals use a body part as an object, for example they use a finger for brushing their teeth. Finally, in the late stage, many AD patients present with dressing apraxia: they are unable to dress properly and look at their clothes with strangeness.

VISUOSPATIAL SKILLS – SPATIAL ORIENTATION AND WAYFINDING

Difficulties in spatial orientation are among the early manifestations of the cognitive deficits in AD and interfere with independent living, affecting driving abilities in particular[112] and causing patients to get lost. Early studies tended to conceptualize this difficulty exclusively as a spatial representation and cognitive mapping problem. Indeed, various studies showed that Alzheimer's patients have difficulties in spatial representations.[113] More recent studies, however, showed that this problem was in fact frequently accompanied by impaired spatial problem-solving abilities. For this reason, such deficits are now referred to as wayfinding disabilities. Memory deficits also play a significant role in wayfinding difficulties,[114] although spatial disorientation is probably due to a combination of factors including visuoperceptual, visuospatial and memory disturbances. Recent studies have identified several cognitive deficits that can affect wayfinding abilities, including difficulties in planning and organizing behaviour,[115,116] impairment in focused attention and inhibition,[115] deficits in

visual perception[117] as well as distractibility and impulsivity.[118]

COGNITIVE CHARACTERIZATION IN ATYPICAL PRESENTATIONS OF AD

Atyical presentations of AD account for about 15 per cent of all AD cases.[119] Contrary to the typical presentation, which starts by a relatively isolated amnesic syndrome, early manifestations in atypical presentations of AD do not concern memory, but affect rather selectively other cognitive domains such as language and vision.[120] They are generally associated with focal cortical atrophy in specific regions of the brain. Instrumental functions can remain impaired in isolation during several years before the clinical diagnosis of dementia is fully established. Interestingly, these atypical presentations are most often reported in younger people (usually before the age of 65). A major difficulty with such atypical presentations of AD is the overlap in the clinical and neuropsychological presentation of such focal disorders with other progressive neurological diseases, which sometimes makes the diagnosis particularly difficult.

Posterior cortical atrophy

Visual forms of Alzheimer's disease were first reported as a separate clinical entity under the name of posterior cortical atrophy.[121] Clinically, visual presentations of AD are characterized by severe visuospatial difficulties including simultagnosia and visual-field defects. It is not uncommon that many of these individuals are seen by several ophthalmologists before being referred to a neurologist. Other common signs associated with this syndrome affecting predominantly the occipitoparietal region include alexia, agraphia, acalculia, anomia, digital agnosia and sometimes apraxia.[119,122] Aperceptive prosopagnosia and agnosia may also occur. The onset of symptoms starts earlier than in the classic form of AD, around 55–60 years of age. Progression is faster and severe visuospatial disturbances may be present 3 years after onset. Insight is usually preserved during a very long period of time. Memory also appears largely preserved over a long period of time. Anatomo-pathological studies have found that most patients presenting with this syndrome had confirmed AD, with atrophy predominating in the parietal lobes.[122,123] In contrast to individuals presenting with classic AD, patients with posterior cortical atrophy were shown to have a greater neurofibrillary tangle (NFT) density in the primary and associative visual cortices and in the inferior parietal lobes, while a significantly lower NFT density was found in the hippocampus.[122]

Primary progressive aphasia

Language-based forms of AD are less frequent and rarely isolated. As in posterior cortical atrophy, they rarely concern the older subject.[124] Primary progressive aphasia[125] can be subdivided in different subgroups based on the nature of the speech impairment. Logopenic aphasia is probably the form of aphasia most related to AD.[126] Logopenic speech is characterized by a slow rate of speech output and hesitations in spontaneous speech, anomia in picture-naming tasks, impaired syntactic comprehension and impaired sentence repetition. Single-word comprehension and semantics, on the other hand, are preserved. Gorno-Tempini et al[126] suggested that a short-term phonological memory impairment may be the core underlying mechanism that is disrupted in logopenic primary aphasia. Episodic memory is mildly impaired in contrast. Patients remain independent and have a good insight about their condition for a long period of time. Atrophy predominates in the left posterior temporal cortex and inferior parietal lobule.[126]

Pure progressive amnesia

Although memory impairment is the main presenting feature of AD, it can sometimes take a highly unusual course and remain isolated during many years despite a severe amnesic syndrome. Such patients are rare and very few have been described. An isolated memory impairment lasting up to 10 years has been reported in some patients, with memory performance declining very slowly over this length of time before eventually meeting all the criteria of AD.[127] Although not enough cases have been reported to this day in order to pinpoint a specific neuropsychological profile, these patients appear to present with a severe amnesic syndrome despite relatively preserved functions in other domains such as executive functions, praxis and language. A distinctive feature of pure progressive amnesia is that, in spite of the severe and isolated memory defect, patients remain entirely independent in everyday life for many years[128] and appear to remain very well spatially oriented.[129] In one case reported, autobiographical memory remained intact for a long time despite severe semantic disturbances. For instance, the patient could recall with vivid detail some events of the Second World War she had lived through (e.g. airplane bombings) despite having forgotten who Hitler was or who was persecuted during the war.[129] Two anatomo-clinical studies have reported lesions characteristic of AD in such patients.[127,130]

CONCLUSION

Alzheimer's disease is characterized at the outset by difficulty acquiring new information and impaired memory for recent events. Patients may start showing signs of spatial and temporal disorientation. During subsequent stages, patients slowly become impaired within and across domains of cognition, presenting with impairments in semantic and working memory, executive functions, language, praxis and visuospatial abilities. Semantic memory impairments are important in AD and give rise to a range of linguistic, praxic and perceptual difficulties. As the disease progresses, cognitive impairments start having more impact on activities of everyday life and patients gradually lose their functional autonomy. Patients also become less aware of their difficulties. Finally, the presentation and evolution of cognitive deficits in AD can be quite heterogeneous from one individual to another. In certain atypical presentations, the disease may take a highly unusual course and affect selectively language, memory or visuospatial skills during many years.

ACKNOWLEDGEMENTS

Sven Joubert is supported by the Alzheimer Society of Canada and les Fonds de recherche en santé du Québec (FRSQ).

REFERENCES

1. Groupe de travail de l'Étude canadienne sur la santé et le vieillissement. Méthodes d'étude et prévalence de la démence. Can Med Assoc J 1994; 150:899–913.

2. Kawas C, Gray S, Brookmeyer R, Fozard J, Zonderman A. Age-specific incidence rates of Alzheimer's disease: the Baltimore Longitudinal Study of Aging. Neurology 2000; 54:2072–2077.

3. Kukull WA, Higdon R, Bowen JD, et al. Dementia and Alzheimer disease incidence: a prospective cohort study. Arch Neurol 2002; 59:1737–1746.

4. Silverman JM, Ciresi G, Smith CJ, Marin DB, Schnaider-Beeri M. Variability of familial risk of Alzheimer disease across the late life span. Arch Gen Psychiatry 2005; 62: 565–573.

5. Valdois S, Joanette Y, Poissant A, Ska B, Dehaut F. Heterogeneity in the cognitive profile of normal elderly. J Clin Exp Neuropsychol 1990; 12:587–596.

6. Crystal HA, Horoupian DS, Katzman R, Jotkowitz S. Biopsy-proved Alzheimer's disease presenting a right parietal lobe syndrome. Ann Neurol 1981; 12:186–188.

7. Joanette Y, Ska B, Poissant A, Béland R. Neuropsychological Aspects of Alzheimer's Disease: Evidence of Inter- and Intra-functions Heterogeneity. New York: Springer 1992.

8. Martin A, Brouwers P, Lalonde F, et al. Towards a behavioral typology of Alzheimer's patients. J Clin Exp Neuropsychol 1986; 8:594–610.

9. Neary D, Snowden JS, Bowen DM, et al. Neuropsychological syndromes in presenile dementia due to cerebral atrophy. J Neurol Neurosurg Psychiatry 1986; 49:163–174.

10. Joanette Y, Belleville S, Gely-Nargeot M, Ska B, Valdois S. [Plurality of patterns of cognitive impairment in normal aging and in dementia.] Rev Neurol (Paris) 2000; 156: 759–766.

11. Baddeley AD. Working memory: The interface between memory and cognition. In: Gazzaniga MS, ed. Cognitive Neuroscience. Malden, MA: Blackwell 2000; 292–304.

12. Folstein MF, Folstein SE, McHugh PR. 'Mini-mental state'. A practical method for grading the cognitive state of patients for the clinician. J Psychiatr Res 1975; 12:189–198.

13. Brown J. Some tests of the decay theory of immediate memory. J Exp Psychol 1958; 19:215–224.

14. Petersen LR, Petersen MJ. Short-term retention of individual items. J Exp Psychol 1959; 58:193–198.

15. Germano C, Kinsella GJ. Working memory and learning in early Alzheimer's disease. Neuropsychol Rev 2005; 15:1–10.

16. Collette F, Van der Linden M, Salmon E. Executive dysfunction in Alzheimer's disease. Cortex 1999; 35:57–72.

17. Belleville S, Peretz I, Malenfant D. Examination of the working memory components in normal aging and in dementia of the Alzheimer type. Neuropsychologia 1996; 34:195–207.

18. Grossi D, Becker JT, Smith C, Trojano L. Memory for visuospatial patterns in Alzheimer's disease. Psychol Med 1993; 23:65–70.

19. Lee BH, Chin J, Kang SJ, et al. Mechanism of the closing-in phenomenon in a figure copying task in Alzheimer's disease patients. Neurocase 2004; 10:393–397.

20. Grober E, Lipton RB, Hall C, Crystal H. Memory impairment on free and cued selective reminding predicts dementia. Neurology 2000; 54:827–832.

21. Petersen RC. Mild Cognitive Impairment. Aging to Alzheimer's Disease. Oxford: University Press 2003.

22. Buschke H. Selective reminding for analysis of memory and learning. J Verb Learning Verb Behav 1973; 12:543–550.

23. Buschke H, Fuld PA. Evaluating storage, retention, and retrieval in disordered memory and learning. Neurology 1974; 24:1019–1025.

24. Weschler D. Échelle Clinique de Mémoire de Weschler MEM III (WMS-III). Paris: Les éditions du Centre de Psychologie appliquée 2001.

25. Delis DC, Kramer JH, Kaplan E, Ober BA. California Verbal Learning Test: Adult Version Manual. San Antonio, TX: The Psychological Corporation 1987.

26. Warrington EK. Recognition Memory Test Manual. Windsor: NFER-Nelson 1984.

27. Barbeau E, Didic M, Tramoni E, et al. Evaluation of visual recognition memory in MCI patients. Neurology 2004; 62: 1317–1322.

28. Small BJ, Fratiglioni L, Viitanen M, Winblad B, Backman L. The course of cognitive impairment in preclinical Alzheimer disease: three- and 6-year follow-up of a population-based sample. Arch Neurol 2000; 57:839–844.

29. Ivanoiu A, Adam S, Van der Linden M, et al. Memory evaluation with a new cued recall test in patients with mild cognitive impairment and Alzheimer's disease. J Neurol 2005; 252:47–55.

30. Pasquier F, Grymonprez L, Lebert F, Van der Linden M. Memory impairment differs in frontotemporal dementia and Alzheimer's disease. Neurocase 2001; 7:161–171.

31. Tulving E. Episodic and semantic memory. In: Tulving E, Donaldson W, eds. Organization of Memory. New York: Academic Press 1972; 381–403.

32. Ribot T. Diseases of Memory. New York: Appleton 1882.

33. Graham KS, Hodges JR. Differentiating the roles of the hippocampal complex and the neocortex in long-term memory storage: evidence from the study of semantic dementia and Alzheimer's disease. Neuropsychology 1997; 11:77–89.

34. Piolino P, Desgranges B, Belliard S, et al. Autobiographical memory and autonoetic consciousness: triple dissociation in neurodegenerative diseases. Brain 2003; 126(part 10): 2203–2219.

35. Snowden JS, Griffiths HL, Neary D. Semantic–episodic memory interactions in semantic dementia: implications for retrograde memory function. Cogn Neuropsychol 1996; 13: 1101–1137.

36. Mummery CJ, Patterson K, Price CJ, et al. A voxel-based morphometry study of semantic dementia: relationship between temporal lobe atrophy and semantic memory. Ann Neurol 2000; 47:36–45.

37. Snowden JS, Goulding PJ, Neary D. Semantic dementia: a form of circumscribed cerebral atrophy. Behav Neurol 1989; 2:167–182.

38. Kopelman MD, Wilson BA, Baddeley AD. The autobiographical memory interview: a new assessment of autobiographical and personal semantic memory in amnesic patients. J Clin Exp Neuropsychol 1989; 11:724–744.

39. Crovitz HF, Schifmann H. Frequency of episodic memories as a function of their age. Bull Psychonom Soc 1974; 4:517–518.

40. Snodgrass JG, Vanderwart M. A standardized set of 260 pictures: norms for name agreement, image agreement, familiarity, and visual complexity. J Exp Psychol [Hum Learn] 1980; 6:174–215.

41. Chertkow H, Bub D. Semantic memory loss in dementia of Alzheimer's type. What do various measures measure? Brain 1990; 113(part 2):397–417.

42. Hodges JR, Salmon DP, Butters N. Differential impairment of semantic and episodic memory in Alzheimer's and Huntington's diseases: a controlled prospective study. J Neurol Neurosurg Psychiatry 1990; 53:1089–1095.

43. Rosser A, Hodges JR. Initial letter and semantic category fluency in Alzheimer's disease, Huntington's disease, and progressive supranuclear palsy. J Neurol Neurosurg Psychiatry 1994; 57:1389–1394.

44. Hodges JR, Salmon DP, Butters N. Semantic memory impairment in Alzheimer's disease: failure of access or degraded knowledge? Neuropsychologia 1992; 30:301–314.

45. Silveri MC, Daniele A, Giustolisi L, Gainotti G. Dissociation between knowledge of living and nonliving things in dementia of the Alzheimer type. Neurology 1991; 41:545–546.

46. Warrington EK, McCarthy RA. Categories of knowledge. Further fractionations and an attempted integration. Brain 1987; 110(part 5):1273–1296.

47. Warrington EK, Shallice T. Category specific semantic impairments. Brain 1984; 107(part 3):829–854.

48. Garrard P, Patterson K, Watson PC, Hodges JR. Category specific semantic loss in dementia of Alzheimer's type. Functional–anatomical correlations from cross-sectional analyses. Brain 1998; 121(part 4):633–646.

49. Gonnerman LM, Andersen ES, Devlin JT, Kempler D, Seidenberg MS. Double dissociation of semantic categories in Alzheimer's disease. Brain Language 1997; 57: 254–279.

50. Greene JD, Hodges JR. Identification of famous faces and famous names in early Alzheimer's disease. Relationship to anterograde episodic and general semantic memory. Brain 1996; 119(part 1):111–128.

51. Thompson SA, Graham KS, Patterson K, Sahakian BJ, Hodges JR. Is knowledge of famous people disproportionately impaired in patients with early and questionable Alzheimer's disease? Neuropsychology 2002; 16: 344–358.

52. Thompson SA, Graham KS, Williams G, et al. Dissociating person-specific from general semantic knowledge: roles of the left and right temporal lobes. Neuropsychologia 2004; 42:359–370.

53. Dopkins S, Kovner R, Rich JB, Brandt J. Access to information about famous individuals in Alzheimer's disease. Cortex 1997; 33:333–339.

54. Greene JD, Hodges JR. The fractionation of remote memory. Evidence from a longitudinal study of dementia of Alzheimer type. Brain 1996; 119(part 1):129–142.

55. Estévez-Gonzalez A, Garcia-Sanchez C, Boltes A, et al. Semantic knowledge of famous people in mild cognitive impairment and progression to Alzheimer's disease. Dement Geriatr Cogn Disord 2004; 17:188–195.

56. Lambon Ralph MA, Patterson K, Graham N, Dawson K, Hodges JR. Homogeneity and heterogeneity in mild cognitive impairment and Alzheimer's disease: a cross-sectional and longitudinal study of 55 cases. Brain 2003; 126(part 11): 2350–2362.

57. Perry RJ, Watson P, Hodges JR. The nature and staging of attention dysfunction in early (minimal and mild) Alzheimer's disease: relationship to episodic and semantic memory impairment. Neuropsychologia 2000; 38:252–271.

58. Vogel A, Gade A, Stokholm J, Waldemar G. Semantic memory impairment in the earliest phases of Alzheimer's disease. Dement Geriatr Cogn Disord 2005; 19:75–81.

59. Blackwell AD, Sahakian BJ, Vesey R, et al. Detecting dementia: novel neuropsychological markers of preclinical Alzheimer's disease. Dement Geriatr Cogn Disord 2004; 17: 42–48.

60. Patterson MB, Mack JL, Geldmacher DS, Whitehouse PJ. Executive functions and Alzheimer's disease: problems and prospects. Eur J Neurol 1996; 3:5–15.

61. Perry RJ, Hodges JR. Attention and executive deficits in Alzheimer's disease. A critical review. Brain 1999; 122(part 3): 383–404.

62. Royal DR, Mahurin RK, Cornell J. Bedside assessment of frontal degeneration: distinguishing Alzheimer's disease from non-Alzheimer's cortical dementia. Exp Aging Res 1994; 20:95–103.

63. Baddeley AD, Baddeley HA, Bucks RS, Wilcock GK. Attentional control in Alzheimer's disease. Brain 2001; 124(part 8):1492–1508.

64. Pignatti R, Rabuffetti M, Imbornone E, et al. Specific impairments of selective attention in mild Alzheimer's disease. J Clin Exp Neuropsychol 2005; 27:436–448.

65. Rizzo M, Anderson SW, Dawson J, Myers R, Ball K. Visual attention impairments in Alzheimer's disease. Neurology 2000; 54:1954–1959.

66. Slavin MJ, Mattingley JB, Bradshaw JL, Storey E. Local–global processing in Alzheimer's disease: an examination of interference, inhibition and priming. Neuropsychologia 2002; 40:1173–1186.

67. Crossley M, Hiscock M, Foreman JB. Dual-task performance in early stage dementia: differential effects for automatized and effortful processing. J Clin Exp Neuropsychol 2004; 26:332–346.

68. Camicioli R, Howieson D, Lehman S, Kaye J. Talking while walking: the effect of a dual task in aging and Alzheimer's disease. Neurology 1997; 48:955–958.

69. Nebes RD, Brady CB. Phasic and tonic alertness in Alzheimer's disease. Cortex 1993; 29:77–90.

70. Pate SP, Margolin DI, Freidrich FJ, Bentley EE. Decision-making and attentional processes in ageing and in dementia of the Alzheimer's type. Cogn Neuropsychol 1994; 11: 321–339.

71. Binetti G, Magni E, Padovani A, et al. Executive dysfunction in early Alzheimer's disease. J Neurol Neurosurg Psychiatry 1996; 60:91–93.

72. Lezak MD, Howieson DB, Loring DW. Neuropsychological Assessment, 4th edn. Oxford: University Press 2004.

73. Amieva H, Lafont S, Auriacombe S, et al. Analysis of error types in the trial making test evidences an inhibitory deficit in dementia of the Alzheimer type. J Clin Exp Neuropsychol 1998; 20:280–285.

74. Albert MS, Moss MB, Tanzi R, Jones K. Preclinical prediction of AD using neuropsychological tests. J Int Neuropsychol Soc 2001; 7:631–639.

75. Haxby JV, Grady CL, Koss E, et al. Heterogeneous anterior–posterior metabolic patterns in dementia of the Alzheimer type. Neurology 1988; 38:1853–1863.

76. Lafleche G, Albert MS. Executive function deficits in mild Alzheimer's disease. Neuropsychology 1995; 9:313–320.

77. Bayles KA, Tomoeda CK, McKnight PE, Helm-Estabrooks N, Hawley JN. Verbal perseveration in individuals with Alzheimer's disease. Semin Speech Lang 2004; 25:335–347.

78. Bondi MW, Monsch AU, Butters N, Salmon DP, Paulsen J. Utility of a modified version of the Wisconsin Card Sorting Test in the detection of dementia of the Alzheimer type. Clin Neuropsychol 1993; 7:161–170.

79. Mack JL, Paterson MB. Executive dysfunction and Alzheimer's disease: performance on a test of planning ability, the Porteous Maze Test. Neuropsychology 1995; 9:556–564.

80. Wagner MT, Spangenberg KB, Bachman DL, O'Connell P. Unawareness of cognitive deficit in Alzheimer disease and related dementias. Alzheimer Dis Assoc Disord 1997; 11:125–131.

81. Barrett AM, Eslinger PJ, Ballentine NH, Heilman KM. Unawareness of cognitive deficit (cognitive anosognosia) in probable AD and control subjects. Neurology 2005; 64:693–699.

82. Kempler D. Neurocognitive Disorders in Aging. Thousand Oaks, California: Sage Publications, Inc 2005.

83. Kaplan EF, Goodglass H, Weintraub S. The Boston Naming Test. Philadelphia: Lea & Febiger 1983.

84. Hodges JR, Salmon DP, Butters N. The nature of the naming deficit in Alzheimer's and Huntington's disease. Brain 1991; 114(part 4):1547–1558.

85. Nicholas M, Obler LK, Albert ML, Helm-Estabrooks N. Empty speech in Alzheimer's disease and fluent aphasia. J Speech Hear Res 1985; 28:405–410.

86. Almor A, Kempler D, MacDonald MC, Andersen ES, Tyler LK. Why do Alzheimer patients have difficulty with pronouns? Working memory, semantics, and reference in comprehension and production in Alzheimer's disease. Brain Language 1999; 67:202–227.

87. Ehrlich JS. Studies of discourse production in adults with Alzheimer's disease. In: Bloom RL, Obler LK, De Santi S, Ehrlich JS, eds. Discourse Analysis and Applications: Studies in Adult Clinical Populations. Hillsdale, NJ: Lawrence Erlbaum Associates 1994; 149–160.

88. Ehrlich JS, Obler LK, Clark L. Ideational and semantic contributions to narrative production in adults with dementia of the Alzheimer's type. J Commun Disord 1997; 30:79–98; quiz 98–99.

89. Biassou N, Harris C, Marchman WB, Kritchevsky M. Production of complex syntax in normal ageing and Alzheimer's disease. Lang Cogn Process 1995; 10:487–539.

90. Welland RJ, Lubinski R, Higginbotham DJ. Discourse comprehension test performance of elders with dementia of the Alzheimer type. J Speech Lang Hear Res 2002; 45: 1175–1187.

91. Altmann LJ, Kempler D, Andersen ES. Speech errors in Alzheimer's disease: reevaluating morphosyntactic preservation. J Speech Lang Hear Res 2001; 44:1069–1082.

92. Bates E, Harris C, Marchman WB, Kritchevsky M. Production of complex syntax in normal ageing and Alzheimer's disease. Lang Cogn Process 1995; 10:487–539.

93. Croisile B, Ska B, Brabant MJ, et al. Comparative study of oral and written picture description in patients with Alzheimer's disease. Brain Language 1996; 53:1–19.

94. Glosser G, Deser T. Patterns of discourse production among neurological patients with fluent language disorders. Brain Language 1991; 40:67–88.

95. Rochon E, Saffran EM, Berndt RS, Schwartz MF. Quantitative analysis of aphasic sentence production: further development and new data. Brain Language 2000; 72: 193–218.

96. Waters GS, Caplan D, Rochon E. Processing capacity and sentence comprehension in patients with Alzheimer's disease. Cogn Neuropsychol 1995; 12:1–30.

97. Bayles KA, Kaszniak AW, Tomoeda CK. Communication and cognition in normal aging and dementia. Boston, MA: Little Brown 1987.

98. Hier DB, Hagenlocker K, Shindler AG. Language disintegration in dementia: effects of etiology and severity. Brain Language 1985; 25:117–133.

99. Nebes RD. Semantic memory in Alzheimer's disease. Psychol Bull 1989; 106:377–394.

100. Ajurriaguerra J, Muller M, Tissot R. A propos de quelques problèmes posés par l'apraxie dans les démences. Encéphale 1960; 5:375–401.

101. Edwards DF, Baum CM, Deuel RK. Constructional apraxia in Alzheimer's disease: contributions to functional loss. Phys Occup Ther Geriat 1991; 9:53–68.

102. Rosen WG. Neuropsychological investigation of memory, visuoconstructional, visuoperceptual, and language abilities in senile dementia of the Alzheimer type. Adv Neurol 1983; 38:65–73.

103. Moore V, Wyke MA. Drawing disability in patients with senile dementia. Psychol Med 1984; 14:97–105.

104. Kirk A, Kertesz A. On drawing impairment in Alzheimer's disease. Arch Neurol 1991; 48:73–77.

105. Brantjes M, Bouma A. Qualitative analysis of the drawings of Alzheimer patients. Clin Neuropsychol 1991; 5:41–52.

106. Ska B. Fonctions visuo-spatiales et praxiques dans la démence de type Alzheimer. In: Habib M, Joanette Y, Puel M, eds. Démences et Syndromes Démentiels: Approche Neuropsychologique. Paris: Masson 1991.

107. Ska B. Apraxie des membres supérieurs et démence de type Alzheimer. In: Le Gall D, Aubin G, eds. Les Apraxies. Marseille, France: Editions Solal 2003; 219–228.

108. Della Sala S, Lucchelli F, Spinnler H. Ideomotor apraxia in patients with dementia of Alzheimer type. J Neurol 1987; 234:91–93.

109. Tsortzis C, Ruel J, Masure MC. Are there different forms of expression in functional deficits in the early stages of Alzheimer's disease? J Neurolinguist 1986; 2:151–162.

110. Richard J, Constantinidis J, Bouras C. La Maladie d'Alzheimer. Paris: Presses universitaires de France 1988.

111. Ochipa C, Rothi LJ, Heilman KM. Conceptual apraxia in Alzheimer's disease. Brain 1992; 115(part 4):1061–1071.

112. Fitten LJ, Perryman KM, Wilkinson CJ, et al. Alzheimer and vascular dementias and driving. A prospective road and laboratory study. JAMA 1995; 273:1360–1365.

113. Richard J, Bizzini L, Arrazola L, Palas C. De l'actualisation des structures cognitives dans les démences à (ou à prédominance de) plaques séniles (PS) et dégénérescences neurofibrillaires. Med Hyg (Geneve) 1981; 38: 4027–4036.

114. Henderson VW, Mack W, Williams BW. Spatial disorientation in Alzheimer's disease. Arch Neurol 1989; 46:391–394.

115. Passini R, Rainville C, Marchand N, Joanette Y. Wayfinding in dementia of the Alzheimer type: planning abilities. J Clin Exp Neuropsychol 1995; 17:820–832.

116. Rainville C, Passini R, Marchand N. A multiple case of wayfinding in dementia of the Alzheimer type: decision making. Aging Neuropsychol Cogn 2001; 8:54–71.

117. O'Brien HL, Tetewsky SJ, Avery LM, et al. Visual mechanisms of spatial disorientation in Alzheimer's disease. Cereb Cortex 2001; 11:1083–1092.

118. Chiu YC, Algase D, Whall A, et al. Getting lost: directed attention and executive functions in early Alzheimer's disease patients. Dement Geriatr Cogn Disord 2004; 17: 174–180.

119. Galton CJ, Patterson K, Xuereb JH, Hodges JR. Atypical and typical presentations of Alzheimer's disease: a clinical, neuropsychological, neuroimaging and pathological study of 13 cases. Brain 2000; 123(part 3):484–498.

120. Didic M, Felician O, Ceccaldi M, Poncet M. [Progressive focal cortical atrophies.] Rev Neurol (Paris) 1999; 155 (suppl 4):S73–S82.

121. Benson DF, Davis RJ, Snyder BD. Posterior cortical atrophy. Arch Neurol 1988; 45:789–793.

122. Tang-Wai DF, Graff-Radford NR, Boeve BF, et al. Clinical, genetic, and neuropathologic characteristics of posterior cortical atrophy. Neurology 2004; 63:1168–1174.

123. Renner JA, Burns JM, Hou CE, et al. Progressive posterior cortical dysfunction: a clinicopathologic series. Neurology 2004; 63:1175–1180.

124. LeRhun E, Richard F, Pasquier F. Natural history of primary progressive aphasia. Neurology. 2005; 65:887–891.

125. Mesulam MM. Slowly progressive aphasia without generalized dementia. Ann Neurol 1982; 11:592–598.

126. Gorno-Tempini ML, Dronkers NF, Rankin KP, et al. Cognition and anatomy in three variants of primary progressive aphasia. Ann Neurol 2004; 55:335–346.

127. Didic M, Ali Cherif A, Gambarelli D, Poncet M, Boudouresques J. A permanent pure amnestic syndrome of insidious onset related to Alzheimer's disease. Ann Neurol 1998; 43:526–530.

128. Stokholm J, Jakobsen O, Czarna JM, Mortensen HV, Waldemar G. Years of severe and isolated amnesia can precede the development of dementia in early-onset Alzheimer's disease. Neurocase 2005; 11:48–55.

129. Joubert S, Barbeau E, Walter N, Ceccaldi M, Poncet M. Preservation of autobiographical memory in a case of pure progressive amnesia. Brain Cogn 2003; 53: 235–238.

130. Caselli RJ, Couce ME, Osborne D, Deen HG, Parisi JP. From slowly progressive amnesic syndrome to rapidly progressive Alzheimer disease. Alzheimer Dis Assoc Disord 1998; 12:251–253.

15

Functional autonomy

Isabelle Gélinas

INTRODUCTION

Deterioration in functional abilities of daily living (ADL) has a major impact on quality of life of an individual with Alzheimer's disease (AD).[1–4] Feelings of incompetence and loss of control are often expressed by the patient in the earlier stages of the disease. Frustration and the feeling of insult are expressed by patients in the later stages of the disease. Because the decline in functional abilities is such a predominant feature in AD, it is included as a criterion for the diagnosis of 'probable dementia of the Alzheimer's type' as recommended by the NINCDS-ADRDA work group,[5,6] in the DSM-IV[7] criteria for 'Dementia of the Alzheimer's Type' and the International Classification of Disease and Related Health Problems (ICD-10).[8] In addition, the rate of decline in the performance of ADL was identified as being a useful index for following the progression of the disease.[9,10] Furthermore, deterioration in functional activities has been found to be a critical predictor of institutionalization for the cognitively impaired.[11,12]

Changes of functional abilities over the course of AD, their relationship to cognition, the nature of difficulties in performing daily activities, consequences of functional loss and the assessment of functional abilities will be discussed in this chapter.

CHANGES IN FUNCTIONAL ABILITIES OVER THE COURSE OF AD

Changes in functional abilities over the course of AD have been investigated in several studies. Functional deficits usually appear subtly and patients slowly deteriorate over a period of several years.

Reisberg et al[13] and Reisberg[14] described the progressive changes of functioning from normality (no functional change) to severe AD in a seven stage scale, the Functional Assessment Staging (FAST) scale. According to this scale (Table 15.1), functional deficits start to occur subjectively in normal ageing (FAST stage 2). They become apparent in complex occupational tasks such as work or hobbies and in social activities at a stage when cognitive deficits are mild (FAST stage 3). For example, individuals may forget appointments or have difficulty finding their way in unfamiliar environments. When deficits in cognition become moderate, individuals with AD have more difficulties in performing complex instrumental ADL (IADL) such as dealing with finances or meals (FAST stage 4). At this point, independent living is attainable and the AD patient can still adequately perform basic tasks such as dressing or moving around their community, although the ability to drive a car becomes increasingly compromised. When the cognitive deficits become moderately severe, individuals start to experience difficulties with basic activities of daily living (BADL). This usually begins with problems in choosing appropriate clothing. At this point, AD patients are no longer able to live alone safely (FAST stage 5). As the disease progresses into FAST stage 6, individuals increasingly lose the ability to dress, bathe and use the toilet. Urinary and faecal incontinence begins at the end of the sixth FAST stage. In the final seventh stage, speech, as well as ambulation, is lost. Later in the seventh stage, basic motor capacities, including the ability to sit up, to smile and to independently hold up the head, are progressively lost. The seven FAST stages correspond optimally to the seven stages of cognitive and global deterioration which are described in the Global Deterioration Scale (GDS).[15]

The characteristic pattern of progressive functional deterioration described in the FAST was empirically tested by Sclan and Reisberg[16] in a study of 56 individuals diagnosed with probable AD, who were free of other complications. The gradual loss of functional abilities in a hierarchical pattern has also been

Table 15.1 Sequence of functional loss in normal ageing and Alzheimer's disease (Functional Assessment Staging)*

FAST Stage	Clinical characteristics	Clinical diagnosis	Corresponding magnitude of cognitive deficit	MMSE (mean score and standard deviation)**
1	No decrement	Normal adult	None	29.0 ± 1.7 (N = 43)
2	Subjective deficit in word-finding or recalling location of objects	Normal aged adult	Subjective only	28.2 ± 2.7 (N = 120)
3	Deficits noted in demanding employment settings	Compatible with incipient AD	Mild	23.8 ± 4.0 (N = 64)
4	Requires assistance in complex tasks, e.g. handling finances	Mild AD	Moderate	20.0 ± 4.8 (N = 121)
5	Requires assistance in choosing proper attire	Moderate AD	Moderately severe	14.4 ± 4.8 (N = 77)
6a	Requires assistance dressing	Moderately severe AD	Severe	11.1 ± 5.1 (FAST stages 6a and 6b, N = 6)
6b	Requires assistance bathing properly			
6c	Requires assistance with mechanics of toileting (such as flushing, wiping)			6.3 ± 5.2 (FAST stages 6c, 6d and 6e, N = 35)
6d	Urinary incontinence			
6e	Faecal incontinence			
7a	Speech ability limited to about a half-dozen words	Severe AD	Very severe	0.3 ± 0.8 (FAST stages 7a and 7b, N = 21)
7b	Intelligible vocabulary limited to a single word			
7c	Ambulatory ability lost			0.0 ± 0.0 (FAST stages 7c, 7d and 7f, N = 25)
7d	Ability to sit up lost			
7e	Ability to smile lost			
7f	Ability to hold head up lost			

*Adapted from Reisberg B.[27] Copyright © 1984 by Barry Reisberg MD
**From Reisberg et al[34]

substantiated by several longitudinal studies.[10,17–21] Stern et al[20] followed 67 individuals with AD from 6 months to 6 and a half years. They found that the ability to perform higher-level tasks such as doing chores, handling money or remembering short lists of items changed early in the course of the disease and continued to decline as the disease progressed. Changes in basic self-care abilities appeared later in the course of the disease (approximately four or five years after onset) and continued to deteriorate over time. Green et al[19] monitored 104 AD subjects for 31 months using well-established BADL and IADL scales. They observed greater deterioration in IADL over a broad range of cognitive severity levels, as measured by the Blessed Test,[22] than in BADL, where decline was very slight in the mild cases and marked only in the moderate to severe dementias.

Baum et al[23] and Gélinas et al[24] arrived at similar conclusions based on data from cross-sectional studies of community residing individuals with AD at various stages of the disease. Comparisons across stages led the authors to conclude that complex activities and problem-solving skills were lost early in the disease, while no significant deterioration in simple over-learned tasks was found until moderate stages of the disease.

Whether the rate of functional decline over the course of AD follows a linear progression has been questioned in more recent years.[18,21,25] Galasko et al[18] arrived at the conclusion that it follows a non-linear pattern. In a naturalistic observational study with 107 persons with AD, Suh et al[21] observed that performance in IADL started to be impaired early on in the disease process and that the rate of decline was linear as the cognitive score on the MMSE declined. In contrast, performance on BADL started to be significantly diminished when subjects had more severe cognitive deficits. The rate of decline was found to be very rapid at that stage and followed a curvilinear pattern.

Furthermore, Ferm[26] and Reisberg[27] reported that the progressive deterioration in functional abilities follows a reversal of the pattern observed in normal human development. Certain similarities in the time course for both patterns were also noted.

The usefulness of monitoring changes in BADL and IADL has been demonstrated by Galasko et al.[10] Their research identified these activities as constituting important clinical milestones for the progression of AD. The IADL were significant milestones in the early stages of the disease, while BADL were useful at intermediate (dressing and toileting) and late stages (feeding).

COGNITION AND FUNCTIONING

The relationship between cognitive deterioration and decline in functional abilities has been subject to several studies since changes in both domains are criteria for the diagnosis of AD, according to the DSM-IV.[7] There is, however, a controversy in the literature as to whether these changes follow a parallel course. Galasko et al[10] identified a direct correlation between the rate of deterioration in cognitive abilities and the risk of reaching functional milestones in a 3-year longitudinal study of 343 community-dwelling patients with probable AD. Tractenberg et al[28] also found a close relationship between the magnitude of change in cognition and functional ability over a 12-month period in 187 persons with AD living in the community.

On the other hand, Gauthier and Gauthier[29] reported differing results in their study of 38 intermediate stage AD subjects who were followed over a period of 9 months. During that time, the subjects were periodically assessed with a functional measure and a mental status examination. Their findings indicated that the magnitude of change differed between functional and cognitive loss.

Several cross-sectional studies of dementia have also indicated a low to moderate association between cognitive skills and functional abilities in ADL.[17,24,30–33] Teri et al[33] investigated the relationship between cognitive functioning, behavioural problems and functional abilities in 56 AD subjects with moderate cognitive impairments. They found a low but significant correlation ($r = 0.38$) between cognitive scores and IADL scores, while no significant association was found between cognitive scores and BADL scores. Reed et al[32] also investigated the relationship between cognition and functioning in order to assess the adequacy of using mental status tests to estimate functional abilities. They suggested that the MMSE score explained only a small portion of the variance in BADL and IADL and that various factors, such as changes in perceptual, sensory and motor skills, contributed additively with cognitive deficits to the observed performance of functional tasks. Moreover, the association between scores on the mental status and functional tests was found to be significant only for the severely demented subjects ($r = 0.68$ for BADL and $r = 0.51$ for IADL), while non-significant relationships were found for the less demented group. Nygard et al,[31] in a study on the relationship between cognitive skills and the ability to perform IADL in persons with mild AD, came to similar conclusions. The cognitive skills accounted only for 25 per cent of the variability in IADL ability.

One reason for the relatively low correlations observed between mental status and other cognitive assessments and functional measures may be the limited severity range studied in some of these investigations. Reisberg et al[13,34] studied the full range of disease severity (from normality until the very late stages of AD) using the FAST. As noted in the previous section, this measure assesses a range of functional capacity from normality, to incipient to severe IADL deficits, to incipient to severe ADL deficits. The correlation noted between the MMSE and this ordinal functional measure was 0.87 ($p < 0.001$) and 0.83 ($p < 0.001$) in the 1984 and 1992 studies, which respectively investigated 40 and 566 subjects with normal ageing and AD at all magnitudes of severity. Table 15.1 shows the mean and standard deviation of MMSE scores for the FAST functional severity stages as reported in the 1992 study of Reisberg et al.[34] As can be seen from Table 15.1, one problem is that cognition as assessed with measures which have traditionally been applied to dementia patients bottoms out in the late stages of AD. This problem has been addressed in recent years.[35] For instance, a test instrument, the Modified Ordinal Scales of Psychological Development (M-OSPD),[35,36] was developed to assess cognition in even the latest stages of AD. The correlation between this late-stage cognitive instrument and the FAST was examined. A correlation coefficient of -0.77 ($p < 0.001$) between this test battery for severely demented patients and the FAST functional measure was observed.

In summary, it is clear that there is a relationship between cognitive and functional losses in AD. The precise magnitude of this relationship found in various studies has varied, depending in part upon the range of severity studied and the instruments employed to measure cognition and functioning. As discussed subsequently, the magnitude of medical comorbidity in the study population will also strongly influence the observed magnitude of the relationship between cognition and functioning in AD. No studies have observed perfect relationships between these disparate domains of behaviour in AD patients. Hence, it is possible that functional loss in AD may not be entirely dependent upon, or related to, the cognitive losses which occur and that other, cognition-independent, factors may also be relevant in explaining some of the functional losses observed in AD patients.

THE NATURE OF DIFFICULTIES IN PERFORMING ACTIVITIES OF DAILY LIVING IN AD

Some of the fundamental underlying factors relating to functional losses in AD are being elucidated. For example, Franssen et al[37,38] have developed a cognition-independent neurological reflex and release sign measure for assessing the progression of AD. In a study of 135 normal aged and AD subjects, who were free of significant medical comorbidity, scores on this neurological measure correlated strongly with cognition as assessed with the MMSE ($r = 0.74$), and even more robustly with functional changes assessed with the FAST procedure ($r = 0.80$).[39] Interestingly, these investigators have reported that the emergence of particular reflexes (the grasp, sucking and the plantar extensor (Babinski) reflex) at a particular magnitude are very robust indicators of the emergence of incontinence in AD patients. A combinatorial measure of these reflexes differentiated permanently incontinent AD patients in FAST stages 7a and 7b from ADL-deficient, not yet incontinent AD patients in FAST stages 6a to 6c, each with a sensitivity, and specificity, and overall accuracy, of greater than 85 per cent.[40] Consequently, some functional changes seen in AD appear to be strongly associated with basic neurological changes in the patient's brain.

Studies have also uncovered very robust relationships between functional losses and continuing neuropathological changes in affected brain regions.[41,42] These studies indicate linear relationships between neural cell losses, volumetric structural changes and the percentages of cells with neurofibrillary changes, and the functional progression of AD. For example, in severe AD (FAST stage 7), the correlation between the FAST stage 7 substages and the number of neurons in the Ammon's horn region of the hippocampus has been found to be 0.90.[41]

Although they may be rooted in basic brain changes, functional deficits observed in AD often appear to be of multiple origin. Several studies have discussed the nature of the functional changes observed in AD.

Very early on, De Ajuriaguerra et al[43] observed dressing and undressing behaviours in approximately 100 demented subjects. They described difficulties in initiating dressing and undressing. Using a piece of clothing, the authors observed whether the subject was able to recognize the piece of clothing and (1) whether the subject was performing the task in the right sequence, (2) whether the subject was able to position the clothing appropriately with regard to the body or with regard to another piece of clothing and (3) whether the subject was able to complete the task appropriately. Problems with dressing were found to appear prior to difficulties with undressing and were mostly related to deficits in cognition and perception. Impairments in executive functions also had a major impact on the ability to perform these tasks. Similar impairments have also been related to disability in eating and in grocery shopping,[44] meal preparation,[44,45] financial capacity[46] and driving.[47]

These studies suggest that a wide range of deficits in perception and cognition, such as memory, attention and executive function, can affect the ability to perform ADL. As noted in the previous section, the impact of cognitive deficits on functional status has been extensively reported in the literature. The cognitive declines appear to impact particularly on the performance of more complex activities such as IADLs, but to a lesser degree on the ability to do routine or more stereotypical activities.[18,21,33,48]

In recent years, several authors have emphasized more particularly the impact of deficits in executive functions, such as spontaneity, planning and organization, completion of a task, judgment, sequencing and volition on functional changes in ADL.[24,49–53] Indeed, these skills are recognized as being crucial for the performance of complex goal-directed ADL.[52] Skurla et al[50] compared severely demented subjects with AD and normal controls and observed difficulties in performing ADL. They related the problems with ADL to the patient's inability to properly sequence the activity. Moreover, they observed volitional problems such as prolonged staring, refusal to complete a task and lack of initiation. Boyle et al[49] and Stout et al[53] demonstrated a clear relationship between problems in executive functions and IADL, while the association was much smaller with BADL. These findings are consistent with the assumptions that while intact executive skills are necessary for the performance in IADL, these skills may not be as important for BADL that tend to be more stereotypical activities.

In addition, factors other than the cognitive and perceptual abilities can further complicate functioning in an elderly demented population. Indeed, results from studies by Reed et al[32] and Willis et al[52] demonstrated that the cognitive measures explained only a portion of the variance in ADL. Borell,[54] Josephsson[55] and Lévesques et al[3] noted that behaviour alterations, the motivational level of the person and the availability of adequate support influence the performance in daily activities. In fact, behavioural alterations, such as apathy, have been found to directly affect ADL functioning beyond the cognitive impairments.[49,53] The impact on the quality of performance in ADL of deficits in motor abilities, such as increased tone, slowness of movement and reaction time and impaired gait, have also been observed, even in higher functioning individuals with AD.[56] Furthermore, numerous other concomitant medical conditions and social variables may strongly contribute to observed deficits in functional capacity.[3,27]

In conclusion, the studies presented above provide support for the hypothesis that the functional impairments observed in AD may be associated in part with cognitive deficits in areas such as memory, concentration, praxis, gnosia and executive functions, and also associated in part with other factors, such as behaviour alterations and concomitant medical morbidity.

CONSEQUENCES OF FUNCTIONAL LOSS

Deterioration in functional abilities has important effects on the life of the individual with AD as well as on those responsible for their care (e.g. family, friends, nursing staff).[3,57,58] Indeed, functional status is an important predictor of quality of life in persons with AD and their caregivers.[1,2,59,60] For the individual who is confronted with progressive losses, these disabilities can result in various emotional and behavioural reactions, such as frustration, withdrawal, anxiety, humiliation, apathy or aggressiveness. These, in turn, will have an impact on the social functioning of the individual.[17,61] As the disabilities become more apparent, safety may be compromised and it may become dangerous for the person to stay alone at home. Eventually, the person's ability to remain in the community will be affected.

Functional disabilities also have an impact on the caregiver. The progressive losses of abilities, and the resulting changes in roles, may cause various emotional reactions from family members and friends. For example, family members may become overwhelmed, embarrassed or irritated.[62] These emotional reactions in conjunction with the physical, financial and social demands that are occurring as a result of the functional limitations may eventually lead to a feeling of burden in the caregiver.[58] Indeed, as the functional disabilities become more severe, the amount of support needed to maintain the individual in the community increases. These great demands placed on the caregiver may also lead to major health conditions.[63–65] The burden of care may be an important element in the caregiver's decision to institutionalize an individual with AD.[11,66,67]

THE ASSESSMENT OF FUNCTIONAL ABILITIES IN AD

There is general agreement that measures of functional disability form an essential part of the diagnostic process as well as in care-planing for dementia patients.[3–5,10,18,32] Measures of functional disability are crucial for monitoring disease progression, assessing the benefit of interventions and making decisions on legal issues such as guardianship. In addition, they are recognized as constituting important outcome measures in clinical trials[18,68] and have been used in several pharmacological studies (Table 15.2). Therefore, it is essential to choose appropriate tools to measure functional capacities in AD in order to obtain accurate information.

Most studies support the need to test functional abilities separately from mental status when assessing

Table 15.2 ADL scales in pharmacological studies of Alzheimer's disease	
Basic Activities of Daily Living (ADL)[22]	Alpha-tocopherol/selegiline[72]
Disability Assessment for Dementia (DAD)[24]	Metrifonate,[73] donepezil,[74,75] galantamine[76]
Self-maintenance and Instrumental Activities of Daily Living (PSMS & IADL)[69]	Lazabemide,[77] donepezil[74]
Interview for Deterioration in Daily living activities in Dementia (IDDD)[18]	Donepezil[78]
Nurses' Observation Scale for Geriatric patients (NOSGER)[70]	Xanomeline[79]
Progressive Deterioration Scale (PDS)[71]	Tacrine,[80] rivastigmine,[81] galantamine,[82] donepezil[83]
Alzheimer's Disease Cooperative Study – Activities of Daily Living Inventory (ADCS-ADL)[18]	Galantamine[84,85]

severity of dementia.[4,23,24,30,32,52] Authors caution against the tendency to rely only on the results of cognitive tests to predict functional performance of demented patients, as they assess different symptomatic domains. Functional assessments provide a concrete and meaningful way to communicate intervention methods and their realistic successes to families.[17]

Many investigators have emphasized the importance of using functional scales specifically designed for the AD population.[16,86,87] Frequently used scales at the present time include the Lawton and Brody Physical Self-Maintenance and Instrumental Activities of Daily Living Scales,[69] which have been developed for general geriatric and medical patients. These scales may not be ideal for the specific requirements of cognitively impaired populations.

When choosing a functional assessment measure for patients with AD, the following criteria should be considered: (1) the instrument should have a conceptual approach based on the natural course of AD, and (2) the instrument should also be practical and have adequate psychometric properties. In addition to these general properties, the purpose and the content of the functional scale should be relevant to the population assessed (e.g. mild AD, community-dwellers or residents in an institution). The scale should be sufficiently sensitive to allow changes in performance to be documented. The potential usefulness of including both BADL and IADL functions in evaluating functioning for dementia patients has been noted.[10,18,19,58,88,89] It has also been suggested by some authors that a suitable measure for assessing functional disability in the AD population should not only measure whether the individual is able to per-

form activities but should also include information about the nature of the functional difficulties. Such scales could be of clinical usefulness in guiding interventions.[23,86,90]

FUNCTIONAL DISABILITY MEASURES IN AD

Several functional status measures have been developed which fulfil the specific needs of dementia patients, and a number of interesting instruments are in development. A description of selected measures currently used which have been tested to different degrees with regard to their reliability and validity is presented in Table 15.3. Few scales have been assessed on more than one type of validity or reliability or have been tested adequately for sensitivity to treatment.

A number of assessment instruments primarily focus on either ADL or IADL. For example, the Functional Activity Questionnaire (FAQ)[95] and the Everyday Problems Test for the Cognitively Challenged Elderly (EPCCE)[94] primarily evaluate IADLs. These scales may be useful for early detection or for assessment in the early stages of AD,[88,99] but may not adequately measure deficits in functional abilities when used with severely impaired patients who can no longer perform complex activities. In cases when one wants to assess a wide range of disability or capture change over time, instruments which incorporate BADL and IADL dimensions are likely to be particularly useful.[18] For instance, the Disability Assessment for Dementia (DAD),[24] a functional scale developed for the AD population, incorporates several activities in both BADL

Table 15.3 Functional disability measures in Alzheimer's disease

Name of the measure	Domains included				Mode of administration		Psychometric properties tested		
	BADL	IADL	Leisure	Others	Report from an informant	Direct observation/ performance-based	Reliability	Validity	Sensitivity
Activities of Daily Living Situational Test[50]	X	X				X		X	
Alzheimer's Disease Cooperative Study–Activities of Daily Living Inventory[18]	X	X	X	X	X		X	X	X
Bayer Activities of Daily Living Scale[91]	X	X	X		X		X	X	
Dementia Scale[22]	X	X		X	X		X	X	
Dependence Scale[92]	X	X		X	X		XX	XX	
Direct Assessment of Functional Status[93]	X	X				X	XX	X	X
Disability Assessment for Dementia[24]	X	X	X		X		XXX	XX	X
Everyday Problems Test for the Cognitively Challenged Elderly[94]		X				X	XX	X	
Functional Activity Questionnaire[95]		X		X	X		X	X	
Functional Assessment Staging[13]	16 stages of deterioration				X	X	X	XX	X
Functional Performance Measure[96]	X	X		X		X	XX	XX	
Kitchen Task Assessment[45]		X				X	XXX	XX	
Progressive Deterioration Scale[71]	X	X	X	X	X		X	X	
Psychogeriatric Basic ADL Scale[97]	X				X		X	X	
Structure Assessment of Independent Living Skills[98]	X	X		X		X	XXX	X	

and IADL categories. Some functional scales focus on specific areas of functioning such as feeding,[81,100,101] dressing,[102] meal preparation,[45] financial ability[103,104] or driving.[105]

Most functional instruments developed for use with the AD population can be classified as being descriptive/discriminative. These scales aim at identifying or quantifying functional impairments in cognitively impaired populations. A few instruments, such as the FAST,[13] have been developed as a predictive tool to be also used for diagnostic purposes. Although most instruments aim at monitoring progression of therapy or measuring the benefit of specific treatment, few of the instruments presented herein have shown therapeutic sensitivity (to detect change), despite the fact that they may have been used in studies to measure change in functional status over time. Some scales require a categorical judgment from the rater. Items are scored either on a nominal or dichotomous scale, reflective of the person's ability to correctly or incorrectly perform the task, or on an ordinal scale, indicative of the degree of impairment or the type of assistance required. Only two of the performance-based scales reviewed take time into account.[50,98] Time is scored independently from the ability to perform the tasks. Skurla and collaborators,[50] however, question the value of using time as an indicator of disability with this population.

With the exception of the instruments from Baum and Edwards,[45] Carswell et al,[96] Laberge and Gauthier[97] and Gélinas et al,[24] none of the measures reviewed provide information about the nature of the functional deficit. Most of the scales document whether a person can perform an activity or what type of assistance (e.g. physical or verbal) is needed to do specific activities.

There are two categories of assessment measures based on the source of information: (1) informant-based measures and (2) direct observational/performance-based methods. The superiority of instruments which use direct observation versus questionnaires, where information about the patient's functioning is obtained from a caregiver, has been debated. Both methods present advantages and limitations[106] and have been found to be comparable in their psychometric properties, acceptability to respondents and ease of administration or scoring.[107] The decision on which method to use will depend upon the presence of informants and other factors. There may be value in using both methods of evaluation in order to have a better understanding of the patient's condition.

CONCLUSION

Individuals with AD experience progressive deterioration in their ability to perform daily activities. The progressive deterioration in functioning clearly has negative repercussions on the life of the individual with AD and their caregivers. These losses appear to occur in a hierarchical pattern. The deterioration in functional abilities seems to be related to a multitude of deficits in cognition, perception, executive functions and behaviour. The proper description of the decline in functioning in AD provides a useful tool for documentation of disease severity and care planning. Therefore, functional assessment tools are an important part of the diagnostic process and the design of management and care strategies.

Several functional instruments designed specifically for AD populations are available. In judiciously choosing a particular instrument, it is important to consider the purpose of utilization, practicality and psychometric properties of the instrument. Assessment of the functional domain is crucial for obtaining an accurate portrait of the individual's level of overall autonomy.

REFERENCES

1. Albert SM, Del Castillo-Castaneda C, Sano M, et al. Quality of life in patients with Alzheimer's disease as reported by patient proxies. J Am Geriatr Soc 1996; 44:1342–1347.
2. Andersen CK, Wittrup-Jensen KU, Lulk A, Andersen K, Kragh-Sørenson P. Ability to perform activities of daily living is the main factor affecting quality of life in patients with dementia. Health Qual Life Outcomes 2004; 2:52.
3. Lévesque L, Roux C, Lauzon S. Alzheimer: Comprendre pour mieux Aider. (Ottawa: Editions du Renouveau Pédagogique Inc 1990).
4. Teunisse S, Derix MMA, Van Crevel H. Assessing the severity of dementia. Patient and caregiver. Arch Neurol 1991; 48: 274–277.
5. McKhann G, Drachman D, Folstein M, et al. Clinical Diagnosis of Alzheimer's Disease: Report of the NINCDS-ADRDA Work Group Under the Auspice of the Department of Health and Human Services Task Force on Alzheimer's Disease. Neurology 1984; 34:393–394.
6. Tierney MC, Fisher RH, Lewis AJ, et al. The NINCDS-ADRDA Work Group criteria for the clinical diagnosis of probable Alzheimer's Disease: a clinicopathologic study of 57 cases. Neurology 1988; 38:359–364.
7. American Psychiatric Association. Diagnostic and Statistical Manual of Mental Disorders, 4th edn. Washington DC: APA 1994.
8. World Health Organization. International Statistical Classification of Disease and Related Health Problems, 10th revision (ICD-10) Geneva: World Health Organization 1992.
9. Ferris, SH, Mackell, JA, Mohs R, et al. A multicenter evaluation of new treatment efficacy instruments for Alzheimer's disease clinical trials: overview and general results. Alzheimer Dis Assoc Disord 1997; 11:S1–S12.

10. Galasko D, Edland SD, Morris JC, et al. The Consortium to establish a registry for Alzheimer's disease (CERAD). Part XI. Clinical milestones in patients with Alzheimer's disease followed over 3 years. Neurology 1995; 45:1451–1455.

11. Mittelman MS, Ferris SH, Steinberg G, et al. An intervention that delays institutionalization of Alzheimer's disease patients: treatment of spouse-caregivers. Gerontologist 1993; 33:730–740.

12. Riter RN, Fries BE. Predictors of the placement of cognitively impaired residents on special care units. Gerontologist 1992; 32:184–190.

13. Reisberg B, Ferris SH, Anand R, et al. Functional staging of dementia of the Alzheimer's type. Ann NY Acad Sci 1984; 435:481–483.

14. Reisberg B. Functional assessment staging (FAST). Psychopharmacol Bull 1988; 24:653–659.

15. Reisberg B, Ferris SH, DeLeon MJ, et al. The Global Deterioration Scale for assessment of primary degenerative dementia. Am J Psychiatry 1982; 139:623–629.

16. Sclan SG, Reisberg B. Functional Assessment Staging (FAST) in Alzheimer's disease: reliability, validity and ordinality. Int Psychogeriatr 1992; 4(suppl 1):55–69.

17. Carswell A, Eastwood R. Activities of daily living, cognitive impairment and social function in community residents with Alzheimer disease. Can J Occup Ther 1993; 60:130–136.

18. Galasko D, Bennett D, Sano M, et al. An inventory to assess activities of daily living for clinical trials in Alzheimer's disease. The Alzheimer's Disease Cooperative Study. Alzheimer Dis Assoc Disord 1997; 11(suppl 2):S33–S39.

19. Green CR, Mohs RC, Schmeidler J, et al. Functional decline in Alzheimer's disease: a longitudinal study. J Am Geriatr Soc 1993; 41:654–661.

20. Stern Y, Hesdorffer D, Sano M, et al. Measurement and prediction of functional capacity in Alzheimer's disease. Neurology 1990; 40:8–14.

21. Suh G-H, Ju Y-S, Yeon BK, Sahah A. A longitudinal study of Alzheimer's disease: rates of cognitive and functional decline. Int J Geriatr Psychiatry 2004; 19:817–824.

22. Blessed G, Tomlinson BE, Roth M. The association between quantitative measures of dementia and of senile change in the cerebral grey matter of elderly subjects. Br J Psychiatry 1968; 114:797–811.

23. Baum CM, Edwards DF, Morrow-Howell N. Identification and measurement of productive behaviors in senile dementia of the Alzheimer type. Gerontologist 1993; 33:403–408.

24. Gélinas I, Gauthier L, McIntyre MC, Gauthier S. Development of a functional measure for persons with Alzheimer's disease: the Disability Assessment for Dementia. Am J Occup Ther 1999; 53:471–481.

25. Mitnitski AB, Mogilner AJ, Rockwood K. The rate of decline in function in Alzheimer's disease and other dementias. J Gerontol 1999; 54A:M65–M69.

26. Ferm L. Behavioral activities in demented geriatric patients. Gerontol Clin 1974; 16:185–194.

27. Reisberg, B. Dementia: a systematic approach to identifying reversible causes. Geriatrics 1986; 41:30–46.

28. Tractenberg RE, Weiner MF, Cummings JL, Patterson MB, Thal LL. Independence of changes in behavior from cognition and function in community-dwelling persons with Alzheimer's disease: a factor analytic approach. J Neuropsychiatr Clin Neurosci 2005; 17:51–60.

29. Gauthier L, Gauthier S. Assessment of functional changes in Alzheimer's disease. Neuroepidemiology 1990; 9:183–188.

30. Hershey LA, Jaffe DF, Greenough PG, et al. Validation of cognitive and functional assessment instruments in vascular dementia. Int J Psychiatry Med 1987; 17:183–192.

31. Nygard L, Amberla K, Bernspang B, Almkvist O, Winblad B. The relationship between cognition and daily activities in cases of mild Alzheimer's disease. Scand J Occup Ther 1998; 5:160–166.

32. Reed BR, Jagust WJ, Seab JP. Mental status as a predictor of daily function in progressive dementia. Gerontologist 1989; 29:804–807.

33. Teri L, Borson S, Kiyak HA, et al. Behavioral disturbance, cognitive dysfunction, and functional skill. Prevalence and relationship in Alzheimer's Disease. J Am Geriatr Soc 1989; 37:109–116.

34. Reisberg B, Ferris SH, Torossian C, et al. Pharmacologic treatment of Alzheimer's disease: a methodologic critique based upon current knowledge of symptomatology and relevance for drug trials. Int Psychogeriat 1992; 4(supp 1): 9–42.

35. Auer SR, Sclan SG, Yaffee RA, et al The neglected half of Alzheimer's disease: cognitive and functional concomitants of severe dementia. J Am Geriatr Soc 1994; 42:1266–1272.

36. Sclan SG, Foster JR, Reisberg B. Application of piagetian measures of cognition in severe Alzheimer's disease. Psychiatr J Univ Ott 1990; 15:221–226.

37. Franssen E, Reisberg B, Klugger A, et al. Cognitive independent neurologic symptom in normal aging and probable Alzheimer's disease. Arch Neurol 1991; 48:148–154.

38. Franssen E, Klugger A, Torossian C, et al. The neurologic syndrome of severe Alzheimer's disease: relationship to functional decline. Arch Neurol 1993; 50:1029–1039.

39. Franssen E, Reisberg B. Neurologic markers of the progression of Alzheimer disease. Int Psychogeriatr 1997; 9(suppl 1): 297–306.

40. Franssen E, Souren LEM, Torossian C, et al. Utility of developmental reflexes in the differential diagnosis and progression of incontinence in Alzheimer's disease. J Geriatr Psychiatry Neurol 1997; 10:22–28.

41. Bobinski M, Wegiel J, Tarnawski M, et al. Relationships between regional neuronal loss and neurofibrillary changes in the hippocampal formation and duration and severity of Alzheimer's disease. J Neuropathol Exp Neurol 1997; 56: 414–420.

42. Bobinski M, Wegiel J, Wisniewski HM, et al. Atrophy of hippocampal formation subdivisions correlated with stage and duration of Alzheimer disease. Dementia 1995; 6: 205–210.

43. De Ajuriaguerra J, Richard J, Tissot R. De quelques aspects des troubles de l'habillage dans les démences tardives dégénératives ou à lésions vasculaires diffuses. Ann médicopsychol 1967; 125:189–218.

44. Gray GE. Nutrition and dementia. J Am Dietetic Assoc 1989; 89:1795–1802.

45. Baum CM, Edwards DF. Cognitive performance in senile dementia of the Alzheimer's type: the Kitchen Task Assessment. Am J Occup Ther 1993; 47:431–436.

46. Griffith HR, Belue K, Sicola A, et al. Impaired financial abilities in mild cognitive impairment: a direct assessment approach. Neurology 2003; 60:449–457.

47. Donnely RE, Karlinsky H. The impact of Alzheimer's disease on driving ability: a review. J Geriat Psychiatry Neurol 1990; 3:67–72.

48. Bau C, Edwards D, Yonan C, et al. The relation of neuropsychological test performance to performance of functional tasks in dementia of the Alzheimer type. Arch Clin Neuropsychol 1996; 11:69–75.

49. Boyle PA, Malloy PF, Salloway S, et al. Executive dysfunction and apathy predict functional impairment in Alzheimer disease. Am J Geriatr Psychiatry 2003; 11:214–221.

50. Skurla E, Rogers JC, Sunderland T. Direct assessment of activities of daily living in Alzheimer's disease. J Am Geriatr Soc 1988; 36:97–103.

51. Swanberg MM, Tractenberg RE, Mohs RC, Thal LL, Cummings JL. Executive dysfunction in Alzheimer disease. Arch Neurol 2004; 61:556–560.

52. Willis SL, Allen-Burge R, Dolan MM, et al. Everyday problem solving among individuals with Alzheimer's disease. Gerontologist 1998; 38:569–577.

53. Stout JC, Wyman MF, Johnson SA, Peavy GM, Salmon DP. Frontal behavioral syndromes and functional status in probable Alzheimer disease. Am J Geriatr Psychiatry 2003; 11:683–686.

54. Borell L. Supporting functional behavior in Alzheimer's disease. Int Psychogeriatr 1996; 8(suppl 1):123–125.

55. Josephsson S. Supporting everyday activities in dementia. Int Psychogeriatr 1996; 8(suppl 1):141–144.

56. Oakley F, Duran L, Fisher A, Merritt B. Differences in activities of daily living motor skills of persons with and without Alzheimer's disease. Aust Occup Ther J 2003; 50:72–78.

57. Cohen D, Eisdorfer C. The Loss of Self: A Family Resource for the Care of Alzheimer's Disease and Related Disorders. New York: W.W. Norton 1986.

58. Potkin SG. The ABC of Alzheimer's disease: ADL and improving day-to-day functioning of patients. Int Psychogeriatr 2002; 14(suppl 1):7–26.

59. Logsdon RG, Gibbons LE, McCurry SM, Teri L. Assessing quality of life in older adults with cognitive impairment. Psychosom Med 2002; 64:510–519.

60. Wlodarczyk J, Brodaty H, Hawthorne G. The relationship between quality of life, Mini-Mental State Examination, and the Instrumental Activities of Daily Living in patients with Alzheimer's disease. Arch Gerontol Geriatr 2004; 39:25–33.

61. Little AG, Hemsley DR, Volans PJ, et al. The relationship between alternative assessments of self-care ability in the elderly. Br J Clin Psychol 1986; 25:51–59.

62. Mace NL, Rabins PV. The 36-hour Day. Baltimore: The Johns Hopkins University Press 1981.

63. Shaw WS, Patterson TL, Semple SJ, et al. Longitudinal analysis of multiple indicators of health decline among spousal caregivers. Ann Behavior Med 1997; 19:101–109.

64. Shaw WS, Patterson TL, Ziegler MG, et al. Accelerated risk of hypertensive blood pressure recordings among Alzheimer caregivers. J Psychosom Res 1999; 46:215–227.

65. von Kanel R, Dimsdale JE, Ziegler MG, et al. Effect of acute psychological stress on the hypercoagulable state in subjects (spousal caregivers of patients with Alzheimer's disease) with coronary or cerebrovascular disease and/or systemic hypertension. Am J Cardiol 2001; 87:1405–1408.

66. Pruchno RA, Micheals JE, Potashnik SL. Predictors of institutionalization among Alzheimer's disease victims with caregiving spouse. J Gerontol 1990; 25:S259–S266.

67. Stephens MP, Kinney JM, Ogrocki PK. Stressors and well-being among caregivers to older adults and dementia: the in-home versus nursing home experience. Gerontologist 1991; 31:217–223.

68. Gauthier S, Bodick N, Erzigkeit E, et al. Activities of daily living as an outcome measure in clinical trials of dementia drugs. Position paper from the International Working Group on Harmonization of Dementis Drug Guidelines. Alzheimer Dis Assoc Disord 1997; 11(suppl 3):6–7.

69. Lawton MP, Brody EM. Assessment of older people: self-maintaining and instrumental activities of daily living. Gerontologist 1969; 9:179–186.

70. Spiegel R, Brunner C, Phil L. A new behavioral assessment scale for geriatric out- and in-patients: the NOSGER (nurses' observation scale for geriatric patients). JAGS 1991; 39:339–347.

71. DeJong R, Osterlund O, Roy G. Measurement of quality-of-life changes in patients with Alzheimer's disease. Clin Ther 1989; 11:545–554.

72. Sano M, Ernesto C, Thomas R, et al. A controlled trial of seleginline, alpha-tocopherol, or both as treatment for Alzheimer's disease. N Engl J Med 1997; 336:1216–1222.

73. Gélinas I, Gauthier S, Cyrus PA. Metrifonate enhances the ability of Alzheimer's disease patients to initiate, organize and execute instrumental and basic activities of daily living. J Geriatr Psychiatr Neurol 2000; 13:9–16.

74. Feldman H, Gauthier S, Hecker J, Vellas B, Subbiah P, et al. A 24-week, randomised, double-blind study of donepezil in moderate to severe Alzheimer's disease. Neurology 2001; 57:613–620.

75. Feldman H, Gauthier S, Hecker J, et al. Efficacy of donepezil on maintenance of activities of daily living in patients with moderate to severe Alzheimer's disease and the effect on caregiver burden. J Am Geriatr Soc 2003; 51:737–744.

76. Wilcock GK, Lilienfeld S, Gaens E. Efficacy and safety of galantamine in patients with mild to moderate Alzheimer's disease: multicentre randomised controlled trial. Galantamine International-1 Study Group. BMJ 2000; 321:1445–1449.

77. Kumar V, Cameron A, Amrein R. Lazabemide in Alzheimer's disease. Neurobiol Aging 1998; 19:S80.

78. Burns A, Rossor M, Hecker J, et al. The effects of donepezil in Alzheimer's disease – results from a multinational trial. Dementia Geriatr Cog Disord 1999; 10:237–244.

79. Bodick N, Offen W, Levey A, et al. Effects of xanomeline, a selective muscarinic receptor agonist, on cognitive function and behavioral symptoms in Alzheimer's disease. Arch Neurol 1997; 54:465–473.

80. Knapp M, Knopman D, Solomon P, et al. A 30-week randomized controlled trial of high-dose tacrine in patients with Alzheimer's disease. JAMA 1994; 271:985–991.

81. Corey-Bloom J, Anand R, Veach J for the ENA 713 B352 Study Group. A randomized trial evaluating the efficacy and safety of ENA 713 (rivastigmine tartrate), a new acetylcholinesterase inhibitor, in patients with mild to moderately severe Alzheimer's disease. Int J Geriatr Psychopharmacol 1998; 1:55–65.

82. Wilkinson D, Murray J. Galantamine: a randomized, double-blind, dose-comparison in patients with Alzheimer's disease. Int J Geriatr Psychiatry 2001; 16:852–857.

83. Windblad B, Engedal K, Soininen H, et al. A 1-year, randomized, placebo-controlled study of donepezil in patients with mild to moderate AD. Neurology 2001; 57: 489–495.

84. Tariot PN, Solomon P, Morris JC, et al. A 5-month, randomized, placebo-controlled trial of galantamine in AD. The Galantamine US-10 Study Group. Neurology 2000; 54: 2269–2276.

85. Galasko G, Kershaw PR, Schneider L, Zhu Y, Tariot PN. Glantamine maintains ability to perform activities of daily living in patients with Alzheimer's disease. J Am Geriatr Soc 2004; 52:1070–1076.

86. Carswell A, Carson LJ, Walop W, et al. A theoretical model of functional performance in persons with Alzheimer disease. Can J Occup Ther 1992; 59:132–140.

87. Weintraub S. The record of independent living. An informant-completed measure of activities of daily living

and behaviour in elderly patients with cognitive impairment. Am J Alzheimer Care Rel Disord 1986; Spring:35–39.

88. Barberger-Gateau P, Commenges D, Gagnon M, et al. Instrumental activities of daily living as a screening tool for cognitive impairment and dementia in elderly community dwellers. J Am Geriatr Soc 1992; 40:1129–1134.

89. Hill LR, Klauber MR, Salmon DP, et al. Functional status, education and the diagnosis of dementia in the Shanghai survey. Neurology 1993; 43:138–145.

90. Pattersons MB, Mack JL, Neundorfer MM, et al. Assessment of functional ability in Alzheimer disease: a review and preliminary report on the Cleveland Scale for Activities of Daily Living. Alzheimer Dis Assoc Disord 1992; 6:145–163.

91. Hindmarch I, Lehfeld H, de Jongh P, Erzigkeit H. The Bayer Activities of Daily Living Scale (B-ADL). Dement Geriatr Cogn Disord 1998; 9(suppl 2):20–26.

92. Stern Y, Albert SM, Sano M, et al. Assessing patient dependence in Alzheimer's disease. J Gerontol 1994; 49: M216–M222.

93. Loewenstein DA, Anigo E, Ranjan D, et al. A new scale for the assessment of functional status in Alzheimer's disease and related disorders. J Gerontol 1989; 44:114–121.

94. Willis SL. Test Manual for the Everyday Problems Test for Cognitively Challenged Elderly. The Pennsylvania State University: University Park 1993.

95. Pfeffer R, Kurosaki M, Harrah CJ, et al. Measurement of functional activities in older adults in the community. J Gerontol 1982; 37:323–329.

96. Carswell A, Sulberg C, Carson L, Zgola J. The functional performance measure for persons with Alzheimer's disease: reliability and validity. Can J Occup Ther 1995; 62: 62–69.

97. Laberge H, Gauthier L. L'autonomie dans les activités de base chez les personnes avec une démence de type Alzheimer et les personnes avec une dépression majeure. Rev Quebec Ergother 1994; 3:90–95.

98. Mahurin RK, DeBettignies BH, Pirozzolo FJ. Structured assessment of independent living skills: preliminary report of a performance measure of functional abilities in dementia. J Gerontol 1991; 46:P58–P66.

99. Perry RJ, Hodges JR. Relationship between functional and neuropsychological performance in early Alzheimer disease. Alzheimer Dis Assoc Disord 2000; 14:1–10.

100. Athlin E, Norberg A, Axelsson K, et al. Aberrant eating behaviour in elderly parkinsonian patients with and without dementia: analysis of video-recorded meals. Res Nurs Health 1989; 12:41–51.

101. Rogers JC, Snow T. An assessment of the feeding behaviours of the institutionalized elderly. Am J Occup Ther 1982; 36:375–380.

102. Beck C. Measurement of dressing performance in persons with dementia. Am J Alzheimer Care Rel Disord Res 1988; May/June:21–25.

103. Marson D. Loss of financial capacity in dementia: conceptual and empirical approaches. Aging Neuropsychol Cogn 2001; 8:164–181.

104. Marson D, Sawrie S, Snyder S, et al. Assessing financial capacity in patients with Alzheimer's disease: a conceptual model and prototype instrument. Arch Neurol 2000; 57: 877–884.

105. Lucas-Blaustein MJ, Filipp L, Dungan C, et al. Driving in patients with dementia. J Am Geriatr Soc 1988; 36: 1087–1091.

106. Bertrand RM, Willis SL. Everyday problem solving in Alzheimer's patients: a comparison of subjective and objective assessments. Aging Mental Health 1999; 3:281–293.

107. Myers AM, Holliday PJ, Harvey KA, et al. Functional performance measures: are they superior to self-assessments? J Gerontol 1993; 48:M196–M206.

16

Behaviour

Edmond Teng and Jeffrey L Cummings

INTRODUCTION

Alzheimer's disease (AD) is characterized by impairments in cognitive, functional and behavioural domains. Although the formal clinical diagnostic criteria are defined by deficits in cognition and function,[1,2] behavioural symptoms are also a common and problematic manifestation of this disorder. Among the most frequent and troublesome symptoms are apathy, agitation, aggression and delusions.[3] Estimates of the overall prevalence of behavioural symptoms range from 53 to 98 per cent, depending upon the specific assessment tools and populations studied.[4,5]

While cognitive symptoms form the cornerstone of the clinical diagnosis of AD, behavioural symptoms are responsible for a substantial proportion of the morbidity caused by the disease. Studies in various populations of patients with AD have demonstrated that the presence of behavioural pathology correlates with higher rates of institutionalization,[6] increased length of inpatient admissions,[7] increased cost of care[8] and increased caregiver stress and burden.[9,10] When caregivers are surveyed, they report that abnormal behaviours are significantly more troublesome than cognitive deficits.[11]

The overall frequency and severity of behavioural disturbances increase in the later stages of the disease.[3] However, these symptoms are not simply a consequence of worsening cognitive and functional impairment. The clinical course of behavioural symptomatology does not correlate closely with the presence and severity of cognitive or functional disturbances.[12,13] Individual behavioural abnormalities do not always correlate well with other behavioural symptoms.[12] Longitudinal studies have shown that while cognitive and functional decline is gradually but inexorably progressive, individual behavioural symptoms are often episodic and usually exhibit a recurrent or waxing and waning course.[12,14]

While both the cognitive and behavioural symptoms in AD are thought to arise from similar underlying pathological processes, the poor correlation between these two classes of symptoms suggests that they may reflect different underlying anatomical patterns of neurodegeneration.[15] Functional imaging studies using single photon emission computerized tomography have demonstrated that behavioural and cognitive disturbances correlate with different patterns of regional hypoperfusion.[16,17] Likewise, neuropathological studies have shown that, while the severity of cognitive impairment correlates with neurofibrillary tangle density in the temporal lobe,[18] the severity of some specific behavioural symptoms, such as agitation and psychosis, correlates with neurofibrillary tangle density in different regions of frontal and cingulate cortex.[19,20] Taken together, these findings suggest that the behavioural symptoms that develop over the course of AD are independent from the concurrently worsening cognitive symptoms and represent a separate manifestation of the underlying neuropathological processes of the disease.

ASSESSMENT OF BEHAVIOURAL SYMPTOMS

The behavioural disturbances seen in AD comprise a heterogeneous collection of symptoms. While these symptoms are thought to have pathological substrates in separate and disparate regions of the brain, they are often grouped together as 'non-cognitive' in nature. Numerous rating scales have been used to assess and quantify the variety of behavioural pathology that is encountered over the course of the disease; those most commonly used are listed in Box 16.1. Some of these scales focus on specific subsets of abnormal behaviour, such as the Cohen–Mansfield Agitation

---

Box 16.1 Assessment tools used in the evaluation of behavioural symptoms in AD. Adapted from Sink et al [27]

Agitated Behaviour Inventory for Dementia

Agitation–Calmness Evaluation Scale

Alzheimer's Disease Assessment Scale: Non-cognitive Subscale

Apathy Scale

Bech–Rafaelsen Mania Scale

Behaviour Observation Scale for Intramural Psychogeriatric Patients

Behaviour and Emotional Activities Manifested in Dementia

Behavioural Pathology in Alzheimer Disease Rating Scale

Behavioural Rating Scale for Dementia

Behavioural Symptoms Scale for Dementia

Brief Psychiatric Rating Scale

Cohen-Mansfield Agitation Inventory

Columbia University Scale for Psychopathology in Alzheimer's Disease

Comprehensive Psychopathological Rating Scale

Cornell Scale for Depression in Dementia

Dementia Behaviour Disturbance Scale

Dementia Psychosis Scale

Disinhibition Scale

Hamilton Rating Scale for Depression

Hamilton Rating Scale for Anxiety

Irritability Scale

Manchester and Oxford Universities Scale for Psychopathological Assessment of Dementia

Neurobehavioural Rating Scale

Neuropsychiatric Inventory

Overt Aggression Scale

Positive and Negative Syndrome Scale

Present Behaviour Examination

Revised Memory and Behaviour Problem Checklist

Social Dysfunction and Aggression Scale

Troublesome Behaviour Scale

Inventory,[21] the Cornell Scale for Depression in Dementia[22] and the Disinhibition Scale.[23] Other scales attempt to assess the full spectrum of psychopathology seen in dementia, often relying on caregiver reports to quantify the frequency and severity of different classes of symptoms. Three such instruments that are used frequently include the Behavioural Pathology in Alzheimer Disease Rating Scale (BEHAVE-AD),[24] the Behavioural Rating Scale for Dementia (BRSD)[25] and the Neuropsychiatric Inventory (NPI).[3]

The BEHAVE-AD asks caregivers to rate the severity of 25 specific behavioural symptoms grouped into seven clusters: paranoid and delusional ideation; hallucinations; aggressiveness; activity disturbances; diurnal rhythm disturbances; affective disturbances and anxieties and phobias.[24] For the BRSD, caregivers

report on the presence or frequency of 46 different behaviours, which have been grouped using factor analysis to generate six subscales: depressive symptoms; inertia; vegetative symptoms; irritability and aggression; behavioural dysregulation and psychotic symptoms.[25] The NPI examines caregiver ratings of the severity and frequency of 12 categories of behavioural disturbances: delusions; hallucinations; agitation/aggression; depression/dysphoria; anxiety; elation/euphoria; apathy/indifference; disinhibition; irritability; aberrant motor behaviour; night-time behaviours and appetite/eating behaviours.[26] Each of these scales has been shown to have good reliability, validity and sensitivity,[24–26] and all three scales have been used as outcome measures in clinical trials assessing pharmacological treatments of behavioural symptoms in dementia.[27]

Although there is substantial overlap in the behavioural abnormalities assessed by these three scales, no single rating scale is able to efficiently describe all of the dimensions of behavioural dysfunction seen in the demented population. Depending on which scale is used, individual behavioral symptoms may be grouped in different categories, as shown in Table 16.1.

SPECIFIC BEHAVIOURAL SYMPTOMS

The prevalence of the various behavioural symptoms of AD can be seen in Figures 16.1 and 16.2. Studies of community-based populations[5,28] have consistently reported lower frequencies of behavioural abnormalities than studies of memory disorder clinic-based populations.[3,29] This is reflected in the lower overall prevalence of behavioural symptoms in Figure 16.1 relative to Figure 16.2.

Depression/dysphoria

Depressive symptoms are very common in AD. The reported prevalence in community based studies ranges from 20 to 30 per cent.[5,28] The most prominent depressive symptoms are similar to those seen in age-matched depressed elderly control subjects and differ from those seen in younger subjects.[30] Anhedonia, difficulty initiating and sustaining activities and decreased self-esteem and confidence are more pronounced in this population, while sadness, feelings of guilt and suicidality are less prominent.[31] Depressive symptoms in AD can be transient, fluctuate over time and be less intense than those seen in younger populations.[32,33]

Specific diagnostic criteria have been proposed for assessing depression in AD. These criteria differ from the diagnostic criteria for major depression in that fewer symptoms are required and specific depressive symptoms seen in the demented population, such as irritability, withdrawal or social isolation, and decreased pleasure with social contact are included.[34] The spectrum of behavioural abnormalities seen in depression overlaps significantly with other neuropsychiatric symptoms that can be seen independently in dementia, such as apathy, irritability, psychomotor symptoms and sleep and appetite disturbances. In order to increase its specificity for depression in dementia, the NPI focuses on dysphoric symptoms. Other dimensions of depressed mood are independently assessed on separate subscales of the NPI.[26]

Apathy/indifference

Several studies have identified apathy as the most common behavioural disturbance seen in AD. The prevalence in demented subjects in the community is 36 per cent,[28] and rises to 72 per cent in demented subjects recruited from a memory disorders clinic.[3] Despite the significant overlap between depressive and apathetic syndromes, apathy has been shown to be an independent behavioural entity.[35] Behavioural symptoms that are particularly specific in distinguishing apathy from depression include emotional blunting, indifference and lack of social engagement.[36] Symptoms of apathy have been shown to correlate with hypoperfusion and neurofibrillary tangle deposition in the anterior cingulate cortex.[17,20]

Table 16.1 Comparison of specific behavioural symptom categories across the Behavioural Pathology in AD Rating Scale (BEHAVE-AD), Behavioural Rating Scale for Dementia (BRSD) and the Neuropsychiatric inventory (NPI)

BEHAVE-AD	BRSD	NPI
Paranoid/delusional ideation; hallucinations	Psychotic symptoms	Delusions; hallucinations
Aggressiveness	Irritability/aggression	Agitation/aggression; irritability
Affective disturbances	Depressive symptoms	Depression/dysphoria
–	Inertia	Apathy/indifference
Anxieties and phobias	–	Anxiety
Activity disturbances	Behavioural dysregulation	Aberrant motor behaviour
Diurnal rhythm disturbances	Vegetative symptoms	Night-time behaviours; appetite/eating behaviours
–	–	Disinhibition
–	–	Elation/euphoria

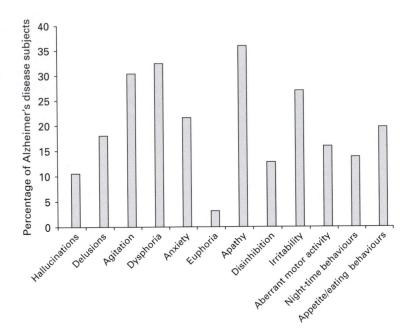

Figure 16.1 Prevalence of NPI behavioural symptoms in a population-based sample of patients with Alzheimer's disease. Data reproduced with permission from Lyketsos et al[28]

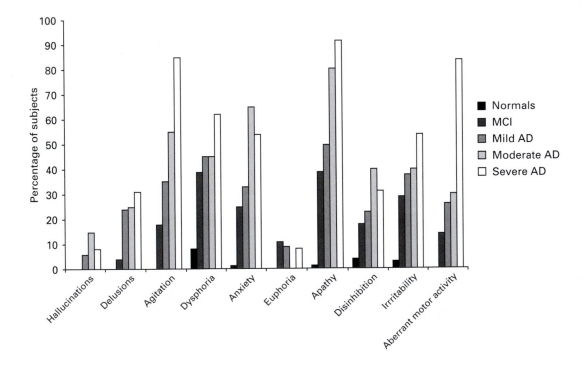

Figure 16.2 Prevalence of NPI behavioural symptoms in a memory disorders clinic based sample of normal aged subjects, subjects with mild cognitive impairment (MCI) and subjects with mild, moderate and severe Alzheimer's disease (AD). Data are derived from Mega et al[3] and Hwang et al[29] with permission from LWW

Elation/euphoria

Symptoms of elevated mood, such as inappropriate happiness, humour and laughter, are relatively rare. Although older studies have suggested a rate of euphoria as high as 17 per cent,[37] more recent studies report euphoric symptoms in only 0.5–3.1 per cent of subjects.[5,28] In smaller studies, 2.2 to 3.5 per cent of subjects meet the clinical criteria for mania.[38,39] Many of the manic patients had a pre-existing diagnosis of bipolar disorder prior to being diagnosed with AD.[39] The frequency of manic symptoms in AD is slightly higher than previously reported estimates of the prevalence of bipolar disorder in the general elderly population, which range from 0.1 to 0.5 per cent.[40] Euphoria is more commonly seen in frontotemporal dementia (FTD) than in AD.[41]

Anxiety

The prevalence of anxiety is variable, ranging from 10 to 70 per cent depending on the specific population studied and instrument used.[5,42] The most common manifestations are excessive worrying, apprehension or fearfulness.[42,43] Patients are most likely to express the fear of being left alone.[44] Caregivers also frequently report the occurrence of the 'catastrophic reaction' in patients with AD. This behaviour, which is characterized by an outburst of generalized anxiety, is often a response to a perceived threat to the subject.[45]

Irritability

Irritability is another common problem, seen in 20 to 60 per cent of demented subjects.[5,46] Behaviours that define irritability include frequent arguments, pouting, sulking and angry loud outbursts. These symptoms typically represent a distinct change in personality, as they do not correlate with premorbid reports of patients having 'a bad temper'.[46]

Agitation/aggression

Cohen-Mansfield has defined agitation as 'inappropriate verbal, vocal, or motor activity not explained by confusion or needs'.[21] Agitation has been reported in 20–60 per cent of subjects with AD, and it is seen with increasing frequency with worsening cognitive impairment, with the prevalence rising to 85 per cent when subjects with severe cognitive impairment are studied.[3,5] Agitated behaviours can be grouped with factor analysis into three categories: physically aggressive behaviour, which includes hitting, biting, spitting and throwing objects; verbally aggressive behaviour, which includes cursing and other verbal abuse, and non-aggressive behaviour, which includes pacing, inappropriate dressing and/or disrobing and constant requests for attention.[21] In the NPI, the agitation subscore focuses on physically and verbally aggressive behaviours. Non-aggressive agitated behaviours are separately addressed in the aberrant motor behaviour subscore of the NPI.

Aberrant motor behaviour

Abnormal motor behaviour also increases markedly with worsening cognitive impairment. While such behaviour is seen in 15–40 per cent of the overall AD population, it is reported in 85 per cent of severely demented patients.[3,28] In addition to the non-aggressive agitated behaviours described above, this category also encompasses motor restlessness and a variety of stereotyped behaviours, such as the repeated use of identical phrases, obsessive hoarding and collecting and strict adherence to customary routines.[47,48]

Disinhibition

Disinhibited behaviour is relatively uncommon in AD. Although different assessment tools identify different symptoms as representative of disinhibition, the overall prevalence across studies is relatively consistent. The NPI focuses upon disinhibition in social settings, such as excessive friendliness, inappropriate comments and violation of interpersonal norms.[26] Using this measure, 10–35 per cent of subjects are disinhibited.[3,28] The Disinhibition Scale measures a wider range of psychopathology, which can be subdivided into four categories: abnormal motor behaviour, egocentrism, poor self-care and hypomania. Subjects must exhibit symptoms from three of these four categories to be classified as disinhibited. Using these criteria, 11 per cent of subjects with AD demonstrate significant disinhibition. The most common disinhibited behaviours reported with this instrument are distractibility, poor awareness of danger, inappropriate social behaviour and loss of insight.[23]

Delusions

Although delusions are reported in only 15–25 per cent of subjects in community-based studies,[5,28] they contribute disproportionately to the overall morbidity of the disease and increase the likelihood of institutionalization.[6] Delusional thinking is typically non-bizarre in content, consisting primarily of misidentifications or paranoid ideation.[49] Misidentifications that are frequently reported include the belief that the patient's house is not their home, that imposters have replaced the patient's friends and relatives (Capgras syndrome) and that the image that the patient sees in the mirror is of someone else. Common paranoid delusions include the belief that someone is stealing the patient's things, that a stranger is living in the patient's house (phantom boarder syndrome) and that the patient's spouse is having an affair.[50]

Hallucinations

Hallucinations are relatively rare, reported in only 10–15 per cent of demented subjects.[3,5] Visual symptoms are more common than auditory symptoms.[51] Frequently reported visual hallucinations include patients seeing people in their room or yard. Common auditory hallucinations include patients hearing voices of persons who are deceased or not in the room.[50] Somatic, olfactory and tactile hallucinations have also been reported, but are significantly less common.[51]

Night-time behaviours

Significant disruptions in sleep/wake cycles are reported in 27 per cent of subjects with AD.[28] Sleep disturbances can be a prominent problem and a major factor leading to increased caregiver distress and rates of institutionalization.[52] Demented subjects have fragmented sleep/wake rhythms, which are characterized by frequent daytime napping, prolonged night-time wakefulness and multiple nocturnal awakenings.[53] Polysomnographic data demonstrate increased latency in rapid-eye movement (REM) sleep onset, decreased overall REM sleep time, decreased total sleep time and decreased sleep efficiency (the proportion of time in bed that the patient is asleep) in demented subjects relative to aged control subjects.[52] These abnormal circadian rhythms often result in increased and inappropriate levels of nocturnal activity, which can be very disruptive to other members of the household.

Appetite/eating behaviours

Changes in eating behaviour are seen in 20 per cent of demented subjects.[28] Both increased and decreased appetite can be seen at different stages in the course of AD. Early in the disease, a minority of patients may experience significant weight gain due to hyperorality, insatiable cravings for sweets and gorging behav-

iour. Later in the disease, patients often experience weight loss, which may be multifactorial in aetiology. Depressive symptoms can lead to decreased nutritional intake and anorexia. Increased motor activity and restlessness can increase daily caloric requirements. Motor apraxias can result in the loss of functional skills required for self-feeding. As the patient's dementia progresses, visual agnosia may result in an inability to identify food items from other objects of similar size and shape. In endstage AD, patients may develop specific eating apraxias and lose the ability to coordinate chewing and swallowing. These patients may require the placement of a gastric tube to achieve adequate nutritional support.[54]

Other behaviours

Although the NPI attempts to comprehensively assess the common behavioural abnormalities seen in dementia, there are a number of behaviours that it does not specifically address, including wandering and aberrant sexual behaviour. Wandering is a term used to describe a broad category of behaviours, including excessive pacing, nocturnal ambulation, attempts to leave the house or nursing home, walking with an inappropriate purpose and/or frequency and walking off during meals. It is difficult to compare the prevalence of wandering across studies due to the inclusion of different behaviours in different studies, but it has been estimated that such behaviours occur in approximately 25 per cent of subjects in the community and 30 per cent of subjects in nursing homes.[55] The prevalence of wandering increases with the severity of dementia, and correlates most robustly with diminished spatial abilities.[55] Changes in sexual behaviour are also seen frequently in AD. The most common change from premorbid behaviour is hyposexuality. Seventy per cent of patients demonstrate an increasing indifference to sexual activity.[56] Hypersexuality is much less common, and has been reported in only 10–15 per cent of patients.[57,58] While relatively uncommon, behaviours such as compulsive masturbation, self-exposure of genitalia and excessive desire for sexual contact can be extremely distressing for caregivers and family members.[59]

EVOLUTION OF BEHAVIOURAL SYMPTOMS

The evolution of behavioural symptoms over the course of AD has been examined with both cross-sectional and longitudinal studies. Although these two approaches offer different perspectives of the changing nature of behavioural pathology over time, both demonstrate that the changes in behaviour seen with worsening dementia are distinct and independent from the decline in cognition and function.[13,60]

Cross-sectional studies have examined the prevalence of different behavioural symptoms at different stages along the continuum that ranges from normal aging to endstage AD. These stages have typically been defined based upon either cognitive function, using the Mini-Mental State Exam (MMSE), or upon more global assessments of cognitive and functional abilities, using the Clinical Dementia Rating (CDR) or the Global Deterioration Scale (GDS).

While older studies have focused on behavioural symptoms in normal control subjects and patients with varying severity of AD, more recent studies have also focused on abnormal behaviours in subjects meeting the diagnostic criteria for mild cognitive impairment (MCI). MCI is conceptualized as a transitional phase between normal ageing and mild dementia. Subjects with amnestic MCI, who have subjective memory complaints and objective memory deficits, but otherwise preserved cognition and functional status, transition to AD at a rate of 10–15 per cent per year and 80 per cent over 6 years, a much higher rate than age-matched control subjects, who develop AD at a rate of 1–2 per cent per year. Thus, amnestic MCI has been proposed as a possible precursor condition to AD.[61] The data from cross-sectional studies demonstrate that the overall frequency and severity of behavioural pathology increase with worsening cognitive impairment. However, specific behavioural symptoms vary in their prominence at different stages of dementia, as can be seen in Figure 16.2.[3,29]

Behavioural symptoms in normal aged controls are uncommon, with only 5–16 per cent of subjects demonstrating any behavioural pathology on the NPI.[5,29,62] The frequency and severity of the behavioural abnormalities in normal elderly subjects are significantly less than that seen in MCI or mild AD. The most commonly reported symptoms are dysphoria (6–8 per cent), abnormal night-time behaviours (8 per cent) and anxiety (1–6 per cent). Other symptoms that can be seen with dementia, such as hallucinations, elation and aberrant motor activity, are almost never reported in this group of subjects.[5,29,62]

Amongst subjects with MCI, the overall pattern of behavioural disturbances becomes more similar to that seen in mild AD, but with a lower prevalence and severity. Some degree of behavioural dysfunction is exhibited by 35–75 per cent of this population. Frequently reported symptoms include dysphoria (9–39 per cent), apathy (11–39 per cent) and irritability (13–29 per cent). Other troublesome symptoms

such as delusions, hallucinations and euphoria remain relatively rare (0–11 per cent).[28,29,62]

Subjects diagnosed with mild AD are more likely to manifest behavioural pathology, with 80–90 per cent of subjects exhibiting significant symptoms when this group is defined by CDR scores of 0.5 to 1[62] or by MMSE scores of 21–30.[29] Dysphoria (50 per cent), apathy (51 per cent) and irritability (38 per cent) continue to be the most prevalent dysfunctional behaviours. However, behaviours that are seen at low frequencies in normal control and MCI subjects, such as agitation (34 per cent), delusions (26 per cent) and aberrant motor activity (27 per cent), begin to become more prominent and problematic at this stage of the disease.[29]

In moderate AD, as defined by an MMSE score of 11–20, the overall frequency of behavioural abnormalities increases only slightly to 95 per cent, but the severity of the symptoms seen in this stage is significantly greater than that seen in mild AD, and the number of symptoms reported for each patient also increases. Apathy (80 per cent), anxiety (65 per cent) and agitation (55 per cent) are the most frequently reported symptoms in this stage of dementia. Despite the increasing overall prevalence of behavioural dysfunction, symptoms such as euphoria and hallucinations remain relatively unusual (0–15 per cent).[3]

Virtually all subjects who are diagnosed with severe AD, defined by an MMSE score less than 11, exhibit some degree of behavioural pathology. Apathy (92 per cent), agitation (85 per cent) and aberrant motor activity (84 per cent) are seen in most patients at this stage of the disease.[3] When patients with advanced disease are classified using the GDS as having moderately severe, severe or very severe dementia (GDS scores of 5–7), the highest frequency of symptoms is seen in the severe stage (GDS 6). The frequency of all symptoms decreases in endstage dementia (GDS 7), possibly because the increasing functional impairment in this group of subjects limits their ability to exhibit abnormal behaviours.[60]

When the frequency of individual behavioural abnormalities is examined across the mild, moderate and severe AD groups, some general patterns related to the severity of cognitive impairment emerge. Delusions, agitation, dysphoria, apathy, irritability and aberrant motor behaviour progressively increase in frequency as cognitive function declines. Hallucinations, anxiety and disinhibition are seen at their highest frequency in moderately demented subjects. The peak prevalence of euphoric behaviour is seen in patients with mild AD and MCI.[3,29]

Cross-sectional studies also illustrate the heterogeneous presentation of behavioural abnormalities.

Different patients demonstrate different behaviours at different points of disease progression. Several symptoms are often present simultaneously in the same patient. Factor, cluster and principal components analyses have been used to statistically group behaviours that are often seen together into specific symptom clusters.[5,25,63–75] McShane has reviewed this literature and has identified five distinct behavioural syndromes: apathy, aggression, depression, psychosis and hyperactivity/agitation.[76] Different investigators have reported slightly different symptom clusters, but the overall patterns of behavioural symptoms are quite similar. Table 16.2 summarizes the different behavioural syndromes that have been proposed and is

Table 16.2 Behavioural symptom clusters in AD. Adapted from Lawlor and Bhriain[94]

Study	Symptom clusters				
	Apathy	Depression	Psychosis	Aggression	Hyperactivity/ agitation
Devanand et al 1992[63]	Apathy	Depression		Aggression	
Sultzer et al 1992[64]	Apathy	Depression	Psychosis		Motor hyperactivity; overactivity
Hope et al 1997[65]			Psychosis	Aggressive behaviour	
Haupt et al 1998[66]	Apathy	Depression	Psychosis/ aggression		Misidentification/ agitation; overactivity
Hope et al 1999[67]		Anxiety/ depression	Psychosis	Aggressive behaviour	
Harwood et al 1998[68]		Depression	Psychosis	Aggression	Agitation/ anxiety; activity disturbance
Frisoni et al 1999[69]	Frontal	Mood	Psychosis		
Mack et al 1999[25]	Inertia; vegetative symptoms	Depression	Psychosis	Irritability/ aggression	Behavioural dysregulation
Lyketsos et al 2000[5]		Depression	Psychosis	Agitation/ aggression	
Fuh et al 2001[70]	Social engagement	Mood and psychosis			Psychomotor regulation; hyperactivity
Aalten et al 2003[71]		Mood/apathy	Psychosis		
Mirakhur et al 2004[72]		Affect	Psychosis		Physical behaviour; hypomania
Spalletta et al 2004[73]		Depression/ apathy	Psychosis		Hyperactivity; anxiety; excitement
Amer-Ferrer et al 2005[74]		Affective	Psychotic		Dyscontrol
Schreinzer et al 2005[75]		Affectivity			Agitation; day/night disturbances

organized around the symptom clusters suggested by McShane.

While investigators have attempted to define behavioural syndromes by identifying specific clusters of symptoms, the utility of these groupings may be limited by the fact that individual patients may exhibit a spectrum of symptoms that are grouped under multiple behavioural syndromes. Another approach is to use latent class analysis to identify different groups of demented patients based upon the behavioural symptoms that they demonstrate. When applied to a population of subjects with mild AD, this strategy defined three distinct groups: patients with a low prevalence of behavioural symptoms, patients with higher frequencies of depressive symptoms and anxiety and patients with predominantly aggressive symptoms.[77]

Longitudinal studies provide additional perspective on the evolution, persistence and recurrence of behavioural symptoms. These studies have been performed both prospectively and retrospectively and analyse the behavioural changes in a given cohort of demented patients over months to years. Subjects are typically stratified by severity of disease at the beginning of the study, which allows investigators to separately analyse behavioural trends that are present at different stages of the disease.

Retrospective longitudinal studies have shown that a number of behavioural symptoms manifest prior to the formal diagnosis of AD. Social withdrawal is the earliest symptom reported and, when present, is seen an average of 33 months prior to formal diagnosis. Other behavioural problems that may precede formal diagnosis include depression, anxiety, paranoid delusions and diurnal rhythm disturbances. Earlier onset of behavioural symptoms correlates with an older age of formal diagnosis.[78] One possible explanation for these results is that there may be a significant subset of patients in which behavioural symptoms precede cognitive and functional decline. Since this study was conducted prior to the development of the distinction between normal ageing and MCI, another possibility is that the patients with early onset of behavioural difficulties met the diagnostic criteria for MCI prior to their formal diagnosis of AD.

Prospective longitudinal studies have confirmed that the evolution of behavioural symptoms is significantly more variable than the gradual and inexorable decline seen in the cognitive and functional domains.[13] Behavioural abnormalities fluctuate over time in both frequency and severity, and individual symptoms tend to demonstrate an episodic course rather than a progressive deterioration.[12,67] Once symptoms appear in the course of AD they tend to recur frequently, even if they are not continuously present.[14]

Over a 1- to 2-year period, the overall frequency and severity of behavioural disturbances increase for subjects with mild or moderate disease. However, amongst subjects with severe or endstage disease, the frequency and severity of behavioural pathology diminish over the same time period.[79,80] Individual symptoms vary in their severity as the disease progresses. The severity of hallucinations and diurnal rhythm disturbances remains essentially stable over this time interval. Mood disturbances, anxiety and delusions are much less stable in individual patients, as the proportion of subjects who report an increase in severity in these symptoms is roughly equal to the proportion of subjects who report a decrease in the severity. Activity disturbances and aggression tend to progressively increase in severity in most subjects as the disease progresses.[81]

Specific symptoms may vary widely in their persistence and recurrence over the course of the disease. Across different longitudinal studies, activity disturbances such as wandering and agitation have been found to be especially persistent. Psychotic symptoms such as paranoid ideation and delusional thinking tend to be moderately persistent. Depressive symptoms, which are often short-lived and episodic in nature, are amongst the least persistent.[81,82] While symptoms such as dysphoria tend to be episodic rather than persistent, they have a very high recurrence rate, as even episodic symptoms that remit have a high probability of re-emerging later in the disease course. Patients who exhibit multiple behavioural abnormalities at the time of initial assessment are more likely to experience the recurrence of individual symptoms.[14]

BEHAVIOURAL SYMPTOMS IN AD RELATIVE TO OTHER DEMENTIAS

Although behavioural abnormalities are an important cause of morbidity in AD, they are not unique to this form of dementia. Behavioural changes are also prominent in other dementias such as vascular dementia (VaD), dementia with Lewy bodies (DLB) and frontotemporal dementia (FTD). Different patterns of behavioural pathology distinguish the behavioural manifestations of AD from those seen in these other common causes of dementia. The different behavioural manifestations seen across different aetiologies of dementia likely reflect the different regional patterns of brain dysfunction characteristic of these diseases.

While the neuropsychological deficits in VaD can be variable, depending on which areas of the brain are preferentially affected by cerebrovascular injury in a particular patient, the overall frequency and severity of behavioural symptoms are similar in both VaD and AD.[83] When individual behaviours are compared, subjects with VaD have been shown to have a higher prevalence of depression,[5,84] anxiety[84,85] and apathy,[83] while subjects with AD have demonstrated a higher prevalence of delusions,[5,83] aberrant motor activity,[83] hallucinations[83] and irritability.[83]

Clinically, DLB can be distinguished from AD by the presence of fluctuating levels of alertness, frequent visual hallucinations and parkinsonian symptoms. The overall prevalence of behavioural abnormalities is higher among patients with DLB than among patients with AD.[86,87] Hallucinations and delusions have consistently been reported at a markedly higher frequency in DLB than AD.[86–88] Some studies have also found that anxiety, anhedonia and decreased energy are more prevalent in DLB than in AD.[85,87]

Personality, emotional and behavioural changes are among the core diagnostic criteria for FTD, and subjects with FTD demonstrate significantly more behavioural pathology than subjects with AD.[41,89] Symptoms such as disinhibition, aggression, apathy, euphoria and aberrant motor activity are seen more often in FTD.[41,86,89,90] Depression and delusions are more frequently reported in AD.[41,86,89] Some investigators have found that anxiety is more common in AD,[89] while others have reported that anxiety is more common in FTD.[85]

TREATMENT OF BEHAVIOURAL SYMPTOMS

Spurred by the significant morbidity caused by the myriad of behavioural symptoms associated with AD, research has been initiated that addresses the treatment of these symptoms. Both pharmacological and non-pharmacological approaches have shown some promise, but specific strategies must be formulated for individual patients, and the combination of these techniques is likely to be more effective than either alone.[91,92] Different treatment approaches will be described briefly in the paragraphs below. A more detailed discussion of this topic can be found in Chapter 22.

Sink et al have systematically reviewed evidence-based approaches to pharmacological treatment options for behavioural symptomatology in dementia, focusing on the conclusions that can be drawn from the limited number of adequate studies that have been performed.[27] A number of different classes of medications have been studied. Typical antipsychotics, particularly haloperidol, have shown specific efficacy for the treatment of aggression, but have not been shown to be beneficial for other behavioural abnormalities, and their use can be limited by significant sedation and extrapyramidal symptoms. The use of atypical antipsychotics such as olanzapine, quetiapine and risperidone has been shown to decrease the frequency and severity of a broader spectrum of symptoms, including agitation, aggression, hallucinations and delusions. While the atypical antipsychotics are less likely to cause extrapyramidal side effects than the older typical antipsychotics, they have been linked to a higher frequency of cerebrovascular events and increased mortality, which limits their use in the elderly population. Serotonin-specific reuptake inhibitors are effective primarily for depressive symptoms, while mood-stabilizing medications, such as carbamazepine and valproic acid, have not been shown to be consistently beneficial for any behavioural syndromes. Multiple studies of cholinesterase inhibitors have demonstrated a small, but statistically robust effect in reducing the overall NPI scores in patients with AD. The evidence for using memantine and other newer medications to reduce abnormal behaviours continues to evolve.[27]

While pharmacological approaches focus on ameliorating the specific behavioural symptoms seen in AD, non-pharmacological approaches have been used to try to address the underlying causes for these symptoms, which may have both psychosocial and environmental dimensions.[93] Cohen-Mansfield has reviewed this literature, and has organized non-pharmacological treatments into eight distinct categories: sensory enhancement/relaxation techniques, increased social contact, behavioural therapies, caregiver education, structured recreational and physical activities, optimized environmental changes, specific medical and nursing interventions and combination therapy.[93] These studies are heterogeneous in design, study population, intervention type and outcome measures. Although 90 per cent report some benefit, only 50 per cent of these studies found statistically significant improvements in behaviour, and most of these studies were not rigorously blinded or controlled. When different non-pharmacological approaches have been compared directly, those that emphasize increased social contact have been found to be the most effective.[93]

SUMMARY

Behavioural symptoms are a significant cause of increased morbidity, caregiver stress and cost of care in AD. The spectrum of abnormal behaviours spans both neuropsychiatric and psychomotor dimensions. While the overall frequency and severity of behavioural dysfunction increase with advancing dementia, specific behavioural syndromes have distinctly different patterns of evolution relative to each other and relative to the progressive cognitive and functional deficits seen over the course of the disease. Individual behavioural symptoms can be heterogeneous in presentation, episodic and recurrent in course and fluctuating in prevalence and severity. Although abnormal behaviours are not limited to AD, the specific patterns of behavioural pathology differ from those seen in other forms of dementia such as VaD, DLB and FTD. Pharmacological and non-pharmacological treatment regimens can help reduce the frequency, severity and impact of these symptoms for both the patient and the caregiver.

ACKNOWLEDGEMENTS

Preparation of this chapter has been supported by the National Institute on Aging (P5Ø AG 16570), the Alzheimer's Disease Research Centers of California and the Sidell–Kagan Foundation.

AUTHORS NOTE

Dr Teng has nothing to disclose. Dr Cummings has provided consultation to the following pharmaceutical companies: AstraZeneca, Aventis, Bristol–Myers Squibb, Eisai, Forest, Janssen, Lilly, Novartis, Ono, Pfizir, Syn–x Pharma, and Wyeth.

REFERENCES

1. McKhann G, Drachman D, Folstein M, et al. Clinical diagnosis of Alzheimer's disease: report of the NINCDS-ADRDA Work Group under the auspices of Department of Health and Human Services Task Force on Alzheimer's Disease. Neurology 1984; 34:939–944.
2. Association AP. Diagnostic and Statistical Manual of Mental Disorders, 4th edn. Washington: APA 1994.
3. Mega MS, Cummings JL, Fiorello T, Gornbein J. The spectrum of behavioral changes in Alzheimer's disease. Neurology 1996; 46:130–135.
4. Chen JC, Borson S, Scanlan JM. Stage-specific prevalence of behavioral symptoms in Alzheimer's disease in a multi-ethnic community sample. Am J Geriatr Psychiatry 2000; 8: 123–133.
5. Lyketsos CG, Steinberg M, Tschanz JT, et al. Mental and behavioral disturbances in dementia: findings from the Cache County Study on Memory in Aging. Am J Psychiatry 2000; 157:708–714.
6. Yaffe K, Fox P, Newcomer R, et al. Patient and caregiver characteristics and nursing home placement in patients with dementia. JAMA 2002; 287:2090–2097.
7. Wancata J, Windhaber J, Krautgartner M, Alexandrowicz R. The consequences of non-cognitive symptoms of dementia in medical hospital departments. Int J Psychiatry Med 2003; 33:257–271.
8. Beeri MS, Werner P, Davidson M, Noy S. The cost of behavioral and psychological symptoms of dementia (BPSD) in community dwelling Alzheimer's disease patients. Int J Geriatr Psychiatry 2002; 17:403–408.
9. Coen RF, Swanwick GR, O'Boyle CA, Coakley D. Behaviour disturbance and other predictors of carer burden in Alzheimer's disease. Int J Geriatr Psychiatry 1997; 12: 331–336.
10. Clyburn LD, Stones MJ, Hadjistavropoulos T, Tuokko H. Predicting caregiver burden and depression in Alzheimer's disease. J Gerontol B Psychol Sci Soc Sci 2000; 55:S2–S13.
11. Deimling GT, Bass DM. Symptoms of mental impairment among elderly adults and their effects on family caregivers. J Gerontol 1986; 41:778–784.
12. Marin DB, Green CR, Schmeidler J, et al. Noncognitive disturbances in Alzheimer's disease: frequency, longitudinal course, and relationship to cognitive symptoms. J Am Geriatr Soc 1997; 45:1331–1338.
13. Tractenberg RE, Weiner MF, Cummings JL, Patterson MB, Thal LJ. Independence of changes in behavior from cognition and function in community-dwelling persons with Alzheimer's disease: a factor analytic approach. J Neuropsychiatry Clin Neurosci 2005; 17:51–60.
14. Levy ML, Cummings JL, Fairbanks LA, et al. Longitudinal assessment of symptoms of depression, agitation, and psychosis in 181 patients with Alzheimer's disease. Am J Psychiatry 1996; 153:1438–1443.
15. Cummings JL. Cognitive and behavioral heterogeneity in Alzheimer's disease: seeking the neurobiological basis. Neurobiol Aging 2000; 21:845–861.
16. Mega MS, Lee L, Dinov ID, et al. Cerebral correlates of psychotic symptoms in Alzheimer's disease. J Neurol Neurosurg Psychiatry 2000; 69:167–171.
17. Benoit M, Koulibaly PM, Migneco O, et al. Brain perfusion in Alzheimer's disease with and without apathy: a SPECT study with statistical parametric mapping analysis. Psychiatry Res 2002; 114:103–111.
18. Haroutunian V, Purohit DP, Perl DP, et al. Neurofibrillary tangles in nondemented elderly subjects and mild Alzheimer disease. Arch Neurol 1999; 56:713–718.
19. Zubenko GS, Moossy J, Martinez AJ, et al. Neuropathologic and neurochemical correlates of psychosis in primary dementia. Arch Neurol 1991; 48:619–624.
20. Tekin S, Mega MS, Masterman DM, et al. Orbitofrontal and anterior cingulate cortex neurofibrillary tangle burden is associated with agitation in Alzheimer disease. Ann Neurol 2001; 49:355–361.
21. Cohen-Mansfield J. Agitated behaviors in the elderly. II. Preliminary results in the cognitively deteriorated. J Am Geriatr Soc 1986; 34:722–727.
22. Alexopoulos GS, Abrams RC, Young RC, Shamoian CA. Cornell Scale for depression in dementia. Biol Psychiatry 1988; 23:271–284.
23. Starkstein SE, Garau ML, Cao A. Prevalence and clinical correlates of disinhibition in dementia. Cogn Behav Neurol 2004; 17:139–147.
24. Reisberg B, Borenstein J, Salob SP, et al. Behavioral symptoms in Alzheimer's disease: phenomenology and treatment. J Clin Psychiatry 1987; 48(suppl):9–15.
25. Mack JL, Patterson MB, Tariot PN. Behavior Rating Scale for Dementia: development of test scales and presentation of

data for 555 individuals with Alzheimer's disease. J Geriatr Psychiatry Neurol 1999; 12:211–223.

26. Cummings JL. The Neuropsychiatric Inventory: assessing psychopathology in dementia patients. Neurology 1997; 48(suppl 6):S10–S16.

27. Sink KM, Holden KF, Yaffe K. Pharmacological treatment of neuropsychiatric symptoms of dementia: a review of the evidence. JAMA 2005; 293:596–608.

28. Lyketsos CG, Lopez O, Jones B, et al. Prevalence of neuropsychiatric symptoms in dementia and mild cognitive impairment: results from the cardiovascular health study. JAMA 2002; 288:1475–1483.

29. Hwang TJ, Masterman DL, Ortiz F, Fairbanks LA, Cummings JL. Mild cognitive impairment is associated with characteristic neuropsychiatric symptoms. Alzheimer Dis Assoc Disord 2004; 18:17–21.

30. Chemerinski E, Petracca G, Sabe L, Kremer J, Starkstein SE. The specificity of depressive symptoms in patients with Alzheimer's disease. Am J Psychiatry 2001; 158:68–72.

31. Lyketsos CG, Lee HB. Diagnosis and treatment of depression in Alzheimer's disease. A practical update for the clinician. Dement Geriatr Cogn Disord 2004; 17:55–64.

32. Katz IR. Diagnosis and treatment of depression in patients with Alzheimer's disease and other dementias. J Clin Psychiatry 1998; 59(suppl 9):38–44.

33. Lee HB, Lyketsos CG. Depression in Alzheimer's disease: heterogeneity and related issues. Biol Psychiatry 2003; 54: 353–362.

34. Olin JT, Schneider LS, Katz IR, et al. Provisional diagnostic criteria for depression of Alzheimer disease. Am J Geriatr Psychiatry 2002; 10:125–128.

35. Starkstein SE, Petracca G, Chemerinski E, Kremer J. Syndromic validity of apathy in Alzheimer's disease. Am J Psychiatry 2001; 158:872–877.

36. Landes AM, Sperry SD, Strauss ME, Geldmacher DS. Apathy in Alzheimer's disease. J Am Geriatr Soc 2001; 49: 1700–1707.

37. Bucht G, Adolfsson R. The Comprehensive Psychopathological Rating Scale in patients with dementia of Alzheimer type and multiinfarct dementia. Acta Psychiatr Scand 1983; 68:263–270.

38. Burns A, Jacoby R, Levy R. Psychiatric phenomena in Alzheimer's disease. III: Disorders of mood. Br J Psychiatry 1990; 157:81–86, 92–94.

39. Lyketsos CG, Corazzini K, Steele C. Mania in Alzheimer's disease. J Neuropsychiatry Clin Neurosci 1995; 7:350–352.

40. Depp CA, Jeste DV. Bipolar disorder in older adults: a critical review. Bipolar Disord 2004; 6:343–367.

41. Levy ML, Miller BL, Cummings JL, Fairbanks LA, Craig A. Alzheimer disease and frontotemporal dementias. Behavioral distinctions. Arch Neurol 1996; 53:687–690.

42. Ferretti L, McCurry SM, Logsdon R, Gibbons L, Teri L. Anxiety and Alzheimer's disease. J Geriatr Psychiatry Neurol 2001; 14:52–58.

43. Teri L, Ferretti LE, Gibbons LE, et al. Anxiety of Alzheimer's disease: prevalence, and comorbidity. J Gerontol A Biol Sci Med Sci 1999; 54:M348–M352.

44. Reisberg B, Auer SR, Monteiro I, Boksay I, Sclan SG. Behavioral disturbances of dementia: an overview of phenomenology and methodologic concerns. Int Psychogeriatr 1996; 8(suppl 2):169–180; discussion 81–82.

45. McLean S. Assessing dementia. Part II: Clinical, functional, neuropsychological and social issues. Aust NZ J Psychiatry 1987; 21:284–304.

46. Burns A, Folstein S, Brandt J, Folstein M. Clinical assessment of irritability, aggression, and apathy in Huntington and Alzheimer disease. J Nerv Ment Dis 1990; 178:20–26.

47. Teri L, Larson EB, Reifler BV. Behavioral disturbance in dementia of the Alzheimer's type. J Am Geriatr Soc 1988; 36:1–6.

48. Nyatsanza S, Shetty T, Gregory C, et al. A study of stereotypic behaviours in Alzheimer's disease and frontal and temporal variant frontotemporal dementia. J Neurol Neurosurg Psychiatry 2003; 74:1398–1402.

49. Schneider LS, Dagerman KS. Psychosis of Alzheimer's disease: clinical characteristics and history. J Psychiatr Res 2004; 38:105–111.

50. Sultzer DL. Psychosis and antipsychotic medications in Alzheimer's disease: clinical management and research perspectives. Dement Geriatr Cogn Disord 2004; 17:78–90.

51. Bassiony MM, Lyketsos CG. Delusions and hallucinations in Alzheimer's disease: review of the brain decade. Psychosomatics 2003; 44:388–401.

52. Bliwise DL. Sleep disorders in Alzheimer's disease and other dementias. Clin Cornerstone 2004; 6(suppl 1A):S16–S28.

53. Vitiello MV, Prinz PN. Alzheimer's disease. Sleep and sleep/wake patterns. Clin Geriatr Med 1989; 5:289–299.

54. Claggett MS. Nutritional factors relevant to Alzheimer's disease. J Am Diet Assoc 1989; 89:392–396.

55. Algase DL. Wandering in dementia. Annu Rev Nurs Res 1999; 17:185–217.

56. Derouesne C, Guigot J, Chermat V, Winchester N, Lacomblez L. Sexual behavioral changes in Alzheimer disease. Alzheimer Dis Assoc Disord 1996; 10:86–92.

57. Zeiss AM, Davies HD, Tinklenberg JR. An observational study of sexual behavior in demented male patients. J Gerontol A Biol Sci Med Sci 1996; 51:M325–M329.

58. Tsai SJ, Hwang JP, Yang CH, Liu KM, Lirng JF. Inappropriate sexual behaviors in dementia: a preliminary report. Alzheimer Dis Assoc Disord 1999; 13:60–62.

59. Kuhn DR, Greiner D, Arseneau L. Addressing hypersexuality in Alzheimer's disease. J Gerontol Nurs 1998; 24:44–50.

60. Reisberg B, Franssen E, Sclan SG, Kluger A, Ferris SH. Stage specific incidence of potentially remediable behavioral symptoms in aging and Alzheimer disease. Bull Clin Neurosci 1989; 54:95–112.

61. Petersen RC, Smith GE, Waring SC, et al. Mild cognitive impairment: clinical characterization and outcome. Arch Neurol 1999; 56:303–308.

62. Geda YE, Smith GE, Knopman DS, et al. De novo genesis of neuropsychiatric symptoms in mild cognitive impairment (MCI). Int Psychogeriatr 2004; 16:51–60.

63. Devanand DP, Brockington CD, Moody BJ, et al. Behavioral syndromes in Alzheimer's disease. Int Psychogeriatr 1992; 4(suppl 2):161–184.

64. Sultzer DL, Levin HS, Mahler ME, High WM, Cummings JL. Assessment of cognitive, psychiatric, and behavioral disturbances in patients with dementia: the Neurobehavioral Rating Scale. J Am Geriatr Soc 1992; 40:549–555.

65. Hope T, Keene J, Fairburn C, McShane R, Jacoby R. Behaviour changes in dementia. 2: Are there behavioural syndromes? Int J Geriatr Psychiatry 1997; 12:1074–1078.

66. Haupt M, Janner M, Ebeling S, Stierstorfer A, Kretschmar C. Presentation and stability of noncognitive symptom patterns in patients with Alzheimer disease. Alzheimer Dis Assoc Disord 1998; 12:323–329.

67. Hope T, Keene J, Fairburn CG, Jacoby R, McShane R. Natural history of behavioural changes and psychiatric

symptoms in Alzheimer's disease. A longitudinal study. Br J Psychiatry 1999; 174:39–44.

68. Harwood DG, Ownby RL, Barker WW, Duara R. The behavioral pathology in Alzheimer's Disease Scale (BEHAVE-AD): factor structure among community-dwelling Alzheimer's disease patients. Int J Geriatr Psychiatry 1998; 13:793–800.

69. Frisoni GB, Rozzini L, Gozzetti A, et al. Behavioral syndromes in Alzheimer's disease: description and correlates. Dement Geriatr Cogn Disord 1999; 10:130–138.

70. Fuh JL, Liu CK, Mega MS, Wang SJ, Cummings JL. Behavioral disorders and caregivers' reaction in Taiwanese patients with Alzheimer's disease. Int Psychogeriatr 2001; 13:121–128.

71. Aalten P, de Vugt ME, Lousberg R, et al. Behavioral problems in dementia: a factor analysis of the neuropsychiatric inventory. Dement Geriatr Cogn Disord 2003; 15: 99–105.

72. Mirakhur A, Craig D, Hart DJ, McLlroy SP, Passmore AP. Behavioural and psychological syndromes in Alzheimer's disease. Int J Geriatr Psychiatry 2004; 19:1035–1039.

73. Spalletta G, Baldinetti F, Buccione I, et al. Cognition and behaviour are independent and heterogeneous dimensions in Alzheimer's disease. J Neurol 2004; 251:688–695.

74. Amer-Ferrer G, de la Pena A, Garcia Soriano MT, Garcia Martin A. [Main components of Neuropsychiatric Inventory in Alzheimer's disease. Definition of behavioral syndromes.] Neurologia 2005; 20:9–16.

75. Schreinzer D, Ballaban T, Brannath W, et al. Components of behavioral pathology in dementia. Int J Geriatr Psychiatry 2005; 20:137–145.

76. McShane RH. What are the syndromes of behavioral and psychological symptoms of dementia? Int Psychogeriatr 2000; 12(suppl 1):147.

77. Moran M, Walsh C, Lynch A, et al. Syndromes of behavioural and psychological symptoms in mild Alzheimer's disease. Int J Geriatr Psychiatry 2004; 19:359–364.

78. Jost BC, Grossberg GT. The evolution of psychiatric symptoms in Alzheimer's disease: a natural history study. J Am Geriatr Soc 1996; 44:1078–1081.

79. Patterson MB, Mack JL, Mackell JA, et al. A longitudinal study of behavioral pathology across five levels of dementia severity in Alzheimer's disease: the CERAD Behavior Rating Scale for Dementia. The Alzheimer's Disease Cooperative Study. Alzheimer Dis Assoc Disord 1997; 11 (suppl 2):S40–S44.

80. McCarty HJ, Roth DL, Goode KT, et al. Longitudinal course of behavioral problems during Alzheimer's disease: linear versus curvilinear patterns of decline. J Gerontol A Biol Sci Med Sci 2000; 55:M200–M206.

81. Eustace A, Coen R, Walsh C, et al. A longitudinal evaluation of behavioural and psychological symptoms of probable Alzheimer's disease. Int J Geriatr Psychiatry 2002; 17: 968–973.

82. Devanand DP, Jacobs DM, Tang MX, et al. The course of psychopathologic features in mild to moderate Alzheimer disease. Arch Gen Psychiatry 1997; 54:257–263.

83. Ikeda M, Fukuhara R, Shigenobu K, et al. Dementia associated mental and behavioural disturbances in elderly people in the community: findings from the first Nakayama study. J Neurol Neurosurg Psychiatry 2004; 75:146–148.

84. Ballard C, Neill D, O'Brien J, et al. Anxiety, depression and psychosis in vascular dementia: prevalence and associations. J Affect Disord 2000; 59:97–106.

85. Porter VR, Buxton WG, Fairbanks LA, et al. Frequency and characteristics of anxiety among patients with Alzheimer's disease and related dementias. J Neuropsychiatry Clin Neurosci 2003; 15:180–186.

86. Hirono N, Mori E, Tanimukai S, et al. Distinctive neurobehavioral features among neurodegenerative dementias. J Neuropsychiatry Clin Neurosci 1999; 11:498–503.

87. Rockwell E, Choure J, Galasko D, Olichney J, Jeste DV. Psychopathology at initial diagnosis in dementia with Lewy bodies versus Alzheimer disease: comparison of matched groups with autopsy-confirmed diagnoses. Int J Geriatr Psychiatry 2000; 15:819–823.

88. Weiner MF, Hynan LS, Parikh B, et al. Can Alzheimer's disease and dementias with Lewy bodies be distinguished clinically? J Geriatr Psychiatry Neurol 2003; 16:245–250.

89. Mendez MF, Perryman KM, Miller BL, Cummings JL. Behavioral differences between frontotemporal dementia and Alzheimer's disease: a comparison on the BEHAVE-AD rating scale. Int Psychogeriatr 1998; 10:155–162.

90. Bozeat S, Gregory CA, Ralph MA, Hodges JR. Which neuropsychiatric and behavioural features distinguish frontal and temporal variants of frontotemporal dementia from Alzheimer's disease? J Neurol Neurosurg Psychiatry 2000; 69:178–186.

91. Cohen-Mansfield J. Use of patient characteristics to determine nonpharmacologic interventions for behavioral and psychological symptoms of dementia. Int Psychogeriatr 2000; 12(suppl 1):373–380.

92. Teri L. Combined therapy: a research overview. Int Psychogeriatr 2000; 12(suppl 1):381–386.

93. Cohen-Mansfield J. Nonpharmacologic interventions for inappropriate behaviors in dementia: a review, summary, and critique. Am J Geriatr Psychiatry 2001; 9:361–381.

94. Lawlor B, Bhriain SN. Psychosis and behavioural symptoms of dementia: defining the role of neuroleptic interventions. Int J Geriatr Psychiatry 2001; 16(suppl 1):S2–S6.

IV Medical management

17

Mild cognitive impairment and very early stage Alzheimer's disease

Howard Chertkow

INTRODUCTION AND DEFINITIONS

The treatment of Alzheimer's disease (AD) can be divided into primary prevention, secondary prevention and treatment of AD itself (Figure 17.1). Treatments can also be divided according to the goal – symptomatic improvement, modulatory and treatments to prevent progression and treatment of behavioural symptoms. A further classification would be medication vs non-pharmacological therapies (including specific therapeutic interventions for the individual, counselling, support for the caregiver and education). In this chapter we will focus on primary prevention and secondary prevention management, all three forms of therapies and both pharmacological and non-pharmacological therapies. Behavioural

symptoms are less common in the very early AD stages and will not be addressed.

Primary prevention refers to therapeutic measures (medications, lifestyle changes) undertaken by healthy or healthy high-risk individuals. The decision to stop smoking by a 30-year-old man with a family history of heart disease would be preventative primary treatment of myocardial infarction. Discontinuation of smoking after a first angina episode would be secondary treatment – after symptoms have begun, but before the objective disease endpoint has occurred. The definition of primary and secondary prevention is somewhat unspecified in the setting of AD. There is considerable evidence[1] that the biological changes of AD begin many years, perhaps decades, before symptoms ensue. That means that primary prevention

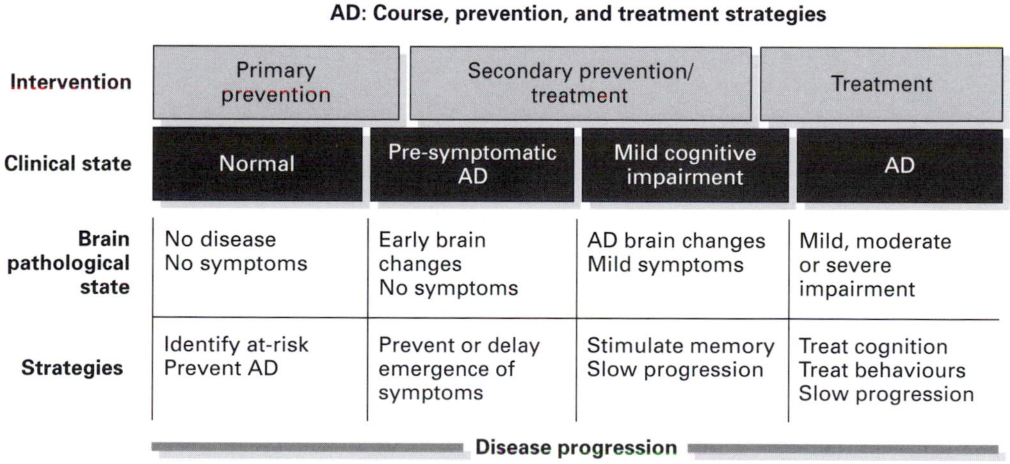

AD: Course, prevention, and treatment strategies

Intervention	Primary prevention	Secondary prevention/ treatment		Treatment
Clinical state	Normal	Pre-symptomatic AD	Mild cognitive impairment	AD
Brain pathological state	No disease No symptoms	Early brain changes No symptoms	AD brain changes Mild symptoms	Mild, moderate or severe impairment
Strategies	Identify at-risk Prevent AD	Prevent or delay emergence of symptoms	Stimulate memory Slow progression	Treat cognition Treat behaviours Slow progression

Disease progression

Figure 17.1 Progression of clinical and pathological states leading from normal to Alzheimer's disease (AD). The taxonomy and timing of therapeutic interventions are also shown

measures of high-risk adults are already targeting individuals who may have the earliest changes of AD present in their brains.

Secondary prevention is relevant to individuals in the very earliest clinical stages of AD who might not meet most clinical diagnostic criteria for AD. Who are these individuals? While multiple labels have been used to designate this group in the past, most would fall into the general current category of mild cognitive impairment (MCI).[2–4] MCI is a clinical label which includes elderly subjects with short term or long term memory impairment, and with no significant daily functional disability. The original diagnosis of MCI required subjective report of cognitive decline from a former level, gradual in onset, and present for at least 6 months. This subjective complaint is supplemented by objective evidence of memory and learning decline, with other cognitive domains remaining 'generally intact'.[5] There was no clear delineation as to how the presence of memory loss was to be established. In all cases, this term excluded individuals with significant depression, delirium, mental retardation or other psychiatric disorders likely responsible for the impairment. If the memory loss was severe and accompanied by significant functional impairment, then the individual met clinical criteria for dementia and was no longer MCI. The concept was intended to capture and classify patients who seem to have a cognitive problem that one would be loath to label as 'normal', and yet clearly are not severe enough to qualify as 'dementia'.[6] The majority of MCI individuals presenting to physicians do so with primarily memory complaints and would be classified as having 'amnestic MCI'.[4,7] Such individuals, when they progress to dementia, almost invariably end with a diagnosis of AD.[8] Many MCI individuals already have significant early AD pathology.[9,10] Indeed, Morris and colleagues have suggested that all MCI goes on to AD and that it should be called 'MCI of the AD type'.[10] We would hasten to add that, in our experience, about a quarter of amnestic MCI patients referred to a memory clinic do not progress to dementia,[11] and in population studies, the non-progressing proportion is even greater.[12] Nevertheless, it is reasonable to rephrase the question of 'how to manage very early AD' into (1) how to manage asymptomatic high-risk individuals (primary prevention), as well as (2) how to manage MCI patients (secondary prevention). Obviously, given our limited clinical data there is great overlap between what can be suggested for the two groups. Concerning medications for MCI for which we have a set of robust, effective and uncontroversial results arising from prospective, randomized, placebo-controlled clinical trials (RCT), there are none at this point.

Nevertheless, we will present an overview of current and potential treatments.

ASSESSMENT OF INDIVIDUALS WITH MILD COGNITIVE IMPAIRMENT

When a patient complains of memory loss, it is advisable to pursue evaluation, in terms of mental status evaluation, to define the presence or not of objective deficits. This may entail a basic office mental status exam, usually with the Mini Mental State Examination (MMSE)[13] and in some countries the 5 word test[14]. More extended clinical testing and neuropsychological brain imaging evaluation are currently carried out in the setting of research studies. A 12-minute screen, the Montreal Cognitive Assessment (MoCA), can adequately document objective cognitive impairment (Figure 17.2): a score below 26 over 30 is abnormal to objective memory loss, detecting 90 per cent of MCI subjects demonstrated on extended testing to have objective impairment.[15] When subjects with mild AD were tested, all scored below the MoCA cut-off, while most normal subjects scored above the cut-off score.

An argument can be made for carrying out a full diagnostic work-up in patients with MCI – since reversibility of memory loss is possible.[16] The neurological exam is generally normal aside from mental status change. Frontal release signs are often not encountered for years after AD diagnosis, and only small subgroups of patients have extrapyramidal signs or myoclonus. At the MCI stage, a broad differential diagnosis must be entertained – for instance, we have seen a number of individuals with a final diagnosis of obstructive sleep apnoea, who first presented complaining of their mild memory loss.[17]

While there has been a flurry of publications regarding new tests and markers for AD, in fact the basic laboratory work-up of patients has not changed – it is still focused on basic blood work to exclude reversible causes of dementia. Molecular genetic analysis is still reserved for those rare individuals with familial AD (or at least with a strong family history). ApoE genotyping has proven an important research tool for exploring the genetics of cognitive decline. It is clear that individuals with an apoE4 genotype (especially homozygous) are at increased risk of developing AD,[18,19] will develop it sooner and will have greater general decline of cognition during ageing than others. Nevertheless, apoE genotyping has insufficient sensitivity or specificity to be used routinely in clinic or in a neurologist's office (see Chapter 27). The same can currently be said of a wide range of other experimental measures (see Chapter 10).

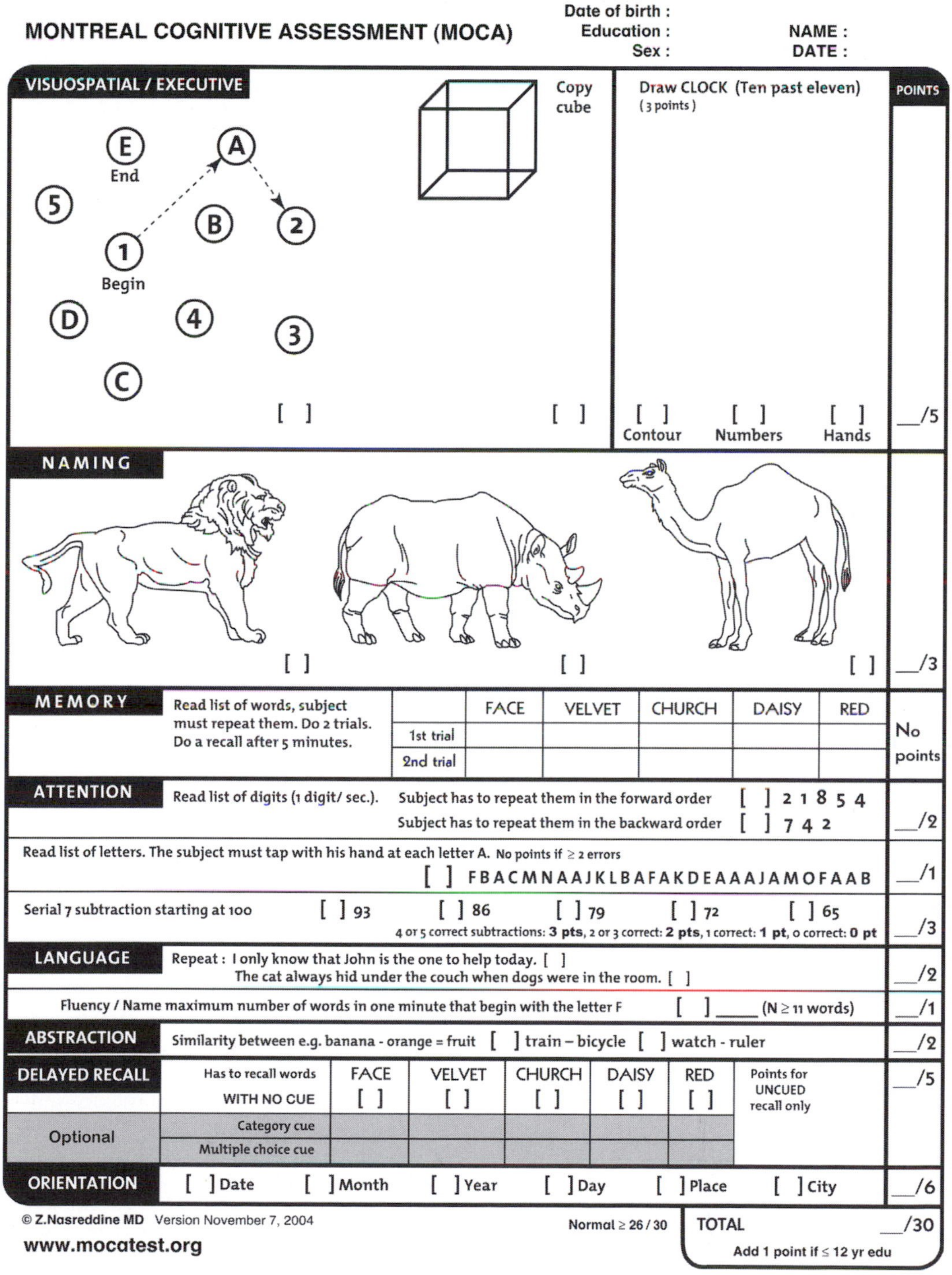

MONTREAL COGNITIVE ASSESSMENT (MOCA)

Date of birth :
Education :
Sex :

NAME :
DATE :

VISUOSPATIAL / EXECUTIVE		POINTS

Copy cube

Draw CLOCK (Ten past eleven)
(3 points)

E
End

A

5

B

2

1
Begin

D

4

3

C

[ ]

[ ]

[ ] [ ] [ ]
Contour Numbers Hands

__/5

NAMING

[ ]   [ ]   [ ]   __/3

MEMORY	Read list of words, subject must repeat them. Do 2 trials. Do a recall after 5 minutes.		FACE	VELVET	CHURCH	DAISY	RED	No points
		1st trial						
		2nd trial						

ATTENTION	Read list of digits (1 digit/ sec.).	Subject has to repeat them in the forward order [ ] 2 1 8 5 4	__/2
		Subject has to repeat them in the backward order [ ] 7 4 2	

Read list of letters. The subject must tap with his hand at each letter A. No points if ≥ 2 errors
[ ] FBACMNAAJKLBAFAKDEAAAJAMOFAAB __/1

Serial 7 subtraction starting at 100 [ ] 93   [ ] 86   [ ] 79   [ ] 72   [ ] 65 __/3
4 or 5 correct subtractions: **3 pts**, 2 or 3 correct: **2 pts**, 1 correct: **1 pt**, 0 correct: **0 pt**

LANGUAGE	Repeat : I only know that John is the one to help today. [ ] The cat always hid under the couch when dogs were in the room. [ ]	__/2

Fluency / Name maximum number of words in one minute that begin with the letter F [ ] _____ (N ≥ 11 words) __/1

ABSTRACTION	Similarity between e.g. banana - orange = fruit [ ] train – bicycle [ ] watch - ruler	__/2

DELAYED RECALL	Has to recall words WITH NO CUE	FACE [ ]	VELVET [ ]	CHURCH [ ]	DAISY [ ]	RED [ ]	Points for UNCUED recall only	__/5
Optional	Category cue							
	Multiple choice cue							

ORIENTATION	[ ] Date [ ] Month [ ] Year [ ] Day [ ] Place [ ] City	__/6

© Z.Nasreddine MD Version November 7, 2004

www.mocatest.org

Normal ≥ 26 / 30

TOTAL __/30
Add 1 point if ≤ 12 yr edu

Figure 17.2 The Montreal Cognitive Assessment (MoCA) test. A score at or below 26 indicates cognitive impairment beyond the normal acceptable level.
Reproduced with permission from Ziad Nasreddine.

What about neuroimaging? Virtually all dementia patients referred to a neurologist will undergo some sort of neuroimaging, and the American Academy of Neurology (AAN) has suggested neuroimaging as part of its guidelines for dementia investigation.[20,21] Nevertheless, in the clinical setting of MCI, there is little evidence that standard CT or MRI will yield useful results that will alter the diagnosis or management. Potentially useful measures such as hippocampal volumetry[22,23] remain as yet limited to research.

Given the lack of clear prognostic markers, an uncertain natural history and lack of proven therapies to prevent decline, there is little consensus on management of MCI patients.[3] The patient should be told that he meets criteria for MCI, which has a real statistical risk (but by no means any certainty) of progressing to dementia. This is vastly preferable to giving no diagnosis or giving false assurances that 'its just normal ageing'. Confronting a patient with MCI, it is best for physicians to acknowledge their current lack of certainty regarding prognosis, as well as the lack of useful tests or proven biomarkers that should be administered.

One important intervention for MCI patients is close follow-up. Baseline mental status (preferably with formal tools such as the MMSE or MoCA) should be carried out. The patient should be seen at 6-month intervals, even over a number of years. It is not appropriate to advise a patient with MCI to immediately stop work, or insist that they stop driving. The studies of Daly and Ritchie both noted that a subset of MCI individuals improved to normal over follow-up, and MCI alone usually will only marginally affect functioning at most workplaces.[24,25]

SYMPTOMATIC TREATMENT OF INDIVIDUALS WITH MILD COGNITIVE IMPAIRMENT

Treatment may be symptomatic in the MCI stage because of the individual's concerns over memory loss and wish for therapy to improve their current memory performance. It is our experience that the majority of patients, however, do not feel 'sick', are not seeking current treatment, but rather request prevention. At the same time, other individuals who do not even meet objective criteria for MCI, complain bitterly of their degree of memory impairment and seek over-the-counter and alternative medications for treatment. Furthermore, the economic results in the marketplace speak to a widespread desire for treatment of the memory loss associated with ageing. Thus, a discussion of treatment approaches for MCI shades into the

'slippery slope' of cognitive enhancement in the elderly.[26] A number of recent publications have seriously examined the coming importance of such memory stimulation, in terms of its ethics, its effect on schools and in the marketplace and the social considerations to come.[27]

There is no current treatment for MCI sufficiently substantiated to have obtained government approval from FDA or Canadian regulatory authorities (see Table 17.1). This contrasts with the situation in Europe, where medications such as *Ginkgo/biloba* have been approved broadly for 'memory impairment'. The three available cholinesterase inhibitors (CI) in North America are approved for treatment of AD, not MCI. Symptomatic treatment of the memory complaints in MCI is, in fact, generally disappointing. The author's own anecdotal experience with MCI patients using CI, *Ginkgo biloba* or stimulants such as ritalin is that none of these usually make a significant clinical impact on their mild memory loss in the majority of patients. Occasionally, however, MCI subjects may have a significant and even a dramatic benefit.

Cholinesterase inhibitors

Symptomatic therapy for AD has already come of age, with the availability in most countries of three CIs: donepezil (Aricept), rivastigmine (Exelon) and galantamine (Reminyl). These all produce modest improvement and stabilization in the majority of patients. A recent meta-analysis[28] concluded that there is modest but significant therapeutic effect from all three, with insufficient evidence to demonstrate that one medication is superior to the others. The medications differ in terms of secondary pharmacological effects, dosing intervals and side effect profiles. All three medications can produce gastro-intestinal side effects initially, but these are rarely intolerable. Starting doses are donepezil 5 mg daily, galantamine 8 mg daily and rivastigmine 1.5 mg bid. Dose escalation for maximum efficacy is recommended in all three medications. The Second Canadian Consensus Conference on dementia supported treatment of AD patients with CIs.[29] We often tell families that we hope to 'roll back the decline by six to twelve months'. Recent studies have reported good results with memantine, an NMDA antagonist available for many years in Germany.[30] Memantine appears most useful for the behavioural symptoms of moderate to severe AD.

Regarding symptomatic treatment of MCI, the results to date have been much less impressive. The theoretical basis for their use arose out of the 'cholinergic hypothesis of AD',[31] which was based on

Table 17.1 Symptomatic and preventative pharmacological therapies for very early AD

Symptomatic therapy

Cholinesterase inhibitors

Ginkgo biloba

Nootropic medications

- phosphatidyl-serine (PS)
- acetyl-L-carnitine
- choline (phosphatidylcholine, citicoline)
- piracetam

Memory stimulants

- ampakines
- NMDA receptor modulation
- CREB modulators

Preventative therapies

Anti-oxidants

- vitamin E
- other anti-oxidants (selegiline, vitamin C)

Homocysteine

Omega fatty acids

Cholinesterase inhibitors

Anti-inflammatory agents

Oestrogen

Statins

Anti-amyloid therapies

- beta and gamma-secretase inhibitors
- GAG-mimetics

Therapy for vascular risk factors

the evidence of a cholinergic deficit in AD that might be amenable to therapy. Recent evidence suggests an absence of cholinergic deficits in MCI or very mild AD.[32,33] The early cholinergic alterations at this stage, however, may also include changes in choline transport, acetylcholine release, nicotinic and muscarinic receptor expression, neurotrophin support and perhaps axonal transport.[34]

Clinicians have anecdotally reported that certain MCI patients benefit from treatment with CI in terms of memory and global function. Salloway et al[35] studied 270 patients across 20 centres meeting Petersen criteria for amnestic MCI. Half were treated with donepezil 10 mg for 6 months and a series of cognitive and global tests were administered. Two-thirds of the donepezil-treated cohort completed the study, and change in a paragraph recall test as well as the Clinical Global Impression of Change-MCI instrument were used as the primary outcome measures. Neither of these measures showed significant beneficial effects of

therapy at the end of 6 months. A major secondary measure, the ADAS-cog, did show a symptomatic benefit, however. Subjectively, subjects treated with donepezil did report greater improvement in memory function than those given placebo. They reported feeling sharper mentally, more organized and more confident of their memory. All of this suggests that at least some MCI individuals will have a significant clinical benefit from donepezil, but overall the effects are mild. Neither, galantamine nor rivastigmine have been demonstrated to have a benefit.

Ginkgo biloba

Ginkgo biloba is commonly prescribed in Europe for all memory-impaired patients, with the idea that ginkgo improves blood and oxygen flow to the brain and supports memory function, mental sharpness and circulation. An anti-oxidant role is also suspected. There are few if any well-designed clinical trials that support this conclusion.[36] There was one placebo-controlled study of *Ginkgo biloba* in AD, with a high drop-out rate. This showed a significant symptomatic benefit in AD, albeit approximately one quarter of the efficacy of CIs.[37] It is notable that in some countries such as Germany, ginkgo is routinely prescribed for AD because of its greater accessibility and lower cost to patients.

A large 24-week study, which was double-blind with placebo controls, compared 123 patients on ginkgo with 44 individuals on placebo.[38] The treated patients included one-third with dementia and two-thirds defined as AAMI, a category with memory impairment compared to young control values (which approximates MCI, but is somewhat different). Neither treated group showed any benefit compared with placebo, and results did not support a role for ginkgo in therapy.

There are ongoing long-term studies in Europe and North America currently testing the hypothesis that *Ginkgo biloba*, as an antioxidant, might prevent onset or slow progression of AD.[39] Data are not yet available.

Nootropics

There are a number of over-the-counter 'dietary supplements' which have been suggested to have the effect of strengthening and protecting neurons of the brain involved in memory, serving as 'memory nutrients'. These 'nootropics' have non-specific mechanisms of action, with putative effects on energy metabolism, cholinergic mechanisms, excitatory amino acid receptor-mediated functions as well as hormonal mechanisms.[40] In this class one would list phosphatidylserine, acetyl-L-carnitine and piracetam. These are available through health food stores as diet supplements, not medications. Evidence for their efficacy is slim, but they have few if any side effects. Presumably these nootropics would have symptomatic rather than preventive effects in MCI.

Phosphatidyl-serine (PS) plays a role in nerve cell membranes. The supplement version is obtained from cows, and more recently a form derived from soy lecithin is being sold. In one randomized controlled trial (RCT), subjects with mild memory loss similar to MCI who took 300 mg of PS for 3 months showed some modest improvement in their memory.[41] The effects tended not to occur in everyone. There was no benefit in AD. There have been no other RCTs of PS in the past 10 years.

Acetyl-L-carnitine, choline (phosphatidylcholine, citicoline) and piracetam: Of these, the most tested has been piracetam, which was tested in a double blind design, in individuals who had some features of MCI.[42] There were mildly positive effects reported on delayed memory during the 3-month study, although groups were not distinguishable by the trial's end. In another multicentre cross-over RCT with non-demented individuals with memory impairment, there was a positive effect reported on tests of attention and memory.[43] A meta-analysis claimed to show positive effects, even for MCI individuals.[44] Evidence for the other two compounds is quite thin in comparison.

Overall, despite claims for the efficacy of nootropics, the proven benefit of each of these agents is modest. One broad review stated in conclusion 'All in all, we believe that the current data do not allow strong scientifically based recommendations for any of these memory nutrients (including PS and ginkgo). However, the data also do not allow us to conclude that these nutrients are ineffective in boosting memory'.[36]

Memory stimulants and future 'smart drugs'

Medications that will attempt to impact on the neurochemical processes of memory itself are currently being tested. These might compensate for the neurochemical deterioration thought to be part of MCI and even AD, without changing or retarding the underlying pathological processes. In addition, they have the potential to even impact on the putative changes we consider to be normal cognitive ageing. The media are already speaking about potential 'Viagra for the brain'.[45] While the clinical trials to come will certainly be aimed at MCI, the future potential for off-label use has been the subject already of a number of serious

discussions.[27] Bioethicists are contemplating the social effects and even dangers of memory enhancement, and potential use of these drugs in lifestyle enhancement.

Enhancement has largely been targeted at memory problems, inasmuch as these are the primary complaints of the elderly. The candidate drugs directed at improving memory fall into one of two categories: those that target the initial induction of long-term potentiation and those that target the later stages of memory consolidation.[46] The first category consists of (1) drugs that modulate NMDA receptors in their response to glutamate-induced depolarization and (2) drugs that modulate AMPA (alpha-amino-3-hydroxy-5-methyl-4-isoxazole propionic acid) receptors to facilitate depolarization. NMDA receptors respond to repeated neuronal signalling by setting up a cascade of molecular events that strengthen the involved synaptic bond. Genetically engineered mice with genetically overreactive NMDA receptors have enhanced memory performance. This represents one molecular approach to memory modification. Drugs using the AMPA mechanism would work through amplification of the AMPA receptor's response to glutamate. Ampakines for MCI treatment are already beginning to enter phase two clinical trials.[47,48] The efficacy and side effect profiles of these cognitive enhancers are unknown.

MANAGEMENT OF ASYMPTOMATIC HIGH-RISK INDIVIDUALS, MCI AND VERY EARLY AD

There have been, up to this point, no successful primary prevention randomized control studies in AD, nor has there been an unequivocally successful prevention/modification study in MCI individuals.[49] Prevention of onset and slowing of progression to AD from MCI would have an enormous benefit to patients, and this has even been operationalized financially as a short term benefit of US$5300 per year for each individual.[50,51] Since primary prevention clinical trials tend to be large and lengthy affairs which require enormous effort,[52] many researchers are turning to MCI as a more 'efficient' means of testing modification/prevention drugs.

Currently we have impressive epidemiological and natural history studies of risk factors in the development of cognitive decline and AD (see Chapter 3), and these may be used to guide therapy and management to some degree. It is important to point out, however, that retrospective observational studies are not the same as prospective randomized intervention studies. This has been brought harshly to the fore by the failure of a number of RCTs to confirm efficacy of interventions derived from epidemiological studies.[53] There are drawbacks in relying on population studies to provide management suggestions: subjects in population studies who are taking some form of therapy are generally healthier and more motivated about their health than other people who are not taking anything. Why otherwise are they taking dietary supplements, for instance? We must also consider the opposite bias – individuals with preclinical dementia might be more likely to stop taking medications or forget to report their taking of supplements. Furthermore, there is a survival bias in population studies – we are, after all, measuring the survivors over time rather than ill individuals presenting to clinics. Finally, a primary prevention trial may inadvertently miss the 'critical period' during which a particular therapy might be effective. There is some suspicion (see the Oestrogens section below) that the Women's Health Initiative Memory Study (WHIMS) on oestrogen, a huge primary prevention study in women, failed to show a benefit of oestrogen in preventing AD because it limited itself to women of age 60 and over, when in fact the critical period when oestrogen is beneficial may be decades earlier.[54–56] Nevertheless, there are sufficient population studies defining risk of AD that management suggestions – pharmacological and non-pharmacological – can be given to high-risk patients, specifically those with a strong family history of AD. Very similar suggestions are appropriate in most instances for MCI individuals. Since a review of causation of AD has already been included in previous chapters, we will focus largely on the clinical data and potential therapy recommendations.

Non-pharmacological therapies

Appropriate advice to MCI individuals and those asymptomatic individuals at high genetic risk primarily involves general non-pharmacological management, for which there is reasonable epidemiological evidence. Much of this revolves around the notion that 'cognitive reserve' may be influenced by lifestyle factors, which are modifiable.[57,58] The current advice given these 'very early AD' patients in the author's Memory Clinic is listed below, along with the evidence to justify it.

'Increase your physical and leisure activities. Exercise frequently, get into shape and get down to a healthy weight'.

Increased physical activities may safely be recommended for MCI individuals, and the theoretical benefits for AD prevention are in addition to the other

health benefits of exercise. Obesity has deleterious effects on both insulin levels and blood pressure, both of which are AD risks.[59,60]

There is thus increasing evidence that engaging in both physical activity and leisure activity, and in mentally stimulating activities, has separate effects in decreasing cognitive decline and reducing AD risk.[61,62]

'Increase your mentally stimulating activities – playing cards and taking classes, for instance.'

The Religious Orders Study in Chicago reported that healthy elderly nuns and priests who scored high on measures of intellectual activities were much less likely to develop AD. On a five-point scale, every one point increase was associated with a striking 33 per cent decrease in the occurrence of clinical dementia.[63] In a separate study based in the Oregon Aging study cohort, involvement in either intellectual activities or heavy physical exercise was independently associated with a decreased risk of normal elderly subjects developing dementia over 5 years of follow-up.[64] The natural assumption that intervention – increasing an individual's intellectual activities – will effectively lower the risk of AD remains to be proven.

'Lower your stress level. Chronic stress (family, finances, home, work) will impact on your concentration and memory at any age, but more so as you get older. '

It is increasingly clear that stress, via cortisol levels, acts as a direct toxin on the hippocampus capable of amplifying disease-related hippocampal dysfunction.[65–67] Only recently have data on emotional factors such as proneness to distress been studied in AD, and this has emerged as a significant risk factor.[68] Attempts to reduce stress levels seem a reasonable goal, although there have not been direct clinical studies.

'Get enough good sleep. Inadequate sleep or sleep disorders such as sleep apnoea will make your memory worse.'

Patients with sleep disorders often present with memory loss,[17,69] and this seems a reasonable factor to modify and control.[17,69,70]

'Treat all medical illnesses early.'

It is now clear that untreated or inadequately treated diseases such as diabetes, heart disease, hypertension (high blood pressure) and high cholesterol represent risk factors for AD, either directly or via vascular mechanisms.[71–74] Encouragement to maximize treatment of these can only be beneficial.

'Get treatment for depression if you are depressed.'

The overlap between dementia and depression continues to be an important area, and untreated depression will exacerbate and amplify memory loss.[75–78] There is little to be lost by closer attention and treatment of depression in MCI and very early AD.

'Focus on friends and your social network.'

An important study in the Kungsholmen district of Stockholm[79] demonstrated that a poor or limited social network increased the risk of dementia by 60 per cent, and a significant gradient was found for increasing degrees of social connections. It appears that an extensive social network seems to protect against dementia. Clearly this requires a lifelong commitment to building social interactions, but this may be a modifiable risk.

'Avoid too much alcohol, or sleeping medications. These all impair memory function.'

The deleterious effects of alcohol on the brain are too many to require explanation of this advice.

Cognitive therapy and directed interventions

Investigation of directed cognitive therapy is in its nascent stages. When found to be effective, it is unclear whether such therapy has a symptomatic benefit or is modifying the disease process itself. Cognitive–motor programmes in patients with MCI and very early AD may include cognitive exercises plus social and psychomotor activities, and appear promising.[50] Rapp and colleagues[81] used a multifaceted intervention that included education about memory loss, relaxation training, memory skills training and cognitive restructuring for memory-related beliefs, compared to a no-treatment control condition in MCI individuals. The treated group had significantly better memory appraisals than controls at the end of treatment and at a 6-month follow-up, but there were no differences between groups on memory performance at post-test, although a trend existed. Interestingly, Poon and colleagues[82] have even shown that such therapy can be given over the internet. Telemedicine is thus a feasible, effective and acceptable means of providing cognitive assessment and intervention to older persons with mild cognitive deficits.

Vitamin E

The evidence for a benefit from vitamin E in preventing or delaying AD derives from a set of epidemiological studies. Individuals in the community eating a high level of dietary vitamin E have been found to have a 36 per cent reduced risk of developing AD when compared to those consuming little dietary vitamin E.[83] In the Rotterdam population study, individuals using supplements of vitamins E and C developed AD at a lower rate than subjects not using supplements.[84] The Cache County population study in Utah is currently examining risk factors for cognitive decline in a cohort of 5677 elderly subjects followed over 10 years. While vitamin E supplementation alone was not found to have impressive results, this study suggests that healthy individuals using vitamin C or E supplements, as well as concurrent anti-inflammatory agents, are indeed at a lower risk of developing dementia.[85]

In a widely cited study of vitamin E in individuals with AD,[86] patients on high-dose vitamin E for up to 24 months reached the functional milestone of institutionalization more slowly than individuals on placebo. The treatment was regarded as safe; vitamin E was not associated with increased risk of death. Indeed, an identical number of subjects on vitamin E died during the course of the trial compared to subjects on placebo. Based on this single study, and the theoretical benefits of anti-oxidants in preventing AD and cognitive decline as well as ageing in general, a large number of MCI and AD patients are currently prescribed vitamin E, or obtain it themselves from pharmacies.

In contrast to this is new evidence from the Memory Impairment Study, an important 3-year trial co-sponsored by the NIA, Alzheimer Disease Cooperative Study group (ADCS) and Pfizer. In this study, individuals with MCI were recruited and randomized into a vitamin E therapy arm, a donepezil therapy arm or placebo. The study was large (240 subjects recruited into each arm), expensive and elaborate. The investigators accepted only more 'advanced' MCI individuals scoring below a memory cut-off score. The crucial primary endpoint was the number of subjects classified as progressing to dementia at the end of 3 years. This study assessed the effects of five daily capsules (2000 IU) of vitamin E and found no overall benefit in the vitamin E group in terms of prevention of progression to AD at the end of 3 years' time.[8]

Is vitamin E safe? A recent publication[87] examined the number of deaths in 19 clinical trials of vitamin E, including a total of 136 000 subjects. None of the individual studies showed an increase in risk of death for subjects on vitamin E alone. Similarly, when all 19 studies were examined together, there was no increase in the risk of death. However, when the studies were arranged by dose of vitamin E (above or below the 400 IU/day median dose), it appeared that individuals on low to moderate doses of vitamin E had a very slight protection against death while those on high dose vitamin E were at a very slightly higher risk of death. There are numerous methodological weaknesses of this analysis, nevertheless, it has led to confusion regarding the risk/benefit ration for vitamin E in MCI. The Cache County population study failed to find any overall increase in mortality in subjects taking vitamin E. However, in subjects with previous cardiovascular incidents (stroke, coronary bypass, myocardial infarction), there might indeed be a small increased risk.[88] In the MCI Memory Impairment Study, there was no increase in risk in the vitamin E group; the death rate was identical in individuals on placebo and vitamin E.[8]

Based on these data from recent publications, it is difficult to draw firm conclusions or make recommendations. The benefits of vitamin E supplements for AD prevention are unproven, and individuals with MCI have not shown benefit from vitamin E in terms of prevention of progression in an RCT. Despite the meta-analysis, the risk of vitamin E also appears minimal. Might a single 400 IU vitamin E tablet be beneficially and safely prescribed for an MCI individual? They receive this in the author's own clinic, albeit with some hesitation.

Alternative antioxidants

The case for antioxidant therapy to prevent onset of AD (as well as other neurodegenerative diseases and ageing in general) is relatively strong, and new evidence continues to accumulate. Oxidative damage can be found in a number of neurodegenerative conditions including AD.[89,90] Oxidative damage in AD is indicated by the presence of elevated levels of nucleic acids, proteins and oxidized lipids. This damage appears to occur early on in the course of the disease, and be most marked in those areas showing earliest AD pathology.[91] In the brains of individuals suffering from MCI at the time of death, there are elevated protein carbonyls, malondialdehyede and TBARS, all indicative of early oxidative damage.[92]

Observational and population studies have largely focused on vitamin E (and vitamin C) as antioxidants.[83,85] The evidence supporting vitamin E was reviewed above. What about other antioxidants? In fact, the objection has been raised that these studies used food questionnaires, and failed to find an effect of vitamin supplements. Furthermore, the interindividual dietary intake of antioxidants is actually quite narrow. High ascorbic acid and beta carotene plasma levels have been associated with better memory performance in the non-demented elderly,[93] but no such data exist in MCI. The protective effects of antioxidants may furthermore be overshadowed by the effect of smoking, which increases the load of free radicals, providing increased oxidative stress.[94] Are there, therefore, RCTs that have tested the antioxidant hypothesis? *Ginkgo biloba*, vitamins A, C and E all act as free radical scavengers. The failure of the Memory Impairment Study to show any effect of vitamin E in MCI is thus a major blow to support antioxidant therapy. A large current study is looking at primary prevention of dementia with selenium and vitamin E,[95] but data are not yet available.

Homocysteine

Analysis of the Framingham study produced the result that higher homocysteine levels were associated with increased risk of sporadic AD.[96] It is known that increased serum homocysteine is associated with histopathological evidence of vascular endothelial injury, vascular smooth muscle proliferation and progressive arterial stenosis. There has been substantial evidence that homocysteine levels correlate with arteriosclerotic vascular disease.[97] What is surprising is the extension to AD as well. The factors in homocysteine levels are well known – vitamin supplements (folate, B_6, B_{12}) lower the levels, while caffeine, smoking and lack of exercise increase levels.[98] Current management of elevated homocysteine has been to increase folate in the diet or treat with supplements when increased homocysteine was greater than 15 μmol/l. Simple treatment with folate (3 mg daily), B_6 (25 mg daily) and B_{12} (250 to 500 μg daily) keeps the homocysteine level low. Treatment of normal elderly as well as MCI individuals with folate, B_6 and B_{12} found in multivitamins (even without monitoring homocysteine levels) is likely to become the norm, even without controlled studies of this intervention.[99–101]

Omega fatty acids

Foods such as meat, butter, olive oil and fish oil contain varying levels of essential fatty acids (EFAs), otherwise known as 'omega' fatty acids, not synthesized by the body. The most important of these is called DHA (docosahexaenoic acid). They are highly concentrated in the human brain and are thought to play a major role in axonal transport and synaptic function.[103,104] Omega fatty acids, particularly DHA, can be obtained by eating cold water fatty fish such as salmon, sardines, mackerel and bluefish. There is evidence from the Framingham study that those with the highest blood levels of DHA were half as likely as those with the lowest levels to develop dementia.

Cholinesterase inhibitors

The Memory Impairment Study described earlier was an important 3-year trial co-sponsored by the NIA, Alzheimer Disease Cooperative Study group (ADCS) and Pfizer. In this study, individuals with MCI were recruited and randomized into a vitamin E arm (2000 IU daily), a donepezil arm (10 mg daily) or placebo. The crucial primary endpoint was the number of subjects classified as progressing to dementia at the end of 3 years. The result was negative – no significant difference between the three groups were found at 3 years.[8] This disappointing result seems to put to rest the possibility of CIs as effective therapies to prevent AD, but there are subanalyses that still seem to offer promise. For instance, it is clear that the group of individuals taking donepezil performed better than the others over the first 18 months, in terms of neuropsychological measures and global outcomes. It is also clear that the majority of individuals progressing to AD had an apoE4 allele, and if the analysis is restricted only to those individuals, there were indeed fewer 'conversions to dementia' on donepezil at the end of 3 years. Currently, debate rages on whether this 'negative study' might be reinterpreted as a positive result for a particular subgroup of patients. There are also the usual methodological concerns (heterogeneity of patients, uncertainty of outcome measures in this population) that make it hard to achieve significant results, even with large numbers of subjects.

The other main CIs are also being assessed for their potential to slow progression to AD. The rivastigmine trial (InDDEX) lasted 4 years; preliminary results indicated a low rate of conversion and no statistically significant effect on the time to clinical diagnosis of AD.[104] Similarly the two galantamine trials of 2-year duration showed no difference in the primary analysis of conversion from amnestic MCI to AD, although there was a reduced rate of whole-brain atrophy in the patients treated with galantamine.[105] However, therapy with this medication was associated with a small but statistically significant increased mortality risk, partly explained by a very low mortality rate in the placebo groups.

From the currently available evidence, there is no benefit for CI in slowing progression to AD, although there may a transient symptomatic effect in MCI using donepezil.[106]

Anti-inflammatory agents

There is clearly an inflammatory component to AD. There is now considerable evidence from observational studies that use of non-steroidal anti-inflammatory drugs (NSAIDs) including ibuprofen and indomethacin as well as prednisone (a steroid) is associated with a decreased risk of AD. These medications appear to protect against the development of AD through their anti-inflammatory properties.[107–110] A meta-analysis of nine observational studies confirmed the fact that NSAIDs protect against development of AD, with a pooled relative reduced risk of 0.72.[111] Those individuals with longer use of NSAIDs seemed to derive a greater protective effect. Nevertheless, a randomized, double-blind, placebo-controlled trial of rofecoxib in patients with MCI was negative, with no evidence of a protective effect.[112,113] Furthermore, results of a study that compared the effects of prednisone versus a placebo on people who had been diagnosed with AD found no difference in cognitive decline between the prednisone and placebo treatment groups. Thus, a low-dose regimen of prednisone does not seem to be useful in treating AD. Again this suggests that there is a (as yet unknown) critical period for treatment, and MCI and early AD are simply too late a stage to intervene with this medication. Another possibility is that doses of NSAIDS used in RCT so far were too small to be effective.

Statins

Statins are a group of drugs widely prescribed to reduce cholesterol. They lower levels of low-density lipoprotein (LDL) cholesterol – the type most strongly linked with coronary artery disease and stroke – by blocking a liver enzyme essential for cholesterol production. Statins are formally known as 3-hydroxy-3-methylglutaryl coenzyme A (HMG CoA) reductase inhibitors. Statins now marketed in the United States include atorvastatin (Lipitor), fluvastatin (Lescol), lovastatin (Mevacor), pravastatin (Pravachol) and simvastatin (Zocor). High LDL levels have been linked to risk of AD.[114,115] In addition, high LDL levels also seem to favour deposition of beta-amyloid, the major component of the senile plaques characteristic of AD. Reduction in cholesterol by statins might alter APP metabolism and thus reduce the production of A-beta.[116] Statins have also been shown to have immunomodulatory effects, blocking the ability of cytokine interferon-gamma (IFN-γ) to activate T-cells. Statins might therefore have a neuroprotective effect by lowering inflammation.

An earlier multicentre analysis of over 60 000 patients indicated a decreased prevalence of AD in patients taking lovastatin and pravastatin.[117,118] In the Canadian Study of Health and Aging, use of statins and other lipid lowering drugs reduced the risk of AD in subjects younger than 80 years, but there was no significant effect in subjects 80 years and older.[119] A pilot study enrolling 63 individuals with normal cholesterol levels and mild to moderate AD found preliminary evidence for some benefit with atorvastatin.[120] There was a difference in the ADAS-cog at the end of one year, and a suggestion that treated individuals had a change in the slope of their cognitive decline over that time. While intriguing, these results have not gone unchallenged,[121] and a large phase two trial of atorvastatin is currently underway for the treatment of AD. Clearly, the same logic in using statins applies to the MCI population. A large scale prevention trial of statins in MCI is warranted and necessary to establish whether these medications can prevent progression to AD.

Anti-amyloid therapies

As noted above, amyloid is considered the most critical part of the pathophysiological cascade of AD. Reduction of A-beta production is theoretically possible through inhibition of two critical enzymes with a role in the cleavage of toxic A-beta fragments and its deposition in the form of plaques. Gamma-secretase inhibitors have been synthesized and are entering clinical testing.[122,123] An APP-specific beta secretase (BACE stands for beta-site APP cleaving enzyme) could be another possible target for anti amyloid AD drugs.[124]

Prevention of amyloid deposition using inhibitors of A-beta aggregation such as GAG-mimetics (Alzhemed, from Neurochem Inc) represents another approach.[125] Alzhemed binds to soluble amyloid-beta (Aβ) protein to prevent and stop the formation and the deposition of amyloid fibrils in the brain, and to reduce the amyloid-induced toxicity on neuronal and brain inflammatory cells associated with amyloid build-up in AD. In a phase two study, 19 mild-to-moderate AD patients received study medication for 20 months, and less decline was noted in the treated group. Approximately 70 per cent of the mild AD patients had stabilized or improved cognitive function tests even after 20 months of enrolment in the Alzhemed open-label phase II extension study.[126] Currently two phase three RCTs of Alzhemed are underway in mild-to-moderate AD. In theory, such an approach should be even more effective at the amnestic MCI level.

Immunotherapy against amyloid has been pursued in the treatment of AD, and could potentially be effective in MCI to prevent progression to AD.[127,128] The unexpected occurrence of meningoencephalitis in a small group of AD patients treated in a phase two trial with active immunization against amyloid beta protein has slowed this approach to therapy. There is still considerable hope, however, that treating amyloid protein deposition via passive immunotherapy using monoclonal antibodies may eventually halt and even prevent the disease.[129]

In the future, there is also the possibility for development of interventions to prevent tau hyperphosphorylation. These have not yet reached the stage of clinical trials. It is hard at the present time to predict when these treatments will reach RCT, nor how effective they will be.[130] One hopes that an effective and safe medication that directly blocks deposition and formation of amyloid protein and tau hyperphosphorylation will be found. This might become the ideal prevention treatment to initiate at the MCI stage.

Therapy for vascular risk factors

As noted above in the section on causation, it is clear that vascular damage impacts on the occurrence of AD and mixed dementia. Risks for vascular disease (diabetes, hypertension, smoking, obesity, hyperlipidaemia) are increasingly being proven to be risk factors for development of dementia. In the Rotterdam Study in the Netherlands, individuals with diabetes had nearly double the risk of dementia,[131] and this finding has been replicated and extended to prediabetes subjects.[59] Presumably the microvascular damage from diabetes is the culprit, although it is possible that higher than normal levels of glucose in the blood might be toxic. The Framingham Heart Study demonstrated an impact of hypertension on cognition 6 years later.[132] The Cardiovascular Health Study showed that cognitive decline occurred even without frank stroke in individuals with vascular risk factors.[133]

These data give us important additional approaches to therapy of MCI, namely aggressively treating vascular risk factors. Note that this therapy is unproven in the sense that no one has yet mounted a long term study that proves that intervention at the MCI stage will be effective in reducing or preventing occurrence of dementia or AD. However, treating these risks makes sense in their own right – a patient with uncontrolled hypertension should be treated anytime. Thus, in recommendations to family physicians, those working to prevent AD are now giving strong advice to 'do what you already do' – namely aggressively treat any risk factors for vascular disease in a patient with MCI.

The risk of dementia thus represents an additional reason to treat the patient.

The MCI diet

Given the factors identified above, it is interesting to note that dietary and nutritional interventions are possible in the treatment of MCI/prevention of dementia. A healthy diet helps prevent hypertension (via reduced saturated fats and sodium), prediabetes (reduce sweets and caloric intake and consume more fibre) and stroke (dietary change to reduce cholesterol). Obesity is to be avoided by dietary limitation and exercise. One study from Chicago reported a higher risk of AD in seniors who ate more saturated and trans fat and less unsaturated fat,[134] but another study did not find a link. Homocysteine levels (high or even normal) can in theory be reduced by a good intake of folic acid, B_6 and B_{12} found in green leafy vegetables. Several multivitamins a day will also supply these amounts. There is evidence that an individual whose diet is high in omega-3 fatty acids, especially DHA, has a 50 per cent reduction in their risk of developing dementia.[85,102] About 180 mg of DHA daily intake is suggested, and this amount can be achieved by eating cold water fatty fish such as salmon, sardines, mackerel and bluefish, about three times a week. Some doctors are now recommending that MCI patients eat such fish (or take two 200 mg DHA capsules) three times weekly.[85,103] Thus there is a theoretical basis for considerable dietary manipulation in MCI, none yet supported by RCTs.

SUMMARY OF THE MANAGEMENT OF MCI AND VERY EARLY AD

Given the lack of clear prognostic markers, the heterogeneity in the natural history of MCI individuals and the lack of proven therapies to prevent decline, the management of MCI patients remains largely non-specific. Education is important – the fact is that some MCI individuals will go on to AD/dementia and patients should be advised that this risk exists. The strongest evidence supports suggestions to 'maintain a healthy lifestyle' with adequate exercise, avoidance of obesity, mental and physical stimulation, control of stress, treatment of medical illnesses and depression and control of vascular risk factors such as diabetes, hypertension and hypercholesterolaemia.

Currently we lack proven pharmacological approaches to prevent cognitive decline or progression from MCI to dementia. Nevertheless, there are therapeutic interventions that the clinician can consider applying. With our increasing appreciation of the degree to which vascular factors interact with AD in symptom onset, it makes good sense to aggressively treat vascular risk factors in MCI individuals using lifestyle interventions and diet, but also medications when necessary. Pharmacological treatment of depression is also indicated when appropriate (see Chapter 13). Drugs with known anticholinergic activity, as well as sleeping pills and sedatives, should be avoided.

Physicians should inform patients that there is no current treatment for MCI sufficiently established to have obtained regulatory approval. Treating MCI individuals (or the healthy elderly) in order to prevent subsequent AD using CIs, anti-inflammatories, oestrogen, statins, various antioxidants or even vitamin E represents prescription beyond proven therapies. It is advisable to refer the eager MCI patient to a research clinic where RCTs of these and other preventative medications are currently underway. Only when the results of MCI drug studies begin to reach the literature will we be in a position to make informed scientific recommendations for such therapies (alone or in combination) for the benefit of our patients.

The ADCS/NIA donepezil study raises significant therapeutic issues. Since there was a delay in progression to AD in MCI individuals with a positive apoE4, then perhaps 'a discussion of therapy' with donepezil is warranted. But what discussion? Should MCI patients be offered genetic testing with apoE prior to a therapy decision? Should donepezil be offered with the hope that the symptomatic benefit will make up for our uncertainty regarding its long term prevention role? Should its role in MCI (and the role of CIs in general) be downplayed as a major part of our therapeutic armamentarium, rather than using them up at the MCI stage?

In the author's clinic, the dietary possibilities noted in the previous section are being exploited as a way to maximize the potential beneficial effects of antioxidants and omega fatty acids, and to control homocysteine levels. Our patients are generally encouraged to take one or two multivitamins daily, which deliver adequate doses of vitamin E (400 IU), along with B_6 and folate supplementation. Furthermore, vascular risk factors are aggressively treated. Other therapies remain in the realm of current research and future possibilities.

ACKNOWLEDGEMENTS

This work was supported by a Chercheur-national award from the Fonds de la Recherche en Santé du Québec (FRSQ) to H. Chertkow, and funding from the CIHR (Canadian Institutes for Health Research).

REFERENCES

1. Reiman EM, Caselli RJ, Yun LS, et al. Preclinical evidence of Alzheimer's disease in persons homozygous for the epsilon 4 allele for apolipoprotein E. N Engl J Med 1996; 334: 752–758.
2. Petersen RC. Mild cognitive impairment: transition between aging and Alzheimer's disease. Neurologia 2000; 15:93–101.
3. Petersen RC, Stevens JC, Ganguli M, Tangalos EG, Cummings JL, DeKosky ST. Practice parameter: early detection of dementia: mild cognitive impairment (an evidence-based review). Report of the Quality Standards Subcommittee of the American Academy of Neurology. Neurology 2001; 56:1133–1142.
4. Winblad B, Palmer K, Kivipelto M, et al. Mild cognitive impairment – beyond controversies, towards a consensus: report of the International Working Group on Mild Cognitive Impairment. J Intern Med 2004; 256:240–246.
5. Petersen RC, Smith GE, Ivnik RJ, et al. Apolipoprotein E status as a predictor of the development of Alzheimer's disease in memory-impaired individuals [published erratum appears in JAMA 1995; 274:538]. JAMA 1995; 273:1274–1278.
6. Chertkow H. Mild Cognitive Impairment. Curr Opin Neurol 2002; 15:401–407.
7. Ganguli M, Dodge HH, Shen C, DeKosky ST. Mild cognitive impairment, amnestic type: an epidemiologic study. Neurology 2004; 63:115–121.
8. Petersen RC, Thomas RG, Grundman M, et al. Vitamin E and donepezil for the treatment of mild cognitive impairment. N Engl J Med 2005; 352:2379–2388.
9. Morris JC, Price AL. Pathologic correlates of nondemented aging, mild cognitive impairment, and early-stage Alzheimer's disease. J Mol Neurosci 2001; 17:101–118.
10. Morris JC, Storandt M, Miller JP, et al. Mild cognitive impairment represents early-stage Alzheimer disease. Arch Neurol 2001; 58:397–405.
11. Bocti C, Whitehead V, Fellow L, Chertkow H. Characteristics of patients with Mild Cognitive Impairment who do not progress to dementia. Neurology 2005; 64:A365.
12. Ritchie K. Mild cognitive impairment: an epidemiological perspective. Dialogues Clin Neurosci 2004; 6:401–408.
13. Folstein MF, Folstein SE, McHugh PR. 'Mini-mental state'. A practical method for grading the cognitive state of patients for the clinician. J Psychratr Res 1975; 12:189–198.
14. McDowell I, Hill G, Lindsay J, et al. Canadian Study of Health and Aging – study methods and prevalence of dementia. CMAJ 1994; 150:899–913.
15. Nasreddine ZS, Phillips NA, Bedrrian V, et al. The Montreal Cognitive Assessment, MoCA: a brief screening tool for mild cognitive impairment. J Am Geriatr Soc 2005; 53: 695–699.
16. Freter S, Bergman H, Gold S, Chertkow H, Clarfield AM. Prevalence of potentially reversible dementias and actual reversibility in a memory clinic cohort. Can Med Assoc J 1998; 159:657–662.
17. Bliwise DL. Is sleep apnea a cause of reversible dementia in old age? J Am Geriatr Soc 1996; 44:1407–1409.
18. Wahlund LO. Biological markers and diagnostic investigations in Alzheimer's disease. Acta Neurol Scand Suppl 1996; 165:85–91.
19. Mosconi L, Perani D, Sorbi S, et al. MCI conversion to dementia and the APO-E genotype: a prediction study with FDG-PET. Neurology 2004; 63:2332–2340.
20. Anon. Practice parameter for diagnosis and evaluation of dementia (summary statement). Neurology 1994; 44: 2203–2206.
21. Knopman D, DeKosky S, Cummings JL, et al. Practice parameter: diagnosis of dementia (an evidence-based review). Report of the Quality Standards Subcommittee of the American Academy of Neurology. Neurology 2001; 56:1143–1153.
22. Jack CR Jr, Petersen RC, Xu Y, et al. Medial temporal atrophy on MRI in normal aging and very mild Alzheimer's disease. Neurology 1997; 49:786–794.
23. Jack CR Jr, Petersen RC, Xu Y, et al. Rates of hippocampal atrophy correlate with change in clinical status in aging and AD. Neurology 2000; 55:484–489.
24. Daly E, Zaitchik D, Copeland M, Schmahmann J, Gunther J, Albert M. Predicting conversion to Alzheimer disease using standardized clinical information. Arch Neurology 2000; 57:675–680.
25. Ritchie K, Artero S, Touchon J. Classification criteria for mild cognitive impairment: a population-based validation study. Neurology 2001; 56:37–42.
26. Rose SP. 'Smart drugs': do they work? Are they ethical? Will they be legal? Nat Rev Neurosci 2002; 3:975–979.
27. Farah MJ, Illes J, Cook-Deegan R, et al. Neurocognitive enhancement: what can we do and what should we do? Nat Rev Neurosci 2004; 5:421–425.
28. Lantot KL, Herrmann N, Yau KK, et al. Efficacy and safety of cholinesterase inhibitors in Alzheimer's disease: a meta-analysis. CMAJ 2003; 169:557–564.
29. Patterson C, Gauthier S, Bergman H, et al. The recognition, assessment and management of dementing disorders: conclusions from the Canadian Consensus Conference on Dementia. Can Med Assoc J 1999; 160(suppl 12):S1–S15.
30. Reisberg B, Doody R, Stoffler A, et al. Memantine in moderate-to-severe Alzheimer's disease. N Engl J Med 2003; 348:1333–1341.
31. Burns A, Whitehouse P, Arendt T, Forsti H. Alzheimer's disease in senile dementia: loss of neurones in the basal forebrain. Science 1982; 215:1237–1239.
32. Davis KL, Mohs RC, Yarin D. Cholinergic markers in elderly patients with early signs of Alzheimer disease [see comments]. JAMA 1999; 281:1401–1406.
33. DeKosky ST, Ikonomovic M, Styrem SD, et al. Cholinergic upregulation in hippocampus in mild cognitive impairment. Relation to Alzheimer neuropathology. Neurology 2002; 58: A239.
34. Terry AV Jr, Buccafusco JJ. The cholinergic hypothesis of age and Alzheimer's disease-related cognitive deficits: recent challenges and their implications for novel drug development. J Pharmacol Exp Ther 2003; 306:821–827.
35. Salloway S, Ferris S, Kluger A, et al. Efficacy of donepezil in mild cognitive impairment: a randomized placebo-controlled trial. Neurology 2004; 63:651–657.
36. McDaniel MA, Maier SF, Einstein GO. 'Brain-specific' nutrients: a memory cure? Nutrition 2003; 19:957–975.
37. Le Bars PL, Katz MM, Berman N, Itil TM, Freedman AM, Schatzberg AF. A placebo-controlled, double-blind, randomized trial of an extract of Ginkgo biloba for dementia. North American EGb Study Group. JAMA 1997; 278: 1327–1332.
38. van Dongen M, van Rossum E, Kessels A, Sielhorst H, Knipschild P. Ginkgo for elderly people with dementia and age-associated memory impairment: a randomized clinical trial. J Clin Epidemiol 2003; 56:367–376.
39. Vellas B, Andrieu S, Ousset PF, et al. A 5 year double blind, randomized trial on EGB 761 efficacy on the prevention of

Alzheimer's dementia in patients over 70 with memory complaint. Guidage study. (P-204). Alzheimer's Dementia J Alzheimer's Assoc 2005; 1:S73.

40. Riedel WJ, Jolles J. Cognition enhancers in age-related cognitive decline. Drugs Aging 1996; 8:245–274.

41. Crook TH, Tinklenberg J, Yesavage J, Petrie W, Nunzi MG, Mussari D. Effects of phosphatidylserine in age-associated memory impairment. Neurology 1991; 41:644–649.

42. Israel L, Melac M, Milinkevitch D, Dubos G. Drug therapy and memory training programs: a double-blind randomized trial of general practice patients with age-associated memory impairment. Int Psychogeriatr 1994; 6:155–170.

43. Fioravanti M, Bergamasco B, Bocola V, et al. A multi-centre, double-blind, controlled study of piracetam vs. placebo in geriatric patients with non-vascular mild-moderate impairment in cognition. New Trends Clin Neuropharmacol 1991; 5:27–34.

44. Montgomery SA, Thal LJ, Amrein R. Meta-analysis of double blind randomized controlled clinical trials of acetyl-L-carnitine versus placebo in the treatment of mild cognitive impairment and mild Alzheimer's disease. Int Clin Psychopharmacol 2003; 18:61–71.

45. Tully T, Bourtchouladze R, Scott R, Tallman J. Targeting the CREB pathway for memory enhancers. Nat Rev Drug Discov 2003; 2:267–277.

46. Squire LR, Kandal ER. Memory: from Mind to Molecules. New York: W.H. Freeman & Co. 1999.

47. Johnson SA, Simmon VF. Randomized, double-blind, placebo-controlled international clinical trial of the Ampakine CX516 in elderly participants with mild cognitive impairment: a progress report. J Mol Neurosci 2002; 19: 197–200.

48. Lynch, G. Memory enhancement: the search for mechanism-based drugs. Nat Neurosci 1999; 5(suppl):1035–1038.

49. Thal LJ. Trials to slow progression and prevent disease onset. J Neural Transm Suppl 2000; 59:243–249.

50. Wimo A, Jonsson B, Karlsson G, Winblad B. Health Economics of Dementia. Chichester: John Wiley and Sons 1998.

51. Wimo A, Winblad B. Pharmacoeconomics of mild cognitive impairment. Acta Neurol Scand Suppl 2003; 179:94–99.

52. Grundman M, Thal L. Clinical Trials to Prevent Alzheimer's Disease in a Population At-Risk in Becker R, Giacobini E (eds). Alzheimer Disease: From Molecular Biology to Therapy. Boston, Birkhauser Verglas. 1996; 375–379.

53. Thal LJ. Therapeutics and mild cognitive impairment: current status and future directions. Alzheimer Dis Assoc Disord 2003; 17(suppl 2):S69–S71.

54. Fillit H. Future therapeutic developments of estrogen use. J Clin Pharmacol 1995; 35(9 suppl):25S–28S.

55. Yaffe K, Sawaya G, Lieberburg I, Grady D. Estrogen therapy in postmenopausal women: effects on cognitive function and dementia. JAMA 1998; 279:688–695.

56. Sherwin BB. Can estrogen keep you smart? Evidence from clinical studies. J Psychiatry Neurosci 1999; 24:315–321.

57. Fratiglioni L, Wang H, Winblad B, et al. Life-course psychosocial factors in relation to dementia in late life (S2-02-02). Alzheimer's Dementia J Alzheimer's Assoc 2005; 1:S93.

58. Stern Y. Lifestyle and other risk factors: cognitive reserve (S2-02-03). Alzheimer's Dementia J Alzheimer's Assoc 2005; 1:S93.

59. Yaffe K, Blackwell T, Kanaya AM, Davidowitz N, Barrett-Connor E, Krueger K. Diabetes, impaired fasting glucose, and development of cognitive impairment in older women. Neurology 2004; 63:658–663.

60. Yaffe K, Kanaya A, Lindquist K, et al. The metabolic syndrome, inflammation, and risk of cognitive decline. JAMA 2004; 292:2237–2242.

61. Laurin D, Verreault R, Lindsay J, MacPherson K, Rockwood K. Physical activity and risk of cognitive impairment and dementia in elderly persons. Arch Neurol 2001; 58:498–504.

62. Scarmeas N, Levy G, Tang M, Stern Y. Influence of leisure activity on the incidence of Alzheimer's disease. Neurology 2002; 57:2236–2242.

63. Wilson R, Bennet D. Participation in cognitively stimulating activities and risk of incident Alzheimer disease. JAMA 202; 287:742–748.

64. Friedman D, Moore M, Quinn J, Howieson D, Kaye J. Use it or lose it: a prospective evaluation of intellectual activity and the development of dementia. Neurology 2002; 58(suppl 3): A103.

65. Sapolsky R, Krey L, McEwen BS. The neuroendocrinology of stress and aging: the glucocorticoid cascade hypothesis. Endocrinol Review 1986; 7:284–301.

66. Issa AM, Rowe W, Gauthier S, Meaney MJ. Hypothalamic–pituitary–adrenal activity in aged, cognitively impaired and cognitively unimpaired rats. J Neurosci 1990; 10:3247–3254.

67. Lupien SJ, Nair NP, Briere S, et al. Increased cortisol levels and impaired cognition in human aging: implication for depression and dementia in later life. Rev Neurosci 1999; 10: 117–139.

68. Wilson RS, Evans DA, Bienias JL, Mendes de Leon CF, Schneider JA, Bennett DA. Proneness to psychological distress is associated with risk of Alzheimer's disease. Neurology 2003; 61:1479–1485.

69. Riemann D, Hohagen F, Bahro M, et al. Cholinergic neurotransmission, REM sleep and depression. J Psychosom Res 1994; 38(suppl 1):15–25.

70. Boeve BF, Silber MH, Ferman TJ, Lucas JA, Parisi JE. Association of REM sleep behavior disorder and neurodegenerative disease may reflect an underlying synucleinopathy. Movement Disorders 2001; 16:622–630.

71. Forette F, Seux ML, Staessen JA, et al. Prevention of dementia in randomised double-blind placebo-controlled Systolic Hypertension in Europe (Syst-Eur) trial. Lancet 1998; 352:1347–1351.

72. Launer LJ, Ross GW, Petrovitch H, et al. Midlife blood pressure and dementia: the Honolulu-Asia aging study. Neurobiol Aging 2000; 21:49–55.

73. Petrovitch H, White LR, Izmirihan G, et al. Midlife blood pressure and neuritic plaques, neurofibrillary tangles, and brain weight at death: the HAAS. Honolulu-Asia Aging Study. Neurobiol Aging 2000; 21:57–62.

74. Kivipelto M, Helkala EL, Hannrnen T, et al. Midlife vascular risk factors and late-life mild cognitive impairment: A population-based study. Neurology 2001; 56:1683–1689.

75. Lockwood K, Alexopoulos G, Kakuma T, Van Gorp W. Heterogeneity and comorbidity in dementia-depression syndromes [editorial]. Am J Geriatr Psychiatry 2000; 8: 201–208.

76. Coen RF, Kirby M, Swanwick GR, et al. Distinguishing between patients with depression or very mild Alzheimer's disease using the delayed-word-recall test. Dement Geriatr Cogn Disord 1997; 8:244–247.

77. Adler G, Bramesfeld A, Jajcevic A. Mild cognitive impairment in old-age depression is associated with increased EEG slow-wave power. Neuropsychobiology 1999; 40:218–222.

78. Reischies FM, Neu P. Comorbidity of mild cognitive disorder and depression – a neuropsychological analysis. Eur Arch Psychiatry Clin Neurosci 2000; 250:186–193.

79. Fratiglioni, L, Wang HX, Ericsson K, et al. Influence of

social network on occurrence of dementia: a community-based longitudinal study. Lancet 2000; 355:1315–1319.

80. Belleville S, Gilbert B, et al. Multifactorial cognitive training in patients with mild cognitive impairment. Proceedings of the Ninth Cognitive Aging Conference 2002: 4.

81. Rapp S, Brenes G, Marsh AP. Memory enhancement training for older adults with mild cognitive impairment: a preliminary study. Aging Ment Health 2002; 6:5–11.

82. Poon P, Hui E, Dai D, Kwok T, Woo J. Cognitive intervention for community-dwelling older persons with memory problems: telemedicine versus face-to-face treatment. Int J Geriatr Psychiatry 2005; 20:285–286.

83. Morris MC, Evans DA, Bienias JL, Tagney CC, Wilson RS. Vitamin E and cognitive decline in older persons. Arch Neurol 2002; 59:1125–1132.

84. Engelhart MJ, Geerling MI, Ruitenberg A, et al. Diet and risk of dementia: Does fat matter?: The Rotterdam Study. Neurology 2002; 59:1915–1921.

85. Fotuhi M, Zandi P, Hayden K, et al. Use of NSAIDs and antioxidant supplements in combination reduces the rate of cognitive decline: The Cache County Study 2002–2005. Alzheimer's Dementia J Alzheimer's Assoc 2005; 1:597–598.

86. Sano M, Ernesto C, Thomas RG, et al. A controlled trial of selegiline, alpha-tocopherol, or both as treatment for Alzheimer's disease. The Alzheimer's Disease Cooperative Study. N Engl J Med 1997; 336:1216–1222.

87. Miller ER 3rd, Pastor-Barriuso R, Dulal D, et al. Meta-analysis: high-dosage vitamin E supplementation may increase all-cause mortality. Ann Intern Med 2005; 142:37–46.

88. Hayden K, Zandi P, Wendgreen H, et al. Does vitamin E use protect against dementia or increase the risk of mortality? (02-02-04). Alzheimer's Dementia J Alzheimer's Assoc 2005; 1:595–596.

89. Markesbery WR. Oxidative stress hypothesis in Alzheimer's disease. Free Radic Biol Med 1997; 23:134–147.

90. Perry G, Nunomura A, Hirai K, et al. Is oxidative damage the fundamental pathogenic mechanism of Alzheimer's and other neurodegenerative diseases? Free Radic Biol Med 2002; 33:1475–1479.

91. Christen Y. Oxidative stress and Alzheimer disease. Am J Clin Nutr 2000; 71:621S–629S.

92. Keller JN, Schmitt FA, Scheff SW, et al. Evidence of increased oxidative damage in subjects with mild cognitive impairment. Neurology 2005; 64:1152–1156.

93. Perrig WJ, Perrig P, Stahelin HB. The relation between antioxidants and memory performance in the old and very old. J Am Geriatr Soc 1997; 45:718–724.

94. Foley DJ, White LR. Dietary intake of antioxidants and risk of Alzheimer disease: food for thought. JAMA 2002; 287:3261–3263.

95. Runyons CR, Schmitt FA, Caban-Holt A, et al. Antioxidants for the prevention of dementia: overview of the preadvise trial (P-208). Alzheimer's Dementia J Alzheimer's Assoc 2005; 1: S74.

96. Seshadri S, Beiser A, Selhub J, et al. Plasma homocysteine as a risk factor for dementia and Alzheimer's disease. N Engl J Med 2002; 346:476–483.

97. Miller JW, Green R, Mungus DM, et al. Homocysteine, vitamin B6, and vascular disease in AD patients. Neurology 2002; 58: 1471–1475.

98. McCaddon A, Davies G, Hudson P, Tandy S, Cutte UH. Homocysteine and cognitive decline in healthy elderly. Dement Geriatr Cogn Disord 2001; 12:309–313.

99. van Asselt DZ, Pasman JW, van Lier HJ, et al. Cobalamin supplementation improves cognitive and cerebral function in older, cobalamin-deficient persons. J Gerontol A Biol Sci Med Sci 2001; 56:M775–M779.

100. Hankey GJ. Is homocysteine a causal and treatable risk factor for vascular diseases of the brain (cognitive impairment and stroke)? [letter; comment]. Ann Neurol 2002; 51: 279–281.

101. Lehmann M, Regland B, Blennaw K, Guttfries CG. Vitamin B12–B6–folate treatment improves blood–brain barrier function in patients with hyperhomocysteinaemia and mild cognitive impairment. Dement Geriatr Cogn Disord 2003; 16:145–150.

102. Engelhart MJ, Geerlings MI, Ruitenberg A, et al. Dietary intake of antioxidants and risk of Alzheimer disease. JAMA 2002; 287:3223–3229.

103. Kalmijn S, Feskens EJ, Launer LJ, Kromhout D. Polyunsaturated fatty acids, antioxidants, and cognitive function in very old men. Am J Epidemiol 1997; 145: 33–41.

104. Feris S, Feldman H, Sfikas N, Macione L, Tekin S, Lane R. Time to clinical diagnosis of dementia in MCI subjects receiving rivastigmine: a randomized, double-blind, placebo-controlled study. Int Psychogeriatr 2005; 17: 242.

105. Scheltens P, Fox NC, Barkhof F, Gold M. Effect of galantamine treatment on brain atrophy as assessed by MRI patients with mild cognitive impairment. Neurobiol Aging 2004; 25:S270–S271.

106. Blacker D. Mild cognitive impairment – no benefit from vitamin E, little from donepezil. N Engl J Med 2005; 352: 2439–2441.

107. Zandi PP, Anthony JC, Hayden KM, Mehta K, Mayer L, Breitner JCS. Reduced incidence of AD with NSAID but not H2 receptor antagonists: The Cache County Study. Neurology 2002; 59:880–886.

108. Breitner JC, Zandi PP. Do nonsteroidal antiinflammatory drugs reduce the risk of Alzheimer's disease? N Engl J Med 2001; 345:1567–1568.

109. Breitner JC, Welsh KA, Helms MJ, et al. Delayed onset of Alzheimer's disease with nonsteroidal anti-inflammatory and histamine H2 blocking drugs. Neurobiol Aging 1995; 16:523–530.

110. Zandi PP, Breitner JC. Do NSAIDs prevent Alzheimer's disease? And, if so, why? The epidemiological evidence. Neurobiol Aging 2001; 22:811–817.

111. Etminan M, Gill S, Samii A. Effect of non-steroidal anti-inflammatory drugs on risk of Alzheimer's disease: systematic review and meta-analysis of observational studies. BMJ 2003; 327:128.

112. Aisen PS, Schafer KA, Grundman M, et al. Effects of rofe-coxib or naproxen vs placebo on Alzheimer disease progression: a randomized controlled trial. JAMA 2003; 289: 2819–2826.

113. Thal LJ, Ferris SH, Kirby L, et al. A randomized, double-blind, study of rofecoxib in patients with mild cognitive impairment. Neuropsychopharmacology 2005; 30: 1204–1215.

114. Hartmann T. Cholesterol, A beta and Alzheimer's disease. Trends Neurosci 2001; 24(11 suppl):S45–S48.

115. Yaffe K, Barrett-Connor E, Lin F, Grady D. Serum lipoprotein levels, statin use, and cognitive function in older women. Arch Neurol 2002; 59:378–384.

116. Das UN. Estrogen, statins, and polyunsaturated fatty acids: similarities in their actions and benefits – is there a common link? Nutrition 2002; 18:178–188.

117. Jick H, Zornberg GL, Jick SS, Seshadri S, Drachman DA.

Statins and the risk of dementia. Lancet 2000; 356: 1627–1631.

118. Wolozin B, Kellman W, Ruosseau P, Celesia GG, Siegel G. Decreased prevalence of Alzheimer disease associated with 3-hydroxy-3-methyglutaryl coenzyme A reductase inhibitors. Arch Neurol 2000; 57:1439–1443.

119. Rockwood K, Kirkland S, Hogan DB, et al. Use of lipid-lowering agents, indication bias, and the risk of dementia in community-dwelling elderly people. Arch Neurol 2002; 59:223–227.

120. Sparks DL, Sabbagh MN, Connor DJ, et al. Atorvastatin for the treatment of mild to moderate Alzheimer disease: preliminary results. Arch Neurol 2005; 62:753–757.

121. Hayden K, Zandi P, et al. Statin use does not reduce cognitive decline in the elderly. The cache county study. (O2-02-04). Alzheimer's Dementia J Alzheimer's Assoc 2005; 1:S97.

122. Moore CL, Leatherwood DD, Diehl TS, Selkoe DJ, Wolfe MS. Difluoro ketone peptidomimetics suggest a large S1 pocket for Alzheimer's gamma-secretase: implications for inhibitor design. J Med Chem 2000; 43:3434–3442.

123. Holtzman D. Amyloid immunotherapy, extra-CNS actions (AM-04). Alzheimer's Dementia J Alzheimer's Assoc 2005; 1:S1.

124. Selkoe DJ. Alzheimer disease: mechanistic understanding predicts novel therapies. Ann Intern Med 2004; 140: 627–638.

125. Tremblay P, Aisen P, Graceuu D, et al. Functional GAG mimetics as an approach for the treatment of amyloid diseases (AM-06). Alzheimer's Dementia J Alzheimer's Assoc 2005; 1:S2.

126. Gervais F. Advances in Alzheimer Therapy: 2004: GAG-mimetics: Potential to modify underlying disease process in AD. 8th International Montreal/Springfield Symposium on Advances in Alzheimer Therapy: Montreal, Canada 2004.

127. Schenk D, Barbour R, Dunn W, et al. Immunization with amyloid-beta attenuates Alzheimer-disease-like pathology in the PDAPP mouse [see comments]. Nature 1999; 400: 173–177.

128. Schenk D. Amyloid-beta immunotherapy for Alzheimer's disease: the end of the beginning. Nat Rev Neurosci 2002; 3:824–828.

129. Schenk D. Advances in Alzheimer Therapy. Advances in A-beta immunotherapy for potential treatment of AD. Eighth International Montreal/Springfield Symposium on Advances in Alzheimer Therapy. Montreal, Canada 2004.

130. Iqbal K. Advances in Alzheimer Therapy Pharmacological approaches of neurofibrillary degeneration. 8th International Montreal/Springfield Symposium on Advances in Alzheimer Therapy. Montreal, Canada 2004.

131. Ott A, Stolk RP, van Harskamp F, Pols HA, Hofman A, Breteler MM. Diabetes mellitus and the risk of dementia: The Rotterdam Study. Neurology 1999; 53:1937–1942.

132. Elias MF, Elias PK, Sullivan LM, Wolf PA, D'Agostino RB. Lower cognitive function in the presence of obesity and hypertension: the Framingham heart study. Int J Obes Relat Metab Disord 2003; 27:260–268.

133. Elkins JS, O'Meera ES, Longstreth WT Jr, Carlson MC, Manolio TA, Johnston SC. Stroke risk factors and loss of high cognitive function. Neurology 2004; 63:793–799.

134. Morris MC, Evans DA, Bienias JL, et al. Dietary fats and the risk of incident Alzheimer disease. Arch Neurol 2003; 60:194–200.

18

Mild to moderate stages

Michael Woodward and Howard Feldman

OVERVIEW

Mild to moderate Alzheimer's disease (AD) is that disease stage where cognitive, functional and increasingly the behavioural symptoms affect everyday life. By this stage the diagnosis can generally be made clinically with considerable confidence. Although biological markers that are in development may help diagnostically in the future, they still have not found their way into routine clinical practice. At this point in the disease continuum, approved AD therapies allow a standard of care for all patients and should be offered to those who have not yet been treated. Many patients will indeed not yet have been commenced on therapy as their clinician has been awaiting a more certain diagnosis.

People with mild to moderate AD are a more homogeneous group than those with mild cognitive impairment, due to greater diagnostic accuracy. The results of therapeutic research in this group can be applied with more certainty.

AIMS OF THERAPY

Symptomatic therapy is directed at both the patient's target symptoms as well as at more general symptoms of the disease. These include cognitive, functional and behavioural symptoms as well as caregiver burden. Effective symptomatic therapy will initially either improve these features or delay their emergence and progression. As AD is a progressive neurodegenerative illness, it cannot be expected that effective symptomatic therapy will continue to control the target features indefinitely, but such therapy may attenuate decline in some domains for up to several years. In the cognitive domain, effective symptomatic therapy might initially improve memory then delay the progression of memory decline for several years. More generally, effec-tive symptomatic therapy at some level should improve the quality of life of the patient and caregiver, and allow a longer time in the community with less reliance on support services and less likelihood of requiring full time residential care.

Currently the only treatments approved by regulatory authorities are those directed at symptoms, however the most effective therapy would be disease modifying or even disease eradicating. These therapies could potentially completely eradicate target symptoms and prevent new features of the disease from developing. Such disease modifying therapies can generally be expected to target the pathological processes underlying the features of AD, including amyloid or tau deposition. Whilst a considerable research effort is being made to develop such therapies, none is currently clinically available.

CHOLINERGIC THERAPY

There is a cholinergic deficit in AD, that is reflected in decreased choline acetyltransferase in the cortex and basal forebrain.[1,2] This cholinergic deficit has been correlated with the clinical manifestation of the disease including cognitive deficits[3] and neuropsychiatric symptoms.[4]

A wide range of cholinomimetic approaches has been tried, however efficacy has only been conclusively demonstrated for the cholinesterase inhibitors (CIs). Drugs in this class that are currently licensed in most countries include donepezil, galantamine and rivastigmine. Other cholinergic therapies for which there is only some preliminary evidence of efficacy include muscarinic agents[5] and phenserine.[6] The activity of these cholinergic agents is shown in Figure 18.1.

These agents increase cholinergic synaptic neurotransmission, however they differ in their mechanism of action, as illustrated in Table 18.1. For the CIs these

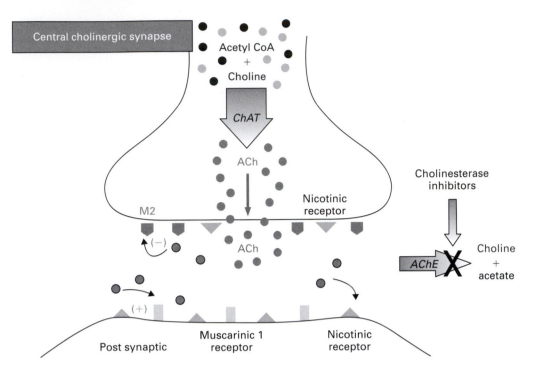

Figure 18.1 Central cholinergic synapse

Table 18.1 Pharmacology of cholinesterase inhibitors			
Property	**Cholinesterase inhibitor**		
	Donepezil	**Rivastigmine**	**Galantamine**
Inhibitor type	Reversible	Mixed pseudoirreversible	Reversible, competitive
Selectivity	AChE >> BuChE	AChE = BuChE	AChE < BuChE
Plasma half life	70 h	1–2 h	6 h
Dosage	Once daily	Twice daily/once daily patch expected soon	Twice daily/once daily (prolonged release formulation)
Dosage strength	5 mg, 10 mg	1.5 mg, 3 mg, 4.5 mg, 6 mg	4 mg, 8 mg, 12 mg (standard); 8 mg, 16 mg, 24 mg (prolonged release)
Plasma protein binding	High (95%)	Low (40%)	Minimal
Metabolism by cytochrome P450 (CYP) system	Yes (CYP2D6 and CYP3A4)	Minimal	Yes (CYP2D6 and CYP3A4)
Potential for drug interactions	Yes	Low	Moderate
Excretion	Urine/faeces	Urine	Urine

AChE = acetylcholinesterase; BuChE = butyrylcholinesterase

differences may be expected to influence efficacy and tolerability. Some individuals who fail to tolerate one agent may tolerate another. However, in mild-to-moderate AD, clinical trials have not shown any substantial differences in efficacy between agents.[7–9]

Donepezil is a second-generation reversible CI given once daily at either 5 or 10 mg. It exhibits high selectivity for neuronal AChE as opposed to BuChE.[10] Both doses have been shown to be effective in trials in mild-to-moderate AD, but greater efficacy has been associated with 10 mg. The dose should be increased no more frequently than 4-weekly, to reduce side effects.

Rivastigmine is a slowly-reversible (pseudoirreversible) CI that targets both AChE and BuChE. There is some evidence that in severe AD, BuChE becomes a more predominant pathway for acetylcholine breakdown, so inhibiting this enzyme may boost acetylcholine levels proportionally more in severe AD.[11] Rivastigmine appears to show brain region selectivity for the areas most affected by AD pathology.[12] It is given as two divided doses, daily doses ranging from 3 to 12 mg, with slow titration upwards (4 weeks between dose increases) recommended to reduce adverse effects. Doses of 6, 9 and 12 mg daily have shown efficacy in trials in mild-to-moderate AD. A once-daily rivastigmine patch is under development and, if approved, will increase the convenience of administration.

Galantamine is a specific, competitive and reversible CI that is also an allosteric modulator at nicotinic receptors. This additional mechanism may provide additional cholinergic effects beyond that of the drug's relatively weak inhibition of AChE.[13] It is administered at a starting dose of 8 mg a day with slow titration upwards (4 weeks between dose increases) recommended to reduce adverse effects. An increasing number of countries have a once daily prolonged-release preparation available, otherwise it is given as two divided daily doses. The starting dose of 8 mg a day has not shown efficacy in trials in mild to moderate AD, whereas 16 and 24 mg daily have been proven effective. Doses of 32 mg daily have been associated with a significantly increased risk of adverse effects and are not recommended.

Adverse effects of CIs are predominantly gastrointestinal and associated with their peripheral and central cholinergic activity. These include nausea, anorexia, weight loss, dyspepsia and diarrhoea. With slow titration, the prevalence of these effects is around 20 per cent[14] and is dose-related. Other adverse effects occuring less commonly include bradycardia and syncope, exacerbation of asthma or peptic ulcer disease. Adverse effects occur mainly at initiation or dose increases and frequently resolve or become less severe with time. In a meta-analysis of 14 studies compared with those receiving placebo, significantly more subjects receiving CI treatment had adverse events (8 per cent), dropped out (8 per cent) and dropped out because of adverse events (7 per cent).[7] Adverse events can be attenuated by less frequent dose increases and may not recur with a switch to a different CI.[15]

As would be expected of effective symptomatic therapy, CIs can improve the cognitive, behavioural, functional and global effects of AD in some patients. They have been subject to numerous meta-analyses and reviews,[7,8] which have generally supported their effectiveness and role in the management of mild-to-moderate AD, though in the recent past there has been some controversy on their efficacy (see below). Most trials have been of 6 months' duration, but two randomised, placebo-controlled 12-month trials have also shown benefits.[16,17] The primary endpoints in these trials are usually a measure of cognition, the Alzheimer's Disease Assessment Scale Cognitive Subscale (ADAS-cog), as well as a global independent clinician-rated assessment, the Clinicians' Interview Based Impression of Change (CIBIC). Whilst these endpoints usually show a statistically significant change, the clinical significance of this change can be more difficult to evaluate. Other (usually secondary) endpoints in these trials include functional and behavioural measures such as the Disability Assessment in Dementia (DAD) scale and the Neuropsychiatric Inventory (NPI).

The cognitive effects of CIs are exemplified by the effects of galantamine, with a mean 6-month improvement in the 70-point ADAS-cog scale of 3.8 points compared to placebo.[18] Similar effects are found with donepezil[19] and rivastigmine.[20] It is generally agreed that a 4-point improvement on the ADAS-cog is clinically apparent. This cognitive improvement is associated with a mean 6- to 12-month period before cognition deteriorates back to baseline – i.e. back to how it was before treatment was commenced (Figure 18.2). Some patients, however, may have a more sustained benefit.

The cognitive benefits of CIs are generally dose-related. The recommended starting dose of 5 mg a day for donepezil can be associated with a clinically significant cognitive benefit, whereas rivastigmine must be titrated up to 6 mg daily (as 3 mg bid) and galantamine up to 16 mg daily (as 8 mg bid or 16 qd). For each agent, doses higher than the minimum effective dose are available, but may be associated with an increased risk of adverse effects. It is, however, recommended that these higher doses be used (e.g. daily doses of 10 mg donepezil, 9 mg rivastigmine and 24 mg galantamine) if there is an inadequate cognitive response. A

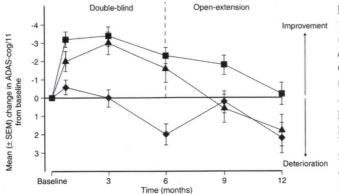

Figure 18.2 Mean change from baseline in 11-item AD Assessment Scale cognitive subscale (ADAS-cog/11) scores over 12 months (observed cases analysis). Black small square = Galantamine 24 mg/galantamine 24 mg; black up pointing small triangle = galantamine 32 mg/galantamine 24 mg; white diamond suit = placebo/galantamine 24 mg. (Reproduced with permission from Raskind MA, Peskind ER, Wessel T, Yuan W and the Galantamine USA-1 Study Group. A 6-month randomised, placebo-controlled trial with a 6-month extension, Neurology, 2000;54:2261–2268)[18]

dose–response relationship has, however, not been consistently demonstrated for cognitive endpoints such as the ADAS-cog using galantamine.[21]

Functional benefits of CIs are highly regarded by caregivers, perhaps even more so than cognitive benefits, and are seen with each of the agents that are available. For instance, a secondary analysis of a 5-month, randomised, placebo-controlled trial with galantamine showed more improvement in an ADL scale (AD Cooperative Study ADL Inventory – ADCS/ADL) with galantamine treatment than with placebo, with the greatest differences occurring in patients with more severe disease. The month five scores favoured galantamine over placebo in three of six basic ADLs and six of 17 instrumental ADLs.[22] Unlike cognition, function is more likely to be maintained rather than improved with CI therapy.

CIs have demonstrated some efficacy in the treatment of neuropsychiatric symptoms in patients with AD. A number of the pivotal trials utilised the NPI as a secondary endpoint. CI therapy generally reduced the emergence of new unwanted behavioural symptoms, and had an effect of attenuating some symptoms if already present. For instance, in a 21-week trial of galantamine, patients treated with 16 or 24 mg per day of this agent had no overall change in behaviour, whereas patients taking placebo had significantly worsened scores. These behavioural differences were associated with a concomitant reduction in reported caregiver distress.[23]

More recently, other trial designs have been used to demonstrate behavioural efficacy. In a randomised withdrawal study of patients selected for marked behavioural symptoms at baseline, withdrawing donepezil was associated with a marked deterioration in total NPI (22 versus 13 for those withdrawn, $p < 0.0001$). All domains of the NPI, with the exception of elation, were improved (all $p < 0.05$ after Bonferroni correction) in those who remained on donepezil.[24] The

behavioural benefits of CI therapy may be related to cholinergic deficits, which contribute to these disturbances.[25] Similarly, psychosis in AD has been associated with changes in cortical muscarinic cholinergic binding.[26]

In several studies caregiver burden, and time spent in caregiving, have been shown to be reduced by therapy with CIs. Pooled data from two concurrent, multicentre, randomised, double-blind, placebo-controlled, 6-month trials of galantamine, involving 825 patients, showed that caregivers of galantamine-treated patients were more likely to report reductions (41 per cent vs 37 per cent), maintenance (19 per cent vs 14 per cent) or smaller increases (26 per cent vs 34 per cent reporting an increase of above 30 minutes a day) in time assisting with daily activities compared with the placebo group ($p = 0.026$, Wilcoxon rank – sum test). The mean daily time difference was 32 minutes ($p = 0.011$). Significant differences were also reported in the time left unsupervised, favouring galantamine therapy over placebo.[27] Donepezil has also been associated with a reduced caregiver burden, as estimated by a self-administered survey of AD caregivers, although selection factors may influence results with this research design.[28]

In eight studies that included a clinical global assessment as the endpoint, the pooled mean proportion of global respondents to CI treatment in excess of that for placebo treatment, where this response was defined as 'improved' (but not 'unchanged'), was 9 per cent.[7] The numbers needed to treat for one additional patient to benefit were 7 for stabilization or better and 12 for minimal improvement or better. The absolute proportion demonstrating a global response (improved) is around 20–30 per cent.[29] These data reflect well the clinical experience with these medications – not all respond, but many do, and as a result they are regarded as a standard of care in published guidelines.[30]

The clinical trials of CIs have used standard psychometric tools which may not capture all clinically demonstrable beneficial treatment effects. A physician focus group, followed by a survey, identified a range of other potential beneficial treatment effects including attentional capacity, initiative, social interactions and involvement in domestic activities. Of the top ten symptomatic treatment effects, only four appeared to be readily identified by the usual trial endpoints.[31]

There has been one randomised prospective trial of a CI in mild, as opposed to mild-to-moderate, AD. This 24-week trial enrolled patients with only early-stage AD (MMSE 21–26 inclusive and diagnosis made within the last 12 months). Significant improvements favouring the agent used, donepezil, were found for the ADAS-cog (treatment difference, compared to placebo, of 2.3 points at endpoint, $p = 0.001$) and the MMSE (1.8 points difference at endpoint, $p = 0.002$).[32] A post-hoc analysis of galantamine data, confined to patients in trials in mild-to-moderate AD who had an MMSE of 21–24 inclusive, showed similar benefits. There was an ADAS-cog difference of 1.7 (treatment versus placebo, $p < 0.001$) as well as significantly more galantamine-treated patients showing improvement on the CIBIC compared with placebo-treated patients (26.9 per cent versus 14.3 per cent, $p = 0.001$).[33] These studies suggest significant treatment benefits of CI therapy in early-stage AD, and support the initiation of therapy early in the disease to improve functioning and cognition.

There have been two prospective, randomised trials over 12 months in mild-to-moderate AD – both with donepezil. One showed benefit, compared to placebo, in a global assessment scale,[17] and the other showed a 36 per cent reduction in the risk of functional decline in the donepezil-treated group.[16] Longer term data are also available, but these are analyses of extension trials where patients initially randomised to active therapy or placebo are then all treated with the active drug with neither patient nor clinician being blinded. These suffer from a number of biases including selective drop-out and survivor effects. Nevertheless, they do offer some evidence of sustained benefits of CI therapy. In a 36-month trial with galantamine, cognition decline on the ADAS-cog was 10.2 points, some 50 per cent below that predicted for a placebo group over the same period.[34] Similarly, an extension study of up to 98 weeks with donepezil showed an ADAS-cog decline of 6.6 points per year compared to a predicted 11 points per year in a placebo-treated group.[35] Also, a 2-year study with rivastigmine has shown sustained cognitive benefits in those remaining on active therapy.[36] In a meta-analysis of published longer term data of those on treatment for up to 5 years, sustained benefits

were found across a range of domains, including cognition.[37] These findings suggest that the benefits of CI therapy may continue beyond 6 to 12 months and provide a rationale for continuing therapy beyond this period.

GLUTAMATERGIC THERAPY

Abnormal and sustained increases in glutamate may produce central nervous system excitotoxic injury which may underlie some of the features of AD.[38] One class of glutamate receptors is the N-methyl-D-aspartate (NMDA) receptor family. Memantine is a low- to moderate-affinity uncompetitive antagonist of this receptor which has demonstrated efficacy in the treatment of AD. Most data have been for benefits in moderate to severe AD, but there is unpublished but recently presented evidence for reported efficacy and safety of memantine in mild-to-moderate AD. In a 24-week placebo-controlled trial of memantine 10 mg bid in 400 people with AD, those on active therapy improved on ADAS-cog by 0.8 points compared to a 1.1 point deterioration in the placebo group (Last Observation Carried Forward (LOCF) analysis, $p = 0.003$). In this trial the difference at 24 weeks between the placebo and the memantine-treated groups on CIBIC was 0.3 (placebo 4.5, memantine 4.2, $p = 0.004$ on an LOCF analysis). Behaviour also improved in the memantine-treated group, as measured by the NPI, but there was no difference in function, as measured by the ADCS-ADL.[39] In a similar 26-week trial in 470 people with AD, non-significant improvements in favour of memantine over placebo were seen in the ADAS-cog and the CIBIC. The differences were significant at 12 and 18 weeks (data from Forest Laboratories reviewed in a meta-analysis[40]).

There are several other classes of glutamate receptors including the amino-3-hydroxy-5-methyl-isoxazelopropionic (AMPA) receptor, and medications that interact with this receptor are being investigated.[41] Evidence of efficacy of these agents is still awaited.

DISEASE-MODIFYING THERAPIES

Cholinesterase inhibitors

An important aim of therapies for mild-to-moderate AD is slowing or reversing disease progression. There is only limited indirect evidence that CIs may have this effect. In an analysis of 135 matched pairs of patients, half of whom were taking CIs and half of whom were not, disease progression was defined using a number of parameters including Mini-Mental State Examination score change and an ADL scale. Some 81 (60 per cent) of the patients on CIs were considered slow progressers at 1-year follow-up, compared to 53 (39 per cent) of the patients who never used CIs.[42] However, this was not a fully prospectively randomised trial so the conclusions need to be regarded with some caution.

Immunotherapy

Perhaps the most exciting prospect in recent times for disease-modifying therapy for mild to moderate AD comes from the trials of immunisation against amyloid. It has been hypothesised that injecting the $A\beta$ peptide would incite an immune response that could remove amyloid from the brain of those with AD.[43] After success in animal models, this approach was tested in 300 patients. Unfortunately, this human trial was prematurely terminated in the face of a subacute meningoencephalitis in 18 patients (6 per cent of those treated).[44] One of the efficacy endpoints in the trial was MRI measures of cerebral volume and it was expected that immunotherapy would reduce the loss of brain volume seen longitudinally in AD. In fact, the opposite was seen, with an accelerated loss of brain volume in the immunised group who were classified clinically and by antibody response as responders.[45] The reason for this MRI result is uncertain, with some speculation that this resulted from the removal of amyloid plaques, or alternatively a reduction of glial and inflammatory response leaving a lower-volume 'purified' brain.[45] Of potentially greater concern, immunotherapy did not lead to any discernible improvement on the ADAS-cog, the other primary efficacy endpoint, although there was a suggestion that those who responded with anti-$A\beta$ antibodies did demonstrate a clinical benefit.[46] More encouragingly, an autopsy on one patient who died after $A\beta$ immunotherapy demonstrated an almost complete removal of amyloid plaques from her brain.[47]

Other immunotherapy approaches are being investigated. Intravenous immunoglobulins containing antibodies against amyloid show potentially beneficial effects.[48] Another approach is immunising with fragments of $A\beta$, which may avoid the encephalomeningitis.

Other amyloid-modifying therapies

Other approaches that may modify disease progression through modification of amyloid deposition in mild-to-moderate AD are shown in Table 18.2. Whilst

Table 18.2 Other potential amyloid modifying therapies

Therapeutic approach	Target
Gamma-secretase inhibitors	Reduction of Aβ-peptide production
Beta-secretase inhibitors	Reduction of Aβ-peptide production
Alpha-secretase promotion	Reduction of Aβ-peptide production
Anti-amyloid aggregants	Decrease aggregation of beta-amyloid

each of these approaches has promising preliminary evidential support, much more research is required before they enter clinical practice.

Non-steroidal anti-inflammatory drugs

The use of non-steroidal anti-inflammatory drugs (NSAIDs) has been associated with a lower risk of AD,[49,50] although this apparent benefit may relate to bias within the epidemiological association studies where it has been examined.[51] The putative benefits of NSAIDs may result from either their anti-inflammatory effect or their effect on amyloid processing. As laboratory evidence suggests that inflammatory mechanisms contribute to neuronal injury in AD,[52] NSAIDs might be predicted to be efficacious in the treatment of mild-to-moderate AD. This hypothesis has been tested with a range of anti-inflammatory drugs including prednisone, rofecoxib and naproxen in prospective randomised placebo-controlled trials which, to date, have all been negative.[53–55] NSAIDs cannot be recommended for the treatment of established AD at this time. They may yet, however, have a role in the prevention of AD, though it would be premature to recommend such treatment presently.

Hormone replacement therapy

Animal models have indicated that oestrogen can enhance cholinergic activity, improve neuronal survival and dendritic sprouting and protect neurones from ischaemia.[56] Epidemiological studies have suggested that users of hormone replacement therapy (HRT) are less likely to develop AD.[57–59] There may be a selection bias, with those less likely to ever develop AD being more likely to use HRT.[60] In turn, these data have been hypothesis-generating. Unfortunately, as with the NSAID epidemiological evidence, when this hypothesis was subject to prospective randomised controlled trials HRT has not provided evidence of efficacy in either preventing or treating AD. In the Women's Health Initiative, a prospective randomised trial, HRT was associated with a nearly double risk of developing dementia.[61] There have been a number of negative trials of oestrogens for the treatment of mild-to-moderate AD.[62] As with NSAIDs, HRT cannot be recommended as a therapy for mild-to-moderate AD at this time.

Cholesterol-lowering therapies

Cholesterol is an essential brain lipid fundamental to neuronal survival and brain repair mechanisms. There is evidence that it can influence β-amyloid production.[63] Epidemiological trials have demonstrated a potentially protective effect of statin use against the development of dementia,[64] however this is currently controversial. To date there have been a limited number of prospective randomised placebo-controlled trials in the treatment of mild-to-moderate AD. A study reported that there were benefits both in cognitive and global function with the use of atorvastatin over 12 months.[65] The need for additional confirmatory studies is identified before this can be adopted as a therapy for AD, although the treatment of vascular risk factors continues to be a long term general medical goal. Further trials are in progress, including a longer term study of atorvastatin versus placebo in those stabilised on 10 mg of donepezil. In summary, at the present time cholesterol-lowering drugs including statins cannot be recommended for the treatment of mild-to-moderate AD.

Antioxidant therapy

The generation of reactive oxygen species may increase the damage that deposition of Aβ exerts on the brain.[66] Antioxidants available as supplements or in foods include vitamins E and C, and their use may prevent these damaging reactions. Epidemiological studies have been mixed, with some suggesting a lower risk of AD in those with higher intakes of vitamin E and/or vitamin C,[67–69] and other studies showing no protective effect.[70] There has been a negative treatment trial of vitamin E in mild cognitive impairment,[71] while a study on vitamin E and selegeline in moderate-to-severe AD demonstrated efficacy at the delay on a number of prespecified outcome measures for each

therapy, but not for the combination of these therapies.[72] Some concerns have been raised recently about the potential toxicity of vitamin E. Higher doses of vitamin E, above 400 mg daily, have been shown in a meta-analysis to increase cardiovascular risk.[73] In consideration of the above, at this stage, antioxidant use cannot be recommended for the treatment of mild-to-moderate AD. If vitamin E supplements are used, the dose should be 400 mg or less daily.

OTHER DRUGS WITH POTENTIAL SYMPTOMATIC OR DISEASE-MODIFYING EFFECTS

There have been numerous trials of other medications as shown in Table 18.3, but to date none have demonstrated sufficient efficacy to enter into routine clinical practice. *Ginkgo biloba* may offer modest therapeutic efficacy, but less than the CIs. Its place in routine therapy for AD is not clear.[74] There are over 25 drugs currently being tested for AD and it is very possible that some may prove efficacious, but at this stage the only therapies with sufficient evidence remain the CIs and memantine.

PRACTICAL ISSUES IN MEDICAL MANAGEMENT OF MILD-TO-MODERATE AD

When to start therapy

Once AD has been diagnosed, CI therapy should be offered to patients without significant contraindications such as active peptic ulcer disease, asthma or significant bradyarrhythmias. These drugs have proven efficacy in mild-to-moderate AD and it is not appropriate to withhold them. In countries or regions where the drugs are not subsidised the cost may prevent a patient accepting them, but they should be offered.

Monitoring response

It is best first to agree on goals of therapy. These may be determined by regulatory authorities – for instance, in Australia, ongoing government subsidisation after the first 6 months is only provided if the score on the MMSE has improved by at least 2 points. Treatment goals should be developed through discussion framed around realistic expectations between patients, carers and doctors.[90] Progress on therapy should be monitored against these goals and if there is an insufficient

Table 18.3 Other drugs tested in the past or currently for Alzheimer's disease	
Drug	**Mechanism**
L-Deprenyl[75]	Monoaminergic neurotransmitter
l-α-glyceryl-phosphoryl choline[76]	Lecithin derivative
Piracetam[77]	Nootropic
Aniracetam[78]	Nootropic
Dihydro-ergotoxine mesylate[79]	Ergot
Nicergoline[80]	Ergot
D-Cycloserine[81]	Glycine agonist
Acetyl-L-carnitine[82]	Enhances mitochondrial energy production
Idebenone[83]	Unknown – may reduce ischaemic nerve cell damage.
Insulin[84]	Stimulates insulin brain receptors, GSK stimulant
Lu 25-109[85]	Muscarinic agent
Cerebrolysin[86]	Neurotrophic
Roziglitasone[87]	Peroxisome proliferator activated receptor (PPAR) agonist
Dehydroepiandrosterone (DHEA)[88]	Unknown – adrenal and gonadal steroid; deficiencies associated with ageing processes
Doxycycline/rifampicin[89]	Antibiotics against *Chlamydia pneumoniae*

Table 18.4 Options if insufficient response to therapy with CIs

- Increase of dose of CI
- Switch to another CI
- Add memantine
- Consider participation in a research trial
- Cease therapy

the CI, especially if others have been tried and not tolerated or also found to be ineffective.

Predictors and modifiers of response to CIs

A number of factors may predict response to CI therapy. Neuropsychological testing in combination with neuroimaging findings was found to predict 60 per cent of good responders in a Scottish study,[92] but this requires further validation. Those already established on antihypertensive therapy may respond better to CIs.[93] The presence of vascular disease has not shown a consistent effect on response to CI therapy.[94] Cigarette smoking seems to attenuate response to a CI.[95]

Concurrent use of anticholinergic drugs may reduce response to a CI, and such co-administration is not uncommon.[96] Wherever possible, drugs with anticholinergic effects should be stopped in patients with all forms of dementia. Those with a more rapid rate of AD progression may respond better to a CI.[97] The apolipoprotein E (apoE) and BuChE genotypes may affect response to a CI, although results from trials have varied[98–100] and at this stage genotyping cannot be recommended solely to predict response.

Managing disease progression

In the absence of timely disease-modifying therapies, AD will inevitably progress. Whilst the therapeutic approaches outlined in Table 18.4 can be considered, it is important that caregivers and patients have realistic expectations and understand that progression is inevitable. Alzheimer's Associations and other organisations can provide appropriate information and counselling as needed.

A sudden decline is unusual in AD and may be due to an intercurrent medical condition such as infection, electrolyte and fluid disturbances, stroke, acute cardiac disease or the effects of a concurrently used medication. These should be sought for before the change is attributed to AD progression (see Chapter 21).

response therapy can be altered as outlined in Table 18.4. If the dose is increased, patients should again be warned of the possibility of adverse effects as these are more common at higher doses. If switching from one CI to another, the new agent is best started at the lowest dose. There is no evidence to support combining CIs, unless overlapping low doses during a switch. Memantine has proven efficacy as monotherapy or add-on to CIs in later stages of AD.[91] Clinical trials allow patients to be exposed to new therapies which may prove efficacious, and often provide the CI as 'standard treatment' to which the new drug or placebo is added. On occasion it is simply appropriate to cease

When to cease therapy

The benefits of CI therapy may be maintained as AD progresses through a slower rate of symptom progression. Where there has been a satisfactory initial response it is often inappropriate to cease this therapy as the disease progresses. As benefits have also been demonstrated in nursing home populations, therapy should be continued if the patient is admitted to residential care, at least during the first few weeks of adjustment to the new environment and routine. It is appropriate to consider cessation when the patient enters the final stages of dementia, characterised by immobility, mutism and incontinence.

Cost-effectiveness of therapy

Several studies have concluded that CI therapy is cost-effective, although these data are not always sufficiently robust to convince regulatory authorities. A study modelling healthcare costs in seven countries (Australia, Canada, Finland, New Zealand, Sweden, the Netherlands and the United Kingdom) demonstrated cost savings from galantamine use over 10 years.[101] Cost savings have also been demonstrated for 12 months of donepezil therapy in mild to moderate AD,[102] although the modelling used in cost effectiveness studies may be imperfect.[103] From a patient/caregiver perspective, these medications can be expensive, especially if not subsidised, and overall cost savings may not influence the individual prescriber.

Current controversies in trial designs and interpretations

Recently, the utility of the CIs as symptomatic treatment for mild-to-moderate AD became the subject of some controversy. The AD 2000 trial[104] set out to address the longer term efficacy of donepezil in mild-to-moderate AD. As a non-pharmaceutically sponsored placebo-controlled trial, this study generated significant attention, particularly as the reported results on the outcomes of nursing home placement and ADLs were negative in the longer term. However, this study was seriously limited by methodological issues including high loss to follow-up rates and by some unusual design issues, such as repeated drug wash-outs. On this basis the long term utility of the CIs remains unsettled. This study set off controversy that has been taken up by others who have added their criticisms about the design of randomised controlled trials of CI.[104,105] As the heat of the controversy has developed, there have been arguments over the limitations of existing studies and other methodological considerations. Unfortunately this has moved the focus away from the patients benefiting from the therapy and in whose lives there has been significant impact. A revisiting of the cost-effectiveness of the CIs has been raised in the UK by the National Institute for Health and Clinical Excellence (NICE), with a final report still pending at the time of this publication.[106]

Despite this controversy, for the authors and for clinicians involved in the care of AD the availability of CIs and memantine represents a significant improvement in caring for this disease. Clinicians are regularly rewarded for their engagement in therapy of AD with these symptomatic medications and consider them as a standard of clinical care.

CONCLUSIONS

At this time the only approved therapy for mild-to-moderate AD is the CIs. A CI should thus be offered once the diagnosis is made, with current evidence that memantine is best used as monotherapy or add-on therapy as the disease progresses. All other therapies, including *Ginkgo biloba*, vitamins and statins, need further evidence before being offered.

REFERENCES

1. Davies KL, Maloney AJ. Selective loss of central cholinergic neurones in Alzheimer's disease. Lancet 1976; 2:1403.
2. Whitehouse PJ, Price DL, Struble RG, et al. Alzheimer's disease and senile dementia: loss of neurones in the basal forebrain. Science 1982; 215:1237–1239.
3. Bohnen NI, Kaufer DI, Hendrickson R, et al. Cognitive correlates of alterations in acetylcholinesterase in Alzheimer's disease. Neurosci Lett 2005; 380:127–132.
4. Minger SL, Esiri MM, McDonald B, et al. Cholinergic deficits contribute to behavioural disturbance in patients with dementia. Neurology 2000; 55:1460–1467.
5. Bodic NC, Offen WW, Levey AI, et al. Effect of xanomeline, a selective muscarinic receptor agonist, on cognitive function and behavioural symptoms in Alzheimer disease. Arch Neurol 1997; 54:465–473.
6. Greig NH, De Micheli E, Holloway HW, et al. The experimental Alzheimer drug phenserine: preclinical pharmacokinetics and pharmacodynamics. Acta Neurol Scand Suppl 2000; 176:74–84.
7. Lanctot KL, Herrman N, Yau KK, et al. Efficacy and safety of cholinesterase inhibitors in Alzheimer's disease: a meta-analysis. CMAJ 2003; 169:557–564.
8. Ritchie GW, Ames D, Clayton T, Lai R. Metaanalysis of randomised trials of the efficacy and safety of donepezil, galantamine, and rivastigmine for the treatment of Alzheimer Disease. Am J Geriatr Psychiatry 2004; 12:358–369.
9. Brodaty H, Ames D, Boundy KL, et al. Pharmacological treatment of cognitive deficits in Alzheimer's disease. Med J Aust 2001; 175:324–329.
10. Waldemar G. Donepezil in the treatment of patients with Alzheimer's disease. Expert Rev Neurother 2001; 1:11–19.

11. Greig NH, Utsuki T, Qian-sheng Y, et al. A new therapeutic target in Alzheimer's disease treatment: attention to butyrylcholinesterase. Curr Med Res Opin 2001; 17:1–7.

12. Poirier J. Evidence that the clinical effects of cholinesterase inhibitors are related to potency and targeting of action. Int J Clin Pract 2002; 127(suppl):6–19.

13. Schrattenholz A, Pereira EFR, Roth U, et al. Agonist responses of neuronal nicotinic receptors are potentiated by a novel class of allosterically acting ligands. Mol Pharmacol 1996; 49:1–6.

14. Gauthier S. Cholinergic adverse effects of cholinesterase inhibitors in Alzheimer's disease. Epidemiology and management. Drugs Aging 2001; 18:853–862.

15. Mintzer J E, Kershaw P. The efficacy of galantamine in the treatment of Alzheimer's disease: comparison of patients previously treated with acetylcholinesterase inhibitors to patients with no prior exposure. Int J Geriatr Psychiatry 2003; 18:292–297.

16. Mohs RC, Doody RS, Morris JC, et al. A 1-year, placebo-controlled preservation of function survival study of donepezil in AD patients. Neurology 2001; 57:481–488.

17. Winblad B, Engedal K, Soininen H, et al. A 1-year, randomised, placebo-controlled study of donepezil in patients with mild to moderate AD. Neurology 2001; 57:489–495.

18. Raskind MA, Peskind ER, Wessel T, Yuan W and the Galantamine USA-1 Study Group. Galantamine in AD. A 6-month randomised, placebo-controlled trial with a 6-month extension. Neurology 2000; 54:2261–2268.

19. Rogers SL, Friedhoff LT and the Donepezil Study Group. The efficacy and safety of donepezil in patients with Alzheimer's disease: results of a US multicentre, randomised, double-blind, placebo-controlled trial. Dementia 1996; 7:293–303.

20. Corey-Bloom J, Anand R, Veach J for the ENA 713 B352 Study Group. A randomized trial evaluating the efficacy and safety of ENA 713 (rivastigmine tartrate), a new acetyl-cholinesterase inhibitor, in patients with mild to moderately severe Alzheimer's disease. Int J Geriatr Psychiatry 1998; 1: 55–65.

21. Loy C, Schneider L. Galantamine for Alzheimer's disease. Cochrane Database Syst Rev 2004; 18(4):CD001747. Review.

22. Galasko D, Kershaw PR, Schneider L, Zhu Y, Tariot PN. Galantamine maintains ability to perform activities of daily living in patients with Alzheimer's disease. J Am Geriatr Soc 2004; 52:1070–1076.

23. Cummings JL, Schneider L, Tariot P, Kershaw P, Yuan W. Reduction of behavioural disturbances and caregiver distress by galantamine in patients with Alzheimer's disease. Am J Psychiatry 2004; 161:532–538.

24. Holmes C, Wilkinson D, Dean C, et al. The efficacy of donepezil in the treatment of neuropsychiatric symptoms in Alzheimer disease. Neurology 2004; 63:214–219.

25. Minger SL, Esiri MM, Mc Donald B, et al. Cholinergic deficits contribute to behavioural disturbance in patients with dementia. Neurology 2000; 55:1460–1467.

26. Lai MKP, Lai O-F, Keene J, et al. Psychosis in Alzheimer's disease is associated with elevated muscarinic M_2 binding in the cortex. Neurology 2001; 57:805–811.

27. Sano M, Wilcock GK, van Baelen B, Kavanagh S. The effects of galantamine treatment on caregiver time in Alzheimer's disease. Int J Geriatr Psychiatry 2003; 18:942–950.

28. Fillit HM, Gutterman EM, Brooks RL. Impact of donepezil on caregiving burden for patients with Alzheimer's disease. Int Psychogeriatr 2000; 12:389–401.

29. Rogers SL, Farlow MR, Doody RS, Mohs R, Friedhoff LT. A 24-week, double-blind, placebo-controlled trial of donepezil in patients with Alzheimer's disease. Donepezil Study Group. Neurology 1998; 50:136–145.

30. Doody RS, Stevens JC, Beck C, et al. Practice parameter: management of dementia (an evidence-based review). Report of the Quality Standards Subcommittee of the American Academy of Neurology. Neurology 2001; 56:1154–1166.

31. Rockwood K, Black SE, Robillard A, Lussier I. Potential treatment effects of donepezil not detected in Alzheimer's disease clinical trials: a physician survey. Int J Geriatr Psychiatry 2004; 19:954–960.

32. Seltzer B, Zolnouni P, Nunez M, et al. Efficacy of donepezil in early-stage Alzheimer disease. A randomised placebo-controlled trial. Arch Neurol 2004; 61:1852–1856.

33. Orgogozo JM, Small GW, Hammond G, Van Baelen B, Schwalen S. Effects of galantamine in patients with mild Alzheimer's disease. Curr Med Res Opin 2004; 20:1815–1820.

34. Raskind MA, Peskind ER, Truyen L, Kershaw P, Damaraju CRV. The cognitive benefits of galantamine are sustained for at least 36 months. Arch Neurol 2004; 61:252–256.

35. Rogers SL, Friedhoff LT. Long-term efficacy and safety of donepezil in the treatment of Alzheimer's disease: an interim analysis of the results of a US multicentre open label extension study. Europ Neuropsychopharm 1998; 8:67–75.

36. Grossberg G, Irwin P, Satlin A, Mesenbrink P, Spiegel R. Rivastigmine in Alzheimer's disease: efficacy over two years. Am J Geriatr Psychiatry 2004; 12:420–431.

37. Bullock R, Dengiz A. Cognitive performance in patients with Alzheimer's disease receiving cholinesterase inhibitors for up to 5 years. Int J Clin Pract 2005; 59:817–822.

38. Le DA, Lipton SA. Potential and current use of N-Methyl-D-Aspartate (NMDA) receptor antagonists in diseases of aging. Drugs Aging 2001; 18:717–724.

39. Peskind ER et al. Presentation at CINP congress, Paris, 20–24 June 2004.

40. McShane R, Schneider LS. Meta-analysis of memantine: summary and commentary on the Cochrane Collaboration's systematic review. Alzheimer's Dement 2005; 1:67–71.

41. Ingvar M, Ambros-Ingerson J, Davis M, et al. Enhancement by an ampakine of memory encoding in human. Exp Neurol 1997; 146:553–559.

42. Lopez OL, Becker JT, Saxton J, et al. Alteration of a clinically meaningful outcome in the natural history of Alzheimer's disease by cholinesterase inhibition. J Am Geriatr Soc 2005; 53:83–87.

43. Schenk D, Hagen M, Seubert P. Current progress in beta-amyloid immunotherapy. Curr Opin Immunol 2004; 16: 599–606.

44. Orgogozo J-M, Gilman S, Dartigues J-F, et al. Subacute meningoencephalitis in a subset of patients with AD after A [beta] 42 immunization. Neurology 2003; 61:46–54.

45. Fox NC, Black RS, Gilman S, et al. Effects of A [beta] immunization (AN 1792) on MRI measures of cerebral volume in Alzheimer disease. Neurology 2005; 64:1563–1572.

46. Gilman S, Koller M, Black RS, et al. Clinical effects of A [beta] immunization (AN 1792) in patients with AD in an interrupted trial. Neurology 2005; 64:1553–1562.

47. Nicoll JAR, Wilkinson D, Holmes C, et al. Neuropathology of human Alzheimer disease after immunization with amyloid-[beta] peptide: a case report. Nat Med 2003; 9:448–452.

48. Dodel RC, Du Y, Depboylu C, et al. Intravenous immuno-globulins containing antibodies against β-amyloid for the treatment of Alzheimer's disease. J Neurol Neurosurg Psychiatry 2004; 75:1472–1474.

49. In'T Veld BA, Ruitenberg A, Hofman A, et al. Nonsteroidal antiinflammatory drugs and the risk of Alzheimer's disease. N Engl J Med 2001; 345:1515–1521.

50. Etminan M, Gill S, Samii A. Effect of non-steroidal anti-inflammatory drugs on risk of Alzheimer's disease: systematic review and meta-analysis of observational studies. BMJ 2003; 327:128–132.

51. de Craen AJM, Gussekloo J, Vrijsen B, Westendorp RG. Meta-analysis of nonsteroidal antiinflammatory drug use and risk of dementia. Am J Epidemiol 2005; 161:114–120.

52. McGeer PL, McGeer EG. The inflammatory response system of brain: implications for therapy of Alzheimer and other neurodegenerative diseases. Brain Res Brain Res Rev 1995; 21:195–218.

53. Reines SA, Block GA, Morris JC, et al. Rofecoxib. No effect on Alzheimer's disease in a 1-year, randomised, blinded, controlled study. Neurology 2004; 62:66–71.

54. Scharf S, Mander A, Ugoni A, Vajda F, Christophidis N. A double-blind, placebo-controlled trial of diclofenac/misoprostol in Alzheimer's disease. Neurology 1999; 53:197–201.

55. Aisen PS, Davis KL, Berg JD, et al. A randomised controlled trial of prednisone in Alzheimer's disease. Neurology 2000; 54:588–593.

56. Yaffe K, Grady D, Pressman A, et al. Serum oestrogen levels, cognitive performance, and risk of cognitive decline in older community women. J Am Geriatr Soc 1998; 46:816–821.

57. Zandi PP, Carlson MC, Plassman BL, et al. Hormone replacement therapy and incidence of Alzheimer disease in older women. The Cache County Study. JAMA 2002; 288:2123–2129.

58. Tang M-X, Jacobs D, Stern Y, et al. Effect of oestrogen during menopause on risk and age at onset of Alzheimer's disease. Lancet 1992; 348:429–432.

59. Baldereschi M, Di Carlo A, Lepore V, et al. Estrogen-replacement therapy and Alzheimer's disease in the Italian longitudinal study on aging. Neurology 1998; 50:996–1002.

60. Almeida OP, Flicker L. Association between hormone replacement therapy and dementia: is it time to forget? Int Psychogeriatrics 2005; 17:155–164.

61. Shumaker SA, Legault C, Rapp SR, et al. Estrogen plus progestin and the incidence of dementia and mild cognitive impairment in postmenopausal women. The Women's Health Initiative Memory Study: a randomized controlled trial. JAMA 2003; 289:2651–2662.

62. Cholerton B, Gleason CE, Baker LD, Asthana S. Estrogen and Alzheimer's disease. The story so far. Drugs Aging 2002; 19:405–427.

63. Wolozin B. Cholesterol and the biology of Alzheimer's disease. Neuron 2004; 41:7–10.

64. Rockwood K, Kirkland S, Hogan DB, et al. Use of lipid-lowering agents, indication bias, and the risk of dementia in community-dwelling elderly people. Arch Neurol 2002; 59:223–227.

65. Sparks DL, Sabbagh MN, Connor DJ, et al. Atorvastatin for the treatment of mild to moderate Alzheimer disease. Arch Neurol 2005; 62:753–757.

66. Halliwell B. Role of free radicals in the neurodegenerative diseases. Therapeutic implications for antioxidant treatment. Drugs Aging 2001; 18:685–716.

67. Masaki KH, Losonezy KG, Izmirlian G, et al. Association of vitamin E and C supplement use with cognitive function and dementia in elderly men. Neurology 2000; 54:1265–1272.

68. Engelhart MJ, Geerlings MI, Ruitenberg A, et al. Dietary intake of antioxidants and risk of Alzheimer disease. JAMA 2002; 287:3223–3229.

69. Morris MC, Evans DA, Bienias JL, et al. Dietary intake of antioxidant nutrients and the risk of incident Alzheimer disease in a biracial community study. JAMA 2002; 287:3230–3237.

70. Luchsinger JA, Tang M-X, Shea S, Mayeux R. Antioxidant vitamin intake and risk of Alzheimer disease. Arch Neurol 2003; 60:203–208.

71. Petersen RC, Thomas RG, Grundman M, et al. Vitamin E and donepezil for the treatment of mild cognitive impairment. N Engl J Med 2005; 352:2379–2388.

72. Sano M, Ernesto C, Thomas RG, et al. A controlled trial of selegeline, alpha-tocopherol, or both as a treatment for Alzheimer disease. N Engl J Med 1997; 336: 216–222.

73. Miller ER 3rd, Pastor-Barriuso R, Dalal D, et al. Meta-analysis: high-dosage vitamin E supplementation may increase all-cause mortality. Ann Intern Med 2005; 142:37–46.

74. Kurz A, Van Baelen B. Ginkgo biloba compared with cholinesterase inhibitors in the treatment of dementia: a review based on meta-analyses by the Cochrane collaboration. Dement Geriatr Cogn Disord 2004; 18:217–226.

75. Burke WJ, Roccaforte WH, Wengel SP, et al. L-Deprenyl in the treatment of mild dementia of the Alzheimer type: results of a 15-month trial. J Am Geriatr Soc 1993; 41:1219–1225.

76. Parnetti L, Abate G, Bartorelli L, et al. Multicentre study of 1-α-glyceryl-phosphorcholine versus ST200 among patients with probable senile dementia of Alzheimer's type. Drugs Aging 1993; 3:159–164.

77. Vernon MW, Sorkin EM. Piracetam. An overview of its pharmacological properties and a review of its therapeutic use in senile cognitive disorders. Drugs Aging 1991; 1:17–35.

78. Lee CR, Benfield P. Aniracetam. An overview of its pharmacodynamic and pharmacokinetic properties, and a review of its therapeutic potential in senile cognitive disorders. Drugs Aging 1994; 4:257–273.

79. Thienhaus OJ, Wheeler BG, Simon S, Zemlan FP, Hartford JT. A controlled double-blind study of high-dose dihydroergotoxine mesylate (Hydergine®) in mild dementia. J Am Geriatr Soc 1987; 35:219–223.

80. Battaglia A, Bruni G, Ardia A, Sacchetti G, Italian nicergoline study group. Nicergoline in mild to moderate dementia. A multi-centre, double-blind, placebo-controlled study. J Am Geriatr Soc 1989; 37:295–302.

81. Schwartz BL, Hashtroudi S, Herting RL, Schwartz P, Deutsch SI. D-Cycloserine enhances implicit memory in Alzheimer patients. Neurology 1996; 46:420–424.

82. Brooks JO, Yesavage JA, Carta A, Bravi D. Acetyl L-carnitine slows decline in younger patients with Alzheimer's disease: a reanalysis of a double-blind, placebo-controlled study using the trilinear approach. Int Psychogeriatr 1998; 10: 193–203.

83. Gillis JC, Benfield P, McTavish D. Idebenone. A review of its pharmacodynamic and pharmacokinetic properties, and therapeutic use in age-related cognitive disorders. Drugs Aging 1994; 5:133–152.

84. Craft S, Asthana S, Newcomer JW, et al. Enhancement of memory in Alzheimer disease with insulin and somatostatin, but not glucose. Arch Gen Psychiatry 1999; 56: 1135–1140.

85. Thal LJ, Forrest M, Loft H, Mengel H, for the Lu25-109 study group. Lu 25-109, a muscarinic agonist, fails to improve cognition in Alzheimer's disease. Neurology 2000; 54:421–426.

86. Bae C-Y, Cho C-Y, Kyunghee C, et al. A double-blind, placebo-controlled, multicenter study of cerebrolysin for Alzheimer's disease. J Am Geriatr Soc 2000; 48:1566–1571.

87. Probing PPAR agonists. Could anti-diabetic drugs improve Alzheimer's disease? 1996, Available at http://www.alzforum. org [accessed 27 October, 2005].

88. Wolkowitz OM, Kramer JH, Reus VI, et al. DHEA treatment of Alzheimer's disease. A randomised, double-blind, placebo-controlled study. Neurology 2003; 60:1071–1076.

89. Loeb MB, Molloy DW, Smieja M, et al. A randomised, controlled trial of doxycycline and rifampin for patients with Alzheimer's disease. J Am Geriatr Soc 2004; 52:381–387.

90. Rockwood K, Graham J, Fay S. Goal setting and attainment in Alzheimer's disease patients treated with donepezil. J Neurol Neurosurg Psychiatry 2002; 73:500–507.

91. Tariot PN, Farlow MR, Grossberg GT, et al. Memantine treatment in patients with moderate to severe Alzheimer disease already receiving donepezil. JAMA 2004; 291: 317–324.

92. Connelly PJ, Prentice NP, Fowler KG. Predicting the outcome of cholinesterase inhibitor treatment in Alzheimer's disease. J Neurol Neurosurg Psychiatry 2005; 76:320–324.

93. Rozzini L, Chilovi BV, Bellelli G, et al. Effects of cholinesterase inhibitors appear greater in patients on established antihypertensive therapy. Int J Geriatr Psychiatry 2005; 20:547–551.

94. Erkinjuntti T, Skoog I, Lane R, Andrews C. Rivastigmine in patients with Alzheimer's disease and concurrent hypertension. Int J Clin Pract 2002; 56:791–796.

95. Connelly PJ, Prentice NP. Current smoking and response to cholinesterase inhibitor therapy in Alzheimer's disease. Dementia Geriatr Cogn Disord 2005; 19:11–14.

96. Roe CM, Anderson MJ, Spivack B. Use of anticholinergic medications by older adults with dementia. J Am Geriatr Soc 2002; 50:836–842.

97. Farlow MR, Hake A, Messina J, et al. Response of patients with Alzheimer disease to rivastigmine treatment is predicted by the rate of disease progression. Arch Neurol 2001; 58:417–422.

98. Macgowan SH, Wilcock GK, Scott M. Effect of gender and apolipoprotein E genotype on response to anticholinesterase therapy in Alzheimer's disease. Int J Geriatr Psychiatry 1998; 13:625–630.

99. Farlow MR, Cyrus PA, Nadel A, et al. Metrifonate treatment of AD. Influence of APOE genotype. Neurology 1999; 53: 2010–2016.

100. Visser PJ, Scheltens P, Pelgrim E, Verhey FR, Dutch ENA-NL-01 study group. Medial temporal lobe atrophy and APOE genotype do not predict cognitive improvement upon treatment with rivastigmine in Alzheimer's disease patients. Dement Geriatr Cog Disorders 2005; 19:126–133.

101. Caro J, Salas M, Ward A, et al. Assessing the health and economic impact of galantamine treatment in patients with Alzheimer's disease in health care systems of different countries. Drugs Aging 2004; 21:677–686.

102. Wimo A, Winblad B, Engedal K, et al. An economic evaluation of donepezil in mild to moderate Alzheimer's disease: results of a 1-year, double blind, randomized trial. Dement Geriatr Cogn Disord 2003; 15:44–54.

103. Wimo A. Cost effectiveness of cholinesterase inhibitors in the treatment of Alzheimer's disease. A review with methodological considerations. Drugs Aging 2004; 21: 279–295.

104. AD2000 Collaborative Group. Long-term donepezil treatment in 565 patients with Alzheimer's disease (AD2000): randomised double-blind trial. Lancet 2004; 363: 2105–2115.

105. Kaduszkiewicz H, Zimmermann T, Beck-Bornholdt H-P, van den Bussche H. Cholinesterase inhibitors for patients with Alzheimer's disease: systematic review of randomised clinical trials. BMJ 2005; 331:321–327.

106. National Institute for Health and Clinical Excellence. 2006 [accessed 10 January, 2006]. Available at www.nice.org.uk.

19

Care of patients in the severe stage of dementia

Per-Olof Sandman, David Edvardsson and Bengt Winblad

The proportion of people with Alzheimer's disease (AD) and related disorders cared for in different settings in Sweden has increased during the last 25 years. For example, while in 1975 about one-third of all beds were occupied by a person with dementia in Sweden, this proportion had increased to about two-thirds in 2000 (Table 19.1). The data in Table 19.1 are drawn from eight different sample times, performed with the same instrument[1] and in the same county in Sweden. The only purpose-built institutions for care of people with severe symptoms of dementia in Sweden are so-called group livings. These are small units with 6 to 10 persons living together and cared for in a homelike environment. The prevalence of patients with dementia is of course high in these institutions. However, a vast majority of the patients with severe dementia are cared for in non-purpose-built environments such as nursing homes and service houses. These settings often consist of a physical environment, a staff/patient ratio and a competence among the staff not quite adequate to meet the needs of people with severe dementia.

Data from the above described investigations also shows an increased mean age among the patients and increased dependency of their caregivers to manage their daily life. As shown in Table 19.2, when comparing patients cared for in 1982, 1988, 1994 and 2000 (Sandman & Karlsson, unpublished data), the proportion of patients who can manage their basic activities of daily living (ADL) has decreased rather dramatically. This means, for example, that the proportion of patients who can eat independently has decreased from 74 to 43 per cent.

VIEWS OF THE PATIENT WITH SEVERE DEMENTIA

A patient with severe dementia does not only suffer from a decreased ability to perform ADL, they are also often described as having reduced capability to communicate, reduced mobility, apraxia, agnosia, psychological and behavioural symptoms. This means that

Table 19.1 Prevalence of dementia (%) in different kinds of settings at different periods of time (county of Västerbotten, Sweden)								
	1975	1982	1986	1988	1993	1994	1996	2000
Homes for the aged	17	19	32	40	53	53	60	
Service houses			10		23		30	41
Nursing homes	57	61		80	83	79	87	78
Group livings for persons with dementia					89	96	99	92
Total	33	41				67		60

Table 19.2 Proportion of patients (%) cared for in different settings in the county of Västerbotten, Sweden, with preserved ability to manage their ADL functions

	1982	1988	1994	2000
Ability to dress independently	38	22	15	10
Independent (bladder)	58	40	30	24
Independent (bowel)	79	64	58	50
Ability to manage hygiene independently	39	20	12	6
Ability to eat independently	74	60	55	43

people in this stage of the disease are dependent on others to manage their daily life. There is a risk that a person with severe functional and cognitive decline may be regarded as an 'empty shell' or as the 'living dead'. However, another way of looking upon patients with severe dementia is trying to see the person 'behind the disease', i.e. attempting to see the individual 'encapsulated' by his/her progressive inability. Metaphorically speaking, the thickness of the 'capsule' increases as the disease progresses, making it increasingly difficult for the person to come and stay in contact with the outer world (for example staff and relatives), and for the outer world to come in contact with the person. If supporting such a view, i.e. that there is still an 'I' behind the symptoms and functional decline, it would be of the utmost importance to create a caring environment where the patient is seen as a person. In such an environment one objective for the caregiver is to be open and sensitive, trying to impute meaning to the increasingly fragmented and weakening signals from the patient. These signals from the person with severe dementia evoke questions about how they experience the surrounding world, and themselves within that world (personal identity). Within sociology, for example, identity is seen as a socially constructed phenomenon, i.e. our identity is constructed in relation to context, situation and in relation to how we are understood and approached by other people. Thus, if we as caregivers understand and approach people with severe dementia as 'living dead', this is likely to influence the patients' construction of their own identity as severely demented; it may also affect the construction of my identity as a caregiver.

Providing care for the 'living dead' (and an experience of offering meaningless care) might evoke the question from the caregiver: 'who am I, having chosen this meaningless work?'. This reasoning illuminates that patients with dementia and their caregivers are mutually dependent on each other.[2]

Jansson et al[3] conducted a study aiming to describe facial expressions of patients in the terminal stage of AD (bedridden, no speech) when interacting with caregivers during different kinds of activities. It was shown that it was possible to see patients as still having capacity to experience the activities performed, and that they were also able to communicate their experiences back to the caregivers by facial expressions. It seemed as if the patients' reactions were adequate, even if they were fragmented and vague in relation to the activity performed. The patients also expressed more frequent reactions by the end of the study in comparison to the beginning. One conclusion was that it is only possible to understand the fragmented communication from the patient if caregivers have the understanding that there is still a person behind the symptoms trying to communicate in a meaningful way. This is congruent with findings from Athlin et al,[4] describing that caregivers seeing the person with dementia as an object did not seem committed, and were more focused on performing tasks rather than focusing on the patient's experiences.

Another phenomenon of interest with regard to patients with severe dementia and their ability to perceive the surrounding world is 'moments of lucidity'. Norman[5] interviewed caregivers who were asked to narrate episodes where persons with severe dementia, normally lacking conversational abilities, suddenly spoke and/or acted with an unexpected adequacy. Moments of lucidity were most often described in situations where the patients were met in a supporting and accepting way and thus a close relation seemed to be a prerequisite. In moments of lucidity, in spite of all symptoms of the disease, these patients were interpreted to have a preserved individual self that became visible for caregivers. It was also concluded that a person-centred care approach facilitated lucidity, i.e. care based on an interest in the 'person behind the disease', showing a confirming and listening approach without demanding and correcting the patient.

PROMOTING WELL-BEING IN PERSONS WITH SEVERE DEMENTIA

Involving patients with severe dementia in everyday activities, such as watering the plants or drinking coffee together with other patients and staff, can promote well-being. Zingmark et al[6] showed that such activities could facilitate experiences of 'at-homeness', i.e. moments when the patient was interpreted to experience meaningfulness and him/herself as a whole. This was seen in situations when the patient seemed related to self, others, time, objects, event and place. Thus, experiences of at-homeness were promoted in situations when patients experienced themselves as present, part of and related to themselves.

Care of people with severe dementia consists of two inseparable parts, the doing and being of caregivers. Doing consists of the tasks that are to be performed, for example feeding, showering, changing diapers, and being consists of the relationship that is formed between the caregiver and the person with dementia. The being of caregivers can be understood as the quality marker of the tasks performed, i.e. the way these tasks are carried out. For example, one can serve an old lady coffee in a careful and loving way, making her feel like a queen, or in a stressful and neglecting manner, making her feel like a burden. In the first case, the lady's experience of the situation is in focus, and in the latter merely completing the task. These examples intend to show that the subtle qualities of people's way of being when doing what they do are of the utmost importance for the care of patients with dementia. It could also be described as adding thoughtfulness and concern to the action, drying an older woman off in a patient, gentle and caring fashion after a shower, instead of stressfully rubbing water from a wet body.

As the section above is intended to illuminate, nursing care is an area of great importance for the well-being of patients with severe dementia. Good nursing care aims to create an environment facilitating experiences of being safe, secure and at home, in spite of suffering from a severe disability that threatens the foundations of existence. Good nursing care comprises an inherent value in itself. Good nursing care can and should be seen as something more than 'non-pharmacological treatment', since caring does not necessarily have a certain target or an anticipated outcome. This means that the person's subjective experience is sometimes more relevant than objective measures.

Zingmark et al[7] interviewed caregivers in special care units for patients with severe dementia, aiming to clarify the meaning of offering care to these people. Ten aspects of care were presented, describing how to promote the good life (well-being) for patients cared for in a group living environment (Table 19.3). The authors summarized their findings as follows: good nursing care involves trying to create a good life for patients where they can experience acceptance, com-

munication, familiarity, a place where they can feel at home.[7]

One prerequisite to facilitate a caring environment for patients with severe dementia is the staff's knowledge. One can reflect about what kind of knowledge is needed for that purpose. First of all the staff need knowledge about facts, i.e. knowledge about the different diseases, their natural progression, symptoms, risk factors, how to diagnose and how to treat. Secondly, they need knowledge about the meaning of being a person with severe symptoms of a dementing disease, for example knowledge about persons experiencing apraxia, agnosia, loss of memory, longing for home. This could be understood as a more experience-based knowledge, making it possible for the caregiver to have a 'feel for' the life of a person with severe dementia. A third type of knowledge needed could be labelled as knowledge of action, i.e. knowledge about how to act in different caring activities, for example how to change a diaper when the patient resists, feed a patient with difficulty in swallowing or convince a patient who is longing for home to stay. Finally, in order to provide a caring environment where tasks are performed in a close relationship with the patient, the caregivers also need to be aware of their own personal ethical reasoning, i.e. an ethical 'knowledge' about their morale as expressed in doing and being. One prerequisite for developing this kind of knowledge is that there are opportunities for the caregivers to reflect upon and discuss their doing and being in relation to the person with severe dementia. Edberg[8] has shown that participation in supervision groups increased the caregivers' job satisfaction and decreased their risk for burn-out.

ENVIRONMENT AND BEHAVIOUR

A frequent and often distressing complication related to dementia is the occurrence of behavioural and psychological symptoms in dementia (BPSD). These symptoms are described as manifestations of disrupted perceptions of reality with altered mood and distorted behaviour as expressed through anxiety, hallucinations and delusions, agitation and aggression such as physical or verbal outbursts, activity disturbances such as restlessness, wandering, rummaging and other socially/sexually deviant behaviours.[9,10] The aetiology of BPSD involves biological, social and psychological factors,[11] and as many as 90 per cent of patients with dementia have been said to show behavioural symptoms at some point during the course of the disease.[12] However, the prevalence of behavioural symptoms among patients with dementia cared for in

Table 19.3 Caring aspects promoting the good life for patients with severe dementia[7]

Subthemes	
Viewing dignity and striving to promote a sense of self in the resident	Promoting the resident's rights and worth, their right to be respected. Providing individual care based on knowledge about the person behind the disease
Accepting the resident's way of being	An acceptance of the person's way of being, allowing them to be just as they are as long their behaviour doesn't harm themselves or others
Sharing everyday life in a sense of nearness	Promoting a close, relaxed relationship facilitating the possibilities to meet the person's individual needs.
Encouraging a sense of belonging	Trying to create an atmosphere of 'we', not 'they and us'. Bringing the past into the present by, for example, becoming familiar with the person's life history, letting them bring personal belongings as a mean to establish familiarity in a home-like environment
Adjusting oneself to the resident and striving for mutual understanding	Grasping the moment, striving for synchronizing in tempo and rhythm, adapting oneself to the person's way of living (for example speech, sound, light) and trying to avoid corrections
Offering relief	Striving to relieve the burden of the disease. For example, promoting emotional safety by being close, substituting for losses in functional capacity, being a 'third hand' trying to initiate, prevent and perform
Providing space for occupation	Trying to not become bound to routines, striving to find a balance between activity and rest. Providing activities where the person could participate actively or passively, just joining
Promoting power and control in the resident	Promoting but not pushing them in decision-making. Providing and respecting their private space, but not letting them feel alone. Balancing the person's need to express feelings and preventing outbursts of, for example, aggression

different settings in Sweden, based on ratings by the staff, is surprisingly low (Table 19.4). For example, on a daily basis 9.3 per cent shriek and shout continuously, 3.1 per cent hit patients/staff and 6.7 per cent exhibit aggressive threats to patients and staff. Psychiatric symptoms, occurring every day, like disturbed and restless (19.7 per cent), easily annoyed (11.8 per cent) and suspicious are more prevalent. One explanation for the relatively low prevalence of behavioural symptoms could be that the patients are in a late phase of the disease when institutionalized, and as a consequence of the progress of the disease show fewer behavioural symptoms than in the earlier stages (see Chapter 16).

Another interesting finding is that the prevalence of depressive symptoms is rather low and unchanged when comparing Swedish data from the years 1982 and 2000 (Table 19.5). In 1982, the proportions who were never experienced by staff as being sad or crying were 42.7 per cent and 66 per cent, respectively. In 2000, the corresponding proportions were 46.4 per cent and 72.9 per cent. During the same period, the prevalence of patients prescribed antidepressants increased from 7 to 42 per cent (Table 19.6). Bains et al[13] concluded in a Cochrane report that 'available evidence offers weak support to the contention that antidepressants are effective for patients with depression and dementia'. They also concluded that there is a

Table 19.4 Prevalence (%) (every day, sometimes per week, never) of behavioural symptoms in patients living in different kinds of settings in Sweden (county of Västerbotten)

	1982			2000		
	Every day	Sometimes per week	Never	Every day	Sometimes per week	Never
Takes things from fellow patients' drawers and cupboards	2.6	10.1	87.3	2.8	7.6	89.6
Picks up his/her things, is often on the way home	3.4	11	85.6	3.6	9.8	89.6
Often stands at the outer door and wants out	3.2	11.7	85.1	5.1	10.5	84.4
Mixes up food	7.2	13.4	79.4	9.1	12.6	78.3
Eats potted soil, cigarette butts, etc.	0.9	2.7	96.3	0.4	2.4	97.1
Undresses in the dayroom	0.8	6.9	92.3	0.5	6.9	92.6
Wanders alone or with other patients back and forth	17.4	11.8	70.8	17.2	11.9	71.0
Unruly in bed, throws bedclothes onto the floor	6.2	16.5	77.3	6.1	14.3	79.6
Piles up chairs, pushes tables, upends furniture, etc.	1.8	4.8	93.4	3.2	5.0	91.9
Urinates in wastepaper basket, washbasin or on the floor	3.7	10.4	85.9	2.1	7.2	90.7
Spits out medicine	4.5	20.7	74.8	3.0	19.5	77.5
Speaks spontaneously with staff and patients	29.3	25.6	45.1	27.8	17.3	54.9
Shrieks and shouts continuously	7.6	15.8	76.6	9.3	12.7	78.0
Smears faeces on clothes, furniture, etc.	1.3	16.7	82.0	0.9	11.7	87.4
Constantly seeks attention of the staff	16.4	31.5	52.1	26.9	27.5	45.7
Eats others' food	1.9	7.2	90.9	1.5	7.0	91.5
Will not go to sleep	3.6	20.3	76.1	2.5	19.5	78.0
Disturbed sleep at night	5.2	44.7	50.0	10.3	46.1	43.7
Goes and lies in other patients' bed	2.2	9.8	88.0	0.7	4.7	94.6
Hits patients/staff	2.6	14.3	83.1	3.1	13.9	83.0
Aggressive threats (words and gesture) to patients, staff	5.9	30.8	63.3	6.7	29.3	64.0
Tears up newspapers, etc.	2.0	6.2	91.8	1.9	8.4	89.8
Hides things	6.2	14.4	79.4	8.5	15.2	76.4
Rolls up table cloths	5.6	11.8	82.6	5.7	15.0	79.3
Resists being dressed and undressed	14.4	23.2	62.4	14.5	22.0	63.5

Table 19.5 Prevalence (%) (every day, sometimes per week, never) of psychiatric symptoms in persons living in different kinds of settings in Sweden (county of Västerbotten)

	1982			2000		
	Every day	Sometimes per week	Never	Every day	Sometimes per week	Never
Sad	6.3	51.1	42.7	7.2	46.4	46.4
Cries	3.1	30.9	66.0	3.4	23.7	72.9
Disturbed and restless	21.9	40.4	37.8	19.7	37.8	42.5
Easily annoyed	12.1	31.0	56.9	11.8	30.9	57.3
Suspicious	8.4	25.5	66.1	8.8	26.1	65.2
Hallucinates (visual)	4.9	15.5	79.6	5.2	18.3	76.5
Hallucinates (auditory)	3.9	13.3	82.8	3.9	12.3	83.8
Fearful	12.0	36.4	51.7	10.1	33.3	56.6
Speaks to him/her self	18.0	24.3	57.6	19.6	21.9	58.5
Complaining	11.8	27.7	60.5	12.1	29.6	58.3
Takes initiative	63.9	23.6	12.5	55.7	23.9	20.4
Cooperates	33.1	31.7	35.1	25.2	29.2	45.6
Seeks help	21.5	32.9	45.5	26.1	27.8	46.1
Overactive ('manic')	3.4	8.1	88.5	4.7	10.6	84.7

Table 19.6 Proportion of patients living in different settings prescribed different types of psychotropic drugs (%). A comparison between people cared for in the years 1988, 1994 and 2000 (county of Västerbotten, Sweden)

	1988	1994	2000
Psychotropics	65	66	68
Neuroleptics	29	33	33
Bensodiazepines	47	21	30
Antidepressants	6	20	43

lack of studies in this area, and that those studies included in their meta-analysis had small samples and newer classes of antidepressants such as selective noradrenergic reuptake inhibitors were not evaluated.

Another finding is that the prevalence of behavioural symptoms is rather stable over time. When comparing data from the year 2000 with data from 1982 (collected in the same county in Sweden and with the same instrument, MDDAS[1]) it was found, when comparing the two sets of data, that the prevalence was relatively unchanged. On the other hand it has also been shown that the prevalence of BPSD varies between contexts and countries[14] (Sandman and Karlsson, unpublished data) and that actions to manage behavioural symptoms, such as the use of physical restraints and neuroleptics, also vary. Karlsson et al[15] and Karlsson and Sandman (unpublished) investigated 45 similar units for care of patients with dementia and found that the prevalence of physical restraints varied between 0 and 40 per cent, and the use of neuroleptics varied between 0 and 70 per cent. Some of the variance could be explained by patients' characteristics, but also by staff characteristics such as attitude, knowledge and their experience of the ward climate. There was a higher use of physical restraints and neuroleptics in units where staff rated their ward climate less positive. These findings reveal that factors other than patients' characteristics contribute to explaining the difference in the use of physical restraints and neuroleptics. In another study[16] a significant association was found between the time patients in group livings spent together with staff and the staff's ratings of their ward climate. In units rated as 'stagnated', about 25 per cent of the patients' total time during the day was spent with staff, and in units rated as having a 'more creative climate', 45 per cent of the patients' time was spent with staff. In conclusion, this means that dimensions other than patients' characteristics must be taken into consideration when trying to improve the care of people in later stages of dementia.

The occurrence of behavioural symptoms creates suffering for patients, significant others and healthcare staff, and is a strong predictor for institutionalization of patients with dementia.[17] For staff, behavioural symptoms impose a burden upon their work[18] and evoke feelings of uselessness, rejection and powerlessness.[2,19,20] Behavioural symptoms are explained by anatomical and neurochemical damage to the brain[21] and by earlier personality traits,[22] but can also be interpreted as a form of meaningful communication.[2] The view of healthcare staff towards the patient with dementia and whether behavioural symptoms are seen as just originating from a damaged brain or as a form of communication will determine the care provided and the actions taken. The primary focus of care can, for instance, be to use strategies that eliminate the behaviour, but it is of interest to try to understand the underlying experiences that might evoke the behaviour classified as disturbing. These assumptions will influence care in somewhat different directions.

If behavioural symptoms are interpreted as unwanted biomedical symptoms only, care will focus upon finding suitable pharmacological strategies, often by using neuroleptics and/or antidepressants.[23] Behavioural symptoms may also be considered to originate only within the patient and the staff may not reflect on how their interaction with the patient influences or even causes this behaviour. This reasoning is intended to demonstrate that, depending on the caregiver's interpretation of the behavioural symptoms, the patient's behaviour can become a medical problem which should be solved with pharmacological interventions. If, instead, the presence of behavioural symptoms is interpreted as a form of communication, pharmacological treatment might not be the first option. Rather, care might focus upon trying to interpret and understand this manifestation from the perspective of the person with dementia: what does this behaviour mean and what can possibly trigger this behaviour?

It has been reported that living with dementia means being surrounded by disorganization[24] and that behaviours experienced as inappropriate by the caregiver can be interpreted as one way to maintain one's self.[25] Furthermore, aggression has been related to experience of invasion of the personal space,[26] wandering interpreted as a manifestation of homesickness[6] and screaming understood as expression of anxiety about abandonment.[27] In acknowledging that the 'demented' is a person who lives in an increasingly unfamiliar world of chaos and disorganization, expression of behaviours such as anxiety, agitation and restlessness might not be that surprising. From such a perspective, care shifts focus towards identifying trigger factors in the environment and using the life history of the person to interpret how to understand and approach the expression of behavioural symptoms.[28] There also seems to be a reason for the negative connotation of the term 'behavioural disturbances' and one should consider what this concept means in terms of negative labelling. For example, for a lady with AD who aggressively accuses other patients of stealing her purse, is the behaviour inappropriate per se or merely disturbing from the carer's perspective? As the lady is convinced that she knows where she placed the purse, the explanation that someone stole the purse is reasonable from her perspective, and the reaction – aggression – is also understandable. The behaviour per se does not seem inappropriate, e.g. the term 'disturbance' might rather signify the effect this behaviour has on the surroundings. Thus, it is easy to generalize the behaviour of patients with dementia as behavioural disturbance, but such a label is not always correct. At times, such behaviour can be understood as a consequence of making too great a demand of the person in relation to his/her competence.

CARING ENVIRONMENTS FOR PATIENTS WITH SEVERE DEMENTIA

The theory of the person–environment fit[29] conceptualizes behaviour as a product of demands of the environment and the level of personal competence available to meet these demands. The diminishing competence (intellectual, emotional and physical ability) inevitable with the progression of AD and related dementias makes it increasingly difficult for the person to interpret the demands of the environment (physical and psychosocial). Thus when environmental demands exceed the person's competence, behaviour will seem inadequate. In light of this theory, caring interventions can be employed to lower the environmental demands and thus the risk for misinterpretation and inadequate behaviour. Such interventions can be used as a complement to medical interventions targeted to reduce behavioural symptoms. Some claim that the environment is more accessible to change than many other factors that relate to outcome among patients with dementia, such as diagnosis, disease stage, age and comorbid conditions.[30] For example, it has been described how the presence of symbols of home-like and familiar places supporting interaction in the environment can compensate for the intellectual decline and help to promote adequate behaviour and feelings of safety and at-homeness in patients with dementia.[7,31–34] It has also been shown that a home-like environment slowed the progression of intellectual deterioration, positively affected interaction and behaviour, lowered confusion and anxiety and improved eating behaviour among patients with dementia.[35,36] Moreover, enriching the environment with nature scenes, sounds and smells, and non-institutional chairs, tables and pictures was associated with positive effects on the behaviour and mood of residents with dementia,[37] and access to outdoor areas was associated with decreased agitated behaviour.[38]

A review of 70 empirical research studies from 1981 to 1995 on the physical design of environments for people with dementia suggested that supportive environments are of small size with a non-institutional design, in which cognitively unimpaired residents are separated from patients with dementia, where accessible outdoor areas are incorporated and where moderate levels of environmental stimulation occur.[39] However, even though evidence has accumulated that various parameters in the environment influence behaviour and well-being among people with dementia, there is still little consensus about which parameters are the most salient.[40,41] There are also some methodological weaknesses to studies conducted, such as small sample size, few control groups, difficulties in isolating the environmental variable under study from confounders and not taking into account variation between stages of dementia.[39] Thus, careful interpretation of these studies is recommended.

Research into environments for dementia care has focused on identifying and designing supportive physical environments, but the psychosocial dimension of the environment has remained largely unexplored.[42] It has been reported that, for people with dementia, emotional memories are more lasting than cognitive memories, and they use their emotional memories to interpret and communicate their experiences of the present.[43] This means that, when it is difficult to understand the surroundings due to diminished cognitive ability, the person with dementia can act according to their emotional perception of their environment. Thus, whether the atmosphere, i.e. the emotional quality or 'feeling tone' of the environment, is characterized as calm, friendly and inviting or stressful, hostile and unwelcome can influence the emotional well-being and perhaps also the prevalence of behavioural symptoms among patients with dementia. The environment is considered as supporting well-being when people experience a calm pace, recognize themselves as persons and where there is communication. There should be a shared philosophy of care, the possibility of creating and maintaining social relations, available and trustworthy staff with a

willingness to serve and strategies to make people feel welcome.[42,44,45]

It has also been shown that environments can convey symbolic meanings to patients and relatives.[46] For example, an environment experienced as unclean and run down can evoke feelings of being in a place where people are unable to care. In other words, not caring for the environment can symbolize not caring for people either. Seemingly negligible aspects in the environment such as dust balls on the floors, for example, symbolize an absence of caring for patients, and thereby evoke mistrust about care at the ward. For instance, a bedridden woman cared for at an oncology unit with nothing else to look at but an empty hook for a painting on the wall described how her interpretation of this situation led to her decision to stop treatment and leave the unit. Not hanging anything on the hook for her to look at symbolized negligence from staff towards her needs in this situation.[46] There are reasons to believe that when patients with severe dementia and their relatives come to a dementia care unit, they are also searching for cues to help them understand what kind of care is performed in that environment. For example, a home-like environment may communicate something about the philosophy predominant at the place, in comparison to a hospital-like environment. We also know that if environments contain objects and/or conversations of interest to patients, this can provide opportunities to shift focus from one's situation and suffering to the consoling powers of, for example, the latest game of hockey or the everyday experience of being able to see and enjoy birds feeding outside a window. The following field note, derived from a project exploring experiences of environments of care, illustrates how the placement of a container with bird seeds outside a dying patient's window provided a meaningful content to the day and facilitated a shift of focus from self to the environment for a patient:

'Today when I entered Nigel's room, he sat there on his bed with a big smile on his face, and he told me that this had been a most happy day – today already six different types of birds had visited the container for bird seeds that the art therapist had put up yesterday. He said, "It is fantastic, I can stay here in bed and watch and hear the birds – they are just so beautiful".'

In this example, shifting focus from oneself to the environment does not imply that the sorrow and darkness connected to living with an incurable disease have vanished, but rather the environment has, for a shorter or longer moment, made darkness bearable and living possible. Another example of shifting focus is when a child or a dog visits a dementia care unit, it will evoke emotions and actions by the patients. These examples are used to illustrate the point of including the whole environment in the concept of care, and show that environmental interventions can be fairly easy to achieve. Actions such as placing a container for bird seeds outside a patient's window or hanging a painting of personal preference on the wall can be caring measures tremendously meaningful for patients.

ASSESSMENT OF TREATMENT RESPONSE IN SEVERE DEMENTIA

The cholinesterase inhibitors donepezil, galantamine and rivastigmine enhance cholinergic neurotransmission and provide cognitive, functional and behavioural benefits in mild-to-moderate AD.[47–49] Further data show donepezil to be effective in moderate-to-severe disease.[50–51] Memantine, an NMDA-receptor antagonist, has been shown to be efficacious in moderate-to-severe AD[52,53] and severe AD.[54] Memantine positively influenced both cognitive and functional impairment. Memantine is, so far, the only drug approved on the indication for severe AD. Furthermore, memantine was recently approved in Europe for moderate AD.

When treating patients with severe dementia using antidementia drugs, there are obstacles in evaluating the effects of treatment, whether pharmacological or not, for the individual patient. In later stages of the disease, patients will be limited or unable to assess and report treatment effects due to their reduced ability for verbal communication, decline in memory and comprehension, and reduced ability for abstract thinking. Clinical experience indicates that effects of drug treatment can often be observed through more or less subtle changes in the person, for example an improved ability to manage ADL, increased attention, better ability to understand or to be understood and/or an improved walking ability. Such changes might be very difficult for the patient's physician to observe when briefly meeting the patent on an occasional basis. Arguably, those closest to the patient are the ones most familiar with the person, and thus also most sensitive to changes, for example in functional ability, mood, communication and/or the presence of behavioural symptoms. This means that, in evaluating treatment effects, physicians will to some extent be dependent on assessments made by others such as staff and relatives.

When being forced to rely on others' evaluation of treatment effects, it is important that these are assessed and reported in such a way that makes the information trustworthy for the physician. A common language is needed to increase the trustworthiness of this important information and there is a need to establish domains guiding the assessment, and to develop concepts facilitating reporting of these assessments. Traditional instruments have some shortcomings in that they often focus on cognition and symptoms of the disease, containing concepts not always easy to interpret for staff and relatives. Thus there seems to be a need for developing an assessment guide for staff and relatives that is easy to interpret and use, but at the same time covers areas regarded as significant in detecting treatment effects.

A two-phase project was carried out aiming to establish a tool to help physicians to evaluate effects of antidementia drug treatment. This project was based on the assumption that staff and relatives closest to the person with dementia are the most sensitive to change, and thus best suitable to assess whether or not a drug has had an observable effect. It was decided that such a tool needed to meet four criteria: being based on domains identified as most important for staff and relatives' observations, i.e. aspects that staff and relatives use to focus their assessment on when expecting a drug to be of importance, being sensitive to change, being based on concepts easy to interpret and communicate and not being extensively time consuming.

First, interview data were collected from nursing staff and physicians with extensive experience of working in psycho-geriatric care, as well as from nurses with vast experience of clinical trials of antidementia drugs and from relatives of patients with severe dementia. In the interviews, participants were asked to identify and describe areas they focus upon when evaluating treatment effects of antidementia drugs. The interviews were analysed using a content analysis[55] and five domains were identified: functional ability, communication, mood, interaction and imposed burden. Second, those five domains laid the foundation for the development of 20 items covering the domains described by informed participants as most essential when evaluating treatment effect (see Table 19.7).

The SWE Tool (Sandman, Winblad, Edvardsson Assessment Tool) is presented in Figure 19.1 and Table 19.8. As shown in the figure and table, the final tool consists of one sheet (A4) with a front and a back page. In the front, the user is provided with a short instruction on how to use the tool, together with the 20 items assessing change. All 20 items need to be accounted for. Each item is to be assessed on a five-grade scale: much worse (−2), worse (−1) unchanged (0), better (+1) and much better (+2). The items are not weighted and the tool is not to be summarized in

Table 19.7 Items included in the SWE Tool	
Orientation to person	Mood
Orientation to place	Sadness
Orientation in time	Anxiety
Speed	Aggressiveness
Presence	ADL
Memory	Mobility
Initiative	Comprehension
Interest	Verbal communication
Stress tolerance	Well-being
Concern	Burden of care

a total score. The back page provides the user with a short description of each item. For example, 'Presence' is described as: 'The perception of to what extent the patient is emotionally present when spoken to or activated, degree of awakeness and contactability.'

When using the SWE Tool for the first assessment after prescribing an antidementia drug, observation about the patient's current clinical status is the departure for comparison. The assessment tool in its present form cannot and should not be used to fill in baseline data. It might be used merely as a guide in assessing the patient's present clinical status. In the clinical setting, those who are instructed to use the assessment tool must be very familiar with the patient. They are to be informed to base their assessments on *changes* in the patient's status and base their assessment of the patient's status during the last week. This assessment should then be compared to the clinical status of the patient when the drug was prescribed.

It is a clinical decision whether a treatment should be continued or not. The SWE Tool functions as an aid in making an informed decision based on high-quality data as reported by those having the closest everyday contact with the patient and who are therefore seemingly the most sensitive to change in the patient's status. When a drug is prescribed, the physician provides the SWE Tool, along with information about the drug, to the person who will perform the assessment. Short information is given about the SWE Tool, and the staff member or the relative is asked to make the assessment before the next visit to the physician.

In clinical practice, a global assessment must guide the physician in continuing or discontinuing the prescription. For example, the patient's status can be assessed as being slightly worsened in certain items but at the same time significantly improved in another, for example in communication, mobility and/or ADL functions. It is up to the physician to decide how to value the information gathered with the assessment tool.

The SWE Tool is not a quantitative scale and has not been formally tested for validity and reliability. On the other hand, the SWE Tool has been proven to be of clinical value, especially for primary care physicians. Clinical experience suggests that it enhances the physician's ability to make informed decisions about continuing/discontinuing treatments.

CONCLUSION

For people with dementia suffering from a progressive disease that affects their competence in a broad sense, care can be organized either from a biomedical model of behaviour as a disturbing symptom or from a humanistic/communicative model of behaviour as a form of communication. Which model is adopted depends upon how behavioural symptoms are viewed. In these two models, the content as well as the provision of care will rest upon different assumptions and thus interventions and the doing and being of staff will also differ. This is not to say that the two models necessarily are in conflict, but should rather be seen as complementary. Nevertheless, it is of therapeutic importance not only to develop strategies on how to use and adapt the environment to compensate for the diminished competence of people with dementia, but also to identify instruments and outcome measures to follow these adaptations.[29] To date there are few indicators by which it is possible to evaluate whether or not the environment of dementia care supports well-being among patients with dementia and there is little consensus about which factors are the most important.[41] The SWE Tool is a significant contribution in this regard. In the severe stage of dementia, interventions should target not only the physical environment but also the whole human environment in care settings for patients with dementia.

Name of rater: .... Name and age of the patient: ....

SWE TOOL
(Sandman PO, Winblad B, Evardsson D)[c]

> Instruction: The form consists of 20 questions. The assessment of effect of treatment is based upon an interview with the caregiver and/or relative and their perception of the patient during the latest week. Each question is described in detail on the back of the form. Ask these questions to the relative or caregiver. The rating is based on the observed abilities of the patient. The rating is an assessment of change and should be evaluated in relation to the latest assessment.

Date of rating .... | Actual MMSE score ....

Treatment started (date) .... | Information obtained from:

Medication (mg/day) ....(...................) | ❏ Carer (name, title) ....

Medication (mg/day) ....(...................) | ❏ Relative (name, rel.) ....

Type of dementia .... | Assessment no:

Residential status .... | ❏ 1   ❏ 2   ❏ 3   ❏ 4   ❏ 5
                                                              ❏ 6   ❏ 7   ❏ 8   ❏ 9   ❏ 10

Much worse	Worse	Unchanged	Improved	Much improved		Much worse	Worse	Unchanged	Improved	Much improved
1. Person recognition ability						**11. Mood**				
❏ −−	❏ −	❏ 0	❏ +	❏ ++		❏ −−	❏ −	❏ 0	❏ +	❏ ++
2. Spatial orientation						**12. Sadness**				
❏ −−	❏ −	❏ 0	❏ +	❏ ++		❏ −−	❏ −	❏ 0	❏ +	❏ ++
3. Orientation in time						**13. Anxiety**				
❏ −−	❏ −	❏ 0	❏ +	❏ ++		❏ −−	❏ −	❏ 0	❏ +	❏ ++
4. Speed						**14. Aggressiveness**				
❏ −−	❏ −	❏ 0	❏ +	❏ ++		❏ −−	❏ −	❏ 0	❏ +	❏ ++
5. Presence						**15. ADL**				
❏ −−	❏ −	❏ 0	❏ +	❏ ++		❏ −−	❏ −	❏ 0	❏ +	❏ ++
6. Memory						**16. Mobility**				
❏ −−	❏ −	❏ 0	❏ +	❏ ++		❏ −−	❏ −	❏ 0	❏ +	❏ ++
7. Initiative						**17. Perception**				
❏ −−	❏ −	❏ 0	❏ +	❏ ++		❏ −−	❏ −	❏ 0	❏ +	❏ ++
8. Interest						**18. Verbal communication**				
❏ −−	❏ −	❏ 0	❏ +	❏ ++		❏ −−	❏ −	❏ 0	❏ +	❏ ++
9. Stress tolerance						**19. Well-being**				
❏ −−	❏ −	❏ 0	❏ +	❏ ++		❏ −−	❏ −	❏ 0	❏ +	❏ ++
10. Caring						**20. Burden of care**				
❏ −−	❏ −	❏ 0	❏ +	❏ ++		❏ −−	❏ −	❏ 0	❏ +	❏ ++

Figure 19.1 SWE Tool to follow up on treatment of dementia (front page).

Table 19.8 SWE Tool to follow up on treatment of dementia (back page)

1. Person recognition ability
   The patient's ability to know who he/she is, recognize close relatives (spouse, children, grandchildren), friends, neighbours or other persons important to the patient

2. Spatial orientation
   The patient's ability to navigate in his/her own home (toilet, kitchen, bedroom), navigate outdoors in close vicinity of own home

3. Orientation in time
   The patient's ability to differentiate seasons, day and night, knowing the year, weekday, date, and time

4. Speed
   Perception of the speed with which the patient is performing activities of daily living, e.g. dressing and undressing, eating and moving from, for instance, chair to bed

5. Presence
   The perception of to what extent the patient is emotionally present when spoken to or activated, degree of awakeness and contactability

6. Memory
   The ability to remember relevant things in daily life

7. Initiative
   Perception of the patient's spontaneous initiative. More or less alert. Initiative could be to watch TV, pick up the newspaper, make a sandwich or start a conversation

8. Interest
   The patient's interest in, for instance, his or her looks, clothes, hairstyle or the food being served. Asking for persons or belongings

9. Stress tolerance
   The patient's ability to cope in stressful situations

10. Caring
    The patient's interest in others, ability to care emotionally for others

11. Mood
    A comprehensive evaluation of the patient's mood status

12. Sadness
    A comprehensive evaluation of verbal or behavioural expression of sadness, crying or despair

13. Anxiety
    A comprehensive evaluation of verbal or behavioural expression of anxiety or being worried

14. Aggressiveness
    A comprehensive evaluation of verbal or behavioural expression of aggression

15. ADL
    The patient's ability to dress, wash and eat, and continence. Doing more or less by him- or herself, contributing more, less resistance

16. Mobility
    Ability to move, balance

17. Perception
    The patient's ability to understand other people. Perceive situations correctly, know what is going on

18. Verbal communication
    The patient's ability to make him- or herself understood

19. Well-being
    A comprehensive evaluation of how the rated person feels. Expressions of peacefulness, calmness and satisfaction

20. Burden of care
    A global evaluation of the carer or relative's perception of the burden of care. Includes physical and psychological stress

Name of rater: . . . . Name and age of the patient: . . . .

REFERENCES

1. Sandman PO, Adolfsson R, Norberg A, Nyström L, Winblad B. Long-term care of the elderly. A descriptive study of 3600 patients living in different institutions in the county of Västerboten, Sweden. Compr Gerontol 1988; 2:120–133.
2. Graneheim UH. The meaning of interaction between persons with dementia and disturbing behaviour and their care providers [in Swedish]. Umeå University Medical Dissertations, New Series No 906, Umeå, Sweden 2004.
3. Jansson L, Norberg A, Sandman PO, Athlin E, Asplund K. Interpreting facial expressions in patients in the terminal stage of the Alzheimer disease. OMEGA 1993; 26:309–324.
4. Athlin E, Norberg A, Asplund K. Caregivers' perceptions and interpretations of severely demented patients during feeding in a task assignment system. Scand J Caring Sci 1990; 4:147–156.
5. Normann HK. Lucidity in people with severe dementia as a consequence of person-centered care. Umeå University Medical Dissertations, New series no 753, Department of Advanced Nursing.
6. Zingmark K, Norberg A, Sandman PO. Experience of at-homeness and homesickness in patients with Alzheimer's disease. Am J Alzheimer's Care Relat Disord Res 1993; 8:10–16.
7. Zingmark K, Sandman PO, Norberg A. Promoting a good life among people with Alzheimer's disease. J Adv Nurs 2002; 38:50–58.
8. Edberg A-K. The nurse–patient encounter and the patient's state. Effects of individual care and clinical group supervision in dementia care. Medical dissertation, The Medical Faculty, Lund University, Sweden. Bulletin No 2 from the Center of Caring Sciences and Department of Clinical Neuroscience.
9. Finkel SI, Costa e Silva J, Cohen G, Miller S, Sartorius N. Behavioral and psychological signs and symptoms of dementia: a consensus statement on current knowledge and implications for research and treatment. Int Psychogeriatr 1996; 8(suppl 3):497–500.
10. Reisberg B, Oppenheim G. Alzheimer's disease – clinical course: methodologic implications for pharmacologic trials. Int Psychogeriatr 1992; 1:5–7.
11. Purundare N, Allen NPH, Burns A. Behavioural and psychological symptoms of dementia. Rev Clin Gerontol 2000; 10:245–260.
12. Grossberg GT, Desai AK. Management of Alzheimer's disease. J Gerontol Series A Biol Sci Med Sci 2003; 58:331–353.
13. Bains J, Birks JS, Dening TD. Antidepressants for treating depression in dementia. Cochrane Database of Systematic Reviews 2002 Issue 4: CD003944. DOI: 10.1002/14651858. CD003944.
14. Homma A. Parameters considered in multinational clinical drug trials. Int Psychogeriatr 1996; 8:165–167.
15. Karlsson S, Bucht G, Eriksson S, Sandman PO. Factors relating to the use of physical restraints in geriatric care settings. J Am Geriatr Soc 2001; 49:1722–1728.
16. Norberg KG, Hellzén O, Sandman PO, Asplund K. The relationship between organizational climate and the content of daily life for people with dementia living in a group-dwelling. J Clin Nurs 2002; 11:137–146.
17. Wimo A, Gustafsson L, Mattson B. Predictive validity of factors influencing the institutionalization of elderly people with psycho-geriatric disorders. Scand J Prim Health Care 1992; 10:185–191.
18. Clyburn LD, Stones MJ, Hadjistavropoulos T, Tuokko H. Predicting caregiver burden and depression in Alzheimer's disease. J Gerontol Series B Psychol Sci Social Sci 2000; 55:2–13.
19. Norberg A. Ethics in the care of the elderly with dementia. In: Gillion R, ed. Principles of Health Care Ethics, Chichester: Wiley, 1994 721–731.
20. Hallberg IR, Norberg A. Nurses' experiences of strain and their reactions in the care of severely demented patients. Int J Geriatr Psychiatry 1995; 10:757–766.
21. Miller BL, Darby A, Benson DF, Cummings JL, Miller MH. Aggressive, socially disruptive and antisocial behaviour associated with fronto-temporal dementia. Br J Psychiatry 1997; 170:150–155.
22. Holst G, Hallberg IR, Gustafson L. The relationship of vocally disruptive behaviour and previous personality in severely demented institutionalized patients. Arch Psychiatr Nurs 1997; 11:147–154.
23. Eriksson S, Minthon L, Moksnes KM, et al and the BPSD reference group. BPSD from a Nordic Perspective. Behavioural and Psychological symptoms in Dementia. A State-of-the-Art Document. Västra Frölunda, Sweden: Janssen Cilag AB 2000.
24. Robinson P, Giorgi B, Wahlund LO, Ekman SL. The experience of early dementia: a three-year longitudinal phenomenological case study in younger persons with suspected and early stage dementia: their experiences, concerns and need for support. Licentiate thesis, Department of Clinical Neuroscience, Occupational Therapy and Elderly Care Research, Division of Geriatric Medicine, Karolinska Institutet, Stockholm, Sweden.
25. Graneheim UH, Isaksson U, Persson Ljung I–M, Jansson L. Balancing between contradictions. The meaning of interaction with people suffering from dementia and 'behavioural disturbances'. Int J Aging Hum Dev. In press.
26. Graneheim UH, Norberg A, Jansson L. Interaction relating to privacy, identity, autonomy and security. An observational study focusing on a woman with dementia and 'behavioural disturbances' and on her care providers. J Adv Nurs 2001; 36:256–265.
27. Hallberg IR, Norberg A. Staff's interpretation of the experience behind vocally disruptive behaviour in severely demented patients and their feelings about it. An explorative study. Int J Aging Hum Develop 1990; 31:295–305.
28. Desai AK, Grossberg GT. Recognition and management of behavioural disturbances in dementia. J Clin Psychiatry 2001; 3:93–109.
29. Lawton MP. Environment and Aging. Albany: Center for the Study of Aging 1986.
30. Carp FM. Assessing the environment. Ann Rev Gerontol Geriatr 1994; 14:302–314.
31. Diaz Moore K. Dissonance in the dining room: a study of social interaction in a special care unit. Qual Health Res 1999; 9:133–155.
32. McAllister CL, Silverman MA. Community formation and community roles among persons with Alzheimer's disease: a comparative study of experiences in a residential Alzheimer's facility and a traditional nursing home. Qual Health Res 1999; 9:65–85.
33. Morgan DG, Stewart NJ. The physical environment of special care units: needs of residents with dementia from the perspective of staff and family caregivers. Qual Health Res 1999; 9:105–119.
34. Zeisel J, Silverstein N, Hyde J, et al. Environmental correlates to behavioral health outcomes in Alzheimer's special care units. Gerontologist 2003; 43:697–711.
35. Bråne G, Karlsson I, Kihlgren M, Norberg A. Integrity-promoting care of demented nursing home patients:

psychological and biochemical changes. Int J Geriatr Psychol 1989; 4:165–172.

36. Götestam KG, Melin L. Improving well-being for patients with senile dementia by minor changes in the ward environment. In: Levi L, ed. Society, Stress and Disease. Oxford: Oxford University Press 1987, 295–297.

37. Cohen-Mansfield J, Werner P. The effects of an enhanced environment on nursing home residents who pace. Gerontologist 2000; 38:199–208.

38. Mooney P, Nicell PL. The importance of exterior environment for Alzheimer residents: effective care and risk management. Healthcare Mgmnt Forum 1992; 5:23–29.

39. Day K, Carreon D, Stump C. The therapeutic design of environments for people with dementia: a review of the empirical research. Gerontologist 2000; 40:397–416.

40. Sloane PD, Mitchell CM, Weisman G, et al. The therapeutic environment screening survey for nursing homes (TESS-NH): an observational instrument for assessing the physical environment of institutional settings for persons with dementia. J Gerontol Social Sci 2002; 57B:69–78.

41. Grant LA. Conceptualizing and measuring social and physical environments in special care units. Alzheimer Dis Assoc Disord 1994; 8:321–327.

42. Werezak LJ, Morgan DG. Creating a therapeutic psychosocial environment in dementia care. A preliminary framework. J Gerontol Nursing 2003; 29:18–25.

43. Norberg A. Interaction with people suffering severe dementia. In: Wimo A, Jönsson B, Karlsson G, Winblad B, eds. Health Economics of Dementia. Chichester: Wiley, 1998 113–121.

44. Edvardsson D. Atmosphere in care settings – towards a broader understanding of the phenomenon. Umeå University Medical Dissertations, New Series No 941, Umeå, Sweden 2005.

45. Edvardsson D, Sandman PO, Rasmussen B. Sensing an atmosphere of ease – a tentative theory of supportive ward environments. Scand J Caring Sci in press.

46. Edvardsson D, Sandman PO, Rasmussen B. Meanings of being in the physical environment of an oncology clinic. J Adv Nursing in press.

47. Whitehead A, Perdomo C, Pratt RD, et al. Donepezil for the symptomatic treatment of patients with mild to moderate Alzheimer's disease: a meta-analysis of individual patient data from randomised controlled trials. Int J Geriatr Psychiatry 2004; 19:624–633.

48. Ritchie CW, Ames D, Clayton T, Lai R. Metaanalysis of randomized trials of the efficacy and safety of donepezil, galantamine, and rivastigmine for the treatment of Alzheimer disease. Am J Geriatr Psychiatry 2004; 289:358–369.

49. Trinh NH, Hoblyn J, Mohanty S, Yaffe K. Efficacy of cholinesterase inhibitors in the treatment of neuropsychiatric symptoms and functional impairment in Alzheimer disease: a meta-analysis. JAMA 2003; 289:210–216.

50. Feldman H, Gauthier S, Hecker J, et al. A 24-week, randomized, double-blind study of donepezil in moderate to severe Alzheimer's disease (published erratum appears in Neurology 2001; 57:2153). Neurology 2001; 57:613–620.

51. Feldman H, Gauthier S, Hecker J, et al. Efficacy and safety of donepezil in patients with more severe Alzheimer's disease: a subgroup analysis from a randomized, placebo-controlled trial. Int J Geriatr Psychiatry 2005; 20:559–569.

52. Reisberg B, Doody R, Stoffler A, et al. Memantine in moderate to severe Alzheimer's disease. N Engl J Med 2003; 348:1333–1341.

53. Tariot PN, Farlow MR, Grossberg GT, et al. Memantine treatment in patients with moderate to severe Alzheimer disease already receiving donepezil: a randomized controlled trial. JAMA 2004; 291:317–324.

54. Winblad B, Poritis N. Memantine in severe dementia: results of the 9M-Best Study (Benefit and efficacy in severely demented patients during treatment with memantine). Int J Geriatr Psychiatry 1999; 14:135–146.

55. Graneheim UH, Lundman B. Qualitative content analysis in nursing research: concepts, procedures and measures to achieve trustworthiness. Nurse Ed Today 2004; 24:105–112.

20

Terminal stage

Ladislav Volicer

There are several issues that need to be addressed when providing care for individuals with advanced dementia. These issues include appropriate management of symptoms such as pain and behavioural problems, decisions regarding various medical interventions and involvement in programmes such as hospice. A crucial component of this care is providing information about benefits and burdens of these interventions to the proxy of the individual with dementia and supporting development of a care plan that takes into consideration previous wishes of the individual, if any, and his/her best interest as interpreted by the proxy decision-maker. The care plan should consider the goals of care and priority order of the three possible goals – survival, maintenance of function and comfort.[1]

It should be recognized that advanced dementia is a terminal illness similar to incurable cancer because there is no treatment that will stop or reverse its progression. The terminal stage can be defined as a state when patient is unable to ambulate even with assistance and is unable to communicate with the environment.[2] However, even this stage of dementia is often not perceived as a terminal illness and the prognosis is vastly overestimated. At nursing home admission, only 1 per cent of individuals with advanced dementia were perceived to have a life expectancy of less than 6 months, while 71 per cent died during that period.[3] Therefore, it is often not recognized that palliative approach is the optimal care for these individuals and non-palliative interventions are quite common: tube feeding in 25 per cent, laboratory tests in 49 per cent, restraints in 11 per cent and intravenous therapy in 10 per cent of the individuals with advanced dementia.[3] Individuals with advanced dementia do not understand the need and purpose of medical interventions and may be disturbed by discomfort induced by these procedures. Therefore, there is a need for a careful evaluation of the balance betweens benefits and burdens before any medical procedure is initiated. Some of the medical procedures routinely performed for cognitively intact individuals may not be appropriate for individuals with advanced dementia.

CARDIOPULMONARY RESUSCITATION

Cardiopulmonary resuscitation (CPR) is rarely successful in individuals who reside in an institution as many individuals with advanced dementia do. The survival to discharge from an acute care hospital after cardiac arrest in a nursing home ranges from 0 to 5 per cent, and is even lower when the arrest is unwitnessed.[4] In a sample of 114 nursing home individuals, 10 per cent of individuals were discharged from hospitals alive but no one with an unwitnessed cardiac arrest was successfully resuscitated.[5] Similarly, in a community sample, survival rate after unwitnessed arrest is much lower (0.8 per cent) than after witnessed arrest (5.3 per cent).[6] Dementia further decreases the probability that CPR will be successful. Even in a hospital, CPR is three times less likely to be successful in patients with dementia than in patients who are cognitively intact, and the success rate is almost as low as in metastatic cancer.[7]

The benefits of successful resuscitation are further diminished by other factors. CPR is a stressful experience for those who survive, often associated with injuries such as broken ribs and necessitating mechanical respiration. Those who initially survive CPR are taken to an intensive care unit, where most die within 24 hours.[4] The intensive care unit environment produces additional confusion and, almost invariably, delirium. In samples from other populations, approximately one-third of those who survive hospitalization will suffer increased dependence and some will have severe mental impairment.[4] Furthermore, the CPR experience is often sufficiently traumatic for the patient's families that they will request a Do Not Resuscitate (DNR) order to prevent repetition of CPR.

Considering the balance of benefits and burdens, it was suggested that CPR in a nursing home setting should be an optional procedure that should be specifically requested instead of depending on the presence of DNR orders.[4] This would be a difference from the current status where CPR is considered a default option. However, the CPR is currently used relatively rarely in individuals dying in a nursing home, ranging from 2 to 5.6 per cent of deaths.[4] A survey of 36 nursing home facilities showed that less than 30 per cent of them had performed CPR in the past 6 months, and 23 per cent had not written DNR policies. A majority of facilities (79 per cent) required CPR in witnessed arrests of non-DNR individuals, while a minority (24 per cent) required CPR even in unwitnessed arrest.[8]

HOSPITALIZATION

Hospitalization may not be a necessary and an optimal strategy for management of intercurrent diseases in individuals with advanced dementia. Transfer from a nursing home to a hospital results in decline of psychophysiological functioning including mobility, transfer, toileting, feeding and grooming, and none of these functions improve significantly at discharge. Risk factors for this functional decline are cognitive impairment, previous functional impairment, low social activity level and decubitus ulcers.[9] Patients often develop confusion, anorexia, incontinence and falls. These symptoms are often managed by aggressive medical interventions, even in patients with advanced dementia.[10] Similar consequences of hospitalization would be expected in individuals with advanced dementia who are hospitalized from home.

Transfer of individuals to an acute care setting may not be optimal for management of infections and other conditions. A study found that 36 per cent of emergency room transfers and 40 per cent of hospital admissions were inappropriate for medical reasons and this number increased to 44 per cent of emergency room transfers and 45 per cent of hospital admissions when advance directives were considered.[11] The occurrence of hospitalization is reduced if a nursing home has a dementia special care unit, greater physician-to-patient ratio and a physician extender[12] indicating that better care could be provided in a nursing home if resources are available.

Immediate survival and mortality rates are similar whether treatment for pneumonia is provided in a long-term care facility or hospital[13,14] and long-term outcomes are better in individuals treated in a nursing home. The 6-week mortality rate was 18.7 per cent in non-hospitalized individuals and 39.5 per cent in hospitalized individuals, despite no significant differences between the hospitalized and non-hospitalized groups before diagnosis.[15] Similarly, 2 months after the onset of pneumonia, a greater proportion of hospitalized individuals had declined in their functional status or died. However, this improved outcome was seen only in individuals with lower respiratory rate during infection and in those who were independent or mildly dependent at the baseline.[16]

INTERCURRENT INFECTIONS

The most common infections in individuals with dementia are urinary tract infection (UTI), upper respiratory infection, lower respiratory tract infection, cutaneous infection, gastrointestinal infection and eye infection.[17] These infections are almost an inevitable consequence of advanced dementia for several reasons. There is an evidence that immune responses are reduced in advanced dementia,[18] decreasing the ability to resist development of an infection. Risk of development of UTIs is increased by incontinence, especially in women, and by urinary retention in men.[19] Swallowing difficulties with bronchoaspiration present an increasing risk of developing respiratory infections[20] and inability to ambulate independently is increasing risk of urinary and respiratory infections, deep vein thrombosis and infected pressure ulcers.[21] It is also more difficult to diagnose infections in individuals with dementia because of aphasia and because even individuals with mild dementia are less likely to report cough, rash, gastrointestinal symptoms and joint pain than cognitively intact controls.[22] Functional impairment is also an important factor because dependence for feeding and for oral care is the most significant factor predicting development of aspiration pneumonia in institutionalized elderly.[23]

Pneumonia is the most common type of infection among individuals of long-term care facilities, with a median reported incidence of 1 per 1000 patient-days.[24] Risk of pneumonia is increased in individuals who are confined to bed, have a debilitating neurological disease and who are fed by a tube.[9] Other risk factors include older age, male sex, swallowing difficulties and inability to take oral medications.[25] Very often, the pneumonia recurs and patients discharged from hospital after pneumonia have a 5 times higher risk for recurrence of pneumonia than patients admitted for other conditions.[9] Actually, 43 per cent of nursing home individuals who survive an episode of pneumonia develop another episode within 12 months.[24] The mortality rate from pneumonia is increased by altered mental status[26] and cognitive impairment increases the risk of mortality almost 7 times.[27] Pneumonia mortality is also increased by functional impairment, even in individuals living in the community,[28] and that would probably be true also for individuals in assisted living facilities.

Some strategies are available for decreasing the risk of development of intercurrent infections. Avoidance of internal urinary catheters is the most important prevention strategy for UTIs because the bladder is usually colonized with bacteria within 30 days after indwelling catheter insertion. Antimicrobial prophylaxis is effective in decreasing the recurrence of UTIs but is potentially toxic and leads to the development of antibiotic-resistant bacteria. Administration of oestrogen for atrophic vaginitis decreases the frequency of symptomatic cystitis in elderly women prone to this recurrent disease.[21] Oestrogen deficiency causes a lack of lactobacilli in the vaginal flora, but oral intake of yogurt was not found to increase vaginal colonization by lactobacilli.[29] Administration of cranberry juice decreased the number of symptomatic UTIs in women but the optimum dosage and method of administration are not clear.[30] In contrast, attempts to acidify urine by administration of ascorbic acid did not change the urinary pH and did not decrease UTIs in patients with spinal cord injury[31] and, therefore, would also not be effective in individuals with advanced dementia.

Residual urine in the bladder after voiding, caused by bladder outlet obstruction, an underactive detrusor or detrusor hyperactivity with impaired contractility, promotes bacteriuria. The residual volume may be reduced by massaging the abdomen (Crede manoeuvre) and by straight catheterization on a regular basis. Discontinuation of anticholinergic medications that inhibit bladder contraction can decrease bladder volume. Administration of doxazosin or finasteride may improve bladder emptying in patients with outlet obstruction. In individuals who are still surgical candidates, prostatectomy may resolve obstruction resulting in decreased residual volume.[21]

Incidence of upper respiratory infections and pneumonia may be reduced by vaccinations. Evidence for effectiveness of pneumococcal vaccination is highly controversial,[20] but a study in an institutionalized population showed that vaccination decreased significantly the risk of pneumonia, risk of death due to pneumonia and risk of all deaths.[32] Current recommendation is to vaccinate with pneumococcal vaccine all individuals over the age of 65 and repeat the vaccine every 5–10 years.[20] Influenza vaccine is effective in community-living[33] and institutionalized elderly,[34] even though it does not provide complete protection against influenza epidemics.[35] It is recommended that influenza vaccination should be given annually.

Swallowing difficulty with resulting aspiration is a major risk for development of aspiration pneumonia. Aspiration of nasopharyngeal secretions occurs during sleep in half of healthy adults, but a low burden of virulent bacteria in normal saliva together with a normal cough reflex and ciliary transport and normal immune mechanisms protect the airways from repeated infections.[20] Silent aspiration is present in a large percentage of individuals who develop pneumonia in the community.[36] With development of swallowing difficulties during progression of dementia, aspiration extends to food and liquids and results in choking during food intake. Choking during eating usually starts with thin liquids because swallowing of thin liquids requires the best coordination of muscles involved in swallowing. Choking can be prevented by switching from thin liquids to thick liquids, e.g. from milk to yogurt.[37]

Other strategies to prevent aspiration pneumonia include oral hygiene, avoidance of smoking and endotracheal intubation and potentiation of the cough reflex. Periodontal disease and dental plaques are risk factors for development of pneumonia. In dentate individuals, risk factors for development of aspiration pneumonia included requiring help with feeding, chronic obstructive pulmonary disease, diabetes mellitus, number of decayed teeth, number of functional teeth and presence of specific microbes in the saliva.[38] Oral care was shown to decrease incidence of pneumonia, number of febrile days and death from pneumonia.[39] Decreased salivary production increases colonization of the oral cavity by pathogens and is often caused by drugs with anticholinergic effects.[40]

The cough reflex protects against aspiration and its enhancement decreases the risk of aspiration pneumonia. The cough reflex is enhanced by angiotensin converting enzyme inhibitors because they also inhibit metabolism of substance P that is an important mediator of cough reflex.[41] Another mechanism to increase the cough reflex is potentiation of the dopaminergic system by administration of amantadine.[42] Both of these strategies significantly decrease the incidence of aspiration pneumonia. Tube feeding is not useful for prevention of aspiration pneumonia because it actually increases the rate of pneumonia development and the pneumonia death rate in individuals who had evidence of aspiration on videofluoroscopy.[43] Tube feeding will be further discussed below.

Antibiotic therapy of intercurrent infections

Antibiotic therapy is quite effective in the treatment of single episodes of intercurrent infections in individuals with dementia. However, its effectiveness is limited by the recurrent nature of infections in advanced dementia. Dementia severity increases the mortality after pneumonia because of aspiration and weight loss.[44] Antibiotic therapy does not prolong survival in individuals with severe dementia who are unable to communicate and unable to ambulate alone or with assistance.[45–47] Antibiotic therapy is not necessary for maintenance of symptom control during an infection episode because the observed comfort levels are similar in individuals who receive antibiotic therapy and in individuals who receive palliative care only (analgesics, antipyretics, oxygen).[48,49]

If antibiotics are administered they should be given orally because this route is as effective as parenteral administration and results in less discomfort. Intravenous therapy is difficult in cognitively impaired individuals who do not understand the need for this intervention and often try to remove the intravenous catheters. In patients with poor oral intake, intramuscular administration of cephalosporins offers a reasonable alternative. When antibiotics are used, they may cause significant adverse effects, such as diarrhoea, gastrointestinal upset, allergic reaction, hyperkalemia and rarely agranulocytosis. Diagnostic procedures, such as blood drawing and sputum suctioning, which are necessary for the rational use of antibiotics, cause confusion and discomfort in a individual who does not understand their need and do not reveal the source of infection in 30 per cent of cases.[45]

NUTRITIONAL ISSUES

Nutritional issues in progressive degenerative dementias include weight loss, apraxia that makes use of utensils difficult, chewing difficulties and food refusal. In the severe and terminal stages of dementia individuals also develop swallowing difficulties and may be unable/unwilling to open their mouths.[37] Weight loss may be caused by decreased food intake or by intensive pacing that can result in a significant increase of energy expenditure.[50] It is always important to determine whether the weight loss is being caused because the individuals are not fed correctly. Poor professional supervision and inadequate staffing can result in decreased intake of food and liquids in an institu-

tion.[51] The target weight for individuals with advanced dementia should take into consideration their functional impairment. If they are unable to ambulate even with assistance, the individuals experience atrophy of their leg muscles from disuse. In that case, their ideal body weight may be much lower than the weight listed in tables that consider only height and frame and this lower weight is not an indication of malnutrition.[52]

Apraxia results in inability to use utensils but the individuals may be still able to feed themselves finger food. With the progression of dementia, the individuals will be ultimately unable to feed themselves or drink without assistance. However, adequate nutrition can be provided by hand feeding utilizing a modified diet that is adapted to the ability of individuals to chew and to their swallowing difficulties.[37] Hand feeding can be provided until the beginning of the dying process, when all physiological processes shut down and individuals do not feel hunger and thirst. Voluntary refusal of food and liquids is often initiated by hospice patients and does not result in discomfort. Hospice nurses reported that such individuals usually die within two weeks and rated their death experience as 8 on the scale from 0 (bad death) to 9 (a very good death).[53] Unfortunately, quite often the hand feeding is replaced by feeding through a nasogastric tube or through a percutaneous endoscopic gastrostomy (PEG) tube. Although no randomized control trials investigating the effectiveness of tube feeding were performed, the current evidence indicates that tube feeding does not prevent aspiration pneumonia and might actually increase its incidence, and does not prevent consequences of malnutrition.[54] Tube feeding also does not increase survival in most studies, does not prevent or improve pressure ulcers, does not reduce the risk of infections and does not improve functional status or comfort of the patient. No recent study challenged these conclusions.

Providing nutrition by a tube has many adverse consequences, including discomfort from the tube and restraints that are often necessary to prevent tube removal, lack of enjoyment of oral intake of food, lack of contact with care providers during the feeding process and medical complications of tube placement. It is also not recognized that it is possible to convert tube feeding into hand feeding and, in some cases, individuals may be able to feed themselves again.[55] Tube feeding can be prevented if family members and the healthcare team recognize advanced dementia as a terminal illness and strive for maintaining quality of life instead of maximal survival. It is easier to reach agreement that tube feeding should not be used if this option is discussed earlier in the course of dementia, before the patient starts choking on food and liquids or losing weight. At that time, it is easier for families to understand that tube feeding would not provide any benefit and that hand feeding can be used to maintain nutrition until the dying process.[56] Formation of a palliative care team, which had to be consulted whenever a feeding tube was being considered, and an educational programme resulted in a significant decrease in the number of all patients given feeding tubes as well as in the number of patients with dementia given feeding tubes.[57]

DECISIONS ABOUT END-OF-LIFE CARE

Individuals with advanced dementia cannot make decisions about their end-of-life care and, therefore, these decisions have to be made by their surrogates. The decisions should be made either on the basis of the individual's previous wishes or, when these wishes are not known, on the basis of the individual's best interest as perceived by the surrogate. An individual's previous wishes could be made formal by a living will that was completed before the individual became demented or may be just verbal communication expressing the individual's philosophy regarding end-of-life care. The problem with living wills is that they are very often quite general and do not cover advanced dementia. Advance directive forms often contain inconsistent language and vague conditions for implementation. As a result of that, few individuals with advance dementia receive hospice services, and many die without family present and with little documented evidence of pain or symptom management.[58]

Most individuals (93–95 per cent) would not want cardiopulmonary resuscitation if they were severely demented.[59] However, the decision depends on the way the scenario is presented and depends very much on the person's knowledge of or experience with Alzheimer's disease (AD). Those who had this knowledge refused CPR more often, while knowledge of CPR did not make any difference.[60] About two-thirds of normal older adults would want additional treatment limitations; no hospitalization and no antibiotics, if they were severely demented.[61]

The end-of-life care decision that is most often discussed and made is a 'do not resuscitate' (DNR) status. DNR orders in nursing populations are associated with advanced age, cognitive dysfunction, physical dependency, presence of advance directives or durable power of attorney for health care, absence of Medicaid and daily visitors.[4] A DNR order is sometimes used by the care providers as a proxy for palliative care and results in more care limitations than just CPR.[62] Individuals with DNR orders are also less likely to be hospitalized during an acute illness episode than individual with a full code.[63] However, that is not the intent of the DNR order and all other treatment limitations should be discussed separately.

Decisions about tube feeding are highly emotional and often elicit court involvement. However, there is broad legal consensus that tube feeding is a medical procedure, which may be discontinued if the patient/proxy so desires, both in the United States and Australia.[64] Discontinuation of tube feeding is also supported by most religious ethicists.[65] The orthodox Jewish position is that tube feeding should be given as long as it does not constitute undue danger, arouse serious opposition or cause suffering to the patient.[66] A recent papal statement, supporting the use of tube feeding, was primarily targeted at maintaining tube feeding in individuals in a persistent vegetative state, who cannot perceive any suffering from tube feeding.[67] Since individuals with AD very rarely if ever progress into the persistent vegetative state,[68] this statement may not affect their care, although there could be differing opinions.[69]

Decisions about the end-of-life care may be made easier by the use of guidelines for clinicians and family members. Guidelines for palliative care in dementia resulted in a decrease in antibiotic prescriptions and increased use of analgesics, including opiates.[70] A checklist of considerations for decisions regarding treatment of pneumonia has been developed.[71] There are also two guidelines that specifically address the issue of tube feeding;[72,73] professional societies also developed guidelines,[74] or published illustrative cases.[75] Existing guidelines were recently reviewed and their end-of-life care content evaluated.[76] In the area of dementia, out of 56 possible guidelines, 24 were reviewed and 7 accepted for the study. The best four guidelines were issued by the American Medical Association,[77] American Psychiatric Association,[78] California Workgroup on Guidelines for Alzheimer's Disease Management[79] and American Medical Directors Association.[80]

HOSPICE CARE

Hospice organizations are able to provide palliative care for individuals with advanced dementia living in assisted living or nursing home facilities. The utilization of hospices for individuals with a primary diagnosis of dementia increased significantly from 1 per cent in 1995[81] to 9.6 per cent of patients in 2003.[82] This percentage is now similar to the percentage of deaths from AD estimated from epidemiological data in 1999 (7.1 per cent)[83] and the percentage of reported deaths from AD and cerebrovascular diseases (9 per cent).[84] Despite that, there is evidence that only 11 per cent of individuals with advanced dementia are referred to hospice.[85]

The main barrier to more widespread use of hospice care for individuals with advanced dementia is the requirement of a prognosis of 6 months or less in US Medicare program certified hospice programmes. The current Medicare guidelines are difficult to apply[46,47] and are not valid predictors of survival in hospice patients with dementia.[86] Other criteria for hospice eligibility were proposed but were not accepted by Medicare. Most recently, an estimation of prognosis based on the Minimum Data Set evaluations, was developed.[87] A risk score derived by this method is directly proportional to the number of individuals who die within 6 months, ranging from 2.7 per cent at a score of 0 to 75 per cent at a score of 12 or more. The problem is that the mortality increase is gradual with no clear cut-off point that could be used to eliminate hospice services from individuals with advanced dementia who will live longer than 6 months without excluding many individuals who die within 6 months. For instance, if the cut-off score is 9 or greater, 63 per cent of individuals will die within 6 months but 26 per cent or individuals with lower scores will also die within 6 months. Thus, a significant number of individuals is deprived of hospice services even though they die within the 6-month period. Applying strict criteria for hospice eligibility may be counterproductive because most studies showed that Medicare costs are lower for individuals enrolled in hospice care than for non-hospice individuals.[88,89]

Hospices provide important services to both the individual and his/her family. Involvement in a hospice improves management of pain. Hospice residents are twice as likely as non-hospice residents to receive regular treatment for daily pain, although the pain management is not always optimal even in hospice individuals.[90] Hospice involvement improves documentation of pain assessment and hospice individuals are more likely to receive opioid treatment than non-hospice individuals.[91] Management of pain in individuals with advanced dementia is complicated by the difficulty in assessment of pain presence and intensity because of the language and comprehension deficits. These individuals are unable to complete any pain assessment tools[92] and the pain assessment relies on observation of pain signs by a caregiver. Two observational scales were recently proposed,[93,94] but a study comparing them is not yet available.

Hospice services are also important for the family members and caregivers of individuals with dementia. Caregivers more often say that the hospice involve-ment benefits them than they would say that it benefits the patient. Caregivers value the continuous involvement of the patient's primary physician in his/her care, and an emphasis on avoiding hospitalization.[95] Hospices also provide social support and bereavement services that are not available in nursing homes.[96] Social support for caregivers of institutionalized individuals with dementia is very important because depressive symptoms and anxiety have been reported to be as high in caregivers after they institutionalized their relative as when they were in-home caregivers. The use of antidepressants does not change and the use of anxiolytics increases in caregivers after placement.[97] Caregivers of individuals with dementia involved in a hospice programme continue to be at risk for depression and having lower life satisfaction and physical health than non-caregivers.[98]

CONCLUSION

Current evidence clearly indicates that the palliative care approach is the optimal strategy for management of terminal dementia. Some medical procedures, such as cardiopulmonary resuscitation and tube feeding, are inappropriate in individuals with terminal dementia. Caution should be exercised when transfer to an emergency room or hospital is contemplated because this may not be the optimal strategy. Similarly, use of antibiotics in intercurrent infection should recognize the limitations of this treatment and be congruent with the goals of care.

REFERENCES

1. Gillick M, Berkman S, Cullen L. A patient-centered approach to advance medical planning in the nursing home. J Am Geriatr Soc 1999; 47:227–230.
2. Mahoney EK, Volicer L, Hurley AC. Management of Challenging Behaviours in Dementia. Baltimore: Health Professions Press 2000.
3. Mitchell SL, Kiely DK, Hamel MB. Dying with advanced dementia in the nursing home. Arch Intern Med 2004; 164:321–326.
4. Zweig SC. Cardiopulmonary resuscitation and do-not-resuscitate orders in the nursing home. Arch Fam Med 1997; 6:424–429.
5. Ghusn HF, Teasdale TA, Pepe PE, Ginger VF. Older nursing home residents have a cardiac arrest survival rate similar to that of older persons living in the community. J Am Geriatr Soc 1995; 43:520–527.
6. Lombardi G, Gallagher J, Gennis P. Outcome of out-of-hospital cardiac arrest in New York City. The pre-hospital arrest survival evaluation (PHASE) study. JAMA 1994; 271:678–683.
7. Ebell MH, Becker LA, Barry HC, Hagen M. Survival after in-hospital cardiopulmonary resuscitation. A meta-analysis. J Gen Int Med 1998; 13:805–816.

8. Ryden MB, Brand K, Weber E, Oh HL, Gross C. Nursing home resuscitation policies and practices for residents without DNR orders. Geriatr Nurs 1998; 19:315–319.

9. Volicer L, McKee A, Hewitt S. Dementia. Neurol Clin North Am 2001; 19:867–885.

10. Ahronheim JC, Morrison RS, Baskin SA, Morris J, Meier DE. Treatment of the dying in the acute care hospital. Advanced dementia and metastatic cancer. Arch Intern Med 1996; 156:2094–2100.

11. Saliba D, Kington R, Buchanan J, et al. Appropriateness of the decision to transfer nursing facility residents to the hospital. J Am Geriatr Soc 2000; 48:154–163.

12. Intrator O, Castle NG, Mor V. Facility characteristics associated with hospitalization of nursing home residents: results of a national study. Med Care 1999; 37:228–237.

13. Fried TR, Gillick MR, Lipsitz LA. Whether to transfer? Factors associated with hospitalization and outcome of elderly long-term care patients with pneumonia. J Gen Int Med 1995; 10:246–250.

14. Mylotte JP, Naughton B, Saludades C, Maszarovics Z. Validation and application of the pneumonia prognosis index to nursing home residents with pneumonia. JAGS 1998; 46:1538–1544.

15. Thompson RS, Hall NK, Szpiech M, Reisenberg LA. Treatments and outcomes of nursing-home-acquired pneumonia. J Am Board Fam Pract 1997; 10:82–87.

16. Fried TR, Gillick MR, Lipsitz LA. Short-term functional outcomes of long-term care residents with pneumonia treated with and without hospital transfer. JAGS 1997; 45:302–306.

17. Perls TT, Herget M. Higher respiratory infection rates on an Alzheimer's special care unit and successful intervention. J Am Geriatr Soc 1995; 43:1341–1344.

18. Ahluwalia N, Vellas B. Immunologic and inflammatory mediators and cognitive decline in Alzheimer's disease. Immunol Allergy Clin North Am 2003; 23:103.

19. Brown S. Systematic review of nursing management of urinary tract infections in the cognitively impaired elderly client in residential care: is there a hole in holistic care? Int J Nurs Pract 2002; 8:2–7.

20. Janssens JP, Krause KH. Pneumonia in the very old. Lancet Infect Dis 2004; 4:112–124.

21. Volicer L, Brandeis G, Hurley AC. Infections in advanced dementia. In: Volicer L, Hurley A, eds. Hospice Care for Patient with Advanced Progressive Dementia. New York: Springer Publishing Company 1998, 29–47.

22. McCormick WC, Kukull WA, Van Belle G, et al. Symptom patterns and comorbidity in the early stages of Alzheimer's disease. J Am Geriatr Soc 1994; 42:517–521.

23. Langmore SE, Terpenning MS, Schork A, et al. Predictors of aspiration pneumonia: how important is dysphagia? Dysphagia 1998; 13:69–81.

24. Muder RR, Brennen C, Swenson DL, Wagener M. Pneumonia in a long-term care facility. A prospective study of outcome. Arch Intern Med 1996; 156:2365–2370.

25. Loeb M, McGeer A, McArthur M, Walter S, Simor AE. Risk factors for pneumonia and other lower respiratory tract infections in elderly residents of long-term care facilities. Arch Intern Med 1999; 159:2058–2064.

26. Naughton BJ, Mylotte JM, Tayara A. Outcome of nursing home-acquired pneumonia: derivation and application of a practical model to predict 30 day mortality. J Am Geriatr Soc 2001; 48:1292–1299.

27. Medina-Walpole AM, McCormick WC. Provider practice patterns in nursing home-acquired pneumonia. J Am Geriatr Soc 1998; 46:187–192.

28. Covinsky KE, Palmer RM, Counsell SR, et al. Functional status before hospitalization in acutely ill older adults: validity and clinical importance of retrospective reports. J Am Geriatr Soc 2000; 48:164–169.

29. Colodner R, Edelstein H, Chasan B, Raz R. Vaginal colonization by orally administered Lactobacullus rhamnosus GG. Israel Med Assoc J 2003; 5:812–813.

30. Jepson RG, Mihajlevic L, Craig J. Cranberries for preventing urinary tract infections. Cochrane Database Syst Rev 2004; CD001321.

31. Castello T, Girona L, Gomez MR, Mena Mur A, Garcia L. The possible value of ascorbic acid as a prophylactic agent for urinary tract infection. Spinal Cord 1996; 34:592–593.

32. Wagner C, Popp W, Posch M, Vlasich C, Rosenberg-Spitzy A. Impact of pneumococcal vaccination on morbidity and mortality of geriatric patients: a case-controlled study. Gerontology 2003; 49:246–250.

33. Voordouw BC, van der Linden PD, Simonian S, et al. Influenza vaccination in community-dwelling elderly: impact on mortality and influenza-associated morbidity. Arch Intern Med 2003; 163:1089–1094.

34. Pregliasco F, Mensi C, Serpilli W, et al. Immunogenicity and safety of three commercial influenza vaccines in institutionalized elderly. Aging 2001; 13:38–43.

35. Brandeis GH, Berlowitz DR, Coughlin N. Mortality associated with an influenza outbreak on a dementia care unit. Alzheimer Dis Assoc Disord 1998; 12:140–145.

36. Kikuchi R, Watabe N, Konno T, et al. High incidence of silent aspiration in elderly patients with community-acquired pneumonia. Am J Resp Crit Care Med 1994; 150:251–253.

37. Morris J, Volicer L. Nutritional management of individuals with Alzheimer's disease and other progressive dementias. Nutr Clin Care 2001; 4:148–155.

38. Terpenning MS, Taylor GW, Lopatin DE, et al. Aspiration pneumonia: dental and oral risk factors in an older veteran population. J Am Geriatr Soc 2001; 49:557–563.

39. Yoneyama T, Yoshida M, Ohrui T, Mukaiyama H. Oral care reduces pneumonia in older patients in nursing homes. J Am Geriatr Soc 2002; 50:430–433.

40. Palmer LB, Albulak K, Fields S, et al. Oral clearance and pathogenic oropharyngeal colonization in the elderly. Am J Resp Crit Care Med 2001; 164:464–468.

41. Sekizawa K, Matsui T, Nakagawa T, Nakayama K, Sasaki H. ACE inhibitors and pneumonia. Lancet 1998; 352:1069.

42. Nakagawa T, Wada H, Sekizawa K, Arai H, Sasaki H. Amantadine and pneumonia. Lancet 1999; 353:1157.

43. Croghan JE, Burke EM, Caplan S, Denman S. Pilot study of 12-month outcomes of nursing home patients with aspiration on videofluoroscopy. Dysphagia 1994; 9:141–146.

44. Van der Steen JT, Ooms ME, Mehr DR, Van der Wal G, Ribbe MW. Severe dementia and adverse outcomes of nursing home-acquired pneumonia: evidence for mediation by functional and pathophysiological decline. J Am Geriatr Soc 2002; 50:439–448.

45. Fabiszewski KJ, Volicer B, Volicer L. Effect of antibiotic treatment on outcome of fevers in institutionalized Alzheimer patients. JAMA 1990; 263:3168–3172.

46. Luchins DJ, Hanrahan P, Murphy K. Criteria for enrolling dementia patients in hospice. J Am Geriatr Soc 1997; 45:1054–1059.

47. Hanrahan P, Raymond M, McGowan E, Luchins DJ. Criteria for enrolling dementia patients in hospice: a replication. Am J Hospice Pall Care 1999; 16:395–400.

48. Hurley AC, Volicer B, Mahoney MA, Volicer L. Palliative fever management in Alzheimer patients: quality plus fiscal responsibility. Adv Nurs Sci 1993; 16:21–32.

49. Van der Steen JT, Ooms ME, Van der Wal G, Ribbe MW. Pneumonia: the demented patient's best friend? Discomfort after starting or withholding antibiotic treatment. J Am Geriatr Soc 2002; 50:1681–1688.

50. Rheaume Y, Riley ME, Volicer L. Meeting nutritional needs of Alzheimer patients who pace constantly. J Nutr Elderly 1987; 7:43–52.

51. Kayser-Jones J, Schell ES, Porter C, Barbaccia JC, Shaw H. Factors contributing to dehydration in nursing homes: inadequate staffing and lack of professional supervision. J Am Geriatr Soc 1999; 47:1187–1194.

52. Khodeir M, Conte EE, Morris JJ, Frisoni GB, Volicer L. Effect of decreased mobility on body composition in patients with Alzheimer's disease. J Nutr Health Aging 2000; 4:19–24.

53. Ganzini L, Goy ER, Miller LL, et al. Nurses' experiences with hospice patients who refuse food and fluid to hasten death. N Engl J Med 2003; 349:359–365.

54. Finucane TE, Christmas C, Travis K. Tube feeding in patients with advanced dementia: A review of the evidence. JAMA 1999; 282:1365–1370.

55. Volicer L, Rheaume Y, Riley ME, Karner J, Glennon M. Discontinuation of tube feeding in patients with dementia of the Alzheimer type. Am J Alzheim Care 1990; 5:22–25.

56. Volicer L. Strategies for prevention of tube feeding in advanced dementia. AAHPM Bull 2001; 1:1–18.

57. Monteleoni C, Clark E. Using rapid-cycle quality improvement methodology to reduce feeding tubes in patients with advanced dementia: before and after study. BMJ 2004; 329: 491–494.

58. Happ MB, Capezuti E, Strumpf NE, et al. Advance care planning and end-of-life care for hospitalized nursing home residents. J Am Geriatr Soc 2002; 50:829–835.

59. Schonwetter RS, Walker RM, Solomon M, Indurkhya A, Robinson BE. Life values, resuscitation preferences, and the applicability of living wills in an older population. J Am Geriatr Soc 1996; 44:954–958.

60. Griffith CH 3rd, Wilson JF, Emmett KR, Ramsbottom-Lucier M, Rich EC. Knowledge and experience with Alzheimer's disease. Relationship to resuscitation preferences. Arch Fam Med 1995; 4:780–784.

61. Gjerdingen DK, Neff JA, Wang M, Chanoler K. Older persons' opinions about life-sustaining procedures in the face of death. Arch Fam Med 1999; 8:421–425.

62. Holtzman J, Pheley AM, Lurie N. Changes in orders limiting care and the use of less aggressive care in a nursing home population. J Am Geriatr Soc 1994; 42:275–279.

63. Zweig SC, Kruse RL, Binder EF, Szafara KL, Mehr DR. Effect of do-not-resuscitate orders on hospitalization of nursing home residents evaluated for lower respiratory infections. J Am Geriatr Soc 2004; 52:51–58.

64. Ashby MA, Medelson D. Gardner; re BWV: Victorian Supreme Court makes landmark Australian ruling on tube feeding. Med J Aust 2002; 181:442–444.

65. Gillick MR. Sounding board – rethinking the role of tube feeding in patients with advanced dementia. N Engl J Med 2000; 342:206–210.

66. Rosin AJ, Sonnenblick M. Autonomy and paternalism in geriatric medicine. The Jewish ethical approach to issues of feeding terminally ill patients, and to cardiopulmonary resuscitation. J Med Ethics 1998; 24:44–48.

67. Barry R. The papal allocution on caring for person in a 'vegetative state'. Issues Law Med 2004; 20:155–164.

68. Volicer L, Berman SA, Cipolloni PB, Mandell A. Persistent vegetative state in Alzheimer disease – does it exist? Arch Neurol 1997; 54:1382–1384.

69. Shannon TA. Implications of the papal allocution on feeding tubes. Hastings Cent Rep 2004; 34:18–20.

70. Lloyd-Williams M, Payne S. Can multidisciplinary guidelines improve the palliation of symptoms in the terminal phase of dementia? Int J Pall Care Nurs 2002; 8:370–375.

71. Van der Steen JT, Ooms ME, Ribbe MW, Van der Wal G. Decisions to treat or not to treat pneumonia in demented psychogeriatric nursing home patients: evaluation of a guideline. Alzheimer Dis Assoc Disord 2001; 15:119–128.

72. Rabeneck L, McCullough LB, Wray NP. Ethically justified, clinically comprehensive guidelines for percutaneous endoscopic gastrostomy tube placement. Lancet 1997; 349: 496–498.

73. Mitchell SL, Tetroe JM, O'Connor AM. A decision aid for long-term tube feeding in cognitively impaired older adults. J Am Geriatr Soc 2001; 49:313–316.

74. Fisk JD, Sadovnick AD, Cohen CA, et al. Ethical guidelines of the Alzheimer society of Canada. Can J Neurol Sci 1998; 25:242–248.

75. Karlawish JHT, Quill T, Meier DE. A consensus-based approach to providing palliative care to patients who lack decision-making capacity. Ann Intern Med 1999; 130: 835–840.

76. Mast KR, Salama M, Silverman GK, Arnold RM. End-of-life content in treatment guidelines for life-limiting diseases. J Pall Med 2004; 7:754–773.

77. American Medical Association. Diagnosis, Management and Treatment of Dementia: A Practical Guide for Primary Care Physicians. Chicago, IL: AMA, 1999.

78. American Psychiatric Association. Practice guideline for the treatment of patients with Alzheimer's disease and other dementias of late life. Am J Psychiatry 1997; 154:1–39.

79. California Workgroup on Guidelines for Alzheimer's Disease Management. Guidelines for Alzheimer's Disease Management. Alzheimer's Association of Los Angeles, Riverside and San Bernardino Counties, Los Angeles, CA 2002.

80. Dementia: Clinical Practice Guideline 1998. Columbia, MD: American Medical Directors Association 1998.

81. Hanrahan P, Luchins DJ. Access to hospice programs in end-stage dementia: a national survey of hospice programs. J Am Geriatr Soc 1995; 43:56–59.

82. National Hospice and Palliative Care Organisation. Available at http://www.nhpco.org/files/public/Facts_Figures_ for2004data.pdf 2005 [accessed 06 April, 2006].

83. Ewbank DC. Deaths attributable to Alzheimer's disease in the United States. Am J Publ Health 1999; 89:90–92.

84. Hoyert DL, Kung H-C, Smith BL. Deaths: preliminary data for 2003. Nat Vital Stat Rep 2005; 53:1–48.

85. Mitchell SL, Morris JN, Park PS, Fries BE. Terminal care for persons with advanced dementia in the nursing home and home care settings. J Pall Med 2004; 7:808–816.

86. Schonwetter RS, Han B, Small BJ, et al. Predictors of six-month survival among patients with dementia: an evaluation of hospice Medicare guidelines. Am J Hospice Pall Care 2003; 20:105–113.

87. Mitchell SL, Kiely DK, Hamel MB, et al. Estimating prognosis for nursing home residents with advanced dementia. JAMA 2004; 291:2734–2740.

88. Pyenson B, Connor S, Fitch K, Kinzbrunner B. Medicare cost in matched hospice and non-hospice cohorts. J Pain Sympt Mgmnt 2004; 28:200–210.

89. Miller SC, Intrator O, Gozalo P, et al. Government expenditures at the end of life for short- and long-stay nursing home

residents: differences by hospice enrollment status. J Am Geriatr Soc 2004; 52:1284–1292.

90. Miller SC, Mor V, Wu N, Gozalo P, Lapane K. Does receipt of hospice care in nursing homes improve the management of pain at the end of life? J Am Geriatr Soc 2002; 50:507–515.

91. Miller SC, Mor V, Teno J. Hospice enrollment and pain assessment and management in nursing homes. J Pain Sympt Mgmnt 2003; 26:791–799.

92. Krulewitch H, London MR, Skakel VJ, et al. Assessment of pain in cognitively impaired older adults: a comparison of pain assessment tools and their use by nonprofessional caregivers. J Am Geriatr Soc 2000; 48:1607–1611.

93. Warden V, Hurley AC, Volicer L. Development and psychometric evaluation of the PAINAD (Pain Assessment in Advanced Dementia) Scale. JAMDA 2003; 4:9–15.

94. Villanueva MR, Smith TL, Erickson JS, Lee AC, Singer CM. Pain assessment for the dementing elderly (PADE): reliability and validity of a new measure. JAMDA 2003; 4:1–8.

95. Casarett D, Takesaka J, Karlawish J, Hirschman KB, Clark CM. How should clinicians discuss hospice for patients with dementia? Anticipating caregivers' preconceptions and meeting their information needs. Alzheimer Dis Assoc Disord 2002; 16:116–122.

96. Murphy K, Hanrahan P, Luchins D. A survey of grief and bereavement in nursing homes: the importance of hospice grief and bereavement for the end-stage Alzheimer's disease patient and family. J Am Geriatr Soc 1997; 45:1104–1107.

97. Schulz R, Belle SH, Czaja SJ, et al. Long-term placement of dementia patients and caregiver health and well being. JAMA 2004; 292:961–967.

98. Haley WE, LaMonde LA, Han B, Burton AM, Schonwetter R. Predictors of depression and life satisfaction among spousal caregivers in hospice: application of a stress process model. J Pall Med 2003; 6:215–224.

21

Co-existent medical problems and concomitant diseases

Roy Jones

INTRODUCTION

It is important to remember that everything that occurs in people with dementia is not necessarily due to dementia. Most people with Alzheimer's disease (AD) are elderly and are therefore likely to suffer from other significant illnesses, both acute and chronic. One prospective study[1] of 200 elderly outpatients with dementia identified 248 other medical diagnoses in 124 patients; 92 of the diagnoses were new.

Co-existent medical problems and concomitant diseases are very common in persons with AD and require careful and skilled management. A clinician caring for persons with AD must be alert to these possibilities and review the situation frequently, particularly if there has been deterioration in a patient's general health or an increase in their confusion. Other illnesses can increase confusion either temporarily or chronically. Drugs used to treat other conditions (even those the patient has been taking for some time) may be responsible for worsening cognition. These other medical problems can have an adverse effect on the quality of life of patients and their families, although overzealous treatment can also be distressing, particularly if the patient is at the terminal stage of AD.

Regular review is essential, partly because medical problems may be aggravated by the inability of patients with AD to report their own symptoms. Common conditions can present atypically or in a non-specific way. An example of this is the significant association between an impaired mental test score and an atypical presentation of myocardial infarction.[2] It is also easy to overlook standard health measures, such as annual immunisation to protect against influenza and regular eye checks including measurements of intraocular pressure to identify glaucoma.

The present chapter will consider some of the more important concomitant diseases and related problems that are likely to be encountered in people with AD. Emphasis has been placed on those conditions where good management may contribute to the maintenance of health and quality of life for the person with AD or where the management of the concomitant disease may be complicated by the presence of dementia.

COST OF CONCOMITANT DISEASES

Concomitant diseases are not only important to the quality of life of people with dementia but they are also costly. The medical management problems of Alzheimer's disease and related disorders (ADRD) patients result in higher costs in both fee-for-service and Medicare managed care organisations (MCOs) in the USA.[3] However, ADRD may also increase costs for co-existing conditions such as congestive heart failure, since it is more difficult to obtain good patient self management for things such as diet and drugs. The negative effects of this might include increased risk of hospitalisation and increased risk of complications such as pneumonia.

In view of the potential burden of chronic diseases in healthcare, MCOs have developed disease management programmes for conditions like heart failure and diabetes.[4] Yet there are few disease management programmes for ADRD, despite the high prevalence and costs. Strategies such as patient education for diabetes, monitoring congestive heart failure by telephone or reminders by mail or phone to improve compliance with medications are more difficult to implement successfully in people with cognitive impairment.

A retrospective analysis of administrative data for a 2-year period from an MCO in the north-eastern USA of 3934 patients with ADRD and 19 300 age/sex-matched controls (five controls for each case) without dementia has been carried out.[3] For the 10 most prevalent comorbidities in ADRD patients, costs were higher than with controls. Higher costs were attributable to higher inpatient and skilled nursing facility utilisation. The 10 comorbidities were cerebrovascular disease, congestive heart failure, chronic pulmonary disease, diabetes, peripheral vascular disease, myocardial infarction, malignancy, renal disease, chronic complications of diabetes and peptic ulcer disease. Of particular interest was that ADRD patients with congestive heart failure and diabetes – two conditions of high prevalence and cost in the Medicare population – had substantially higher costs relative to control patients with these conditions (US$4756 more for uncomplicated diabetes and US$6134 for congestive heart failure).

The study only measured costs from the MCO perspective and did not include costs for informal and formal caregivers or for nursing home care. Nevertheless, the findings suggest that better treatment and care management of AD could reduce the costs of comorbid illnesses commonly experienced by frail elderly people.

Support for the view that drug treatment of AD, for example with a cholinesterase inhibitor, might reduce the costs to a Medicare managed care plan comes from a recent paper from the same group.[5] In a case-control study, use of donepezil in people with predominantly mild-to-moderate ADRD was associated with a mean reduction of US$2500. This reduction was largely due to lower hospital and postacute skilled nursing facility costs and partly offset by higher prescriptions, physician's office and outpatient hospital costs.

MORTALITY

The relation between comorbidity and survival has been investigated in an 8-year follow-up study of 606 nursing home dementia patients in the Netherlands.[6] The data were collected retrospectively and comorbidity was identified if it occurred during the first 6 weeks after admission. Two-year survival rates for 437 women and 169 men were 60 per cent and 39 per cent respectively. Parkinsonism, atrial fibrillation, pulmonary infection and the malignancies were powerful predictors which more or less doubled the mortality chances. Stroke patients with a pulmonary infection had a particularly poor prognosis. More severely demented patients had more comorbidity than less severely demented patients, but the impact of comorbidity on survival did not depend on severity of

dementia. Patients admitted from a hospital had more comorbidity and were more severely demented than patients coming from home, but this did not modify the effects of age, gender and comorbidity in the multivariate survival model. The authors concluded that comorbidity and severity of dementia independently influence mortality.[6]

SPECIFIC CONDITIONS

Diabetes

Like dementia, non-insulin dependent diabetes mellitus is highly prevalent in elderly people. A number of studies have suggested that diabetes affects cognition, but the relationship with dementia has been uncertain. Increasingly it appears that diabetes is a risk factor, particularly for vascular dementia but also for AD.[7,8] Interestingly, one study examining diabetes and dementia in long-term care[9] found that AD and adult onset diabetes (AODM) did not co-occur, whereas AODM was associated with vascular dementia diagnosed clinically. AD may be more frequent in elderly diabetic patients treated with insulin.[7]

The specifics of how best to manage elderly people with diabetes are not clear.[8] For example, glycaemic control, management of blood pressure and hyperlipidaemia could all potentially affect cognitive decline but few data exist to inform clinicians.[8] There is quite extensive evidence to suggest that too strict glycaemic control, with the risk of recurrent and severe hypoglycaemia, can cause cognitive impairment in insulin-dependent diabetics.[10]

On the other hand, the management of diabetes, whether insulin-dependent or non-insulin dependent, may be especially challenging in the presence of impaired cognition or dementia. Management of diabetes preferably requires an informed and cooperative patient. Poor diabetic control may lead to a number of problems including further cognitive damage. Keeping tight control of the blood sugar may reduce the risk of further cognitive deterioration and other complications of diabetes,[11,12] but it is important to avoid hypoglycaemia. Missed or inadequate meals will increase the risk, and this is more likely in people with cognitive impairment. For this reason, it is usually safer to accept only moderately good control of the blood sugar.

Ideally, newly diagnosed non-insulin-dependent diabetics should be given a few months of dietary restriction together with encouragement to take more physical activity. Such advice may be impractical for persons with AD, particularly if they are elderly. There is an increased risk of hypoglycaemia in older individuals receiving long-acting sulphonylureas and chlorpropamide and glibenclamide should be avoided. Shorter-acting drugs such as gliclazide, glipizide and tolbutamide are preferable. It is also better to avoid insulin if possible.

Hypertension

Hypertension is another common condition in elderly people. It may be relevant in the management of the person with dementia but also represents a risk factor for the development of dementia including AD. High blood pressure is a major risk factor for cerebrovascular disease and is also correlated closely with cognitive decline and dementia.[13] Several epidemiological studies have found that cognitive function is inversely proportional to blood pressure values measured 15 or 20 years ago in mid-life.[13]

Treatment of hypertension has been demonstrated to reduce cardiovascular risk substantially in elderly people, yet clinicians often seem reluctant to do so. Elderly patients with AD and asymptomatic hypertension are a particular dilemma because of concerns about compliance and the risk of adverse drug effects such as postural hypotension and incontinence (from diuretics). Yet for blood pressure levels of systolic greater than 160 mm Hg or diastolic greater than 90 mm Hg there is good evidence for intervention; this is probably more to prevent the risk of stroke rather than for any perceived benefits on its effects in dementia.[14]

Successful control of blood pressure can improve cognitive performance, at least in patients with multi-infarct dementia.[15] Antihypertensive treatment is also associated with a reduced incidence of dementia in elderly people with isolated systolic hypertension.[16] Nevertheless, it may be both impractical and unreasonable to treat hypertension aggressively, particularly in patients with moderately severe and severe AD.

In general, it is satisfactory to treat hypertension conventionally in patients with AD. A low dose of thiazide diuretic such as bendroflumethiazide, 2.5 mg daily, is an appropriate starting point. If necessary, and providing there are no contraindications, a low dose of a beta-blocker such as atenolol, 25 mg daily, can then be added. Beta-blockers can occasionally cause confusion and also cause bradycardia, which is also seen with the cholinesterase inhibitors prescribed for AD. Patients who cannot tolerate beta-blockers and diabetic patients are probably better managed with an angiotensin-converting enzyme inhibitor. There are contradictory information concerning calcium-channel blocking agents such as nitrendipine. There are limited data that suggest they are associated

with a lower incidence of dementia (but only relatively few patients in either the calcium-channel group or the placebo group developed dementia),[16] while another study suggested that they were more likely to be linked with cognitive decline.[17]

Atrial fibrillation

Atrial fibrillation (AF) increases in prevalence with age, affecting 5 per cent of people over 65 and around 10 per cent of those over 75.[18] It is associated with a significant risk of mortality and morbidity from heart failure, stroke and thromboembolic complications. In particular, non-valvular AF accounts for 10–15 per cent of all ischaemic strokes and almost a quarter of strokes in people aged >80 years.[19] Guidelines concerning the management of permanent AF are clear and recommend the use of anticoagulant and antiplatelet drugs that reduce the risk of stroke. Anticoagulation therapy with aspirin reduces stroke by 22 per cent (95 per cent CI, 2–38 per cent), whilst warfarin in conventional doses (to maintain the International Normalized Ratio between 2.0 and 3.0) reduces stroke by 62 per cent (95 per cent CI, 48–72 per cent).[20] The risk of stroke is highest in people with a previous stroke, those over the age of 75 and those with hypertension, coronary artery disease, heart failure or diabetes.[18]

Despite elderly people having the highest risk of stroke yet the potential to gain most, studies confirm that older patients with AF have the lowest frequency of anticoagulant use[21] because of the perceived increase in risks associated with interactions with other medications, comorbidity and bleeding. Dementia is a significant independent determinant of non-treatment with aspirin or warfarin when otherwise indicated for the prevention of recurrent stroke.[21] Underutilisation of aspirin and warfarin in older stroke patients with dementia may be responsible for their increased risk of recurrent stroke and death and is therefore potentially modifiable.[21] Although the reluctance to use warfarin in persons with AD is understandable because of the potential difficulty with compliance, decisions should be made on a case by case basis. Individual risk–benefit assessment is important, with personal circumstances (for example, whether a patient lives alone or with someone who can supervise medication) and biological age more important than chronological age when assessing the benefits of anticoagulation versus the risks.

In many cases it is wiser to select the less effective but usually safer alternative of aspirin, 75–300 mg/day or an alternative antiplatelet drug such as clopidogrel 75 mg. At present it is still not clear whether the combination of clopidogrel and aspirin is as effective as warfarin in people with AF.[22]

In terms of the more general management of AF, then all patients with permanent AF and those who are difficult to keep in sinus rhythm (with recurrent or persistent AF) should receive treatment to control their heart rate.[23] Drugs used to control heart rhythm include flecainide, propafenone and sotalol in patients with good left ventricular function.[24] Amiodarone can be used to maintain sinus rhythm in patients with heart failure whilst beta-blockers are the drugs of choice for people with coronary artery disease.[24]

Rate control drugs in patients without heart failure include the non-dihydropyridine calcium antagonists (verapamil, diltiazem) or beta-blockers (metoprolol, propranolol and atenolol). The combination of digoxin with a beta-blocker may be better than either used alone in improving control of the ventricular rate and left ventricular function.[24] In addition, beta-blockers may be considered in patients with stable heart failure.

GENERAL HEALTH ISSUES

The following section will consider some more general problems and symptoms that are not necessarily specifically associated with any one disease, but which can be of immense importance in maximising the quality of life of the person with AD.

Delirium

Delirium (acute confusional state) is an acute fluctuating mental disorder of impaired consciousness, alertness, awareness and global impairment of cognition.[25] Age and prior cognitive impairment are significant risk factors for delirium, especially in response to medication,[26] so delirium is a common concomitant problem in persons with AD. Whenever someone with AD deteriorates suddenly then a cause should be sought before concluding that it is due to the underlying dementia. Some common causes of delirium are shown in Table 21.1.

In elderly people, the commonest cause of delirium is adverse drug effects. The list of drugs that may theoretically cause confusion is long and particularly includes drugs with anticholinergic properties. These drugs can cause acute or chronic confusion. Table 21.2 shows the more commonly used drugs that can cause confusion.[27]

A clinician should pay careful attention when introducing any new medication to someone with AD, especially if the drug is listed in the table. Ideally,

Table 21.1 Some causes of delirium in elderly people

Drugs including drug withdrawal: see Table 21.2	
Metabolic causes	Electrolyte imbalance; endocrine disorders; hypothermia; renal, hepatic or pulmonary failure
Structural causes	Stroke; subarachnoid or cerebral haemorrhage; subdural haematoma; primary or secondary brain tumour; brain abscess
Infections	Urinary tract, chest, wound and intravenous sites
Seizure	
Trauma	

Table 21.2 Drugs that can cause acute confusion[27]

Drugs with anticholinergic properties

Antihistamines (such as diphenhydramine)

Antispasmodics

Tricyclic antidepressants

Antipsychotics

Antiparkinsonian drugs

Oxybutynin

Other drugs

Benzodiazepines

Alcohol

Trazodone and other antidepressants

Narcotic analgesics

Lithium carbonate

Digoxin

Diuretics

Antihypertensives (?especially calcium-channel blockers)

Anticonvulsants

Cimetidine

Steroids

Indomethacin and other non-steroidals

Drug withdrawal

Alcohol

Benzodiazepines

changes in medication should be made to occur serially, rather than introducing or stopping several drugs at the same time. All drug therapy for people with AD should be reviewed regularly and unnecessary or ineffective medications withdrawn. It is still possible for a long established drug to cause problems, for example electrolyte imbalance can occur with a diuretic if the patient develops other problems such as diarrhoea.

Medication

Drug therapy used wisely can bring enormous benefits to the quality of life for many older people but adverse effects can lead to serious problems, misery and even premature death. The use of any medication in AD requires even more consideration. Apart from drugs that can increase cognitive impairment, other adverse effects include problems such as sedation, postural hypotension and falls.

It is important to consider the size and biological, rather than chronological, age of the person. Standard doses of drugs may not be appropriate. There is an inevitable decline in renal and hepatic function with increasing age and weight loss is common, especially in people with AD. Doses of drugs for chronic conditions such as hypertension or epilepsy that were previously satisfactory may be excessive for an older, frailer person with AD. All drugs should be reviewed regularly particularly for older people in care homes who are known to take more medications than older people in the wider community[28] and to be particularly at risk. In the UK, the National Services Framework for older people recognises the special medication needs of older people and the need for regular review of medications (6-monthly in patients taking four or more medications) to help avoid inappropriate prescribing and drug-related morbidity.[29,30] Yet, a recent study from the UK revealed that only 30 per cent of nursing home residents had had a medication review in the previous 12 months.[28]

There is a particular risk from neuroleptic and other drugs that are frequently prescribed for the management of behavioural problems such as agitation in AD. Adverse effects such as sedation can lead to problems including immobility and incontinence. It has previously been suggested that neuroleptics may also hasten cognitive decline in dementia;[31] this was confirmed in a recent study using quetiapine for agitation in AD, where the drug caused significantly greater cognitive decline than placebo.[32]

Hearing and vision

The initial registration of information is especially important for a person with memory problems or AD. For most older people, a deterioration in hearing and vision is the norm. Every older person should have a regular test of hearing and vision and this should include the measurement of intraocular pressure to check for glaucoma. It is easy to overlook these regular checks in a person with AD but these should be continued for as long as possible. It is important that the person carrying out hearing and vision tests is aware that they are testing someone with cognitive impairment who may be less able to cooperate. Tests such as examination of visual fields may be more difficult but are still important.

There are almost no formal studies looking at the combined problems of visual impairment and dementia. Both conditions are prevalent in elderly people. Although there are no studies that have assessed the size of the population with both dementia and significant sight loss, estimates based on figures derived for each condition separately suggest that a minimum of 2 per cent of elderly people will have both dementia and significant visual impairment. The actual figure is likely to be higher than this, partly because of the difficulties in accurately quantifying visual loss in people with dementia. A study of vision impairment in nursing-home residents in Australia[33] concluded that residents with dementia had a slightly higher prevalence of blindness (13 per cent) than those without dementia (9 per cent). However, there were only small numbers in the study and the results should be interpreted cautiously, particularly since blind people with dementia are probably more likely to require nursing-home care.

Assessment of cognitive function in people with significant visual or hearing problems is difficult. Research is needed to investigate methods of assessing vision in people who may be 'untestable' by conventional means. Similarly it is easy to overestimate a person's cognitive problems if they have not heard the question that they are being asked. It is essential therefore to consider potential difficulties with vision and hearing in anyone undergoing tests of memory and cognitive function. If the patient uses a hearing aid or requires reading glasses then these should be used whenever testing is carried out. This is easy to overlook in patients who arrive at clinics without either their reading glasses or their hearing aid. Keeping spare pairs of reading glasses and making available a personal amplifying device with a stethoscope headset for use when people have forgotten their hearing aid can overcome some of these difficulties. It is also essential that the testing room is reasonably quiet.

A lot of practical advice may be given to the person with AD and their family to allow them to overcome some of these problems. For example, people with hearing problems usually prefer one-to-one conversations in a quiet room and may find it more difficult to engage in conversations involving several people. Examination of the ears to remove wax can sometimes solve much of the problem. Vision will usually be improved by using brighter lighting and sometimes merely by cleaning the glasses of a person with AD.

Since people with AD are likely to misplace their glasses, it has been suggested that the number of pairs of glasses should be minimised.[34] However, a study of more able older people has suggested that multifocal glasses may impair edge-contrast sensitivity and depth perception, and thereby increase the risk of falls.[35] It is suggested that older people may benefit from wearing non-multifocal glasses when negotiating stairs and in unfamiliar settings outside the home. Although this study was in healthier older people, it seems likely that the conclusions will apply to people with AD and should be borne in mind.

Glaucoma is common in older people and its treatment is important to maintain good vision. Topical eye drops to treat glaucoma can still cause untoward systemic effects in older people. Bradycardia from drops containing the β-blocker timolol may be of particular relevance in patients receiving cholinesterase inhibitors, which can also cause bradycardia.

Nutrition, weight loss and dental problems

There is an important link between good nutrition and general health and well-being in persons with AD, especially if living alone. Persons with dementia are often underweight and may have feeding problems.[36] Indeed, weight loss has been considered as almost inevitable with AD and related dementias. This is not always the case[37,38] and some patients with AD may overeat and binge.[39] An important and often overlooked problem in older people, especially those with dementia, is the importance of oral and dental hygiene. Regular tooth brushing is important to prevent gum and tooth disease and yet may be performed poorly or not at all by the person with AD. Regular dental check-ups are important whether the patient has their own teeth or dentures. Ill-fitting dentures can be a cause of problems with eating and speaking.

Insufficient attention is placed on oral health and hygiene in older people, particularly those residing in institutions and nursing homes.[40] In a US survey, over 25 per cent of the population aged 65 and older had not seen a dental professional in the previous 5 years.[41] Older people with dentures and no remaining teeth of their own were four times less likely to visit a dentist. Moreover because of improved oral health earlier in life and the fact that more people now retain their teeth, the dental needs of older people in the future are likely to increase.[40]

There are a number of procedures that can help maintain oral health in older people. For individuals with their own teeth, the use of fluoridated toothpaste, toothbrushes, dental floss and antimicrobial mouth rinses can be useful. For edentate adults then denture cleansers and brushes should be used. In general, dental hygiene can be improved by relatively simple measures and more attention should therefore be paid to these issues by carers of people with AD and staff in residential and nursing facilities.

Undernutrition can contribute to other problems such as muscle and weight loss, anaemia and constipation. It is important to encourage and, if necessary, help a person with AD to eat nutritious, balanced meals. Using common sense and creativity can often help, for example by providing access to snacks and drinks and by feeding patients at times during the day when they are at their best.

Feet, falls and fractures

Problems with the feet often cause discomfort and disability in older people and may be one of the reasons why an older person is 'off their legs'. Walking safely and effectively is important if one is to remain independent and socially active. Degenerative changes in the feet can occur as a result of chronic diseases such as diabetes with peripheral neuropathy, rheumatoid arthritis and osteoarthritis. However, it is not uncommon for the problems to be caused by simpler problems such as curved or hypertrophied nails or fungal infections and this is more likely in persons with AD who may be inattentive to their own physical needs and hygiene. When examining an older patient it is important to inspect the feet and to remove socks or stockings so that this is done properly. The regular attention of a chiropodist can be important, particularly in people such as diabetics who are at higher risk of problems.

Foot problems can increase the risk of falls. Persons with AD are at increased risk of falls and fractures, particularly of the neck of the femur, and these are associated with admission to long-term care.[42,43] Although the risk of injury after falls in persons with AD is related to disease severity,[44] the risk of injury tends to decline in very severe dementia, probably because they are relatively immobile. Persons with dementia who fall are more likely to sustain a fracture than older people in general.[44]

Many patients with AD have reduced self-confidence and the psychological consequences of falling may exacerbate this. This can lead to a cycle of restricted activity, increased dependence and reduced mobility followed by further falls. Eventually this will lead to patients moving to a more supervised environment.[45] Interestingly, a recent study assessing the value of a multifactorial intervention on 196 subjects in 20 residential care homes in the UK showed a trend towards a greater effect size in subjects with cognitive impairment;[46] this emphasises the importance of continuing to offer persons with AD access to appropriate care and rehabilitation.

As with other problems in persons with dementia, it is important to try and identify why the person is falling and not merely to assume it is as a result of the dementia. Falls may arise from problems with vision and balance, agitation, environmental hazards and conditions such as postural hypotension, whether drug-induced or not. Persons with AD may have poor judgment, poor concentration to avoid environmental hazards and abnormalities of gait. Psychotropic medication can certainly increase the risk of falls [47] and it has been suggested that cholinesterase inhibitors might also potentially increase the risk, possibly as a result of the bradycardia that these drugs cause.[48] Reducing or avoiding psychotropic medication may be of benefit whilst hip protectors may be considered for those at higher risk to protect them from hip fractures.[47]

Management of pain

Pain is a common and unpleasant symptom that can occur as a result of a multitude of conditions. Persons with AD may not be able to explain satisfactorily that they are in pain[49] and pain can significantly affect their ability to function normally. Acute pain due to a fracture, retention of urine or some other cause may only be noted as a change in behaviour, agitation or increased confusion. A range of verbal and non-verbal behaviours may occur as a result of pain and it is essential that people caring for someone with AD maintain a high index of suspicion that the person they are looking after may be in pain.

Painful conditions are both underdetected and undertreated in persons with dementia living in institutions.[49] Persons with dementia in nursing homes and residential settings are less likely to be prescribed analgesics than cognitively intact residents.[50] Older persons with dementia must be encouraged to report their pain and such reports should be trusted.[51]

When assessing pain, then the most obvious causes should be excluded. If a diagnosis cannot be made but pain is still suspected then it is reasonable to give a therapeutic trial of an analgesic.

The American Geriatrics Society has published recommendations for the management of persistent pain in older people.[52] The guidelines emphasise the prevention of problems such as opioid-related constipation, sedation and impaired cognitive performance and these are especially relevant in patients with AD. As with all medication in people with AD, the situation should be re-evaluated frequently, both to check for efficacy, particularly in persistent pain, and to minimise adverse effects.

CONCLUSION

Co-existent medical problems and concomitant diseases are very common in persons with AD and require careful and skilled management. A clinician caring for such patients must be alert to these possibilities and review the situation frequently, particularly if there has been deterioration in a patient's general health or an increase in their confusion.

REFERENCES

1. Larson EB, Reifler BV, Sumi SM, et al. Diagnostic tests in the evaluation of dementia: a prospective study of 200 elderly outpatients. Arch Intern Med 1986; 146:1917–1922.
2. Black DA. Mental state and presentation of myocardial infarction in the elderly. Age Ageing 1987; 16:125–127.
3. Hill JW, Futterman R, Duttagupta S, et al. Alzheimer's disease and related dementias increase costs of co-morbidities in managed Medicare. Neurology 2002; 58:62–70.
4. Leider HL. Heart failure and disease management. Am J Manag Care 1998; 4:S343–S346.
5. Lu S, Hill J, Fillit H. Impact of donepezil use in routine clinical practice on healthcare costs in patients with Alzheimer's disease and related dementias enrolled in the large Medicare-managed care plan: a case-control study. Am J Geriatr Pharmacother 2005; 3:92–102.
6. Van Dijk PTM, Dippel DWJ, van der Meulen JHP, Habbema JDF. Co-morbidity and its effect on mortality in Nursing Home patients with dementia. J Nerv Ment Dis 1996; 184: 180–187.
7. Ott A, Stolk RP, Hofman A, et al. Association of diabetes mellitus and dementia: the Rotterdam Study, Diabetologia 1996; 39:1392–1397.
8. Gregg EW, Engelgau MM, Narayan V. Complications of diabetes in elderly people. BMJ 2002; 325:916–917.
9. Tariot PN, Ogden MA, Cox C, Williams TF. Diabetes and dementia in long-term care. J Am Geriatr Soc 1999; 47: 423–429
10. Gold AE, Deary IJ, Jones RW, et al. Severe deterioration in cognitive function and personality in five patients with long-standing diabetes: a complication of diabetes or a consequence of treatment? Diabet Med 1994; 11:499–505.
11. The Diabetes Control and Complications Trial Research Group. The effect of intensive treatment of diabetes on the

development and progression of long-term complications in insulin-dependent diabetes mellitus. N Engl J Med 1993; 329:977–986.

12. UK Prospective Diabetic Study (UKPDS) Group 33. Intensive blood-glucose control with sulphonylureas or insulin compared with conventional treatment and risk of complications in patients with type 2 diabetes. Lancet 1998; 352: 837–853.

13. Hanon O, Forette F. Treatment of hypertension and prevention of dementia. Alzheimer's Dementia 2005; 1: 30–37.

14. Qizilbash N. Blood pressure reduction. In: Qizilbash N, Schneider LS, Chui H et al, eds. Evidence-based Dementia Practice. Oxford: Blackwell Science 2002 593–595.

15. Meyer JS, Judd BW, Tawaklna T, et al. Improved cognition after control of risk factors for multi-infarct dementia. JAMA 1986; 256:2203–2209.

16. Forette F, Seux M-L, Staessen JA, et al. Prevention of dementia in randomised double-blind placebo-controlled Systolic Hypertension in Europe (Syst-Eur) trial. Lancet 1998; 352: 1347–1351.

17. Dinsdale H. Searching for a link between calcium-channel blockers and cognitive function. Can Med Assoc J 1999; 161: 534–535.

18. Hampton JR. The management of atrial fibrillation in elderly patients. Age Ageing 1999; 28:249–250.

19. Lane D, Lip YH. Anti-thrombotic therapy for atrial fibrillation and patients' preferences for treatment. Age Ageing 2005; 34:1–3.

20. Hart RG, Benavente O, McBride R, Pearce LA. Antithrombotic therapy to prevent stroke in patients with atrial fibrillation: a meta-analysis. Ann Intern Med 1999; 131:492–501.

21. Moroney JT, Tseng C-L, Paik MC, et al. Treatment for the secondary prevention of stroke in older patients: the influence of dementia status. J Am Geriatr Soc 1999; 47:824–829.

22. Lorenzoni R, Lazzerini G, Cocci F, et al. Short-term prevention of thromboembolic complications in patients with atrial fibrillation with aspirin plus clopidogrel: the Clopidogrel–Aspirin Atrial Fibrillation (CLAAF) pilot study. Am Heart J 2004; 148:e6.

23. Page RL. Newly diagnosed atrial fibrillation. N Engl J Med 2004; 351:2408–2416.

24. Iqbal MB, Taneja AK, Lip GYH, Flather M. Recent developments in atrial fibrillation. BMJ 2005; 330:238–243.

25. American Psychiatric Association. Diagnostic and Statistical Manual of Mental Disorders, 4th edn. Washington DC: APA 1994.

26. Schor JD, Levkoff SE, Lipsitz LA, et al. Risk factors for hospitalized elderly. JAMA 1992; 267:827–831.

27. Jones RW. Drug Treatment in Dementia. Oxford: Blackwell Science 2000.

28. Alldred DP, Zermansky A, Petty DR, et al. Clinical medication review by a pharmacist for older people in care homes: preliminary report. Int J Pharm Pract 2003; 11:R90.

29. Department of Health. National Services Framework for Older People. London: Department of Health 2001.

30. Howard R, Avery T. Inappropriate prescribing in older people. Age Ageing 2004; 33:530–532.

31. McShane R, Keene J, Gedling K, et al. Do neuroleptic drugs hasten cognitive decline in dementia? Prospective study with necropsy follow-up. BMJ 1997; 314:266–270.

32. Ballard C, Margallo-Lana M, Juszczak E, et al. Quetiapine and rivastigmine and cognitive decline in Alzheimer's

disease: randomised double blind placebo controlled trial. BMJ 2005; 330:874–877.

33. Mitchell P, Hayes P, Wang J. Visual impairment in nursing home residents: the Blue Mountains Eye Study. Med J Aust 1997; 166:73–76.

34. Mace NL, Rabins PV. The 36-Hour Day, 3rd edn. Baltimore: The Johns Hopkins University Press 1999.

35. Lord SR, Dayhew J, Howland A. Multifocal glasses impair H-contrast sensitivity and depth perception and increase the risk of falls in older people. J Am Geriatr Soc 2002; 50: 1760–1766.

36. Sandman TO, Adolfsson R, Nygren C, Hallmans G, Winblad B. Nutritional status and dietary intake in institutionalised patients with Alzheimer's Disease and multi-infarct dementia. J Am Geriatr Soc 1987; 35:31–38.

37. Franzoni S, Frisoni GB, Boffelli S, Rozzini R, Trabucchi M. Good nutrional oral intake is associated with equal survival in demented and non demented very old patients. J Am Geriatr Soc 1996; 44:1366–1370.

38. Wang SY, Sukagawa N, Hossain M, Ooi WL. Longitudinal weight changes, length of survival and energy requirements of long-term care residents with dementia. J Am Geriatr Soc 1997; 45:1189–1195.

39. Hope T, Keene J. Behavioural problems in dementia and biochemistry: clinical aspects. Neurodegeneration 1996; 5: 399–402.

40. Ship JA. Improving oral health in older people. J Am Geriatr Soc 2002; 50:1454–1455.

41. Gift HC, Newman JF. How older adults use oral health care services: results of a National Health Interview Survey. J Am Dent Assoc 1993; 124:89–93.

42. McLennan WJ, Isles FE. Medical and social factors influencing admission to residential care. BMJ 1984; 288: 701–703.

43. Sattin RW. Falls among older persons: public health perspective. Ann Rev Pub Health 1992; 13:489–508.

44. Oleske DN, Wilson RS, Bernard BA, Evans DA, Terman EW. Epidemiology of injury in people with Alzheimer's Disease. J Am Geriatr Soc 1995; 43:741–746.

45. Tinettin E, Powell L. Fear of falling and low self-efficacy: a cause of dependence in elderly persons. J Gerontol 1993; 48(special issue):35–38.

46. Dyer CAE, Taylor GJ, Reed M, et al. Falls prevention in residential care homes: a randomised controlled trial. Age Ageing 2004; 33:596–602.

47. American Geriatrics Society, British Geriatrics Society and American Academy of Orthopedic Surgeons Panel on Falls Prevention. Guideline for the prevention of falls in older persons. J Am Geriatr Soc 2001; 49:664–672.

48. Schneider LS. Treatment of Alzheimer's disease with cholinesterase inhibitors. Clin Geriatr Med 2001; 17:337–358.

49. Cook AKR, Niven CA, Downs MG. Assessing the pain of people with cognitive impairment. Int J Geriatr Psychiatry 1999; 14:421–425.

50. Brummel-Smith K, London MR, Drew N, et al. Outcomes of pain in frail older adults with dementia. J Am Geriatr Soc 2002; 50:1847–1851.

51. Ferrell BA, Ferrell BR, Rivera L. Pain in cognitively impaired nursing home patients. J Pain Symptom Mgmnt 1995; 10:591–598.

52. AGS Panel on Persistent Pain in Older Persons. The management of persistent pain in older persons. J Am Geriatr Soc 2002; 50:S205–S224.

22

Management of neuropsychiatric symptoms

Nathan Herrmann

INTRODUCTION

The neuropsychiatric symptoms of dementia include agitation, aggression, delusions, hallucinations, apathy and depression. These disturbances, also referred to as behavioural and psychological symptoms of dementia (BPSD)[1] are common serious problems that can impair the quality of life for both patient and caregiver. The epidemiology of BPSD varies depending on the type of dementia and the stage of the illness, but studies suggest that over 90 per cent of dementia patients will exhibit one or more of these behaviours at some point in their illness.[2] For example, in a large community sample of elderly individuals with dementia, 61 per cent suffered from at least one symptom of BPSD and 32 per cent experienced at least moderate to severe symptoms.[3] BPSD are even more common in long-term care residents[4] and these behaviours are frequently significant risk factors for institutionalization.[5,6] Studies which have focused on the correlates of BPSD suggest they are associated with more rapid cognitive and functional decline and possibly increased mortality.[7–11] They are also associated with stress, burden and increased rates of depression in the caregiver.[12–14] Finally, in addition to increasing the risk of institutionalization (the largest driver of total dementia care costs), BPSD, by themselves, may account for up to 30 per cent of the cost of care.[15]

Given the prevalence and significance of BPSD, evidence-based treatment strategies are essential. While various reviews and clinical practice guidelines have been published,[16–20] their conclusions and recommendations occasionally conflict, and more recent concerns about the safety and efficacy of pharmacological interventions have left many clinicians wondering if there are any truly effective treatments for these disturbances. As this review will highlight, more randomized controlled trials for both pharmacological and non-pharmacological treatments are desperately needed.

This chapter will review the assessment and treatment of BPSD. Treatment strategies will include both pharmacological and non-pharmacological approaches and, wherever possible, comments will focus on the strength and weakness of the available evidence. The chapter will conclude with a synthesis and recommendations based on the best available evidence at the present time.

ASSESSMENT

The management of BPSD must include elements such as assessment and diagnosis, identifying and monitoring appropriate target symptoms, and consideration for the safety of the patient, their caregivers and co-residents if they reside in long-term care. Because BPSD can be precipitated by underlying medical conditions and concomitant medications,[21,22] a history, physical examination and appropriate laboratory investigations are necessary for the diagnostic process. For example, an acute urinary tract infection can cause delirium in patients with dementia and result in agitated aggressive behaviours with hallucinations and delusions. Chronic medical conditions must also be considered as symptoms such as constipation, pain and shortness of breath can cause or exacerbate BPSD. Sensory impairment must be assessed as auditory and visual impairment have been associated with agitation, persecutory ideation and hallucinations.[23,24] In one study, visual hallucinations were significantly more common in AD patients with visual impairment, and hallucinations improved by refraction in some of these patients.[25] In a small prospective non-randomized study of the effects of improving hearing in dementia patients, while ratings of BPSD did not improve, hearing disability and speech intelligibility did improve significantly.[26] Finally, studies suggest 5–16 per cent of BPSD is attributable to concomitant medications including psychotropics.[27,28] Unfortunately, there are no randomized controlled trials to support the efficacy of medical assessment and optimization, though few could argue with the need for these approaches, and all available practice guidelines recommend their use.

Numerous rating scales for BPSD are available, all characterized by relative strengths and weaknesses.[29] Some scales describe the wide range of neuropsychiatric symptoms while others focus on individual symptoms. For example, one of the most frequently used scales for BPSD in intervention studies is the Neuropsychiatric Inventory,[30] which measures the frequency and severity of 12 behaviours: delusions, hallucination, agitation, depression/dysphoria, anxiety, euphoria/elation, apathy/indifference, disinhibition, irritability/lability, aberrant motor behaviours, sleep and appetite/eating disturbances. Individual symptom-focused scales include the Cornell Depression Rating Scale[31] and the Cohen-Mansfield Agitation Inventory.[32] Rating scales can be used for both screening and monitoring of treatment outcome. For example, one study suggested that nursing home staff use of depression rating scales increased the sensitivity of the diagnosis of depression from 32 to 50 per cent.[33] The systematic use of rating scales can also highlight specific target symptoms for treatment and help to actively engage the caregiver in the management plan. Finally, there is some evidence that use of structured observation with some rating scales can actually improve BPSD.[34]

NON-PHARMACOLOGICAL INTERVENTIONS

Non-pharmacological interventions include a wide, diverse range of treatments which can be categorized under the following headings: environmental (e.g. wandering tracks), behavioural (e.g. differential reinforcement), sensory (e.g. music), physical activity (e.g. walking), social contact (e.g. simulated presence), psychotherapeutic (e.g. reminiscence therapy), staff training and health service delivery models. These categorizations are clearly arbitrary as some interventions could be considered under a variety of these labels (e.g. bright light can be both an environmental and sensory intervention). Proponents of non-pharmacological interventions have argued that many

forms of BPSD are a result of unmet needs (e.g. physical or social contact, activity, relief of pain or discomfort), the patients' inability to express these needs and their environment's inability to meet these needs.[35] In this context, the interventions described above can be seen as components of 'good care' for all patients with dementia.

A variety of systematic reviews have attempted to evaluate critically the evidence for non-pharmacological approaches.[36,37] Opie et al[38] found 43 studies which included at the very least some measure of behaviour pre- and postintervention. The methodology of only one study was rated highly and only five studies utilized a randomized, controlled design. In a more recent review, Verkaik et al[39] evaluated the evidence for behaviour-, emotion-, cognition- and stimulation-oriented psychosocial methods for the treatment of depression, aggression and apathy in dementia. Including both randomized and non-randomized controlled trials, these authors found 177 studies, only 19 of which met the authors' minimal criteria for inclusion. The authors concluded that there is some evidence that multisensory stimulation ('Snoezelen') reduces apathy in severe dementia, limited evidence that behaviour therapy reduces depression in community-dwelling AD patients and limited evidence that psychomotor therapy groups reduce aggression in nursing home residents. Of note, of the 19 studies reviewed, only seven were highly rated randomized controlled trials (RCTs).

Reviews have also attempted to examine the evidence for a variety of specific approaches including aromatherapy[40] (two studies; more studies required before effectiveness can be determined), light therapy[41] (five studies; insufficient evidence to assess value of treatment) and music therapy[42] (five studies; methodology too poor to draw useful conclusions). These and other reviewers all conclude that more research is necessary to determine the efficacy of non-pharmacological approaches, despite the fact that studies of these approaches clearly outnumber the published pharmacological studies.

Cohen-Mansfield and others have described the reasons for the limitations of the available research, but also the barriers to utilization of these approaches in clinical practice.[35] The latter include lack of financial resources and reimbursement for these approaches, lack of caregiver knowledge and the perception that medication is easier to administer. Despite these concerns, organizations such as the American Geriatrics Society and the American Association for Geriatric Psychiatry have recently concluded that, after the assessment and treatment of associated medical conditions, the initial treatment of BPSD, in the absence of psychosis or immediate danger to self or others, should be non-pharmacological approaches.[19]

PHARMACOTHERAPY

General principles

The use of psychotropics for BPSD is a common treatment approach despite the recommendations noted previously, which suggest their use should only be considered after assessment and non-pharmacological treatments have been implemented first. This had led to concerns about overuse and inappropriate use, and attempts to regulate their use by health care legislation (e.g. OBRA-87).[43,44] Staff in long-term care facilities are frequently poorly trained in their use and are unaware of their expected benefits and potential side effects.[45] More recently, serious adverse events associated with a number of these agents have led some health regulatory authorities to recommend that their use for the treatment of BPSD be avoided completely.[46] For all these reasons, knowledge of the efficacy and safety of pharmacological interventions for BPSD is essential.

Pharmacological management begins with the identification of target symptoms for treatment. Whether this is done by utilizing one of the behavioural rating scales mentioned previously, or in conjunction with discussions with caregivers, this process is essential because some target symptoms will respond to these interventions and others will not. Examples of symptoms more likely to respond to pharmacotherapy include apathy, depression, anxiety, delusions, hallucinations, agitation, aggression and insomnia. BPSD, which are more likely to be resistant to pharmacological management, include wandering, exit seeking, screaming and perseverative verbalizations, inappropriate voiding and some inappropriate sexual behaviours. Severe depressive symptoms, psychosis and aggression, which place the patient and others at risk of harm, might be considered indications for first-line use of pharmacotherapy,[19] though studies comparing the relative efficacy of pharmacological and non-pharmacological approaches are almost totally lacking.

Knowledge of the natural history of individual BPSD can be helpful in determining how long treatment will be necessary. For example, depression tends to occur early in the illness and is rarely persistent. Delusions and hallucinations tend to occur somewhat later and tend to be more persistent. Wandering and agitation tend to be very persistent, while aggression increases in frequency throughout the disease course and becomes more persistent in the moderate to severe stages of the illness.[47]

All pharmacological interventions must be monitored carefully for effectiveness and adverse events. After a period of symptom improvement and stability, it is important to consider tapering and withdrawing psychotropics. There are now several randomized double-blind, placebo-controlled withdrawal studies.[48–51] These studies have consistently demonstrated that most patients on psychotropic medications for BPSD could be successfully withdrawn without exacerbating behaviours which required treatment initially. For example, in the largest trial to date, 82 patients were randomized to either ongoing treatment with an antipsychotic or withdrawal with a placebo, and followed for three months.[50] There were no differences in the rate of behavioural worsening between the two groups overall, though patients with higher levels of baseline behavioural symptoms were significantly more likely to experience relapse compared to patients with lower levels. In a smaller recent double-blind, randomized placebo-controlled withdrawal study, the majority of patients' behaviours remained stable or improved after withdrawal, though withdrawal was associated with significantly reduced sleep time.[51] In summary, evidence clearly supports attempts to withdraw psychotropics after a period of stability with the caveats that monitoring for behavioural exacerbation and sleep disturbances is essential, and that patients with ongoing severe BPSD may be less likely to tolerate withdrawal.

A variety of approaches for choosing specific medications have been proposed. The 'rational approach' to management attempts to match individual BPSD with psychotropic effects that have been documented in non-demented patient populations (e.g. aggression with psychosis treated with antipsychotics, aggression with mood symptoms treated with lithium or SSRIs, etc.).[52] Unfortunately, while this approach appears rational, there are few data available to support this. Another approach is based on the knowledge of the underlying neurobiology of specific BPSD.[53–56] Using this approach, investigators have attempted to determine if behaviours such as aggression, associated with serotonergic or noradrenergic dysfunction, will respond preferentially to serotonergic or noradrenergic therapies.[57,58] While this approach appears promising, more efficacious therapies and better understanding of the neurobiology of BPSD are still required. Finally, an evidence-based approach which weighs the relative risks and benefits of these interventions based on RCT data can be utilized and will form the basis of the following recommendations, summarized in Table 22.1.

Table 22.1 Pharmacological interventions for BPSD*

Drug	Possible indicators	Suggested dose/range	Comments
Antipsychotics			
Risperidone	Agitation, aggression, psychosis	$\simeq$ 1 mg/day	Increased risk of CVAEs and mortality
Olanzapine	Agitation, aggression, psychosis	5–10 mg/day	Increased risk of CVAEs and mortality
Quetiapine	Agitation, aggression, psychosis	100–200 mg/day	Increased risk of mortality; few published efficacy data
Antidepressants			
Citalopram	Depression, irritability, anxiety, agitation	20–40 mg/day	Possible similar benefits with other SSRIs
Trazodone	Sundowning, sleep disturbance Agitation, aggression	25–50 mg hs 50–300 mg/day	Possible excessive sedation, orthostatic hypotension
Anticonvulsants			
Carbamazepine	Agitation, aggression	300 mg/day	Possible drug–drug interactions
Cognitive enhancers			
Donepezil	Depression, apathy, anxiety agitation, psychosis	10 mg/day	Likely similar benefits with galantamine and rivastigmine
Memantine	Agitation Aggression	10–20 mg/day	Benefit in moderate to severe AD

* Based on randomized controlled trials

Antipsychotics

The best studied medications for the treatment of BPSD are the antipsychotics, which may, in part, account for the fact that they are among the most frequently used medications for control of most types of BPSD including psychosis, aggression and agitation.[59] Antipsychotics have preferentially been recommended as first-line pharmacotherapy for BPSD by various reviews and guidelines.[16,18,60] The symptoms which are most likely to respond to antipsychotics include delusions, hallucinations, aggression, agitation and sleep disturbance.[61]

The largest number of published RCTs compare typical antipsychotics (e.g. haloperidol) with placebo. Seventeen RCTs enrolled approximately 500 patients treated with typical antipsychotics and 235 controls treated with placebo. Meta-analyses of these trials suggest a response rate >60 per cent for the antipsychotic with a significant therapeutic effect of 18–26

per cent compared to placebo.[62,63] While these meta-analyses suggest the efficacy rate is approximately equivalent to the side effect rate, patients with dementia are at significant risk of developing parkinsonism and tardive dyskinesia, even when treated with low doses of typical antipsychotics.[64,65] There is also some evidence that typical antipsychotics may increase the rate of cognitive decline in patients with AD[66] and hasten mortality in patients with dementia with Lewy Bodies.[67]

While there are fewer published trials of the atypical antipsychotics, over 2000 patients were included in the seven RCTs of risperidone,[68–71] olanzapine[72,73] and quetiapine.[74] The studies of risperidone and olanzapine demonstrated efficacy greater than placebo. There was some evidence for a dose–response effect, and two studies which utilized an active haloperidol-treated arm suggested equal efficacy with less tendency to cause extrapyramidal symptoms (EPS). In the only published quetiapine RCT, quetiapine, up to 100 mg/day, was no more effective than placebo and was associated with worsening of cognition.[74] The lack of efficacy may have been due to the low dose of quetiapine as unpublished data suggest that only doses of approximately 200 mg per day are associated with efficacy greater than placebo.[75]

After reviewing data from published and unpublished BPSD RCTs, health regulatory agencies have recently raised concerns about serious adverse events including cerebrovascular adverse events (CVAEs) and death. For example, in 11 RCTs of olanzapine and risperidone (five published, six unpublished), 48 of 2187 (2.2 per cent) drug-treated patients experienced CVAEs compared with 10 of 1190 (0.8 per cent) placebo-treated patients for a relative risk of 2.7 (95 per cent CI, 1.4–5.3).[76] The FDA (Food and Drug Administration of the USA) recently warned that analyses of 17 placebo-controlled trials of olanzapine, aripiprazole, risperidone and quetiapine with 5106 dementia patients with BPSD suggested a 4.5 per cent mortality rate in drug-treated patients compared with 2.6 per cent of placebo-treated patients.[77] The publication of these warnings must be concerns for clinicians from two perspectives: (1) Are these drugs truly safe? (2) How can clinicians be assured of their efficacy given that the majority of the studies reviewed by the FDA have not been published? The latter is a question that plagues evidence-based practitioners of all aspects of medicine. The question would probably equally apply to non-pharmacological interventions as there is no reason to assume there is not an equal proportion of unpublished studies of these modalities. Clinical trial registration and access to study data submitted for drug registration, available to all researchers and clinicians, would significantly advance the cause of evidence-based medicine.

With respect to the safety of antipsychotics for BPSD, the increased incidence of CVAEs appears to be accounted for by non-specific vascular events rather than completed strokes. For example, in a review of the risperidone trials, while the percentage of patients with any CVAEs was statistically greater in risperidone-treated patients compared with placebo, there were no significant differences in the rates of serious CVAEs (defined as death, life threatening, requiring hospitalization, leading to persistent disability, etc.).[76] Furthermore, large observational administrative health database studies also suggest no differences in the rates of hospitalization for strokes when comparing olanzapine to risperidone and typical antipsychotics.[78,79] Because many patients in the RCTs had numerous treated and untreated vascular risk factors, clinical recommendations might include avoiding the use of atypicals in AD patients with vascular risk fac-

tors. While this recommendation appears reasonable, data from a study of over 32 000 elderly dementia patients treated with either typical or atypical antipsychotics suggested no differences in the risk of stroke associated with either class of drugs when analysed for other stroke risk factors such as history of previous stroke and atrial fibrillation.[79]

Similar data from RCTs led health regulatory agencies to issue warnings about increased mortality in atypical AP-treated dementia patients compared to placebo.[77] In a meta-analysis of 15 published and unpublished BPSD trials, 118/3353 (3.5 per cent) atypical AP-treated patients died compared with 40/1757 (2.3 per cent) placebo-treated patients.[80] There was no evidence that risk varied by drug, severity or diagnosis. In two studies that included haloperidol arms, a similar increased magnitude of risk was noted. These results conflict with four observational studies which suggested there was no increased risk of mortality compared with untreated patients or patients treated with typical antipsychotics.[81–84]

In summary, as a class, the antipsychotics are the best studied of any intervention for BPSD with numerous, relatively small, high quality studies of the typical antipsychotics, and a smaller number of high quality RCTs of atypical agents with much larger sample sizes supporting their efficacy. Use of typical antipsychotics is plagued by concerns about the tendency to cause EPS (both acute EPS and tardive dyskinesia), while use of atypical antipsychotics appears to increase the risk of CVAEs and mortality. Given that emerging data suggest no differences between typical and atypical antipsychotics with respect to stroke risk and increased mortality, there is no rationale for clinicians to return to the use of typical antipsychotics. If pharmacological management in BPSD is required, use of atypicals would still appear to be the most reasonable first-line pharmacological intervention for psychosis, agitation and aggression, especially when patient and caregiver safety are concerns. Full disclosure of the relative risks and benefits with substitute decision-makers is clearly essential.

Cholinesterase inhibitors and memantine

The currently available cognitive enhancer agents, the cholinesterase inhibitors (CIs) and memantine, appear to modestly improve not only cognition and function, but behaviour as well. In a meta-analysis of the pivotal CI RCTs, Trinh et al[85] found small but statistically significant benefits for behavioural measures. The studies reviewed in this analysis included AD subjects with mostly mild-to-moderate illness and very little in the way of behavioural disturbances at baseline, potentially limiting the ability to demonstrate a robust drug effect. In fact, in an RCT of donepezil in moderate-to-severe AD patients, with much more severe BPSD at baseline, behavioural improvements were significant and much larger.[86] In the best study to address the issue to date, Holmes et al[87] conducted a double-blind, placebo-controlled withdrawal study in moderately disturbed AD patients who had been treated with open-label donepezil for 12 weeks. Patients randomized to placebo experienced a significant worsening of behaviours, while patients on donepezil continued to improve in the ensuing 12-week double-blind phase. These investigators concluded that the benefit with donepezil for BPSD was not only statistically significant but also clinically important. Not all of the RCTs, however, have demonstrated positive effects on behaviour.[74,88] Specific behaviours which appear to improve with the CIs include hallucinations, delusions, apathy, anxiety, agitation, depression, disinhibition and aberrant motor behaviours.[89,90] CIs may also reduce the emergence of BPSD and can reduce caregiver stress.[91]

The effects of memantine, an NMDA receptor antagonist, on behaviour have been studied in two RCTs with moderate to severe AD[92,93] and one study of patients with severe AD or VaD.[94] In a post-hoc analysis of two of these studies, behavioural improvements favoured memantine in both studies and reached statistical significance in the study in which memantine was added to pre-existing treatment with donepezil.[95] In both studies, agitation/aggression improved significantly with memantine therapy.

In summary, there are emerging data that the CIs and memantine can improve BPSD. It would, therefore, appear reasonable that given their effects on cognition and function, first-line use in patients with mild-to-moderate BPSD can be recommended. Whether these agents are affective in severe BPSD, and how effective they are relative to the antipsychotics, has not yet been determined.

Antidepressants

Antidepressants have been used to treat depression in AD patients as well as other BPSD such as agitation and aggression. The concept of depression and depressive symptoms in patients with AD has received increasing attention, and specific criteria for depression of AD have recently been proposed.[96] Treatment of depression in placebo-controlled RCTs has resulted in mixed conclusions.[97] Some studies with imipramine, citalopram, sertraline and fluoxetine have not demonstrated improvements beyond placebo, while other studies with citalopram, clomipramine, moclobemide and sertraline did demonstrate significant drug effects. Furthermore, these studies suggest that treatment with tricyclic antidepressants may worsen cognition (likely secondary to anticholinergic effects) and improvements can be significant, even in the placebo-treated patients (likely an effect of a psychosocial/environmental impact of an RCT). In the most rigorous study to date, Lyketsos et al[98] treated 44 AD patients with major depression in a randomized placebo-controlled trial with sertraline. Sertraline demonstrated significant overall depressive symptom reduction and more patients being judged as responders compared to placebo.

In summary, AD patients with depression appeared to respond well to both antidepressant and psychosocial interventions. It is unclear which type of therapy works better for which type of patient (or severity of depression). If an antidepressant is chosen, clinicians should avoid the use of tricyclic antidepressants.

Trazodone, a triazolopyridine antidepressant, has been studied for BPSD such as agitation and aggression. There have been three RCTs which include a small cross-over trial,[99] a comparison study with haloperidol[100] and a larger, well-designed placebo-controlled trial. Terri et al compared trazodone, haloperidol and behavioural therapy to placebo in 149 moderately disturbed AD patients with agitation.[101] There were no statistically significant benefits associated with trazodone therapy (nor with haloperidol or behavioural therapy) and the most frequent reason for dropouts from the trazodone arm was actually an increase in agitation. While there were methodological problems associated with the study,[102] the investigators concluded that the three studied treatments have only marginal efficacy and other forms of therapy should be considered. A recent meta-analysis of trazodone for BPSD also concluded that there is insufficient evidence to recommend the use of trazodone for BPSD at the present time.[103]

In a large RCT comparing citalopram to placebo, Nyth and Gottfries[104] noted significant improvement in symptoms such as confusion, irritability, anxiety, fear and restlessness in patients treated with citalopram. Because these patients had only mild BPSD at baseline, the study was replicated in a more severely disturbed patient population. Pollock et al[105] treated 85 patients with moderate to severe BPSD with either citalopram, perphenazine or placebo in a blinded RCT. While the patients treated with both citalopram and perphenazine improved significantly, only citalopram-treated patients experienced statistically more improvement compared to placebo. Specific behavioural improvements were noted in agitation, aggression, psychosis, lability/tension and retardation. There is some evidence of efficacy from RCTs for the use of sertraline for BPSD as well.[57]

In summary, there are emerging data supporting the use of SSRIs especially citalopram for BPSD such as agitation, aggression and irritability. The results of the recently completed CATIE study,[106] an RCT comparing three atypical antipsychotics and citalopram, will hopefully help clarify the role of citalopram in the treatment of BPSD.

Anticonvulsants

Carbamazepine and valproate have been studied for BPSD treatment. Four RCTs have been reported with carbamazepine suggesting a significant benefit compared to placebo.[107–110] For example, in a study of 51 nursing home residents with significant agitation and aggression, global improvement was noted in 72 per cent of carbamazepine-treated patients compared with 21 per cent of placebo-treated patients, representing the largest drug–placebo difference of all BPSD therapeutic trials.[109] Because of concerns about tolerability and drug–drug interactions with carbamazepine, valproic acid was investigated for the treatment of BPSD. The four RCTs with valproate did not show any significant benefit compared with placebo in the primary outcome measures, though some secondary measures of agitation and aggression did seem to improve in some of these studies.[111–114] A recent meta-analysis of these studies suggested that lower doses of valproate were ineffective and higher doses were associated with an unacceptable rate of adverse effects including excessive sedation.[115] Valproate also appears to be associated with thrombocytopenia, which is more common in the elderly.[116,117] Open-labelled studies of gabapentin suggest some benefit for BPSD including agitation and aggression though no RCT data are available at the present time.[118,119]

In summary, though RCT data suggest efficacy for the use of carbamazepine for BPSD, side effects and potential drug interactions will probably make its use limited to a second-line agent. There is currently insufficient evidence to recommend the use of valproate for BPSD, and potential safety concerns appear to attenuate demonstrated benefit.

Benzodiazepines

Benzodiazepines have been studied for many years for the treatment of BPSD. Unfortunately, the early double-blind RCTs suffered from a lack of standardized diagnostic criteria and poorly defined outcome measures.[120–122] Several older RCTs suggest that agitation, anxiety, irritability and insomnia respond to treatment with benzodiazepines and efficacy may be similar to that of the antipsychotics.[123–129] While these short-term studies suggest reasonable efficacy and tolerability, concerns with long-term use include tolerance and dependence. Even with short-term use, adverse effects such as excessive sedation, falls and increased cognitive impairment have limited recommendations to use as pro re nata agents.[130] In this context, a double-blind placebo-controlled study compared intramuscular lorazepam to intramuscular olanzapine.[131] Both active treatments were equally effective and significantly better than placebo for managing acute agitation, though the effects of olanzapine appeared to be slightly longer lasting. More importantly, there were no differences in the adverse events between the active treatments and placebo including sedation.

In summary, benzodiazepines appear to be effective in managing BPSD. Given concerns about short-term and long-term adverse events, however, their use should be limited to managing acute behavioural exacerbations as pro re nata agents. This recommendation has been supported by one high quality RCT.

Beta-blockers

Several small RCTs have examined the use of beta-blockers including propranolol and pindolol for BPSD such as agitation and aggression.[132,133] A small double-blind cross-over study found limited efficacy for pindolol in aggressive AD patients with severe dementia,[58] and a recent, slightly larger RCT found that, while propranolol was more effective than placebo initially, the benefit appeared to diminish over a subsequent 6-month open-label phase.[134] These studies have also raised questions about the frequency of contraindications to use the beta-blockers in this medically frail population, as well as the potential for adverse events.

In summary, while there is some RCT evidence for the efficacy of beta-blockers for BPSD, more evidence, especially with respect to their safety, is required before recommendations for their use can be made.

Other pharmacological approaches

A number of other pharmacotherapies have undergone RCTs for treatment of BPSD. Buspirone, a non-benzodiazepine serotonergic anxiolytic, has been studied in two RCTs.[99,135] In the only trial which included a placebo control, efficacy was found to be no better than placebo.[99] Two small placebo-controlled trials have suggested that oral conjugated oestrogens reduced agitation and aggression in both men and women with BPSD.[136,137] In a small RCT of a transdermal oestrogen patch, there were no significant improvements noted in aggression.[138] A small, double-blind placebo-controlled trial suggested dronabinol, a chemical compound of marihuana, decreased BPSD and increased body weight in anorexic AD patients.[139] In a partially blinded non-randomized trial, long-acting opioids appeared to have some benefit in a subset of agitated dementia patients >85 years of age.[140] Finally, two double-blind placebo-controlled trials failed to demonstrate any efficacy for melatonin for sleep disorders in patients with AD.[141,142] In summary, while a variety of other pharmacological interventions have been tested with RCTs for BPSD, there is insufficient evidence to recommend any of these at the present time.

RECOMMENDATIONS AND DISCUSSION

The management of BPSD should include assessment and diagnosis, optimization of concomitant medical conditions and medications, institution of non-pharmacological interventions and medication management with psychotropics when indicated. The author acknowledges the following caveats to these recommendations: (1) there is little in the way of controlled data to provide evidence for the recommendations of assessment/diagnosis and medical optimization; (2) evidence for individual non-pharmacological interventions, while plentiful, is poor at best; (3) the efficacy for the best studied pharmacological intervention, the antipsychotics, is counterbalanced by infrequent, but potentially serious adverse events. Given these caveats, how can the preceding recommendations be made with any degree of confidence? Recommendations about assessment, diagnosis and medical optimization not only have face validity but are critical elements of good humane care for elderly individuals. It has also been argued that non-pharmacological interventions for BPSD are crucial parts of 'structured good care' and should take precedence over pharmacological treatment.[35] This stance is based on a humanitarian framework that assumes BPSD represents unmet physical and emotional needs. In this context, treatment with psychotropic medication may sedate the patient and 'rob' them of their abilities to express or address these needs.[35] Regardless of whether one is sympathetic to this philosophy, and in spite of the inherent difficulties in studying non-pharmacological approaches, these therapies still require confirmatory trials, at the very least, to provide clinicians with some guidance as to which of the myriad of therapies should be used for which patients, and for what types of BPSD. With respect to the balance between efficacy and safety of the pharmacological interventions, once again, a theo-retical framework might be helpful. Perhaps clinicians should view the treatment of AD with a palliative care approach, whereby quality of life takes precedence over quantity of life. Proponents have argued forcibly for this type of approach for advanced dementia,[143] though earlier disease may benefit from this philosophy as well. If this approach was more widely adopted, researchers would need to focus on evidence for changes in the quality of life for their patient and caregiver, something that is sorely lacking in the current pharmacotherapy literature.

REFERENCES

1. Finkel SI, Costa e Silva J, Cohen G, Miller S, Sartorius N. Behavioral and psychological signs and symptoms of dementia: a consensus statement on current knowledge and implications for research and treatment. Int Psychogeriatr 1996; 8(suppl 3):497–500.
2. Teri L, Rabins P, Whitehouse P, et al. Management of behavior disturbance in Alzheimer disease: current knowledge and future directions. Alzheimer Dis Assoc Disord 1992; 6:77–88.
3. Lyketsos CG, Steinberg M, Tschanz JT, et al. Mental and behavioral disturbances in dementia: findings from the Cache County Study on Memory in Aging. Am J Psychiatry 2000; 157:708–714.
4. Rosenblatt A, Samus QM, Steele CD, et al. The Maryland Assisted Living Study: prevalence, recognition, and treatment of dementia and other psychiatric disorders in the assisted living population of central Maryland. J Am Geriatr Soc 2004; 52:1618–1625.
5. Ryden MB. Aggressive behavior in persons with dementia who live in the community. Alzheimer Dis Assoc Disord 1988; 2:342–355.
6. Chenoweth B, Spencer B. Dementia: the experience of family caregivers. Gerontologist 1986; 26:267–272.
7. Miller TP, Tinklenberg JR, Brooks JO 3rd, Fenn HH, Yesavage JA. Selected psychiatric symptoms associated with rate of cognitive decline in patients with Alzheimer's disease. J Geriatr Psychiatry Neurol 1993; 6:235–238.
8. Moritz DJ, Fox PJ, Luscombe FA, Kraemer HC. Neurological and psychiatric predictors of mortality in patients with Alzheimer disease in California. Arch Neurol 1997; 54:878–885.
9. Walsh JS, Welch HG, Larson EB. Survival of outpatients with Alzheimer-type dementia. Ann Intern Med 1990; 113:429–434.
10. Lopez OL, Wisniewski SR, Becker JT, Boller F, DeKosky ST. Psychiatric medication and abnormal behavior as predictors of progression in probable Alzheimer disease. Arch Neurol 1999; 56:1266–1272.
11. Mortimer JA, Ebbitt B, Jun SP, Finch MD. Predictors of cognitive and functional progression in patients with probable Alzheimer's disease. Neurology 1992; 42:1689–1696.
12. Clyburn LD, Stones MJ, Hadjistavropoulos T, Tuokko H. Predicting caregiver burden and depression in Alzheimer's disease. J Gerontol B Psychol Sci Soc Sci 2000; 55:S2–S13.
13. Coen RF, Swanwick GR, O'Boyle CA, Coakley D. Behaviour disturbance and other predictors of carer burden in Alzheimer's disease. Int J Geriatr Psychiatry 1997; 12:331–336.

14. Donaldson C, Tarrier N, Burns A. Determinants of carer stress in Alzheimer's disease. Int J Geriatr Psychiatry 1998; 13:248–256.
15. Beeri MS, Werner P, Davidson M, Noy S. The cost of behavioral and psychological symptoms of dementia (BPSD) in community dwelling Alzheimer's disease patients. Int J Geriatr Psychiatry 2002; 17:403–408.
16. Alexopoulos GS, Silver JM, Kahn DA, et al. The expert consensus guideline series: treatment of agitation in older persons with dementia. Postgrad Med 1998; 26:1–88.
17. Practice guideline for the treatment of patients with Alzheimer's disease and other dementias of late life. American Psychiatric Association. Am J Psychiatry 1997; 154:1–39.
18. Herrmann N. Recommendations for the management of behavioral and psychological symptoms of dementia. Can J Neurol Sci 2001; 28(suppl 1):S96–S107.
19. Consensus statement on improving the quality of mental health care in U.S. nursing homes: management of depression and behavioral symptoms associated with dementia. J Am Geriatr Soc 2003; 51:1287–1298.
20. Sink KM, Holden KF, Yaffe K. Pharmacological treatment of neuropsychiatric symptoms of dementia: a review of the evidence. JAMA 2005; 293:596–608.
21. Kiely DK, Morris JN, Algase DL. Resident characteristics associated with wandering in nursing homes. Int J Geriatr Psychiatry 2000; 15:1013–1020.
22. Cohen-Mansfield J, Billig N, Lipson S, Rosenthal AS, Pawlson LG. Medical correlates of agitation in nursing home residents. Gerontology 1990; 36:150–158.
23. Corbin SL, Eastwood MR. Sensory deficits and mental disorders of old age: causal or coincidental associations? Psychol Med 1986; 16:251–256.
24. Horowitz A. The relationship between vision impairment and the assessment of disruptive behaviors among nursing home residents. Gerontologist 1997; 37:620–628.
25. Chapman FM, Dickinson J, McKeith I, Ballard C. Association among visual hallucinations, visual acuity, and specific eye pathologies in Alzheimer's disease: treatment implications. Am J Psychiatry 1999; 156:1983–1985.
26. Allen NH, Burns A, Newton V, et al. The effects of improving hearing in dementia. Age Ageing 2003; 32:189–193.
27. Learoyd BM. Psychotropic drugs and the elderly patient. Med J Aust 1972; 1:1131–1133.
28. Lanctot KL, Bowles SK, Herrmann N, Best TS, Naranjo CA. Drugs mimicking dementia. Dementia symptoms associated with psychotropic drugs in institutionalised cognitively impaired patients. CNS Drugs 2000; 14:381–390.
29. Weiner MF, Koss E, Wild KV, et al. Measures of psychiatric symptoms in Alzheimer patients: a review. Alzheimer Dis Assoc Disord 1996; 10:20–30.
30. Cummings JL, Mega M, Gray K, et al. The Neuropsychiatric Inventory: comprehensive assessment of psychopathology in dementia. Neurology 1994; 44:2308–2314.
31. Alexopoulos GS, Abrams RC, Young RC, Shamoian CA. Cornell Scale for Depression in Dementia. Biol Psychiatry 1988; 23:271–284.
32. Cohen-Mansfield J, Billig N. Agitated behaviors in the elderly. I. A conceptual review. J Am Geriatr Soc 1986; 34:711–721.
33. Teresi J, Abrams R, Holmes D, Ramirez M, Eimicke J. Prevalence of depression and depression recognition in nursing homes. Soc Psychiatry Psychiatr Epidemiol 2001; 36:613–620.
34. Nilsson K, Palmstierna T, Wistedt B. Aggressive behavior in hospitalized psychogeriatric patients. Acta Psychiatr Scand 1988; 78:172–175.
35. Cohen-Mansfield J, Mintzer JE. Time for change: the role of nonpharmacological interventions in treating behavior problems in nursing home residents with dementia. Alzheimer Dis Assoc Disord 2005; 19:37–40.
36. Cohen-Mansfield J. Nonpharmacologic interventions for inappropriate behaviors in dementia: a review, summary, and critique. Am J Geriatr Psychiatry 2001; 9:361–381.
37. Snowden M, Sato K, Roy-Byrne P. Assessment and treatment of nursing home residents with depression or behavioral symptoms associated with dementia: a review of the literature. J Am Geriatr Soc 2003; 51:1305–1317.
38. Opie J, Rosewarne R, O'Connor DW. The efficacy of psychosocial approaches to behaviour disorders in dementia: a systematic literature review. Aust NZ J Psychiatry 1999; 33:789–799.
39. Verkaik R, van Weert JC, Francke AL. The effects of psychosocial methods on depressed, aggressive and apathetic behaviors of people with dementia: a systematic review. Int J Geriatr Psychiatry 2005; 20:301–314.
40. Thorgrimsen L, Spector A, Wiles A, Orrell M. Aroma therapy for dementia. Cochrane Database Syst Rev 2003: CD003150.
41. Forbes D, Morgan DG, Bangma J, et al. Light therapy for managing sleep, behaviour, and mood disturbances in dementia. Cochrane Database Syst Rev 2005; 2:CD003946.
42. Vink AC, Birks JS, Bruinsma MS, Scholten RJ. Music therapy for people with dementia. Cochrane Database Syst Rev 2005; CD003477.
43. Semla TP, Palla K, Poddig B, Brauner DJ. Effect of the Omnibus Reconciliation Act 1987 on antipsychotic prescribing in nursing home residents. J Am Geriatr Soc 1994; 42:648–652.
44. Beers MH, Ouslander JG, Rollingher I, et al. Explicit criteria for determining inappropriate medication use in nursing home residents. UCLA Division of Geriatric Medicine. Arch Intern Med 1991; 151:1825–1832.
45. Avorn J, Dreyer P, Connelly K, Soumerai SB. Use of psychoactive medication and the quality of care in rest homes. Findings and policy implications of a statewide study. N Engl J Med 1989; 320:227–232.
46. Committee on Safety of Medicines. Summary of clinical trial data on cerebrovascular adverse events (CVAEs) in randomized clinical trials of risperidone conducted in patients with dementia. Available from URL: http://www.mca.gov.uk/aboutagency/regframework/csm/cshome.htm (accessed 28 June 2004).
47. Devanand DP, Jacobs DM, Tang MX, et al. The course of psychopathologic features in mild to moderate Alzheimer disease. Arch Gen Psychiatry 1997; 54:257–263.
48. Cohen-Mansfield J, Lipson S, Werner P, et al. Withdrawal of haloperidol, thioridazine, and lorazepam in the nursing home: a controlled, double-blind study. Arch Intern Med 1999; 159:1733–1740.
49. van Reekum R, Clarke D, Conn D, et al. A randomized, placebo-controlled trial of the discontinuation of long-term antipsychotics in dementia. Int Psychogeriatr 2002; 14:197–210.
50. Ballard CG, Thomas A, Fossey J, et al. A 3-month, randomized, placebo-controlled, neuroleptic discontinuation study in 100 people with dementia: the neuropsychiatric inventory median cutoff is a predictor of clinical outcome. J Clin Psychiatry 2004; 65:114–119.
51. Ruths S, Straand J, Nygaard HA, Bjorvatn B, Pallesen S. Effect of antipsychotic withdrawal on behavior and sleep/wake activity in nursing home residents with dementia: a randomized, placebo-controlled, double-blinded study.

The Bergen District Nursing Home Study. J Am Geriatr Soc 2004; 52:1737–1743.

52. Yudofsky SC, Silver JM, Hales RE. Pharmacologic management of aggression in the elderly. J Clin Psychiatry 1990; 51(suppl):22–28.

53. Lanctot KL, Herrmann N, Mazzotta P. Role of serotonin in the behavioral and psychological symptoms of dementia. J Neuropsychiatry Clin Neurosci 2001; 13:5–21.

54. Cummings JL. Cholinesterase inhibitors: A new class of psychotropic compounds. Am J Psychiatry 2000; 157:4–15.

55. Herrmann N, Lanctot KL, Khan LR. The role of norepinephrine in the behavioral and psychological symptoms of dementia. J Neuropsychiatry Clin Neurosci 2004; 16:261–276.

56. Lanctot KL, Herrmann N, Mazzotta P, Khan LR, Ingber N. GABAergic function in Alzheimer's disease: evidence for dysfunction and potential as a therapeutic target for the treatment of behavioural and psychological symptoms of dementia. Can J Psychiatry 2004; 49:439–453.

57. Lanctot KL, Herrmann N, van Reekum R, Eryavec G, Naranjo CA. Gender, aggression and serotonergic function are associated with response to sertraline for behavioral disturbances in Alzheimer's disease. Int J Geriatr Psychiatry 2002; 17:531–541.

58. Herrmann N, Lanctot KL, Eryavec G, Khan LR. Noradrenergic activity is associated with response to pindolol in aggressive Alzheimer's disease patients. J Psychopharmacol 2004; 18:215–220.

59. Greve M, O'Connor D. A survey of Australian and New Zealand old age psychiatrists' preferred medications to treat behavioral and psychological symptoms of dementia (BPSD). Int Psychogeriatr 2005; 17:195–205.

60. Alexopoulos GS, Streim J, Carpenter D, Docherty JP. Using antipsychotic agents in older patients. J Clin Psychiatry 2004; 65(suppl 2):5–99.

61. Rabinowitz J, Katz IR, De Deyn PP, et al. Behavioral and psychological symptoms in patients with dementia as a target for pharmacotherapy with risperidone. J Clin Psychiatry 2004; 65:1329–1334.

62. Schneider LS, Pollock VE, Lyness SA. A metaanalysis of controlled trials of neuroleptic treatment in dementia. J Am Geriatr Soc 1990; 38:553–563.

63. Lanctot KL, Best TS, Mittmann N, et al. Efficacy and safety of neuroleptics in behavioral disorders associated with dementia. J Clin Psychiatry 1998; 59:550–561.

64. Sweet RA. Neuroleptic-induced parkinsonism in elderly patients diagnosed with psychotic major depression and dementia of the Alzheimer type. Am J Geriatr Psychiatry 1996; 4:311–319.

65. Caligiuri MP, Rockwell E, Jeste DV. Extrapyramidal side effects in patients with Alzheimer's disease treated with low-dose neuroleptic medication. Am J Geriatr Psychiatry 1998; 6:75–82.

66. McShane R, Keene J, Gedling K, et al. Do neuroleptic drugs hasten cognitive decline in dementia? Prospective study with necropsy follow up. BMJ 1997; 314:266–270.

67. McKeith I, Fairbairn A, Perry R, Thompson P, Perry E. Neuroleptic sensitivity in patients with senile dementia of Lewy body type. BMJ 1992; 305:673–678.

68. Katz IR, Jeste DV, Mintzer JE, et al. Comparison of risperidone and placebo for psychosis and behavioral disturbances associated with dementia: a randomized, double-blind trial. Risperidone Study Group. J Clin Psychiatry 1999; 60: 107–115.

69. De Deyn PP, Rabheru K, Rasmussen A, et al. A randomized trial of risperidone, placebo, and haloperidol for behavioral symptoms of dementia. Neurology 1999; 53:946–955.

70. Chan WC, Lam LC, Choy CN, et al. A double-blind randomised comparison of risperidone and haloperidol in the treatment of behavioural and psychological symptoms in Chinese dementia patients. Int J Geriatr Psychiatry 2001; 16: 1156–1162.

71. Brodaty H, Ames D, Snowdon J, et al. A randomized placebo-controlled trial of risperidone for the treatment of aggression, agitation, and psychosis of dementia. J Clin Psychiatry 2003; 64:134–143.

72. Street JS, Clark WS, Gannon KS, et al. Olanzapine treatment of psychotic and behavioral symptoms in patients with Alzheimer disease in nursing care facilities: a double-blind, randomized, placebo-controlled trial. The HGEU Study Group. Arch Gen Psychiatry 2000; 57:968–976.

73. De Deyn PP, Carrasco MM, Deberdt W, et al. Olanzapine versus placebo in the treatment of psychosis with or without associated behavioral disturbances in patients with Alzheimer's disease. Int J Geriatr Psychiatry 2004; 19: 115–126.

74. Ballard C, Margallo-Lana M, Juszczak E, et al. Quetiapine and rivastigmine and cognitive decline in Alzheimer's disease: randomised double blind placebo controlled trial. BMJ 2005; 330:874.

75. Zhong K, Tariot P, Minkwitz MC, et al. Quetiapine for the treatment of agitation in elderly institutionalized patients with dementia: a randomized double-blind trial. In: American Association of Geriatric Psychiatry Annual Meeting; 5–6 March 2005, San Diego, California, 2005.

76. Herrmann N, Lanctot KL. Do atypical antipsychotics cause stroke? CNS Drugs 2005; 19:91–103.

77. Kuehn BM. FDA warns antipsychotic drugs may be risky for elderly. JAMA 2005; 293:2462.

78. Herrmann N, Mamdani M, Lanctot KL. Atypical antipsychotics and risk of cerebrovascular accidents. Am J Psychiatry 2004; 161:1113–1115.

79. Gill SS, Rochon PA, Herrmann N, et al. Atypical antipsychotic drugs and risk of ischaemic stroke: population based retrospective cohort study. BMJ 2005; 330:445.

80. Schneider LS, Dagerman KS, Insel P. Risk of death with atypical antipsychotic drug treatment for dementia: meta-analysis of randomized placebo-controlled trials. JAMA 2005; 294:1934–1943.

81. Raivio MM, Laurila JV, Strandberg TE, Tilvis RS, Pitkala KH. Psychotropic medication and stroke outcome. Am J Psychiatry 2005; 162:1027; author reply 1027–8.

82. Nasrallah HA, White T, Nasrallah AT. Lower mortality in geriatric patients receiving risperidone and olanzapine versus haloperidol: preliminary analysis of retrospective data. Am J Geriatr Psychiatry 2004; 12:437–439.

83. Suh GH, Shah A. Effect of antipsychotics on mortality in elderly patients with dementia: a 1-year prospective study in a nursing home. Int Psychogeriatr 2005; 17:429–441.

84. Wang PS, Schneeweiss S, Avorn J, et al. Risk of death in elderly users of conventional vs. atypical antipsychotic medications. N Engl J Med 2005; 353:2335–2341.

85. Trinh NH, Hoblyn J, Mohanty S, Yaffe K. Efficacy of cholinesterase inhibitors in the treatment of neuropsychiatric symptoms and functional impairment in Alzheimer disease: a meta-analysis. JAMA 2003; 289:210–216.

86. Feldman H, Gauthier S, Hecker J, et al. A 24-week, randomized, double-blind study of donepezil in moderate to severe Alzheimer's disease. Neurology 2001; 57:613–620.

87. Holmes C, Wilkinson D, Dean C, et al. The efficacy of donepezil in the treatment of neuropsychiatric symptoms in Alzheimer disease. Neurology 2004; 63:214–219.

88. Tariot PN, Cummings JL, Katz IR, et al. A randomized, double-blind, placebo-controlled study of the efficacy and safety of donepezil in patients with Alzheimer's disease in the nursing home setting. J Am Geriatr Soc 2001; 49: 1590–1599.

89. Mega MS, Masterman DM, O'Connor SM, Barclay TR, Cummings JL. The spectrum of behavioral responses to cholinesterase inhibitor therapy in Alzheimer disease. Arch Neurol 1999; 56:1388–1393.

90. Herrmann N, Rabheru K, Wang J, Binder C. Galantamine treatment of problematic behavior in Alzheimer disease: post-hoc analysis of pooled data from three large trials. Am J Geriatr Psychiatry 2005; 13:527–534.

91. Cummings JL, Schneider L, Tariot PN, Kershaw PR, Yuan W. Reduction of behavioral disturbances and caregiver distress by galantamine in patients with Alzheimer's disease. Am J Psychiatry 2004; 161:532–538.

92. Reisberg B, Doody R, Stoffler A, et al. Memantine in moderate-to-severe Alzheimer's disease. N Engl J Med 2003; 348:1333–1341.

93. Tariot PN, Farlow MR, Grossberg GT, et al. Memantine treatment in patients with moderate to severe Alzheimer disease already receiving donepezil: a randomized controlled trial. JAMA 2004; 291:317–324.

94. Winblad B, Poritis N. Memantine in severe dementia: results of the 9M-Best Study (Benefit and efficacy in severely demented patients during treatment with memantine). Int J Geriatr Psychiatry 1999; 14:135–146.

95. Gauthier S, Wirth Y, Mobius HJ. Effects of memantine on behavioural symptoms in Alzheimer's disease patients: an analysis of the Neuropsychiatric Inventory (NPI) data of two randomised, controlled studies. Int J Geriatr Psychiatry 2005; 20:459–464.

96. Olin JT, Schneider LS, Katz IR, et al. Provisional diagnostic criteria for depression of Alzheimer disease. Am J Geriatr Psychiatry 2002; 10:125–128.

97. Lyketsos CG, Olin J. Depression in Alzheimer's disease: overview and treatment. Biol Psychiatry 2002; 52:243–252.

98. Lyketsos CG, DelCampo L, Steinberg M, et al. Treating depression in Alzheimer disease: efficacy and safety of sertraline therapy, and the benefits of depression reduction: the DIADS. Arch Gen Psychiatry 2003; 60:737–746.

99. Lawlor BA, Radcliffe J, Molchan SE, et al. A pilot placebo-controlled study of trazodone and buspirone in Alzheimer's disease. Int J Geriatr Psychiatry 1994; 9: 55–59.

100. Sultzer DL, Gray KF, Gunay I, Berisford MA, Mahler ME. A double-blind comparison of trazodone and haloperidol for treatment of agitation in patients with dementia. Am J Geriatr Psychiatry 1997; 5:60–69.

101. Teri L, Logsdon RG, Peskind E, et al. Treatment of agitation in AD: a randomized, placebo-controlled clinical trial. Neurology 2000; 55:1271–1278.

102. Herrmann N, Black SE. Behavioral disturbances in dementia: will the real treatment please stand up? Neurology 2000; 55:1247–1248.

103. Martinon-Torres G, Fioravanti M, Grimley EJ. Trazodone for agitation in dementia. Cochrane Database Syst Rev 2004:CD004990.

104. Nyth AL, Gottfries CG. The clinical efficacy of citalopram in treatment of emotional disturbances in dementia disorders. A Nordic multicentre study. Br J Psychiatry 1990; 157:894–901.

105. Pollock BG, Mulsant BH, Rosen J, et al. Comparison of citalopram, perphenazine, and placebo for the acute treatment of psychosis and behavioral disturbances in hospitalized, demented patients. Am J Psychiatry 2002; 159:460–465.

106. Schneider LS, Tariot PN, Lyketsos CG, et al. National Institute of Mental Health Clinical Antipsychotic Trials of Intervention Effectiveness (CATIE): Alzheimer disease trial methodology. Am J Geriatr Psychiatry 2001; 9:346–360.

107. Tariot PN, Erb R, Leibovici A, et al. Carbamazepine treatment of agitation in nursing home patients with dementia: a preliminary study. J Am Geriatr Soc 1994; 42:1160–1166.

108. Cooney C, Mortimer A, Smith A, et al. Carbamazepine use in aggressive behaviour associated with senile dementia. Int J Geriatr Psychiatry 1996; 11:901–905.

109. Tariot PN, Erb R, Podgorski CA, et al. Efficacy and tolerability of carbamazepine for agitation and aggression in dementia. Am J Psychiatry 1998; 155:54–61.

110. Olin JT, Fox LS, Pawluczyk S, Taggart NA, Schneider LS. A pilot randomized trial of carbamazepine for behavioral symptoms in treatment-resistant outpatients with Alzheimer disease. Am J Geriatr Psychiatry 2001; 9:400–405.

111. Porsteinsson AP, Tariot PN, Erb R, et al. Placebo-controlled study of divalproex sodium for agitation in dementia. Am J Geriatr Psychiatry 2001; 9:58–66.

112. Sival RC, Haffmans PM, Jansen PA, Duursma SA, Eikelenboom P. Sodium valproate in the treatment of aggressive behavior in patients with dementia—a randomized placebo controlled clinical trial. Int J Geriatr Psychiatry 2002; 17:579–585.

113. Tariot PN, Schneider LS, Mintzer JE, Cutler AJ. Safety and tolerability of divalproex sodium in treatment of signs and symptoms of mania in elderly patients with dementia: results of a double-blind placebo-controlled trial. Curr Ther Res Clin Exp 2001; 62:51–67.

114. Tariot PN, Raman R, Jakimovich L, et al. Divalproex sodium in nursing home residents with possible or probable Alzheimer disease complicated by agitation: a randomized, controlled trial. Am J Geriatr Psychiatry 2005; 13:942–949.

115. Lonergan ET, Luxenberg J. Valproate preparations for agitation in dementia. Cochrane Database Syst Rev 2005; 3.

116. So CC, Wong KF. Valproate-associated dysmyelopoiesis in elderly patients. Am J Clin Pathol 2002; 118:225–228.

117. Trannel TJ, Ahmed I, Goebert D. Occurrence of thrombocytopenia in psychiatric patients taking valproate. Am J Psychiatry 2001; 158:128–130.

118. Herrmann N, Lanctot K, Myszak M. Effectiveness of gabapentin for the treatment of behavioral disorders in dementia. J Clin Psychopharmacol 2000; 20:90–93.

119. Moretti R, Torre P, Antonello RM, Cazzato G, Bava A. Gabapentin for the treatment of behavioural alterations in dementia: preliminary 15-month investigation. Drugs Aging 2003; 20:1035–1040.

120. Beber CR. Management of behavior in the institutionalized aged. Dis Nerv Syst 1965; 26:591–595.

121. Chesrow EJ, Kaplitz SE, Vetra H, et al. Blind study of oxazepam in the management of geriatric patients with behavioral problems. Clin Med 1965; 71:1001–1005.

122. Sanders JF. Evaluation of oxazepam and placebo in emotionally disturbed aged patients. Geriatrics 1965; 20: 739–746.

123. Kirven LE, Montero EF. Comparison of thioridazine and diazepam in the control of nonpsychotic symptoms associated with senility: double-blind study. J Am Geriatr Soc 1973; 21:546–551.

124. Covington JS. Alleviating agitation, apprehension, and related symptoms in geriatric patients: a double-blind com-

parison of a phenothiazine and a benzodiazepien. South Med J 1975; 68:719–724.

125. Stotskey B. Multicenter study comparing thioidazine with diazepam and placebo in elderly nonpsychotic patients with emtoinal and behavioral disorders. Clin Ther 1984; 6: 546–549.

126. Coccaro EF, Kramer E, Zemishlany Z, et al. Pharmacologic treatment of noncognitive behavioral disturbances in elderly demented patients. Am J Psychiatry 1990; 147: 1640–1645.

127. Ancill RJ, Carlyle WW, Liang RA, Holliday SG. Agitation in the demented elderly: a role for benzodiazepines? Int Clin Psychopharmacol 1991; 6:141–146.

128. Christensen DB, Benfield WR. Alprazolam as an alternative to low-dose haloperidol in older, cognitively impaired nursing facility patients. J Am Geriatr Soc 1998; 46: 620–625.

129. Sunderland T, Weingartner H, Cohen RM, et al. Low-dose oral lorazepam administration in Alzheimer subjects and age-matched controls. Psychopharmacology (Berl) 1989; 99:129–133.

130. Stern RG, Duffelmeyer ME, Zemishlani Z, Davidson M. The use of benzodiazepines in the management of behavioral symptoms in demented patients. Psychiatr Clin North Am 1991; 14:375–384.

131. Meehan KM, Wang H, David SR, et al. Comparison of rapidly acting intramuscular olanzapine, lorazepam, and placebo: a double-blind, randomized study in acutely agitated patients with dementia. Neuropsychopharmacology 2002; 26:494–504.

132. Greendyke RM, Kanter DR, Schuster DB, Verstreate S, Wootton J. Propranolol treatment of assaultive patients with organic brain disease. A double-blind crossover, placebo-controlled study. J Nerv Ment Dis 1986; 174:290–294.

133. Greendyke RM, Kanter DR. Therapeutic effects of pindolol on behavioral disturbances associated with organic brain disease: a double-blind study. J Clin Psychiatry 1986; 47:423–426.

134. Peskind ER, Tsuang DW, Bonner LT, et al. Propranolol for disruptive behaviors in nursing home residents with probable or possible Alzheimer disease: a placebo-controlled study. Alzheimer Dis Assoc Disord 2005; 19:23–28.

135. Cantillon M, Brunswick R, Molina D, Bahro M. Buspirone vs. haloperidol. A double-blind trial for agitation in nursing home population with Alzheimer's disease. Am J Geriatr Psychiatry 1996; 4:263–267.

136. Kyomen HH, Hennen J, Gottlieb GL, Wei JY. Estrogen therapy and noncognitive psychiatric signs and symptoms in elderly patients with dementia. Am J Psychiatry 2002; 159:1225–1227.

137. Kyomen HH, Satlin A, Hennen J, Wei JY. Estrogen therapy and aggressive behavior in elderly patients with moderate-to-severe dementia: results from a short-term, randomized, double-blind trial. Am J Geriatr Psychiatry 1999; 7:339–348.

138. Hall KA, Keks NA, O'Connor DW. Transdermal estrogen patches for aggressive behavior in male patients with dementia: a randomized, controlled trial. Int Psychogeriatr 2005; 17:165–178.

139. Volicer L, Stelly M, Morris J, McLaughlin J, Volicer BJ. Effects of dronabinol on anorexia and disturbed behavior in patients with Alzheimer's disease. Int J Geriatr Psychiatry 1997; 12:913–919.

140. Manfredi PL, Breuer B, Wallenstein S, et al. Opioid treatment for agitation in patients with advanced dementia. Int J Geriatr Psychiatry 2003; 18:700–705.

141. Serfaty M, Kennell-Webb S, Warner J, Blizard R, Raven P. Double blind randomised placebo controlled trial of low dose melatonin for sleep disorders in dementia. Int J Geriatr Psychiatry 2002; 17:1120–1127.

142. Singer C, Tractenberg RE, Kaye J, et al. A multicenter, placebo-controlled trial of melatonin for sleep disturbance in Alzheimer's disease. Sleep 2003; 26:893–901.

143. Volicer L, Rheaume Y, Brown J, Fabiszewski K, Brady R. Hospice approach to the treatment of patients with advanced dementia of the Alzheimer type. JAMA 1986; 256:2210–2213.

V Community and institutional management

23

Caregiver support: support of families

Henry Brodaty and Karen Berman

INTRODUCTION

There are currently more than 25 million patients with dementia worldwide, with 63 million expected globally by 2030 and 114 million in 2050, with the majority living in less developed regions of the world.[1] In the USA, more than 15 million adults provide care to ill or disabled relatives,[2] with informal caregivers providing 71 per cent of long-term care and 85 per cent of in-home care.[3] The caregiving career is highly dynamic and evolving, and the kinship relationship between patient and caregiver is extremely important. Family caregivers perform an important service for their relatives and for society, but do so at great cost to themselves. Decline in cognitive abilities, loss of functional capacity, dwindling companionship and increasing demands of physical care and possible behavioural changes in patients with a dementing illness impose escalating stresses on family caregivers.[4]

Medical management of a dementia patient and his/her caregiver should aim to maximize the quality of life of the patient and that of the caregiver.[5] This requires a long-term view and the establishment of partnerships between the patients, families and clinicians. Family caregivers should be recognized as part of the medical team as this accords them status and will ensure more co-operation with medical staff and longer-term care for the patient. Most caregivers today prefer to be included in the management process.[6]

As the dementing illness progresses, usually one person in the family comes forward as caregiver. This is generally a spouse or partner if the patient is married or in a relationship, or a child (more commonly a daughter or daughter-in-law) if the patient has no partner. About 75 per cent of caregivers are women, whom society traditionally views as responsible for nursing sick family members.[4,7,8] Caregivers of dementia patients tend to be older people, so are also prone to the concomitant problems of ageing. The Canadian Study of Health and Aging found the mean age of caregivers of dementia patients to be 62 years, with 36 per cent being 70 years or older.[7]

Recently, cultural and medical practice factors have made the caregiving role more difficult, with increasing numbers of people (particularly females) working outside the home, and decreased family size resulting in fewer people to share the caregiving role.[9] Caregiving often starts as a part-time occupation, but then grows and expands and continues for months if not years.[10] Typically, caregivers offer their services for emotional and economic reasons, not because they are proficient at, or feel comfortable with, the type of care required. They frequently expect to, or are expected to, assume the role of caregiver without regard for the possible emotional, physical and financial consequences.[11] Primary caregivers spend an average of 60 hours per week caring for the patient,[12] however, in many families the caregiving is shared, with other family members taking on a secondary caregiving role and providing periodic caregiving.[13] The mix of formal and informal help varies from country to country.[6] Families tend to keep the caregiving role within the family, but may hire outside help.[14] A hierarchical pattern of caregiver preference exists, with older people turning first to a spouse, then to an adult child, then to another relative and finally to a friend for care.[15–17] A significant majority of patients with chronic illness are cared for at home by family members,[18] however there are major differences between caregivers of dementia patients and caregivers of other elderly patients.[19] Older people who become increasingly dependent generally prefer to receive care at home; this is usually also the least expensive for society.[20]

DEFINITION OF CAREGIVER TERMINOLOGY

Many terms are used for those who provide care for people with dementia. In essence:

- Caregivers = carers = caretakers = informal carers = family and friends
- Formal caregivers = paid caregivers = paid carers
- Care co-ordinators = supervise the (paid) caregivers, but do not necessarily have a role in hands-on care.

Where co-ordination is provided by a family member, that person is more likely to be a male and to be a child of the patient; rarely is it the spouse.[21] Family care co-ordinators are more likely to set limits, delegate and take an objective approach to care. They are less personally involved with the patient and thus have less psychological stress. By taking a broad perspective the care co-ordinator may be able to expand and strengthen the caregiver's social network and help alleviate some of the strain.

WHAT ARE THE EFFECTS OF CAREGIVING ON CAREGIVERS

When a patient is diagnosed with dementia there is almost always a 'second' or 'hidden' patient. The combination of loss, prolonged distress and the physical demands of giving care in older caregivers increases the risk of physical health problems. As well, over one-third of caregivers suffer high levels of distress, objective and subjective burden and depression.[22–25] Caregivers take more medication than noncaregivers of a similar age.[26] Caregivers providing more care have simultaneously been shown to experience more satisfaction with their lives and more burden.[27–29] Frustration and grief are also common, reported as occurring in 81 per cent and 73 per cent of caregivers, respectively, in one study.[30] Hostility and anxiety are also often reported.[31] Some caregivers care for the patient willingly and cheerfully while others do so grudgingly and become more distressed.[21]

CAREGIVER BURDEN

This is defined as 'the negative phenomena associated with caring for an elderly, chronically ill or disabled family member or other person'.[32] This may be further divided into objective and subjective burden.

OBJECTIVE BURDEN

The burden or load borne by a person who cares for an elderly, chronically ill or disabled family member or other person is a multidimensional response to physical, psychological, emotional, social and financial stressors associated with the caregiving experience. It is greatly influenced by the amount of time spent with the patient.[33] Physical and social burden are good predictors of likelihood of institutionalization.[32] Financial burden is also a predictor of likelihood to institutionalize in some, but not in all studies.[32,34]

SUBJECTIVE BURDEN (sometimes called strain)

Subjective burden is defined as the caregiver's perception of the objective burden, and includes emotional reactions such as resentment, worry, frustration, depression, anxiety and fatigue. Feelings of 'being trapped' and 'being manipulated' are common, as is lack of privacy.[10] Indications of subjective burden include an increase in somatic complaints by the caregiver, fatigue, withdrawal and an unkempt appearance.[11]

Physical burden

Caregivers have poorer physical health than noncaregivers,[35–38] with higher rates of chronic conditions, prescription medication use, doctor visits,[25] poorer self-related health[39] as well as a higher mortality rate.[37] Reasons for the association between caregiving and physical morbidity and mortality include caregivers being less likely to get enough rest in general, having less time to rest when they are sick, having less time to exercise and having less time to attend to their own health.[2] The National Alliance for Caregiving in the US[40] reported that the two greatest predictors of caregiver physical strain were poor caregiver health and the caregiver's lack of choice in taking on caregiving responsibilities. Mental or emotional strain is an independent risk factor for mortality among elderly spousal caregivers[2,41] and those with poor psychological health are even more likely to have physical morbidity.[4] Grasel[42] found that the physical health of former caregivers improves in the long term once they cease to provide care. The finding of decreased immunological competence in caregivers of dementia patients[43] has been supported in an elegant study of response to influenza vaccine. Vedhara et al[44,45] reported that elderly caregivers of spouses with dementia have increased activation of the hypothalamic–pituitary axis and a poorer antibody response to the influenza vaccine, which could be enhanced by cognitive-behavioural intervention. They concluded that caregivers may be vulnerable to infectious disease. A meta-analysis of 32 studies of dementia caregivers found that caregiving was associated with a slightly greater risk of health problems and that this risk was moderated by measures of health (e.g. self-rated global health, medication use, antibodies, cardiovascular measures) and was greater in females.[46]

Other indicators of poorer physical health are increased service use, hospitalization, physician visits, drug use and aggregate use of health service; and less healthy behaviours such as increased alcohol intake and smoking more, and poorer sleep patterns, eating behaviour and nutrition.[47] Further, pre-existing conditions such as hypertension are more likely to be exacerbated by the caregiving role.[47] Caregiving has also been associated with a higher mortality rate.[2]

Psychological burden

One-third to one-half of caregivers suffer significant psychological distress[8,28,48] compared to depression rates for non-caregivers of a similar age of 8 per cent.[49] Numerous studies have demonstrated increased psychological morbidity in caregivers.[4,25,39,50–58] For example, Gallagher et al[55] found that amongst caregivers seeking help, 26 per cent met research diagnostic criteria (RDC) for major depression and 18 per cent for minor depression. Rates among non-help seekers were 10 per cent and 8 per cent respectively. In a study by Coope et al[58] of 100 caregivers of research subjects, 29.4 per cent met GMS-AGECAT criteria for major depression and 11.9 per cent met criteria for minor depression. Mittelman et al[56] reported that over 41.7 per cent of caregivers had a Geriatric Depression Scale score of 11 or greater, the rate being higher among women (50 per cent) than men (30 per cent).

A meta-analysis of 84 studies comparing caregivers of the elderly to non-caregivers found that there were significantly higher levels of depression and stress and significantly lower levels of self-efficacy, general subjective well-being and physical health in caregivers. This difference was larger when dementia caregivers were compared to non-caregivers than to heterogenous samples of caregivers of elderly patients.[36] Untreated, depression may lead to psychosocial difficulties, including general social maladjustment and overall discontent.[59]

Social burden

Caregivers become socially isolated.[4,60] Outside friendships dwindle as friends are unable to maintain meaningful contact with the dementia patient. Caregivers leave their homes less frequently due to their caregiving roles and become more isolated.[21,61] Caregivers involved in 'planning' and decision-making sessions with other family members are more satisfied with outcomes,[62] as are caregivers who have larger social support networks.[63]

Financial burden

Caregivers suffer financial hardship directly, through the cost of patient care (e.g. prescriptions, home modifications, transport and support services) and indirectly through loss of earnings by the patient and/or the caregiver.[60,64] The associated additional yearly cost of informal care per case (community dwelling patients aged over 70 years) in Langa's study (researched in 2000 and published in 2001) was US$3630 for mild dementia, US$7420 for moderate dementia and US$17 700 for severe dementia.[65] Caregiver estimations in 1998 for out of pocket expenses were US$15 000 to US$18 000 per year, and US$36 000 per year for loss of productivity.[66] In one study, 59 per cent of caregivers of dementia patients reduced their working hours or stopped working altogether and 89 per cent reported financial problems.[30] A national survey in 1997 found that 6 per cent of employed dementia caregivers turned down a promotion and 10 per cent reported taking early retirement because of their caregiving responsibilities.[67] Of caregivers aged 60 or under who held jobs while being the primary caregiver for a demented relative, 57 per cent reported that their work was disturbed as a result of their caregiving role.[40] Thomas et al[68] found that being forced to alter their working hours in order to look after a dementing parent was a problem specific to daughter caregivers. Caregivers are also faced with the increased financial burden of caring for their own health as they suffer increased rates of depression, distress, substance abuse and illness. However, one Scottish study centred in Dundee found the financial burden on the caregiver to be less than expected.[19]

PREDICTORS OF CAREGIVER EFFECTS

Studies have shown that there are no clear predictors of caregiver effects. Many factors combine to determine how caregivers will respond to caring for a dementing patient. This is reflected by the conflicting results of the many studies quoted below.

Caregiver variables (Table 23.1)

Kinship relationship of caregiver to patient

Spouse caregivers Spouses are the most frequent caregivers, wives twice as often as husbands, accounting for about 60 per cent of domestic caregivers.[69] Elderly unemployed spouse caregivers are more likely to provide continuous in-home care and are most likely to report feeling satisfied with life.[70] Spouses are less likely to institutionalize care recipients than are siblings/children,[61,70,71] and report more areas of satisfaction than do adult children.[26] Caregivers undergo a change in role from that of partner to that of caregiver or surrogate parent; this is no longer an equal partnership, but one where one partner becomes dependent on the other. Sexual difficulties are frequent accompaniments of these role changes.

Adult child caregivers About one in three caregivers are children, almost always the daughters or daughters-in-law of the dementing patient.[21] Henretta et al[72] observed a positive and statistically significant relationship between past financial transfers (from parent to child) and the child's current helping behaviour. This relationship may be a stronger determinant than gender, in deciding which child becomes the principal caregiver. When adult children become caregivers the relationship with the patient is one of role reversal, which may result in caregivers experiencing grief, anger and high levels of stress.[26] Child caregivers often report increased use of social services before finally moving their parent to a nursing home and increased use of stress-reducing drugs after relinquishing care.[70] Children may also harbour an underlying fear that they will later develop Alzheimer's disease.

Gender may affect the level of child caregiver stress, with more conflict reported in mother–daughter relationships than in other parent–child relationships, and daughters' relationships with the care recipients may become more distant as the care progresses.[73] These adult child caregivers are 'caught' between the needs of their own spouse/children and those of their parent. Adult child caregivers who work outside the home may be more vulnerable to 'role overload',[70] though others[74] disagree with this finding and believe that multiple roles may be beneficial to the caregiving role. Competing demands may increase stress. According to Brody et al,[75] problems may multiply when three generations live in one home. Brody compared daughters living in one-, two- or three-generation households and found that daughters whose mothers lived sepa-

Table 23.1 Predictors of depression and/or distress in caregivers of persons with dementia	
Variable	**Result**
Blood kinship	Caregivers with closer blood ties experience more distress
Females	Female caregivers tend to experience more adverse psychological effects of caregiving than do males
Husbands	Husbands experience significant changes in household chores, social interactions, marital relationships and general well-being
Spouses	Spouses tend to experience higher objective burden than adult children though not always.[77] Spouses have fewer physical and psychological coping mechanisms than do adult children
More committed vs conflicted relationship	Caregivers in a more committed relationship experience more distress. Those from a more conflicted relationship are more likely to abuse the patient
Physical health	Good physical health is an important factor in ongoing care of a dementing spouse
Age	Younger caregivers generally experience more distress.
Subjective feelings of caregiver	The subjective feelings of the caregiver (appraisal of problems and self-confidence) are better predictors of their burden than the objective assessment by medical staff
Physical proximity	Caregivers in closer physical proximity to the patient experience more distress

rately fared best. Daughters in two-generation households provided the most care and their mothers were the oldest and most impaired. Daughters in three-generation households reported the most numerous negative mental and emotional effects of caregiving. However, Spitze and Logan[76] argued that the situation described by Brody is fairly uncommon and is not typical of middle-aged men or women in the USA today.

Gender of caregiver

Female caregivers are generally more stressed than male caregivers,[78] reporting more depression, burden,[33] anxiety[79,80] and paranoia.[81] Wives who provided care for a longer time reported less burden, and those who perceived themselves to be in the later stages of caregiving reported a closer relationship with their husbands.[73] These differences are not at all explained by the severity of the patients' dementia, though Li et al's study[82] showed that emotional support for wives buffered the stress emanating from their husbands' behavioural problems. Social participation did not have the same helpful effect. Female caregivers in France were found to be more vulnerable in terms of their own health, to consume more psychotropic drugs and to postpone their own treatment than were male caregivers.[68] However, over time, depression levels in males may increase and become equivalent to women's scores.[57] Other studies[83] found that distress in men, but not in women, was increased by the caregiving role. Men, once in the caregiving role, are more likely to relinquish it than are women.[8]

Quality of the relationship between caregiver and patient

Spouse caregivers The duration and quality of the relationship between the spouse and the patient before the onset of dementia bears on how caregivers fare. Spousal caregivers are more likely to be depressed than non-spousal caregivers,[84] although this was not noted in Waite's study.[48] Caregivers who experienced lower levels of marital intimacy, both at the time of the study and before the onset of the dementia, were found to have higher levels of perceived strain and depression.[4,85] Caregivers who experienced a greater loss of intimacy had a higher level of depression, but did not show evidence of increased perceived strain.[85] Caregivers who are the spouses in second marriages tend to have more problems as marriages of relatively short duration do not accrue the same feelings of spousal obligation and there may be conflict with stepchildren.[21]

Adult child caregivers If the previous relationship with the parent has not been a good one, the caregiving role will be much more difficult for the child caregiver than it would have been had there been a good and close parent–child relationship.

Daughters are three times more likely to be the primary caregivers than sons.[13,86–88] Daughters are more likely to provide higher levels of domestic and personal care than sons,[89] with daughters more likely to provide 'hands on' care and sons more likely to provide assistance with home maintenance and financial management.[90]

In a study comparing siblings who share the care of a mother with dementia, daughters tended to provide more care than sons, and were more stressed by their role.[91] Negative intersibling interactions were associated with greater care needs in the mother. Compared to their unmarried sisters, daughter caregivers who were married had more socio-emotional support, higher incomes and less depression.[92]

In an 18-month longitudinal study, daughter caregivers of aged parents had a relatively low rate of clinical depression, 23.5 per cent, as defined by a CES-D cut-off of 16.[93] However, only 18.3 per cent of caregivers in this study were caring for parents with dementia. Daughter caregivers found problem behaviours to be the most difficult aspect of care. Shared care, even if the care was not equally shared, lessened the stress of the primary caregiver. Li et al reported that emotion-focused coping strategies such as venting frustration or detaching from the problem were high-risk strategies for depression when used frequently.[93]

Daughters-in-law as caregivers This is a special, more vulnerable group, with more difficult caregiver related problems than daughters, and reporting more caregiver related stress.[94] Daughters-in-law are especially susceptible as they receive fewer resources from parents-in-law than do sons-in-law. Daughters-in-law who work outside the home are even more at risk.[94] They have no blood tie with the patient, no feeling of 'reciprocal care' and little real influence in overall management of the patient, which is usually controlled by the child/ren, but are nevertheless burdened with the physical care of the patient. Mizuno and Takashaki[95] found that daughters-in-law who were caregivers perceived their burden as more severe than did daughters, although they took care of less-impaired parents-in-law for fewer hours each day. Despite the fact that in Korean society, filial values and social pressures ensure that demented parents are looked after by the wife of the oldest son, Kim and Lee[96] found that these daughter-in-law caregivers reported high levels of depression and also had high rates of self-reported poor physical health. The lack of a support infrastructure for these caregivers makes their task even more difficult. While daughter-in-law caregivers are frequently involved in providing care for their husband's parents, daughters providing care to their own parents attempt to minimize the involvement of their husbands in the caregiving process.[97]

Caregiver physical health

There is a correlation between the psychological and physical health of caregivers.[4,98] Good physical health of the spouse is an important predictor of the spouse's ability to continue caring for patients,[23] especially as patients are being discharged from hospital sooner, and often required to help with tasks at home that were previously undertaken by nursing staff in hospitals, e.g. managing home oxygen and bladder catheters.

Age of caregiver

There are conflicting reports on the intersection of age and caregiver stress. On the one hand, age is a significant predictor of physical ill-health, with older caregivers reporting significantly poorer health than younger caregivers.[96] Older women have been reported to be more stressed than either older men or younger women.[31] On the other hand, caregivers of younger patients with dementia are young themselves, face special issues (see p284), and may be liable to feel stressed.[99]

Caregiver psychological health

(role enhancement versus role strain)
Two conflicting theories exist regarding busy adults caring for demented elderly parents. One theory, role enhancement, claims that people occupying more roles should experience higher levels of well-being.[86,88,100] This well-being may be mediated by more positive social networks. The other theory, role strain, claims that strain results from the many demands placed on individuals, who feel overloaded.[87,88,101] Studies have found conflicting evidence for these theories; the final answer involving the additive and interactive effects of multiple roles and mental well-being remains unclear.[83,86,87,102]

Other caregiver demographics

Dementia is an expensive illness for both the family of the affected patient and the healthcare system of each country. Higher incomes give caregivers the option of paying for some formal care and thus relieving their own burden somewhat. Family income was noted to be an important predictor of depression in Korean caregivers.[96]

Less well-educated caregivers tend to report slightly more depression than those who are better educated.[103] Caregiver education is an important determinant of the management strategies used by caregivers. De Vugt et al reported that more highly educated caregivers used more successful supportive strategies (34 per cent of caregivers in this group were highly educated) rather than less successful non-adaptive strategies (11.8 per cent of caregivers in this group were highly educated) when dealing with dementia patients.[104] Navaie-Waliser et al found 36 per cent of a cross-section of 1002 caregivers to be 'vulnerable', i.e. more likely to have difficulty providing care, to report a decline in their own physical health, to be older, to be married and to have had less than 12 years of education.[105]

The caregiver's social class did not influence the caregiver burden in Annerstedt's study.[106] Race as a predictor variable is considered below.

Patient variables

Behavioural problems

The non-cognitive features of AD, occurring in up to 80 per cent of patients at some stage of the dementing process,[20] are more stressful for the caregivers than are the cognitive features or dependency;[20,21,57,77,107] they are powerful predictors of caregiver distress,[108,109] especially in spouse caregivers,[110] and of institutionalization.[111] Behavioural changes affect both the physical and the mental functioning of caregivers.[109] Behavioural disturbances, depression, apathy, difficulty with walking, shouting and calling out, sleep disruptions and hallucinations in the patient all caused adverse caregiver outcomes, as does the loss of companionship. It is thought that the unpredictability of behavioural changes is in itself stressful.[109] Decreases in dysfunctional behaviour over a two-month period were a strong predictor of reduced caregiver burden in spouses in Bedard's study.[112] Where the care recipient appeared pleased, content or appreciative, caregivers reported deriving much more satisfaction from their role.[26]

Functional, cognitive and depressive symptoms

Cognitive impairment and functional disability tend to occur earlier in the disease than behavioural problems.[113] Most researchers,[108,114] but not all,[20] do not find an association between the degree of cognitive and functional impairment of the patient and caregiver stress, burden and/or depression. Patient depression, however, has been associated with caregiver distress.[105,115]

Duration of illness

Schulz and Williamson[57] found that although male caregivers exhibited normative levels of depressive symptomatology at the start of their study, they became significantly more depressed over time. As patient disability and care needs increased over time so the ability of some individuals to cope with the caregiving role declined.[57] This finding was confirmed in Pinquart and Sorensen's meta-analysis, with the effect being more marked in spouse caregivers than in adult child caregivers.[110] However, Schulz et al reported inconsistent associations between duration of illness and caregiver outcomes.[84] Confounding factors include the higher likelihood of behavioural problems as the dementia progresses and the possibility of selective attrition so that more stressed caregivers have placed the care recipient in residential care, thereby reducing their stress and removing these dyads from cross sectional survey samples.

Severity of illness

Sleeplessness, incontinence and behavioural symptoms mark the later stages of the illness. These, along with severe cognitive impairment, are often the factors that precipitate nursing home admission.[111,116] The evidence that severity per se, i.e. independent of behavioural symptoms, increases caregiver stress is weak or conflicting.

Patient demographics

Gender differences have been reported: sons being more likely to help fathers with activities of daily living and daughters to help mothers.[94,117] Caregivers both give and receive more help when helping mothers than when helping fathers;[94] however, some fathers expect more assistance than do mothers.[83] Lee et al[117] stated that more daughters become caregivers than do sons, partly because the majority of elderly people requiring care are female. Increasing age is associated with the increased amount[118] and type of help required,[89,119] though there are reports that caregivers of younger patients may have higher levels of stress.[120]

Physical distance from caregiver

Physical proximity matters. Caregivers living with, or close to, the patient, experience a greater sense of obligation,[42,94,121] more burden and elevated levels of depression.[4,96]

SPECIAL GROUPS

Caregivers in minority families

The findings regarding African-American caregivers in the USA have been contradictory. One study reported

that African-American caregivers may be at higher risk than their Caucasian counterparts because of generally poorer health and greater exposure to chronic stressors such as poverty, unemployment, crime and racism.[122] However, they may have unique assets in their use of extended family and high levels of social support. By contrast, Haley et al compared a group of 70 Black and 105 White family caregivers (of AD or other dementia patients) and 70 Black and 105 White non-caregivers in Alabama, USA.[123] The Black and White patients did not differ significantly in gender, co-residence with the caregiver, diagnosis, age, duration of dementia, MMSE scores, self-care impairment or memory or behaviour problems. Family support was similar in both Blacks and Whites. His results suggested that Black caregivers may be more resilient to the stress of caregiving than are White caregivers. White caregivers compared with White non-caregivers showed more than twice the likelihood of a significant increase on depression scores (using CES-D). No significant difference in depression scores was noted when comparing Black caregivers with Black non-caregivers.

In a 3-year prospective follow-up of older (65 years and over) residents and their caregivers (in a defined biracial community) caregivers who were married, younger or white were more likely than their opposite counterparts to be providing care at follow-up.[23]

Pinquart and Sorensen's meta-analysis of caregivers from ethnic backgrounds[124] found worse physical health but better psychological health among ethnic minority caregivers than among White caregivers. Asian-American caregivers were more depressed than White caregivers, which may be due to the fact that daughters-in-law are expected to look after elderly parents-in-law irrespective of their previous relationship. Hispanic caregivers were also more depressed than White caregivers, but reported more 'uplifts' from caregiving. Compared to other ethnic groups in this study, African-Americans fared best psychologically, with lower levels of burden and depression and higher levels of uplifts and subjective well-being.

Caregivers in migrant families

The caregiving process is far more complicated in migrant families who may be multiply isolated by language, culture and dementia. Often patients revert to their 'mother tongue', making communication with outside helpers more difficult. Families may have low levels of education and may be less likely to be aware of, or to avail themselves of, services. The prevailing cultural values may be at odds with the imported ones; for example, accessing community services or placing the patient in a nursing home may be viewed as 'abandonment' in some cultures. In-laws, siblings, nieces or grandchildren may be the primary caregivers in extended migrant families, even if the spouse is living in the home.[125] In some cultures, any mental health problem is viewed as shameful or even the fault of the family. The associated stigma may lead families to hide the person with dementia away or not to seek services.

Lee and Sung[126] noted, when comparing Korean-American adult child caregivers with American adult child caregivers (all caring for family members with dementia), that the low burden of the Korean caregivers was associated with extended family support and high filial responsibility, while that of the American caregivers was related to the use of formal services and high gratification from caregiving. On the other hand, the high burden felt by the Korean caregivers was associated with limited use of formal services and low gratification from caring for in-laws, while that of the Americans was thought to be due to limited extended family support and low filial responsibility. In another study[127] comparing motivations of Korean-Americans with that of Caucasian Americans in caring for parents with dementia, Lee and Sung noted that the American caregivers, usually daughters, had strong bonds of affection with their parents, but expressed low degrees of filial responsibility. Korean-Americans tended to leave the care of the demented patients predominantly to daughters-in-law who had little affection for the patients, but high degrees of filial responsibility.

Caregivers in developing countries

Although 66 per cent of people with dementia live in developing countries, only 10 per cent or less of population-based research has been conducted in these regions.[128] Dementia has a low profile in most developing countries, where families view dementia as a normal part of ageing, neglect patients and tend not to seek help.[128,129] In Goa, India, for example, where the prevalence of dementia is 1.8–5.4 per cent, primary care physicians rarely see dementing patients, but community workers often do.[129] Care for aging parents is almost entirely carried out by the family and is often conditional on the child receiving an inheritance from the dementing parent.[129] However, social and economic changes in developing countries have decreased the availability and willingness of women to become full-time caregivers, and have resulted in adult children moving away from home to 'improve' themselves. Thus caregiving, until recently an integral part of family life in developing countries, is being left to social services, which are not able to cope with the dementing population.[130] The myth that large families and different life-styles and cultures mitigate the distress experienced by family caregivers has been debunked by studies from India, China and Latin America, where rates of caregiver distress are as high as in Western countries.[131,132]

Caregivers of younger persons with dementia

Caregivers of younger people (65 years and younger) with dementia experience significant degrees of burden associated with the higher levels of physical dependency and behavioural disturbance often found in younger patients.[99] A theme of double isolation occurs as families of younger persons with dementia are confronted by services geared to a much older population. There is also the problem of a younger person perhaps having an 'atypical' form of dementia or in encountering difficulty with diagnosis,[30] where more extensive or invasive investigations may be needed.[133] Loss of potential income is greater in this group and is a greater source of anxiety, than in an older patient caregiver group. As well the patient may have elderly dependent parents. Adolescent children facing a parent with dementia have a difficult time coping and have also to face the fact of an increased risk of inheriting the disease.[134]

Caregivers of professionals and VIPs

Professionals and VIPs are very often isolated by their status and the awkwardness that others feel in offering their care. These patients may find it difficult to accept community and residential services,[135] and medical assessments may be delayed for fear of jeopardizing careers and this may place others in danger. Persuading these patients that they can no longer continue working and/or driving can be a problem.[135] Perceived class barriers to care and community service may further increase family burden.

Couples where both patient and caregiver are dementing

Couples where both the patient and caregiver are dementing clearly have special needs[21] and their problems are more than doubled.[135] There is no adequate supervision of the dementing patient/s, no informant to give correct information to medical attendants and poor understanding of, and compliance with, medication.

Friends as caregivers

Sometimes friends become caregivers (20 per cent of female caregivers are friends giving care, 1992–1994 data[17]), most commonly providing help through emotional support, transportation and shopping.[17] In a study of female caregivers (caring for a variety of illnesses, not specifically dementia),[17] women friends providing care were more likely to be older and to be age peers of the patient, and less likely to be employed or to be married than family caregivers. Friends are less likely to take on caregiving responsibilities when those responsibilities conflict with other roles, e.g. paid employment. Himes and Reidy reported that women providing care to a female friend spent a mean of 18 weeks per year and 8.1 hours each week providing care, whereas women providing care for a family member spent 19.7 weeks per year and 14.9 hours per week providing care.[17] This difference was not statistically significant. The quality and duration of the friendships were not measured in the above study.

Caregivers in alternative relationships

Dementing patients who are unmarried and/or childless or have offspring who are incapable of rendering care have less support available. This may also be the case where children have moved away or emigrated, a problem that is becoming more common, or with older gay couples where one partner has dementia.

Gay couples coping with human immunodeficiency virus (HIV) infection associated dementia (HAD) have added burdens. The incidence of HAD is as high as 19 per cent in acquired immune deficiency syndrome (AIDS) patients aged 75 and over.[136] With new therapy, AIDS has become a drawn out disease with a long period of cognitive decline.[137] High rates of depression and caregiver burden have been reported in caregivers of AIDS patients (not necessarily those with HAD).[138] The AIDS population is ageing[139] and relies heavily on friends (who are also ageing) for support. These caregivers have a set of very specific problems: the possibility that they themselves have AIDS (almost 25 per cent in this study), a high rate of illegal drug use and alcohol abuse (almost 50 per cent in this study) and high rates of poverty.[138] Many caregivers of AIDS patients are caring for more than one patient at a time, which adds to their degree of burden.[138] As well, many are fighting the stigma associated with AIDS.[140]

ELDER ABUSE

This is a topic complete in itself. It affects 3.2 per cent of older people in the USA.[14] Abuse may be physical, sexual, psychological, financial or by neglect. Typically the abuser is a family member[21] and more likely to be a son or daughter of the patient than a spouse.[142] Brief mention is made here to point out that ill health in the caregiver may lead to compromized care of the patient, which is often a precursor to abuse.[37] Potentially harmful caregiver behaviour is more likely (in spouse caregiving situations) when care recipients have greater needs for care and when caregivers themselves are more cognitively impaired, have more physical illnesses and are at risk for clinical depression.[37] Care recipient factors likely to lead to abuse include behavioural problems, violence or aggression towards the caregiver and high levels of physical and cognitive impairment with repetitive questioning.

Reported rates of physical aggression by caregivers towards dementing patients range from 5.4 to 20 per cent.[143] Persons with AD are 2.25 times at greater risk of experiencing a physically abusive episode than older (cognitively intact) persons living in the community.[142,143] Caregiver characteristics leading to abuse include personality traits such as anxiety and depression, low self-esteem, substance abuse, longer duration of care of patient long term and a higher number of hours of care each day.[144] The abuser may have a history of being abused, of drug or alcohol use or of psychiatric problems.[145] Caregiver cognitive status is also an important predictor of abuse, with abuse more likely if the caregiver is cognitively impaired.[146] Relationship risk factors include living with the patient and a poor premorbid relationship between patient and caregiver, including unresolved conflicts.[144] Potentially harmful caregiver behaviour can be considered as an early warning sign to full blown elder abuse.[37]

Interventions should be tailored to the situation and may include increased caregiver support, respite care or separation of the older person from the abuser, often under the guise of admission for a medical diagnosis. Legal mechanisms such as guardianship legislation may be needed to effect alternative living arrangements.

POSITIVE ASPECTS OF CAREGIVING

Caregivers may be able to adapt to the stress of caregiving, and caregivers may draw on previously unused strengths and resources.[147] Cohen et al[28] found that over 70 per cent of caregivers reported that they were happy or positive about the caring role.[148–150] Positive aspects included companionship, fulfilment, a rewarding feeling and pride in one's ability to handle problems. Caregivers who reported more positive feelings were less likely to report burden, depression or poor health,[2] and had a decreased risk of patient institutionalization.[115] This finding was not consistent.[109] Caregivers who could not identify any positive aspects of caring may be at risk for depression and poor health outcomes, as well as earlier institutionalization of their care recipients.[28]

CAREGIVERS AS PARTNERS IN CARE

Caregivers are pivotal partners in aged care.[150] Diagnosis relies heavily on caregiver information, though up to 40 per cent of caregivers may be inaccurate in their reports of impairment, particularly when the patient has low education and poor remote memory or when overall cognitive difficulties are mild.[151] Caregivers are usually the decision-makers as regards whether or not to start a treatment or management programme and the ones who request help/support, bear the responsibility of administering medication, act as the informant for drug trials, give informed consent or proxy consent for clinical trials and monitor treatment outcomes.[150] Dementia treatment studies are increasingly focusing on measuring caregiver time, burden and reaction to different behaviours as secondary outcome measures.[150]

NURSING HOME PLACEMENT

Although many families view this as a 'last resort', in Western countries most patients with dementia spend some time in a nursing home. The decision to place a loved one in a nursing home is neither easy nor taken lightly. Institutional placement, when it occurs, may change the nature of the caregiver involvement, but certainly does not end it.[21] Decisions regarding nursing home admission are often influenced by cultural differences, with some cultures regarding nursing home admission as abandonment of the patient.[27]

Increased risk of nursing home placement is associated with severe functional disability,[152] incontinence and immobility,[36] significant cognitive problems,[152] receiving formal community services[153] and caregiver 'burnout'.[153] We found that caregiver stress was a strong predictor of nursing home placement.[154] Patients with male caregivers are at twice the risk of nursing home placement than those with female caregivers. Children and other relatives are more likely to place a patient with dementia than are spouses.[155]

Increasing amounts of formal services may[153] or may not[152] be associated with decreasing risk of nursing home use in cognitively impaired elderly.

END-OF-LIFE CARE

Quality end-of-life care treats the whole person, reflects the choices and values of the individual and is provided in a culturally sensitive manner by well-educated and well-supported family members, who in turn are supported by a team.[156] Gessert et al found that many caregivers were unprepared to face all the decisions that needed to be made at this time and recommended support from health professionals.[157] Many patients express a wish to live as long as possible at home or to die there, and caregivers often feel the need to honour these wishes. There are special challenges to caregivers at this time, due to the patients' inability to communicate and the problems of co-ordinating all the support systems needed to provide adequate in-home care for a terminally ill patient.[158] Patients can be cared for at home longer if they have appropriate pain relief and their behavioural symptoms are treated.[159]

BEREAVEMENT IN THE CONTEXT OF CAREGIVING

The funeral that never ends finally does so. However, caregivers do not feel a sense of relief that their ordeal is now over. Often the care of the patient has become the entire focus of the caregiver's life and the death heralds a black void rather than a new freedom. In the short term, and sometimes longer, the grief can be 'remarkably intense'.[160] For those considering autopsy, usually for scientific reasons to determine hereditary risk, decisions about postmortem examination should be made well before death so that these can be arranged expeditiously.

However, in the long term the effects of bereavement on caregivers appear to be positive.[158,161] Over 90 per cent of caregivers in Schulz's study[158] believed somewhat or very much that death came as a relief to the patient, and 72 per cent reported that the death was somewhat or very much a relief to themselves. Following the death of their spouse, strained caregivers had improved health practices and no further increase in depressive symptoms, antidepressant medication use or significant weight loss.[161] For wives, bereavement was often accompanied by an increase in social activity and personal growth.[61] This supports the hypothesis that the death of a spouse among strained caregivers represents a significant reduction in burden and does not further tax their ability to cope. This is in contrast to widowed non-caregivers who had increased depressive symptoms and increased antidepressant use following their bereavement.[161]

CAREGIVER INTERVENTIONS

Caregivers may benefit from support, education and training for the duration of their time as caregivers, which may be several years. Interventions are many and varied and some are more effective than others.[162] The benefits of specific interventions include decreased caregiver stress,[162,163] improved caregiver coping skills,[162] reduced caregiver psychological morbidity,[164] decreased or delayed nursing home placements,[162,165,166] improved patient survival[168] and improved knowledge of dementia.[163] Education alone appears to be only modestly effective,[79] emotional support alone slightly more effective, and the combination more effective than either support alone.[168] The majority of interventions have shown mixed results.[169] Multicomponent interventions appear to be more effective than narrowly focused ones,[170] and programmes tailored to individual needs appear more effective than generic programmes.[170]

TARGETS OF INTERVENTION

Anecdotally, interventions that occur earlier, i.e. before problems develop, are more effective.[162] As preventative caregiver interventions are unlikely to become available universally, it is desirable to target those most likely to benefit. Pinquart and Sorensen[110] recommended that education about coping with behavioural problems should be a priority as these cause the most stress in caregivers. Female caregivers are known to suffer more psychiatric morbidity and may be more specifically targeted as an 'at risk' group.[8] Women are more likely than men to comply with home environmental modification, to implement recommended strategies and to derive greater benefits from intervention.[171] Also, spouses may benefit more than other caregivers from interventions that reduce objective burden.[110] Different interventions may be required at different times during the course of the illness and all interventions should be flexible and geared to individual patient and/or caregiver needs, taking into account migrant and minority families and other special cases.

ELEMENTS OF INTERVENTION

Information and education

While it is generally agreed that families and caregivers should be made aware of the diagnosis and prognosis of the patient, Thomas et al found that almost half the caregivers were ill informed of the patient's diagnosis and the disease in general.[68] Information, while clearly important, does not by itself decrease caregiver burden or impact significantly on the patient.[172] Once aware of the diagnosis, caregivers can be helped by acquiring the knowledge and skills pertinent to the care of the patient. Education regarding the illness, medication use and care strategies can enhance the quality of care that they are providing, reduce caregiver negative affect[173] and improve communication with the patient. Information about resources, services and training, forward planning, use of advance directives and respite care may be useful. Maintaining their identity, interests and social support networks is important for caregiver welfare.

Caregiver training programmes

Patient-focused programmes have taught caregivers cognitive stimulation techniques aimed to stimulate patient memory, problem solving skills and conversational fluency.[174,175] The outcomes of the many training programmes reported have been generally positive, though some merely report satisfaction.

A Swedish programme[176] trained family caregivers with volunteers, who later relieved the caregivers by providing in-home help. Both caregivers and volunteers expressed satisfaction with this training programme.

Family intervention programmes appear to be acceptable to those involved and can significantly reduce burden in caregivers as well as behavioural disturbances in patients. Intervention programmes involving both patients and families are more intensive, modified to the caregivers' and the families specific needs and may be more successful than counselling alone.[177] They aim to help the caregiver cope better with his or her own emotional state, and to ensure that their own behaviour is more consistent, resulting in positive consequences in dealing with the patient. A prospective randomised controlled trial of family intervention[172] was carried out in the UK on 42 caregiver/patient dyads. Patients were all diagnosed with Alzheimer's disease and were living in the community with a caregiver who provided the main support. Participants were randomly divided into three groups of 14 dyads each. (Groups consisted of two control groups and one intervention group). The family intervention was based on caregiver education, stress management and coping skills training, spread over 14 sessions. Caregivers were assessed on two health measures. Patients were assessed using measures of cognition, depression and behavioural disturbance. There were significant reductions in distress and depression in the intervention group compared with the control groups at post-treatment and at follow-up. No significant difference was found between the two control groups leading the authors to conclude that interview alone had no effect on burden. Behavioural disturbances in the patients were significantly improved post treatment, but were not sustained at follow-up.[172]

We conducted a 10-day intensive, residential, comprehensive and extensive training programme, consisting of counselling, provision of information, practical advice, role play and skills training for groups of up to four carers and their charges.[164,168] For the following year the groups of carers were linked by telephone conference calls second weekly, then fourth weekly and sixth weekly. The programme was part of a randomized controlled trial, with one group of carers receiving training immediately, a second group receiving training after 6 months' delay and a third group receiving no training at all. For the third or control group, patients were admitted for 10 days and participated in a memory retraining programme while their carers had 10 days' respite. All groups of carers had similar telephone conference links over 12 months. At the end of the 12 months, patients declined uniformly on tests of cognition and function regardless of which group they were in. However, the carers in the immediate training programme had a significant decline in their General Health Questionnaire (GHQ) scores, a commonly used measure of psychological morbidity, over the 12 months, while the GHQ scores of control carers rose. The GHQ score of the delayed training carers remained steady. Rates of institutionalization were significantly lower for both carer training groups over 8 years of follow-up. For example, at 4 years 55 per cent of patients in the immediate dementia caregiving training programme, and 40 per cent of those in the delayed programme, were still at home, whereas only 8 per cent of patients whose carers were in the control group were still at home. Although the programme was more costly than necessary, as it was residential and within a hospital setting, it still resulted in savings of about (1987) US$6000 per couple over 39 months, because of the delay in nursing home admission.[156] Over 8 years the odds ratio of surviving patients staying at home was 5.03 (95 per cent confidence intervals 1.73, 14.7) greater if the caregiver had participated in training.

Teaching behavioural strategies

A programme that taught caregivers how to administer one of two behavioural techniques to their spouse or relative with AD demonstrated that caregivers can be trained to become the therapists. 'Pleasant event planning' and problem solving techniques improved depression levels in both patients *and* caregivers.[178] Teri et al[179] found that an exercise training programme for patients with AD, combined with teaching caregivers behavioural management techniques, decreased frailty and improved behavioural problems in the patients.

Counselling

This involves a therapeutic relationship between the caregiver(s) and a trained professional. Counselling needs are different at each stage as caregiving requirements change, including comfort for the family that is mourning the slow death of the dementia patient.[180] Caring for dementia patients is very different from caring for other patients and far more demanding, changing constantly as the disease progresses. In the early stages of the illness, the caregiver is involved in minor day-to-day help, for example cooking, cleaning and banking. Later, personal care is needed as well. Later still, round-the-clock care may be required. Caregivers of dementia patients need to deal with the patients' lack of insight and behavioural problems in addition to their physical needs. Patient resentment, anger and communication difficulties all add to the burden of care. Counselling gives caregivers 'permission' to seek assistance and offers validation,[11] helping to normalize their feelings and to reassure them. The therapist may teach self-monitoring behaviour, challenge negative thoughts and help caregivers develop problem-solving skills. Counselling can offer fresh insight, introduce caregivers to alternatives, provide support, change caregivers' appraisals of and their responses to behavioural disturbances and offer a good opportunity to include other family members in the care of the patient and so distribute the burden more equally between family members.[180] Counselling should also include practical legal and financial advice and should direct attention to the caregiver's physical health.

Whitlatch et al[181] found that caregivers participating in individual and family counselling were more likely to have fewer symptoms, less personal strain and less role strain. Li et al[82] reported that social participation improved depressive symptoms in daughter caregivers, and emotional support buffered the stress emanating from behavioural problems and functional limitations in the parent.

A single blind randomized trial (The Three Country Study) was conducted in Australia, England and the USA. Investigators studied the effects of regular and ad hoc counselling on 77 caregivers whose patients were diagnosed with mild-to-moderate AD (all taking donepezil), compared with similar dyads who received donepezil and 'standard care'. Results showed a significant reduction in caregiver depression scores in the intervention compared with the control group, the effect becoming more pronounced over time. Patients' scores on cognition, behaviour and function over time, or rates of institutionalization, did not differ significantly. The study concluded that psychosocial intervention, in combination with pharmacological intervention, can be of considerable value to caregivers.[182]

Mittelman's programme of counselling and support[183] of 206 spouse caregivers of AD patients substantially increased the time that the caregivers were able to care for the patients at home, particularly during the early to middle stages of the disease. Caregivers in the treatment group had six sessions of individual and family counselling and were required to join support groups. Counsellors were also available for ad hoc sessions at any time. A similar counselling intervention study[184] showed that, although intervention did not influence the frequency of patient behavioural problems, it did significantly reduce the caregivers' reaction ratings to these problems.

Support groups

Support groups for caregivers have been well received.[172] They are effective in reducing caregiver stress and improving caregiver quality of life,[180] but are less effective than highly structured individual interventions.[172,185] Groups may be national associations, self-help groups or telephone/newsletter or computer support services. Support groups teach the caregivers that they are not alone in their daily struggle, decrease caregivers' sense of isolation and are educational. Professionally led groups appear to produce the greater improvement in caregiver's psychological functioning, whereas peer-led groups have been found to increase informal support networks and the extent to which caregivers feel more able to handle the caregiving role.[186,187] Support groups appear to be more effective if they appeal to the local community as far as cultural and ethnic values are concerned.[188] There is an increasingly wide choice of support groups, as these are now also based on gender, age, setting of care and stage of disease.[189] Virtual support groups or computer support networks can decrease strain for some caregivers.[190,191]

Alzheimer's Associations or societies exist in over 75 countries worldwide (www.alz.co.uk). They provide education, support, counselling, telephone help-lines, advocacy and, in many places, direct services such as day centres and even nursing homes. The more developed associations fund research directly and are very effective in lobbying government. At the heart of the Associations are the support groups. Customarily these meetings are held monthly and offer local caregivers the chance to ventilate, to learn from others and to socialize. Empirical data regarding the efficacy of self-help groups are lacking, but anecdotal accounts are positive.[188] Not all caregivers will join an Association or even obtain information from one, for example caregivers with large informal networks are less likely to be members. The commonest reason for caregivers not contacting their local Association is lack of awareness and, implicitly, lack of referral by healthcare professionals.[188]

Home modification

Adjustments to the home environment can create a safer living environment,[180] for example, protection from hot surfaces, unlit gas stoves or sharp objects and perimeter locks to secure wandering patients.

Formal care

Formal care services include meals-on-wheels, home care, day care, in-home care (sitting), residential respite care and permanent care, all of which may be relevant at different stages of the caring process, though it has been suggested[170] that respite care is a middle-to-late service need. The amount of services offered differs by country and within countries, as does the cost of using the services. Some caregivers have limited knowledge of help and/or services available.[19] Many caregivers do not avail themselves of services despite expressing a need for help.[192] The Family Survival Project developed the concept of minimal required hours of respite care. They concluded that 8 hours per week is the minimum number of hours necessary to achieve relief from caregiving work.[193] Many respite programmes may thus not be meeting the respite requirements of caregivers. The use of formal support services is much higher in caregivers of dementia patients than caregivers of other elderly patients,[19] particularly the use of home help, day care and district nursing. Despite this, caregivers of people with dementia are less satisfied with services than caregivers of people with non-dementing illnesses and have more unmet needs.[24]

Service use may not alleviate either caregiver overload or caregiver depression.[112] There is limited evidence that respite care provides long-term benefits to the patient or the caregiver or even improves outcome.[194] Day-care programmes may be cost-effective alternatives for some patients to nursing home care and may delay institutionalization of patients who cannot be managed at home on a full time basis.[180] Thomas et al reported that the commonest difficulty reported by caregivers was lack of time for themselves.[68] Zarit et al[195] found that caregivers of relatives with dementia who used adult day care services at least twice each week for a minimum period of 3 months experienced lower levels of caregiver related stress and better psychological well-being than a control group not using this service. Short-term (3 months) and long-term (12 months) benefits were found, however feelings of 'role captivity' in the caregivers were not improved. Zarit[196] considered that the following groups do not benefit from day care: spouse caregivers, caregivers with less formal education and caregivers who feel trapped. Patients attending day care benefitted as they showed less agitation, were easier to handle, slept better and were less depressed.[196]

OUTCOMES OF CAREGIVER INTERVENTIONS

Interventions can make a difference. All interventions taken together in a meta-analysis produced significant improvements in all modalities measured.[197] Successful interventions have been reported to reduce caregiver stress, depression and psychological morbidity, to delay nursing home placement and to improve patients' psychological well-being.[177]

EFFECTIVENESS OF DIFFERENT FORMS OF INTERVENTION

Unsuccessful interventions are short educational programmes (beyond enhancement of knowledge), support groups alone, single interviews and brief interventions or courses not supplemented with long-term contact.[162,177] Social and health services other than respite care seem to have no consistent impact on caregiver distress.[170]

In a meta-analysis of 30 studies of intervention for caregivers of dementia patients (of the 45 that met criteria for inclusion) we found significant benefits in caregiver psychological distress, caregiver knowledge, caregiver main outcome measures and patient mood, but not in caregiver burden.[177] Success was more likely if patients as well as caregivers were involved and if the dose of intervention was larger.

In a meta-analysis of 78 intervention studies (not exclusively for dementia patients) on six outcome measures, Sorensen et al[197] found that psycho-educational interventions and psychotherapy had a significant effect on all outcome variables. Multicomponent interventions had significant effects on caregiver burden, well-being and ability/knowledge, but not on depression or on the symptoms of the care recipient. Respite and day care interventions were effective for three outcomes: caregiver burden, caregiver depression and caregiver well-being. Supportive interventions reduced caregiver burden and increased ability and knowledge, but had no effect on the other outcome variables. Interventions were generally less effective when the care recipient was suffering from dementia.

Group interventions have been found to be more effective than individual interventions[197] and the length of the intervention is also important in alleviating caregiver depression and patient symptoms.[197] Spouse caregivers benefited less from intervention than did adult child caregivers.[197] In this meta-analysis, the majority of the effects persisted for an average of 7 months post-intervention.

Knight's meta-analysis[170] demonstrated a strong effect for individual psychosocial interventions and for respite care that delivered more respite to the treatment group than to the control group. Group psychosocial interventions showed a small but positive effect on caregiver distress.

CONCLUSIONS

The role of the caregiver in supporting family members with dementia is vital. While demanding and stressful, the role often delivers satisfaction to caregivers. There are many adverse effects on family caregivers – psychological, physical, social and financial. Interventions can be effective but should be tailored to the needs of the caregiver and those of the patient. Predictors of negative consequences can be identified and it may be more effective to target interventions at vulnerable caregivers. General measures such as increased community awareness of dementia, referrals to Alzheimer's Associations and enhancing caregiver knowledge appear useful, but are more difficult to be proven to be empirically efficacious.

REFERENCES

1. Wimo A, Winblad B, Aguero-Torres H, von Strauss E. The magnitude of dementia occurrence in the world. Alzheimer Dis Assoc Disord 2003; 17:63–67.
2. Schulz R, Beach SR. Caregiving as a risk factor for mortality: the Caregiver Health Effects Study [see comment]. JAMA 1999; 282:2215–2219.
3. Whitlatch C, Noelker L. Caregiving and caring. Encyclopaed Gerontol 1996; 1:253–268.
4. Brodaty H, Hadzi-Pavlovic D. Psychosocial effects on carers of living with persons with dementia. Aust NZ J Psychiatry 1990; 24:351–361.
5. Brodaty H, Green A, Lee-Fay L. Vascular dementia: consequences for family carer and implications for management. In: O'Brien J, Ames D, Gustafson L, Folstein M, Chiu E, eds. Cerebrovascular Disease and Dementia: Pathology, Neuropsychiatry and Management, 2nd edn. Trowbridge: Martin Dunitz 2004; 363–378.
6. Lyons KS, Zarit SH. Formal and informal support: the great divide. Int J Geriatr Psychiatry 1999; 14:183–192.
7. Canadian Study of Health and Aging Working Group. Canadian study of health and aging: study methods and prevalence of dementia. CMAJ 1994; 150:899–913.
8. Yee JL, Schulz R. Gender differences in psychiatric morbidity among family caregivers: a review and analysis. Gerontologist 2000; 40:147–164.
9. Zarit SH. Family care and burden at the end of life. CMAJ 2004; 170:1811–1812.
10. Schur D, Whitlatch CJ, Clark PA. Beyond the chi-square: caregivers are more than just faceless statistics. Lippincott's Case Mgmnt 2005; 10:65–71.
11. Kasuya RT, Polgar-Bailey P, Takeuchi R. Caregiver burden and burnout. A guide for primary care physicians. Postgrad Med 2000; 108:119–123.
12. Max W, Webber P, Fox P. Alzheimer's disease. The unpaid burden of caring. J Aging Health 1995; 7:179–199.
13. Stone R, Cafferata GL, Sangl J. Caregivers of the frail elderly: a national profile. Gerontologist 1987; 27:616–626.
14. Brody EM. Parent care as normative stress. Gerontologist 1985; 25:19–29.
15. Antonucci TC, Hiroko A. Convoys of social support: Generational issues. Marriage Fam Rev 1991; 16:103–119.
16. Cantor MH. Neighbours and friends: an overlooked resource in the informal support system. Res Aging 1979; 1: 434–463.
17. Himes CL, Reidy EB. The role of Friends in Caregiving. Res Aging 2000; 22:315–336.
18. Rabins PV, Fitting MD, Eastham J, Zabora J. Emotional adaptation over time in caregivers for chronically ill elderly people. Age Ageing 1990; 19:185–190.
19. Philp I, McKee KJ, Meldrum P, et al. Community care for demented and non-demented elderly people: a comparison study of financial burden, service use, and unmet needs in family supporters. BMJ 1995; 310:1503–1506.
20. Leinonen E, Korpisammal L, Pulkkinen LM, Pukuri T. The comparison of burden between caregiving spouses of depressive and demented patients. Int J Geriatr Psychiatry 2001; 16:387–393.
21. Brodaty H. Dementia and the family. In: Bloch S, Hafner J, Harari E, Szmukler GI, eds. The Family in Clinical Psychiatry. Oxford University Press, Oxford 1994; 224–246.
22. Brodaty H. The Sydney Dementia Carers Training Program. In: Copeland J, Abou-Saleh MT, Blazer DG, eds. Principle and Practice of Geriatric Psychiatry. John Wiley and Sons, West Sussex 2002.
23. McCann JJ, Hebert LE, Bienias JL, Morris MC, Evans DA. Predictors of beginning and ending caregiving during a 3-year period in a biracial community population of older adults. Am J Pub Health 2004; 94:1800–1806.
24. Bedford S, Melzer D, Dening T, Lawton C. What becomes of people with dementia referred to community psychogeriatric teams? Int J Geriatr Psychiatry 1996; 11:1051–1056.
25. Haley WE, Levine EG, Brown SL, Berry JW, Hughes GH. Psychological, social, and health consequences of caring for a relative with senile dementia. J Am Geriatr Soc 1987; 35: 405–411.
26. Oyebode J. Assessment of carer's psychological needs. Adv Psychiatr Treat 2003; 9:45–53.
27. Lawton MP, Rajagopal D, Brody E, Kleban MH. The dynamics of caregiving for a demented elder among black and white families [see comment]. J Gerontol 1992; 47: 5156–5164.
28. Cohen CA, Colantonio A, Vernich L. Positive aspects of caregiving: rounding out the caregiver experience. Int J Geriatr Psychiatry 2002; 17:184–188.
29. Beach SR, Schulz R, Yee JL, Jackson S. Negative and positive health effects of caring for a disabled spouse: longitudinal findings from the caregiver health effects study. Psychol Aging 2000; 15:259–271.
30. Luscombe G, Brodaty H, Freeth S. Younger people with dementia: diagnostic issues, effects on carers and use of services. Int J Geriatr Psychiatry 1998; 13:323–330.
31. Anthony-Bergstone CR, Zarit SH, Gatz M. Symptoms of psychological distress among caregivers of dementia patients. Psychol Aging 1988; 3:245–248.
32. Stuckey JC, Neundorfer MM, Smyth KA. Burden and well-being: the same coin or related currency? Gerontologist 1996; 36:686–693.
33. Bullock R. The needs of the caregiver in the long-term treatment of Alzheimer disease. Alzheimer Dis Assoc Disord 2004; 18:517–523.
34. Stull DE, Kosloski K, Kercher K. Caregiver burden and generic well-being: opposite sides of the same coin? [see comment]. Gerontologist 1994; 34:88–94.
35. Kiecolt-Glaser JK, Dura JR, Speicher CE, Trask OJ, Glaser R. Spousal caregivers of dementia victims: longitudinal changes in immunity and health. Psychosom Med 1991; 53: 345–362.
36. Pinquart M, Sorensen S. Differences between caregivers and noncaregivers in psychological health and physical health: a meta-analysis. Psychol Aging 2003; 18:250–267.
37. Beach SR, Schulz R, Williamson GM, et al. Risk factors for potentially harmful informal caregiver behavior. J Am Geriatr Soc 2005; 53:255–261.
38. Schulz R, Visintainer P, Williamson GM. Psychiatric and physical morbidity effects of caregiving. J Gerontol 1990; 45: 181–191.
39. Baumgarten M, Battista RN, Infante-Rivard C, et al. The psychological and physical health of family members caring for an elderly person with dementia. J Clin Epidemiol 1992; 45:61–70.
40. National Alliance For Caregiving. Family Caregiving in the US: Findings from a National Survey. Washington DC: National Alliance For Caregiving 2004.
41. Vitaliano PP. Physiological and physical concomitants of caregiving: introduction. Ann Behav Med 1997; 19:75–77.
42. Grasel E. When home care ends – changes in the physical health of informal caregivers caring for dementia patients: a longitudinal study. J Am Geriatr Soc 2002; 50:843–849.
43. Kiecolt-Glaser JK, Glaser R, Shuttleworth EC, et al. Chronic stress and immunity in family caregivers of Alzheimer's disease victims. Psychosom Med 1987; 49:523–535.
44. Vedhara K, Cox NK, Wilcock GK, et al. Chronic stress in elderly carers of dementia patients and antibody response to influenza vaccination. Lancet 1999; 353:627–631.

45. Vedhara K, Bennett PD, Clark S, et al. Enhancement of antibody responses to influenza vaccination in the elderly following a cognitive-behavioural stress management intervention. Psychother Psychosom 2003; 72:245–252.

46. Vitaliano PP, Zhang J, Scanlan JM. Is caregiving hazardous to one's physical health? A meta-analysis. Psychol Bull 2003; 129:946–972.

47. Schulz R, Williamson GM. The measurement of caregiver outcomes in Alzheimer disease research. Alzheimer Dis Assoc Disord 1997; 6:117–124.

48. Waite A, Bebbington P, Skelton-Robinson M, Orrell M. Social factors and depression in carers of people with dementia. Int J Geriatr Psychiatry 2004; 19:582–587.

49. Blazer D, Williams CD. Epidemiology of dysphoria and depression in an elderly population. Am J Psychiatry 1980; 137:439–444.

50. Grafstrom M, Winblad B. Family burden in the care of the demented and nondemented elderly – a longitudinal study. Alzheimer Dis Assoc Disord 1995; 9:78–86.

51. Gilleard CJ, Boyd WD, Watt G. Problems in caring for the elderly mentally infirm at home. Arch Gerontol Geriatr 1982; 1:151–158.

52. Poulshock SW, Deimling GT. Families caring for elders in residence: issues in the measurement of burden. J Gerontol 1984; 39:230–239.

53. Morris RG, Morris LW, Britton PG. Factors affecting the emotional wellbeing of the caregivers of dementia sufferers. Br J Psychiatry 1988; 153:147–156.

54. George LK, Gwyther LP. Caregiver well-being: a multidimensional examination of family caregivers of demented adults. Gerontologist 1986; 26:253–259.

55. Gallagher D, Rose J, Rivera P, Lovett S, Thompson LW. Prevalence of depression in family caregivers. Gerontologist 1989; 29:449–456.

56. Mittelman MS, Ferris SH, Shulman E, et al. A comprehensive support program: effect on depression in spouse-caregivers of AD patients. Gerontologist 1995; 35:792–802.

57. Schulz R, Williamson GM. A 2-year longitudinal study of depression among Alzheimer's caregivers. Psychol Aging 1991; 6:569–578.

58. Coope B, Ballard C, Saad K, et al. The prevalence of depression in the carers of dementia sufferers. Int J Geriatr Psychiatry 1995; 10:237–242.

59. Coryell W, Endicott J, Winokur G, et al. Characteristics and significance of untreated major depressive disorder. Am J Psychiatry 1995; 152:1124–1129.

60. Dhooper SS. Caregivers of Alzheimer's disease patients: a review of the literature. J Gerontol Social Work 1991; 18:19–37.

61. Seltzer MM, Li LW. The dynamics of caregiving: transitions during a three-year prospective study. Gerontologist 2000; 40:165–178.

62. Sorensen S, Zarit SH. Preparation for caregiving: a study of multigeneration families. Int J Aging Hum Devel 1996; 42: 43–63.

63. Haley WE, Levine EG, Brown SL, Bartolucci AA. Stress, appraisal, coping, and social support as predictors of adaptational outcome among dementia caregivers. Psychology Aging 1987; 2:323–330.

64. Leung GM, Yeung RY, Chi I, Chu LW. The economics of Alzheimer disease. Dement Geriatr Cogn Disord 2003; 15: 34–43.

65. Langa KM, Chernew ME, Kabeto MU, et al. National estimates of the quantity and cost of informal caregiving for the elderly with dementia. J Gen Intern Med 2001; 16:770–778.

66. Schumock GT. Economic considerations in the treatment and management of Alzheimer's disease. Am J Health Syst Pharm 1998; 55:1.

67. National Alliance For Caregiving. Family caregiving in the US: Findings from a National Survey. Washington DC: National Alliance for Caregiving 1997.

68. Thomas P, Chantoin-Merlet S, Hazif-Thomas C, et al. Complaints of informal caregivers providing home care for dementia patients: the Pixel study. Int J Geriatr Psychiatry 2002; 17:1034–1047.

69. Wells YD, Jorm AF, Jordan F, Lefroy R. Effects on care-givers of special day care programmes for dementia sufferers. Aust NZ J Psychiatry 1990; 24:82–90.

70. Colerick EJ, George LK. Predictors of institutionalization among caregivers of patients with Alzheimer's disease. J Am Geriatr Soc 1986; 34:493–498.

71. Morycz RK. Caregiving strain and the desire to institutionalize family members with Alzheimer's disease. Possible predictors and model development. Res Aging 1985; 7:329–361.

72. Henretta JC, Hill MS, Li W, Soldo BJ, Wolf DA. Selection of children to provide care: the effect of earlier parental transfers. J Gerontol Series B Psychol Sci Social Sci 1997; 52: 110–119.

73. Seltzer MM, Li LW. The transitions of caregiving: subjective and objective definitions. Gerontologist 1996; 36:614–626.

74. Edwards AB, Zarit SH, Stephens MA, Townsend A. Employed family caregivers of cognitively impaired elderly: an examination of role strain and depressive symptoms. Aging Men Health 2002; 6:55–61.

75. Brody EM, Kleban MH, Hoffman C, Schoonover CB. Adult daughters and parent care: a comparison of one-, two- and three-generation households. Home Health Care Serv Quart 1988; 9:19–45.

76. Spitze G, Logan J. More evidence on women (and men) in the middle. Res Aging 1990; 12:182–198.

77. Donaldson C, Tarrier N, Burns A. Determinants of carer stress in Alzheimer's disease. Int J Geriatr Psychiatry 1998; 13:248–256.

78. Collins C. Carers: gender and caring for dementia. In: Arie, T, ed. Recent Advances in Psychogeriatrics 2. Edinburgh: Churchill Livingstone 1992; 173–186.

79. Gitlin LN, Belle SH, Burgio LD, et al. Effect of multicomponent interventions on caregiver burden and depression: the REACH multisite initiative at 6-month follow-up. Psychology Aging 2003; 18:361–374.

80. Parks SH, Pilisuk M. Caregiver burden: gender and the psychological costs of caregiving. Am J Orthopsychiatry 1991; 61:501–509.

81. Fitting M, Rabins P, Lucas MJ, Eastham J. Caregivers for dementia patients: a comparison of husbands and wives. Gerontologist 1986; 26:248–252.

82. Li LW, Seltzer MM, Greenberg JS. Social support and depressive symptoms: differential patterns in wife and-daughter caregivers. J Gerontol Series B Psychol Sci Social Sci 1997; 52:S200–S211.

83. Spitze G, Logan JR, Joseph G, Lee E. Middle generation roles and the well-being of men and women. J Gerontol 1994; 49:S107–S116.

84. Schulz R, O'Brien AT, Bookwala J, Fleissner K. Psychiatric and physical morbidity effects of dementia caregiving: prevalence, correlates, and causes. Gerontologist 1995; 35: 771–791.

85. Morris LW, Morris RG, Britton PG. The relationship between marital intimacy, perceived strain and depression in spouse caregivers of dementia sufferers. Br J Med Psychol 1988; 61(Part 3):231–236.

86. Rozario P, Morrow-Howell N, Hinterlong JE. Role enhancement or role strain. Assessing the impact of multiple productive roles on older caregiver well-being. Res Aging 2004; 26:413–428.

87. Mui AC. Caregiver strain among black and white daughter caregivers: a role theory perspective. Gerontologist 1992; 32:203–212.

88. Chumbler NR. The depressive symptomatology of parent care among the near elderly. Res Aging 2004; 26:330–351.

89. Dwyer JW, Coward RT. A multivariate comparison of the involvement of adult sons versus daughters in the care of impaired parents. J Gerontol 1991; 46:S259–S269.

90. Stoller EP. Males as helpers: the role of sons, relatives, and friends. Gerontologist 1990; 30:228–235.

91. Brody EM, Hoffman C, Kleban MH, Schoonover CB. Caregiving daughters and their local siblings: perceptions, strains, and interactions. Gerontologist 1989; 29:529–538.

92. Brody EM, Litvin SJ, Hoffman C, Kleban MH. Differential effects of daughters' marital status on their parent care experiences. Gerontologist 1992; 32:58–67.

93. Li LW, Seltzer MM, Greenberg JS. Change in depressive symptoms among daughter caregivers: an 18-month longitudinal study. Psychol Aging 1999; 14:206–219.

94. Ingersoll-Dayton B, Starrels ME, Dowler D. Caregiving for parents and parents-in-law: is gender important? Gerontologist 1996; 36:483–491.

95. Mizuno T, Takashaki K. Caring for a Yobiyose-rojin: a comparison of burden on daughters and daughters-in-law. J Gerontol Nursing 2005; 31:15–21.

96. Kim JS, Lee EH. Cultural and noncultural predictors of health outcomes in Korean daughter and daughter-in-law caregivers. Pub Health Nurs 2003; 20:111–119.

97. Horowitz A. Sons and daughters as caregivers to older parents: differences in role performance and consequences. Gerontologist 1985; 25:612–617.

98. Zanetti O, Frisoni GB, Bianchetti A, et al. Depressive symptoms of Alzheimer caregivers are mainly due to personal rather than patient factors. Int J Geriatr Psychiatry 1998; 13:358–367.

99. Freyne A, Kidd N, Coen R, Lawlor BA. Burden in carers of dementia patients: higher levels in carers of younger sufferers. Int J Geriatr Psychiatry 1999; 14:784–788.

100. Moen P, Robison J, Dempster-McClain D. Caregiving and women's well-being: a life course approach. J Health Social Behav 1995; 36:259–273.

101. Marks NF. Does it hurt to care? Caregiving, work–family conflict and midlife well-being. J Marriage Fam 1998 60: 951–966.

102. Brody EM. 'Women in the middle' and family help to older people. Gerontologist 1981; 21:471–480.

103. Buckwalter KC, Gerdner L, Kohout F, et al. A nursing intervention to decrease depression in family caregivers of persons with dementia. Arch Psychiatr Nurs 1999; 13:80–88.

104. de Vugt ME, Stevens F, Aalten P, et al. Do caregiver management strategies influence patient behaviour in dementia? Int J Geriatr Psychiatry 2004; 19:85–92.

105. Navaie-Waliser M, Feldman PH, Gould DA, et al. When the caregiver needs care: the plight of vulnerable caregivers. Am J Pub Health 2002; 92:409–413.

106. Annerstedt L, Elmstahl S, Ingvad B, Samuelsson SM. Family caregiving in dementia – an analysis of the caregiver's burden and the 'breaking-point' when home care becomes inadequate. Scand J Pub Health 2000; 28:23–31.

107. Victoroff J, Mack WJ, Nielson KA. Psychiatric complications of dementia: impact on caregivers. Dement Geriatr Cogn Disord 1998; 9:50–55.

108. Clyburn LD, Stones MJ, Hadjistavropoulos T, Tuokko H. Predicting caregiver burden and depression in Alzheimer's disease. J Gerontol Series B Psychol Sci Social Sci 2000; 55: S2–S13.

109. Hooker K, Bowman SR, Coehlo DP, et al. Behavioral change in persons with dementia: relationships with mental and physical health of caregivers. J Gerontol Series B Psychol Sci Social Sci 2002; 57:453–460.

110. Pinquart M, Sorensen S. Associations of caregiver stressors and uplifts with subjective well-being and depressive mood: a meta-analytic comparison. Aging Ment Health 2004; 8: 438–449.

111. Banerjee S, Murray J, Foley B, et al. Predictors of institutionalisation in people with dementia. J Neurol Neurosurg Psychiatry 2003; 74:1315–1316.

112. Bedard M, Molloy DW, Pedlar D, Lever JA, Stones MJ. 1997 IPA/Bayer Research Awards in Psychogeriatrics. Associations between dysfunctional behaviors, gender, and burden in spousal caregivers of cognitively impaired older adults. Int Psychogeriatr 1997; 9:277–290.

113. Yates ME, Tennstedt S, Chang BH. Contributors to and mediators of psychological well-being for informal caregivers. J Gerontol Series B Psychol Sci Social Sci 1999; 54: 12–22.

114. Pruchno RA, Resch NL. Aberrant behaviors and Alzheimer's disease: mental health effects on spouse caregivers. J Gerontol 1989; 44:S177–S182.

115. Brodaty H, Luscombe G. Depression in persons with dementia. Int Psychogeriatr 1996; 8:609–622.

116. Cohen CA, Gold DP, Shulman KI, et al. Factors determining the decision to institutionalise dementing individuals: a prospective study. Gerontologist 1993; 33:714–720.

117. Lee GR, Dwyer JW, Coward RT. Gender differences in parent care: demographic factors and same-gender preferences. J Gerontol 1993 48:S9–S16.

118. Kivett VR. Consanguinity and kin level: their relative importance to the helping network of older adults. J Gerontol 1985; 40:228–234.

119. Merrill D. Daughters-in-law as caregivers to the elderly. Res Aging 1993; 15:70–91.

120. Schulz R, Gallagher-Thompson D, Haley Q, Czaja S. Understanding the intervention process: a theoretical/conceptual framework for intervention approaches to caregiving. In: Schulz R, ed. Handbook on Dementia Caregiving. Evidence Based Interventions for Family Caregivers. New York: Springer-Verlag 2000; 44–45.

121. Lang A, Brody E. Characteristics of middle-aged daughters and help to their elderly mother. J Marriage Fam 1983; 45: 193–202.

122. Anderson LP. Acculturative stress: a theory of relevance to Black Americans. Clin Psychol Rev 1991; 11:685–702.

123. Haley WE, West CA, Wadley VG, et al. Psychological, social, and health impact of caregiving: a comparison of black and white dementia family caregivers and noncaregivers. Psychology Aging 1995; 10:540–552.

124. Pinquart M, Sorensen S. Ethnic differences in stressors, resources, and psychological outcomes of family caregiving: a meta-analysis. Gerontologist 2005; 45:90–106.

125. Nichols L, Malone C, Tarlow B, Loewenstein D. The pragmatics of implementing intervention studies in the community. In: Schultz R, ed. Handbook on Dementia Caregiving: Springer Publishing Company Inc, New York 2000; 127–150.

126. Lee YR, Sung KT. Cultural influences on caregiving burden: cases of Koreans and Americans. Int J Aging Hum Devel 1998 46:125–141.

127. Lee YR, Sung KT. Cultural differences in caregiving motivations for demented parents: Korean caregivers versus American caregivers. Int J Aging Hum Devel 1997; 44: 115–127.

128. Prince M. Dementia in developing countries. Int Psychogeriatr 2001; 13:389–393.

129. Patel V, Prince M. Ageing and mental health in a developing country: who cares? Qualitative studies from Goa, India. Psychol Med 2001; 31:29–38.

130. Prince M. The need for research on dementia in developing countries. Trop Med Intl Health 1997; 2:993–1000.

131. Prince M, 10/66 Dementia Research Group. Care arrangements for people with dementia in developing countries. Int J Geriatr Psychiatry 2004; 19:170–177.

132. Prince M, Acosta A, Chiu H, et al. Care arrangements for people with dementia in developing countries (conference presentation; Prevention of Alzheimer's Disease. Organised by Alzheimer's Association of USA). Philadelphia USA 2004.

133. Harvey R, Roques PK, Fox NC, Rossor MN. CANDID – Counselling and Diagnosis in Dementia: a national telemedicine service supporting the care of younger patients with dementia. Int J Geriatr Psychiatry 1998; 13: 381–388.

134. Keady J, Matthew L. Younger people with dementia. Elderly Care 1997 9:19–23.

135. Brodaty H. Families of people with dementia. In: Okasha A, ed. Families and Mental Disorders. From Burden to Empowerment. Chichester UK: John Wiley and Sons 2005; 25–54.

136. Valcour VG, Shikuma CM, Watters MR, Sacktor NC. Cognitive impairment in older HIV-1-seropositive individuals: prevalence and potential mechanisms. Aids 2004; 18:1.

137. Anonymous. HIV dementia persists, but now it's a chronic disease. AIDS Alert 2002; 17:46–48.

138. Pirraglia P, Bishop D, Herman D, et al. Caregiver burden and depression among informal caregivers of HIV infected individuals. J Gen Intern Med 2005; 20:510.

139. Shippy RA, Karpiak SE. The aging HIV/AIDS population: fragile social networks. Aging Ment Health 2005; 9: 246–254.

140. Poindexter CC. The lion at the gate: an HIV-affected caregiver resists stigma. Health Social Work 2005; 30:64–74.

141. Pillemer K, Finkelhor D. The prevalence of elder abuse: a random sample survey. Gerontologist 1988; 28:51–57.

142. Paveza GJ, Cohen D, Eisdorfer C, et al. Severe family violence and Alzheimer's disease: prevalence and risk factors. Gerontologist 1992; 32:493–497.

143. Cooney C, Mortimer A. Elder abuse and dementia – a pilot study. Int J Social Psychiatry 1995; 41:276–283.

144. Williamson GM, Shaffer DR. Relationship quality and potentially harmful behaviors by spousal caregivers: how we were then, how we are now. The Family Relationships in Late Life Project. Psychology Aging 2001; 16:217–226.

145. Reay AM, Browne KD. Risk factor characteristics in carers who physically abuse or neglect their elderly dependants. Aging Ment Health 2001; 5:56–62.

146. Miller LS. Cognitive impairment and quality of elder care. In: Symposium paper presented at the Annual Conference of the Gerontological Society of America, San Diego, CA 2003.

147. Stephens MA, Zarit SH. Family caregiving to dependent older adults: stress, appraisal, and coping. Psychology Aging 1989; 4:387–388.

148. Grant G, Ramcharan P, McGrath M, Nolan M, Keady J. Rewards and gratifications among family caregivers: towards a refined model of caring and coping. J Intellect Disab Res 1998; 42(Pt 1):58–71.

149. Kramer BJ. Husbands caring for wives with dementia: a longitudinal study of continuity and change. Health Social Work 2000; 25:97–107.

150. Brodaty H, Low LF. Involvement of carers, consumers and the broader community. In: Draper B, Melding P, Brodaty H, eds. Psychogeriatric Service Delivery. An International Perspective. Oxford: Oxford University Press 2005; 293–307.

151. Kemp NM, Brodaty H, Pond D, Luscombe G. Diagnosing dementia in primary care: the accuracy of informant reports. Alzheimer Dis Assoc Disord 2002; 16:171–176.

152. McFall S, Miller BH. Caregiver burden and nursing home admission of frail elderly persons. J Gerontol 1992; 47: S73–S79.

153. Jette AM, Tennstedt S, Crawford S. How does formal and informal community care affect nursing home use? J Gerontol Series B Psychol Sci Social Sci 1995; 50:S4–S12.

154. Brodaty H, Peters KE. Cost effectiveness of a training program for dementia carers. Int Psychogeriatr 1991; 3:11–22.

155. Horowitz A. Family caregiving to the frail elderly. Ann Rev Gerontol Geriatr 1985; 5:194–246.

156. Hurley AC, Volicer L, Blasi ZV. End-of-life care for patients with advanced dementia. JAMA 2000; 284:2449–2450.

157. Gessert CE, Forbes S, Bern-Klug M. Planning end-of-life care for patients with dementia: roles of families and health professionals. Omega J Death Dying 2000; 42:273–291.

158. Schulz R, Mendelsohn AB, Haley WE, et al. End-of-life care and the effects of bereavement on family caregivers of persons with dementia. N Engl J Med 2003; 349: 1936–1942.

159. Volicer L, Hurley AC, Blasi ZV. Characteristics of dementia end-of-life care across care settings. Am J Hospice Pall Care 2003; 20:191–200.

160. Steele C. Management of the family. In: Burns A, Levy R, eds. Dementia. London: Arnold 1994; 546.

161. Schulz R, Beach SR, Lind B, et al. Involvement in caregiving and adjustment to death of a spouse: findings from the caregiver health effects study. JAMA 2001; 285:3123–3129.

162. Brodaty H, Gresham M. Effect of a training programme to reduce stress in carers of patients with dementia. BMJ 1989; 299:1375–1379.

163. Kahan J, Kemp B, Staples FR, Brummel-Smith K. Decreasing the burden in families caring for a relative with a dementing illness. A controlled study. J Am Geriatr Soc 1985; 33:664–670.

164. Brodaty H, Gresham M, Luscombe G. The Prince Henry Hospital dementia caregivers' training programme. Int J Geriatr Psychiatry 1997; 12:183–192.

165. Mittelman MS, Ferris SH, Steinberg G, et al. An intervention that delays institutionalization of Alzheimer's disease patients: treatment of spouse-caregivers. Gerontologist 1993; 33:730–740.

166. Ferris SH, Steinberg G, Shulman E, Kahn R, Reisberg B. Institutionalization of Alzheimer's disease patients: reducing precipitating factors through family counseling. Home Health Care Serv Quart 1987; 8:23–51.

167. Brodaty H, McGilchrist C, Harris L, Peters KE. Time until institutionalization and death in patients with dementia. Role of caregiver training and risk factors. Arch Neurol 1993; 50:643–650.

168. Rabins PV. The caregiver's role in Alzheimer's disease. Dement Geriatr Cogn Disord 1998; 3:25–28.

169. Brodaty H, Green A. Caregiver interventions. In: Qizibash N, Schneider L, Chui H, et al, eds. Evidence Based

Dementia Practice: A Practical Guide to Diagnosis and Management. Oxford: Blackwell Science 2002; 764–794.

170. Knight BG, Lutzky SM, Macofsky-Urban F. A meta-analytic review of interventions for caregiver distress: recommendations for future research. Gerontologist 1993; 33:240–248.

171. Gitlin L, Corcoran M, Winter L, Boyce A, Hauck W. A randomized, controlled trial of a home environmental intervention: effect on efficacy and ipset in caregivers and on daily function of persons with dementia. Gerontologist 2001; 41:4–14.

172. Marriott A, Donaldson C, Tarrier N, Burns A. Effectiveness of cognitive-behavioural family intervention in reducing the burden of care in carers of patients with Alzheimer's disease. Br J Psychiatry 2000; 176:557–562.

173. Chiverton P, Caine ED. Education to assist spouses in coping with Alzheimer's disease. A controlled trial. J Am Geriatr Soc 1989; 37:593–598.

174. Corbeil RR, Quayhagen MP, Quayhagen M. Intervention effects on dementia caregiving interaction: a stress–adaptation modeling approach. J Aging Health 1999; 11:79–95.

175. Quayhagen MP, Quayhagen M. Differential effects of family-based strategies on Alzheimer's disease. Gerontologist 1989; 29:150–155.

176. Jansson W, Almberg B, Grafstrom M, Winblad B. The Circle Model – support for relatives of people with dementia. Int J Geriatr Psychiatry 1998; 13:674–681.

177. Brodaty H, Green A, Koschera A. Meta-analysis of psychosocial interventions for caregivers of people with dementia. J Am Geriatr Soc 2003; 51:657–664.

178. Teri L, Logsdon RG, Uomoto J, McCurry SM. Behavioral treatment of depression in dementia patients: a controlled clinical trial. J Gerontol Series B Psychol Sci Social Sci 1997; 52:159–166.

179. Teri L, Gibbons LE, McCurry SM, et al. Exercise plus behavioral management in patients with Alzheimer disease: a randomized controlled trial. JAMA 2003; 290:2015–2022.

180. Pioloi SF. Non-pharmacological management of dementia. In: Mendez MF, Cummings JL, eds. Dementia. A Clinical Approach, 3rd edn. Philadelphia: Butterworth Heinemann 2003; 654.

181. Whitlatch CJ, Zarit SH, von Eye A. Efficacy of interventions with caregivers: a reanalysis. Gerontologist 1991; 31:9–14.

182. Brodaty H, Mittelman M, Burns A. The three country study: Added benefits of caregiver intervention to treatment of Alzheimer's Disease with Aricpet. Presented by Mary Miltelmann in: 19th International Conference of Alzheimer's Disease International; Santo Domingo, Dominican Republic 2003.

183. Mittelman MS, Ferris SH, Shulman E, Steinberg G, Levin B. A family intervention to delay nursing home placement of patients with Alzheimer disease. A randomized controlled trial. JAMA 1996; 276: 1725–1731.

184. Mittelman MS, Roth DL, Haley WE, Zarit SH. Effects of a caregiver intervention on negative caregiver appraisals of behavior problems in patients with Alzheimer's disease: results of a randomized trial. J Gerontol Series B Psychol Sci Social Sci 2004; 59:27–34.

185. Gallagher-Thompson D, DeVries HM. 'Coping with frustration' classes: development and preliminary outcomes with women who care for relatives with dementia. Gerontologist 1994; 34:548–552.

186. Toseland RW, Rossiter CM, Labrecque MS. The effectiveness of peer-led and professionally led groups to support family caregivers. Gerontologist 1989; 29: 465–471.

187. Zarit SH, Femia EE, Watson J, Rice-Oeschger L, Kakos B. Memory Club: a group intervention for people with early-stage dementia and their care partners. Gerontologist 2004; 44:262–269.

188. Brodaty H, Green A, Graham N. Alzheimer's (disease and related disorders) associations and societies: supporting family carers. In: O'Brien J, Ames D, Burns A, eds. Dementia, 2nd edn. Arnold, London 2000; 361–367.

189. Gwyther LP. Social issues of the Alzheimer's patient and family. Am J Med 1998; 104:27.

190. Bass DM, McClendon MJ, Brennan PF, McCarthy C. The buffering effect of a computer support network on caregiver strain. J Aging Health 1998; 10:20–43.

191. Brennan PF, Moore SM, Smyth KA. The effects of a special computer network on caregivers of persons with Alzheimer's disease. Nurs Res 1995; 44:166–172.

192. Brodaty H, Thomson C, Thompson C, Fine M. Why caregivers of people with dementia and memory loss don't use services. Int J Geriatr Psychiatry 2005; 20:537–546.

193. Family Survival Project. Annual Reports: Family Survival Program Pilot Project. San Francisco: Family Survival Project; 1984 Survey 1981–1984.

194. Montgomery R, Borgatta E. The effects of alternative support strategies on family caregiving. Gerontologist 1989; 29:457–464.

195. Zarit SH, Stephens MA, Townsend A, Greene R. Stress reduction for family caregivers: effects of adult day care use. J Gerontol Series B Psychol Sci Social Sci 1998; 53:S267–S278.

196. Zarit SH. Interventions for family caregivers: do they work and why. Available at http://www2.uni-jena.de/svw/devpsy/news/2003/download/zarit.pdf Penn State University, 2003 [accessed 06 April, 2006].

197. Sorensen S, Pinquart M, Duberstein P. How effective are interventions with caregivers? An updated meta-analysis. Gerontologist 2002; 42:356–372.

24

Community-based formal support services

Lilly Katofsky

INTRODUCTION

Several phenomena of concern to clinicians are occurring simultaneously: an increase in the number of people afflicted with Alzheimer's disease (AD),[1] the impact of AD on care providers[2] and a trend towards delivering comprehensive, streamlined and cost-effective health care.[1,3-5] There is also a movement on the part of policy-makers to shift the responsibility for long-term caregiving to individuals and their families. In reality, families have always provided most of the care to their frail elderly relatives.[6-8] Families provide 70–80 per cent of the care received by the elderly.[9-11] There is no indication that this pattern is different today than it was in the recent past.[12] As a result, families are bearing the burden of caring for AD patients who have greater functional disabilities at home for longer periods of time.[6,8,11-15]

We recognize that the elderly prefer to remain at home and that, as they become frail, they receive most of their care from their informal network.[2,3,8,13] As the course of caregiving can be long and gradual deterioration in the care recipient is to be expected, families need assistance in this increasingly onerous task.[8,16] It is at this juncture that we need to examine the role that community-based formal support services can play in assisting families in maintaining their loved one at home.

Gerontological literature and clinical practice have underscored families' lack of information about the resources available to them to reduce the burden and stress of caregiving.[1,6,15,17,18] The family's first contact in the health and social care system is with the physician to whom they have come for evaluation and treatment of their relative's illness.[19] The physician is in a position to provide information on AD and its

progress. In collaboration with other healthcare clinicians, the physician can discuss techniques of coping with the deterioration in cognition and physical functioning as well as provide tips on the management of difficult and disruptive behaviour. The team of clinicians can direct the family towards appropriate community resources. The physician must therefore be knowledgeable about what the community offers and how to access these resources.[19-21]

This chapter outlines the goals of the community-based formal support services network, describes the services and their consumers and addresses the barriers to their use. It will also discuss the clinical implications of formal support services and the role of the clinician in promoting their use.

GOALS OF THE FORMAL SUPPORT SYSTEM

The rationale for the development of community-based formal support services is that they are less costly than institutional care and they prevent premature institutionalization of the frail and functionally dependent elderly individual.[22] In reality, the goals of community-based services are many and varied.[23,24] Reduction of costs and delaying premature institutionalization are only two of the objectives. These services can replace more costly in-hospital care by substituting less expensive home care.[4] They cannot, however, replace in a cost-effective way the high level of care required by very severely disabled individuals and those with extreme behaviour problems.[9,13]

In general, community-based services enable the elderly to remain at home as long as possible. They supplement and complement the informal care provided by families.[8,19,23,25,26] As noted above, remaining at home constitutes the most satisfying alternative for the elderly. This desire to live in the community is reflected in social policies which have deinstitutionalized many vulnerable groups, such as the mentally ill, and the physically and mentally handicapped. The challenge, however, is to assure a good quality of life for community-dwelling dependent groups. Community-based resources can contribute significantly to this improvement in quality of life by offering support to vulnerable individuals and to those who care for them.

Community-based services help families to cope with the increased responsibility of caring for a loved one with greater and more complex functional disabilities, memory impairment and behavioural problems. The literature has reported that intervention with formal support services can reduce the stress of caregiving.[8,14,25,27–30] A less stressed, better prepared, more knowledgeable and skilled caregiver can continue to provide care to an ever more demanding care recipient.

Clinicians are concerned that if the stress of caregiving becomes too great,[16] the caregiver may resort to physical abuse or neglect. Therefore, another goal of community services is to moderate this stress and to reduce the possibility or incidence of abuse.

Caregiving exacts a heavy toll on the health and well-being of the care provider. Community services can moderate the deleterious health effects of caregiving by keeping the care provider 'healthy', thereby reducing the dual risks of costly health services utilization by the care provider and institutionalization of the care recipient.[31]

Community services can delay institutionalization but they do not prevent it. The single most common reason for institutionalization is the loss of the primary caregiver.[13] Indeed, use of resources such as a day centre or respite care may give 'permission' to a caregiver to place a relative who actually requires more care than she or he is physically and emotionally able to provide.[32–35] Such resources are also a good opportunity for the caregiver to obtain other important information about relevant services.

To summarize, community-based formal support services can achieve many goals. They are not only more cost-effective, they permit AD patients to remain at home longer by providing assistance to their caregivers. They may reduce the stress and strain of caregiving by offering respite, support and validation of the caregiving role. They can contribute to the quality of life of the caregiver and care recipient by helping to maintain their family life. And, very importantly, they may facilitate the transition to institutionalization by demonstrating that the AD patient can be cared for effectively by people other than the primary informal caregiver.

WHAT ARE COMMUNITY-BASED FORMAL SUPPORT SERVICES?

McPherson[23] describes the support system for the elderly as a series of concentric circles surrounding the elderly person. The closer circles representing family, friends and neighbours are the more intimate (informal) supports; the outer circles are the formal supports representing the objective and bureaucratic system. The formal system comprises a range of health and social services delivered by voluntary groups, government and, increasingly, the private sector.

Community-based formal support services can be defined as those services, paid for with public or private funds, provided to persons living at home to help maintain their maximum level of autonomy and independence. They can be delivered in, or outside of, the home. In the latter, the individual attends the activity, such as a day centre, on a day basis or may be admitted for a short stay, such as in the case of institution-based respite. Community-based services can also include group-type living arrangements resembling home style environments.

RELATIONSHIP BETWEEN INFORMAL AND FORMAL SUPPORT SERVICES

A rich literature exists on the relationship between the informal and formal support system.[17,25,36–38] Different models have been described and researched. Gerontologists question whether the formal support services are substitutes for, complementary to, supplementary to, or a bridge between, the informal and formal support networks.[17,23,36] In the substitution model, the formal support services provide the care either when the elderly have no family or when the family is unavailable or no longer able to provide the care.

In the complementary model, the formal and informal systems provide different types of tasks best suited to each system's capabilities. Both types of care are needed to provide the complete care the individual requires.[36]

The supplementary model provides additional help to the primary caregiver. It recognizes that the caregiver requires help with caregiving tasks. This supplemental assistance eases the burden and stress.

The most prevalent model is the complementary relationship between the formal and informal network. In this model the caregiver and care recipient are assured of a continuum of care.[25] Tasks are shared and not differentiated, as postulated by Litwack.[36]

Regardless of which model is described, it is clear that the two systems are intricately linked. The formal network's major goal is to support the informal network in optimally performing its caregiving duties.

Logan and Spitze[17] propose that family members can be a bridge to the utilization of formal services by the elderly. The elderly may not know about the availability of the services, or if they do, may not know how to access them. Families can act as facilitators by providing information on existing services or by advocating on the elderly person's behalf.

Policy-makers are concerned that family members may withdraw their support when care is provided by the formal system. On the contrary, research does not substantiate this concern.[6–9,39] Family members continue to provide care. Community resources serve as a mediator of stress of caregiving by providing support and respite.[22,37] Low levels of formal help may result in institutionalization if the stressed caregiver sees no other alternative.[40]

USERS OF SERVICES

The study of the utilization pattern of community-based formal support services challenges our commonly held beliefs about caregivers of the frail elderly. Can we predict who will be the consumer of formal support services? Is it the individual who lacks an informal support system or is it the caregiver who has a network of family and friends who will seek out formal services? The answer to a seemingly simple question is quite complex!

Clearly, the individual who lacks informal support relies on the formal system to provide needed care as his level of dependency progresses.[23,25,41]

Amongst those with an informal network, the use of services increases with the level of disability. Several studies report that functional disability is a strong predictor of utilization of the formal system.[8,13,17,25–27,37,38,42] Use of community services was higher among caregivers of patients suffering from dementia than of those who were not.[13] However, when researchers controlled for physical disability, they found that caregivers in the comparison group (non-dementia patients) used more services than caregivers in the dementia group. This finding is consistent with other studies which report that caregivers of patients with AD tend to use formal services less than caregivers of persons with other disabilities.[27,28,43] The Canadian Study on Health and Aging (1994)[13] found that the AD patients who were institutionalized suffered from greater disability than the comparison group who had physical disabilities only. This tendency towards not using formal services will be addressed in greater detail below.

Caregivers seek assistance to relieve the stress of caregiving.[8,13,27,28,33,37,44] These studies concluded that using formal support services did alleviate some of the stress; however, it was only when the care recipient entered into permanent residential care that the mental health of the caregiver may have actually improved.[8]

Female spouses tend to seek assistance less frequently than male spouses. Spouses use less services than sons and daughters,[45] even though users reported satisfaction with the services.[46] Those who are employed seek assistance more frequently than those who are not.[13,47]

Nonetheless, even though caregivers may be emotionally and physically stressed, they continue to cope on their own or with the assistance of their informal network. It is only when the AD patient deteriorates both cognitively and physically that they turn to the formal network for assistance.[28] Levin[8] notes that many care recipients of services were as seriously incapacitated as those in permanent care. What is also very clear is that informal caregivers do not stop providing care when formal support services are available.[25]

TYPES OF AVAILABLE SERVICES

In the last several decades, we have seen a growth in the number and type of community-based formal services. This development is potentially advantageous to AD patients and their caregivers. Service needs, however, vary from one family to another. There is no ideal service package for any individual family.

There are many different kinds of services which may or may not be available in all communities. The services described in this chapter constitute some of those existing in many parts of our countries, but are by no means all the creative programmes designed to improve the lives of AD patients and their families.

Some communities boast a coordinated, integrated network of services accessed through a single entry system.[7,48–51] A centralized comprehensive system facilitates service utilization.

Services can be categorized as follows: in-home services, out-of-the home services, respite services, financial supplementation, information and referral services and complementary and alternative therapies. The services described below do not constitute an exhaustive list but include the principle services.

In-home services

Services, provided in the home, may be delivered by professionals, paraprofessionals or volunteers. They may be publicly funded, organized by not-for-profit voluntary organizations or purchased from private individuals or agencies. They are directed to home-bound functionally and/or cognitively disabled elderly unable to perform activities of daily living (ADL) or instrumental activities of daily living (IADL) or as assistance to the caregiver. They include:

- homemakers;
- home health aides;
- visiting nurses;
- occupational and physical therapist;
- physicians;
- social worker;

- friendly visitors;
- meals-on-wheels;
- assisted transportation;
- telephone buddies/reassurance programme;
- alert programmes;
- telephone support;
- internet/online support services.

The main functions of these services are described in Table 24.1.

Out-of-home services

These are services available outside of the home for those able to leave their homes:

- community health and social services;
- senior centre;

Table 24.1 Community-based formal support services: in-home services

Service	Function
Homemaker	Provides assistance with or performs household tasks
Home health aide	Provides assistance with or performs personal care tasks
Visiting nurse	Coordinates home nursing care; supervises medications, carries out special medical and nursing procedures, supervises homemakers and home health aides, monitors needs and arranges for additional services, as needed
Physician	Provides medical care to homebound elderly
Occupational therapist	Assesses and recommends changes to the home to improve its safety as well as provides therapy and assistive devices to improve functioning
Physical therapist	Assesses mobility problems and either teaches the exercises to the caregiver or provides the therapy directly
Social worker	Assesses psychosocial needs; refers to support services; provides counselling on effects of ageing and impact of acute and chronic illness on patient's and family's emotional and social functioning
Friendly visitors	Volunteers not related to the elderly person visit with the homebound elderly person and provide companionship, leisure activities, etc
Meals-on-wheels	Cooked meals usually at a nominal charge delivered to the homebound elderly. Programme advantage is that it 'keeps an eye' on the person while delivering a hot meal and reports problems. It not only provides nutrition but supervision as well
Assisted transportation	For physically frail elderly unable to use regular transportation or unable to go out on their own. This is the most difficult service to access, as it is very costly, whether publicly or privately funded
Telephone buddies/ Reassurance	Daily hello telephone call to assure that the person is safe
Alert programme	Personal alarm device to signal distress: someone goes to the home to check on the person and takes appropriate action
Telephone support	Automated interactive voice response intervention[52]
Internet/online support	Provides the homebound caregiver with emotional support, practical information and resources;[53–55] seniors fastest growing group of users[56]

- support groups;
- advocacy groups and programmes;
- wheels-to-meals/congregate dining;
- group living arrangements;
- information and referral services;
- case/care management organizations/services.

These services are described in Table 24.2

Respite services

Respite services provide the caregiver with an opportunity to take a break from the task of caregiving. Levin[8] defines respite as any service which gives the caregiver temporary relief from caregiving responsibilities. Respite is of variable duration from a few hours a day, several days at a time, to several weeks. There are different types of respite: (1) in-home, (2) at a day or night centre (the latter offers the caregiver overnight rest; the refreshed caregiver can resume caregiving during daytime hours), (3) in institutional settings such as nursing homes, board or care homes or in hospitals on a temporary basis. Caregivers prefer in-home respite.

They find it less disruptive to the AD patient, who remains at home in a familiar environment while the caregiver spends time away.[17] Caregivers are generally satisfied with in-home respite and report benefits. Some problems reported by caregivers were variability in helper competence and reliability and lack of programme responsiveness to expressed need.[40]

Social policy programmes

These programmes refer to financial resources as well as government sponsored service initiatives available to the caregiver of the AD patient. These include (1) tax credits to compensate for costs associated with caregiving, (2) financial subsidies to purchase services and (3) development of services.

Generally, government-sponsored programmes devise eligibility criteria based on society's determination of need. As demands grows (increase in the number of AD patients) and budgets decrease, criteria may be revised resulting in more limited access.[6,8,9,57] Also, programme eligibility criteria may not reflect need. For example, even though individuals in three of Florida's

Service	Function
Table 24.2 Community-based formal support services: out-of-home services	
Community health and social services	Multi-service agency provides health and social services: physician, occupational therapist, physiotherapist, social worker, leisure activities, support groups, etc
Senior centre	Provides broad range of social activities geared to individual's cognitive and physical abilities
Day centre	Goal is to maintain and improve cognitive and physical functioning of, and provide socialization for the AD patient. The caregiver benefits from respite while the care recipient attends the programme
Support groups	Designed for the caregiver and/or the care recipient. Helps family cope with the emotional impact of caregiving or of being afflicted with the illness by sharing with others in similar situations
Advocacy groups/ Programmes	Not-for-profit or publicly funded to assist in accessing services and programmes; also advocate for the establishment of new services and programmes
Wheels-to-meals/ Congregate dining	Frail elderly are transported to meals for the dual purpose of socialization while partaking of a nutritious meal
Group living arrangements	Family-type/non-institutional living environments for those unable to remain at home
Information and referral	Central number or centre provides information on and referral to available community-based services
Case/care management organizations/services	Model designed to overcome fragmentation of services. Case/care manager assesses, refers to, coordinates and oversees provision of services to the elderly person. 'Person to call' to mediate bureaucratic service maze

community-based programmes were impaired, eligibility criteria, and not necessarily level of need, determined what kind of benefits they would receive.[58] There may also be no congruence between the professional's and the individual's assessment of need.[43,57]

COMPLEMENTARY AND ALTERNATIVE THERAPIES

One can debate whether complementary and alternative therapies constitute part of the continuum of formal community-based support services. However, these areas emerged in a review of the gerontological and geriatric literature as being potentially advantageous to the caregiver and the AD patient. The healthcare practitioner should be aware that the caregiver and/or the care recipient may be a consumer of these services and/or may benefit from them. Gaylord and Crotty[59] define complementary and alternative therapies as those techniques and approaches not conventionally used or taught in mainstream medicine in the United States or other Western countries. They point out that over 40 per cent of Americans now use alternative therapies. Among consumers are older people, cultural minorities, individuals who have limited access to conventional services and those who suffer from chronic or life-threatening conditions. These authors refer to a study by Coleman et al,[60] which found that 55 per cent of caregivers with AD had tried one or more complementary therapies in order to improve memory. Forty per cent noted some benefit. Some selected therapies, such as mind–body, alternative diet, spirituality and music, are described in Table 24.3. The reader is referred to the article by Gaylord and Crotty[59] for an overview of these and other therapies.

DETERMINANTS OF USE OF COMMUNITY-BASED FORMAL SUPPORT SERVICES

The following are some of the factors which encourage service utilization.

Perception of benefits

Researchers[46] studied users and non-users of adult day care. They found users were more likely to perceive that this resource would benefit both the AD patient and themselves: stimulation and socialization for the AD patient and physical and psychological respite for the caregiver. Non-users believed that only the caregiver would benefit by having more time for activities. These authors emphasize that caregivers were less likely to use adult day care if they perceived benefits were only for the caregivers. It is therefore critical to emphasize to the caregiver the potential benefits of this resource to the AD patient as well.[30,40]

Support and encouragement

Studies have indicated that caregivers who have adequate informal support,[66] and who receive encouragement and referral to services from physicians,[67] tend to use formal services more frequently.

Level of impairment

AD patients with fewer ADL impairments are more likely to use out-of-home formal services[66] while those with more functional impairments tend to utilize in-home resources.[8,28,67]

Table 24.3 Community-based formal support services: complementary and alternative therapies

Therapy	Function
Mind–body	Hypnosis, biofeedback, guided imagery, relaxation, mindfulness meditation/exercise (e.g. yoga, tai chi) amongst others[59] to reduce pain and stress[61]
Alternative diet	Partnering with the natural foods movement, emphasizing the importance of organic and whole foods[59]
Spirituality	Helps families cope by drawing on spiritual and religious beliefs and practices;[62,63] may connect the AD patient to his or her faith through e.g. hymns, religious rituals;[63,64] provides emotional, spiritual and instrumental support to families through faith-based care teams[65]
Music therapy	Helps AD patient connect with the past, and may decrease agitation and aggressive behaviour[59]

Perceived availability

If caregivers perceive that services are available, they are more likely to take advantage of them.[26,28]

Psychological health

Cox[28] found that caregivers using respite care were psychologically less anxious than those who did not. She postulates that a certain level of psychological health is required to accept a respite programme. Generally, anxious caregivers are the ones who are reluctant to permit others to care for their loved one.

Adequate amount of assistance

Programmes which provide sufficient amounts of service are of greater interest to caregivers and may contribute to reducing caregiver stress.[40]

BARRIERS TO THE USE OF COMMUNITY-BASED FORMAL SUPPORT SERVICES

In spite of the documented benefits of community-based formal services, such as stress reduction, improved quality of life and delayed institutionalization, these services are not used to advantage by the intended consumer. The reasons are many and have been of keen interest to gerontologists for a long time.[26,28,31,46,68–70] Why do caregivers of AD patients not use community services? This section outlines some of the reasons.

Attitudes

Many elderly people believe in the notion of self-reliance, independence and the obligation to provide all the care themselves.[26,44,71] They also prefer that any help they receive comes from the family group. Caregivers have networks of informal support to which they turn for assistance. Such culturally and socially bound attitudes are difficult to change.[39,43,72] In addition, some professionals adhere to the value that it is the responsibility of the family to look after its frail relatives.[6,9,71] This type of attitude may predispose caregivers to not seek assistance outside of the immediate family. They believe they are not fulfilling their duty to their frail elderly relative if they do.

Social policy

The attitude described above is embodied in the contradictory goals of social policy. Kane and Penrod[39] note that social policy either encourages families to take responsibility for caregiving, relieves them of their responsibility or assists them in the caregiving role. These authors advocate policies which support families in their caregiving efforts. Families are then able to sustain their caregiving for longer periods of time. At the same time their burden and stress are reduced. Indeed, once caregivers begin seeking formal services, it may be too late to avoid institutionalization. Caregivers may have gone beyond their ability to continue to provide care. Offering services to families when they are contemplating permanent residential care is not the way to avert institutionalization. This offer has come too late in the caregiving cycle. Families have reached the end of their ability to continue caregiving when they have made the decision to institutionalize.[27,73] Gottlieb[33] researched the impact of day programmes on family caregivers of persons with dementia. Caregivers described these services as insufficient and offered too late to prolong family care. Almost one-third of the participants were placed in long-term care institutions 5 months after starting the day programme. Clearly these and other types of services must be made available in earlier stages of caregiving. It is imperative to intervene at critical points in the carer's career to be effective.[22] Social policy must reflect these clinical needs.

Knowledge of services

Lack of knowledge about community-based services is another predictor of non-use.[6,9,18,26,30,45,46] People possess insufficient information about the services that exist and how to access them. However, even if they have the information, they do not necessarily avail themselves of them.[27] Mediating factors to utilization are perception of need, functional disability, perceived benefit to the care receiver[46] and perceived helpfulness of the services.[70]

Overall, research has uncovered that the elderly continue to lack information about community services in spite of an extensive network of information and referral services in most communities.[6,9,18,46,57] This finding has major clinical and programme implications for Information and Referral Services. They must develop techniques for reaching the people for whom the services are intended.

Perception of need

In the early stages of AD, caregivers may not perceive that their relative is ill. Family caregivers do not necessarily view the diagnosis of Alzheimer's as a disease and thus do not believe they need assistance. It is only as the disease progresses that this perception may change. The challenge for the clinician is to monitor the caregiving relationship and intervene at the right time to avert avoidable burden and stress.

View of the future

Gerontologists have noted that care providers may have a pessimistic view of the future and therefore may not see in what way services will provide them with relief from the stress of caregiving.[13] Depressed caregivers do not tend to use services.[28,42] Once again, the clinician plays a key role in mediating this situation and offering alternatives which may alleviate the stress and reduce these feelings of despair and hopelessness.

Accessibility

Accessing services can be a challenge, even if the caregiver possesses information about them.[6,9,39,74] Eligibility requirements may not qualify the person for the service. As resources shrink and the demand increases, services devise mechanisms to serve those whom they determine have the greatest needs. Depending upon the social policy perspective, services could be offered to those with greater needs, or those with lighter ones. Service providers may wish to offer a small amount of service to many or a lot to a few. In either scenario, many people requiring services may not be able to receive them.

Application procedures may act as a deterrent if they are too cumbersome, intrusive and bureaucratic. The elderly caregiver, reluctant to apply for assistance, may be discouraged if, having decided to reach out, he or she is unable to receive an immediate response to the request for relief from a caregiving task. Many caregivers do not have the time to spend researching the maze of services. Their wish is to tap into the service right away.

Access to transportation, geographic proximity of the resource and assistance with preparing the AD patient may facilitate or impede utilization of services, such as the adult day centre. Also, patients with disturbed behaviour may be excluded from these programmes.[75]

Availability

The types of resources available locally may not be the ones needed by the caregivers.[30,58] Levin[8] found there were major variations in the types of services developed in different regions of the country. The implica-

tions for care providers are significant: it is not possible to offer the same kind of care for comparable problems.

Appropriateness of services

Given the nature of the illness with its unpredictable course and behaviours, caregivers may be reluctant to expose the AD patient to unknown formal caregivers who may not be able to manage the idiosyncratic behaviour of a loved one. They may be uncertain as to the level of training and understanding of these behaviours this stranger possesses who is coming into their home or providing care at the adult day centre.[46,68,76] Furthermore, they may be reluctant to relinquish control of their loved one to a stranger.[30]

Out-of-home services may be beneficial to the caregiver but not for the AD patient, who may have a difficult time adjusting to a new environment. The few hours or days of respite may not be worth the many hours of re-establishing a fragile routine.

What is offered may not necessarily be the type of service caregivers are requesting or needing.[58] Nursing monitoring may be of the highest calibre, but what the caregiver urgently needs is assistance with functional and concrete tasks, such as bathing and household activities. Most service organizations provide 'assembly-line' rather than 'customized' service packages, that is, everyone receives the same type of service, rather than a package geared to specific needs.[6,8,9]

Cost

Cost is often cited as another barrier to the use of formal services. Private sector services may be beyond the financial means of the individual. Furthermore, carers may be husbanding their resources for a 'rainy day' and may not perceive that it has arrived! On the other hand, many publicly-funded programmes link socio-economic status and service eligibility. However, even in the free services offered in the Quebec model of CLSCs (local community service centres), which has universal access, researchers report underutilization.[6,9]

Emphasis on psychological services

Many services focus on providing psychological assistance. Many elderly caregivers do not perceive that they are in psychological distress, but may instead somatize their stress. They tend to seek instrumental rather than emotional assistance. These types of support programmes need to re-examine their goals in light of these findings.[43]

Lack of coordination among services

Many communities have not developed a 'one stop shopping' or single entry approach to service delivery. The result is a confusing maze of services, both public and private. These services may be difficult to know about and to access both for families and health providers.

UNDERSERVED POPULATIONS

Ethnicity and the use of community-based formal support services

The number of ethnic minority elders is growing faster than among whites and will continue to do so.[77,78] Ethnic minority elders tend to underutilize community services.[20,67,77,79] While many reasons for non-use of formal services are similar to those identified for the general elderly population, there are a number of barriers which are particular to ethnic elderly. Hooyman and Kiyak[77] have summarized these barriers. These include inability to speak the language; services that are not designed for specific ethnic groups (ethnic foods, traditional medicine, culturally appropriate recreational activities); stigma of utilizing services (the family should be the provider, not the mental health services); staff who are not culturally sensitive to differences nor able to communicate in the minority language; geographic distance; fear of Western medicine and distrust of healthcare professionals. In addition there are cultural differences in beliefs and knowledge about AD.[78,80,81] The family may be reluctant to share information about the 'family secret' because it may lose face and suffer shame.[80]

There is a growing literature on the problems faced by cultural communities in developed and developing countries when caring for a loved one with AD. There is a also a debate as to whether to advocate for the development of minority specific services or whether to improve services that will affect all elderly individuals.[77] Healthcare professionals must be sensitive to cultural diversity[80] and encourage referral to community services. Furthermore, policy makers and healthcare providers must include members of the ethnic groups in planning and developing services. Church leaders and community leaders should be involved in reaching out and promoting these services, since research has demonstrated that many of these elders are disadvantaged and will benefit from intervention.

Lesbian and gay elder caregivers and community-based services

Gerontologists are aware that within the elderly population there is a large group of lesbian and gay elders caring for a life partner suffering from AD, yet community support services are structured and provided from a heterosexual perspective.[82] As a result, lesbian and gay caregivers are not receiving services and encounter barriers when they want to access them.[82] Lesbian and gay caregivers have similar but at the same time different challenges and needs to heterosexual couples. Some of the problems they have encountered are assumption by support groups that all couples are heterosexual and that the caregiver is either a spouse or a child and not a life partner; dilemma as to whether to divulge sexual orientation in a support group given the prevalence of homophobia; lack of sensitivity and concern by medical, human service, legal and financial planning professionals; hospital personnel not accepting, in spite of completeness of legal documents, that the caregiver is indeed the person responsible for the AD patient; limited emotional and instrumental support following the illness of the life partner because of the absence of family or friends; no or little employee or conjugal partner benefits necessitating personal financial and legal planning for retirement and long-term health care; loss of the one person who cared about them when family, friends and religious institutions had rejected them; lack of usual sources of support, e.g. family, friends, colleagues, funeral rituals when facing the death of a loved one; loss of a shared life together and the prospect of return to social isolation and loneliness.[82]

The number of elderly lesbian and gay individuals will continue to increase. The benefits of community support services to combat the ill effects of caregiver burden have been well documented. Lesbian and gay caregivers of life partners suffering from AD should have the same access to these services without encountering prejudice and unpleasantness when seeking support for their difficult caregiving role. Research on lesbian and gay caregivers' emotional and supportive needs should inform the design of services so as to acknowledge difference in need and to respond effectively.[82]

STATE OF THE ART

In the more than 30 years since AD has been identified as a major social issue, clinicians, practitioners, social policy makers and researchers have designed and implemented community-based formal support services to assist families and patients with the deleterious effects of the disease. Many studies have been conducted to understand why some people use services while others do not. These professionals have been puzzled that community-based formal support services are underutilized by those for whom they were intended[31] and, when used, the effects on objectives such as stress reduction and delayed institutionalization are moderate.[40] The gerontological and geriatric literature is examining these findings and is proposing approaches to address these questions.[31,83] Some of the issues identified are methodological problems,[31] theoretical assumptions[31] and the intervention itself – have enough services been provided to make a difference[40] and do the goals of the intervention meet the expectations of both the provider and recipient of the service?[30] Researchers recommend, among others, more rigorous attention to research and programme design,[30] an alternate theoretical framework[30,31] and involvement of caregivers and care recipients (to the extent that they can be involved) in a dialogue to explain why an intervention can be helpful. Research should inform programme designers and policymakers in the most effective interventions to mitigate the effects of AD.

PRACTICE IMPLICATIONS

The clinician faces a major challenge in providing comprehensive care to AD patients and their caregivers. He or she must balance the medical care with the social and emotional needs of both the patient and the caregiver, and must listen with the third ear to hear what is actually being expressed. Research has demonstrated that use of formal services, whether in-home respite, participation in support groups or counselling, does reduce the level of stress, burden and depression.[66] The beneficial effect for the care receiver is a less stressed and harried caregiver able to continue in the caregiving role.[8,28,29,84] It was noted above that the stressed caregiver may become abusive if the stress and frustration levels become too great. Therefore the onus is on the clinician to inform and encourage caregivers to utilize services appropriate to the care needs of their loved ones and of themselves.

New techniques of managing disruptive behaviour have been developed and tested[85] to prolong home care and delay institutionalization. The care provider, having learned and applied these techniques in the day-to-day care of the care receiver, could experience a reduction in stress and burden.[86] The clinician has a responsibility to encourage the caregiver and the AD patient when possible to participate in such supportive activities. Indeed, a 'prescription for services' has been found to be effective in promoting utilization.[46,67,87]

The clinician can play a central role in modifying attitudes to accepting assistance by the care provider as well as beliefs held by our society. In addition, the clinician can lobby for the development of and easier access to services for the AD patient and the family.

CONCLUSION

Community-based formal support services can be categorized as society's collective caregiving for the frail elderly. We all contribute financially through our taxes which fund the programmes developed to care for them. Social policies are designed to apportion these services equitably to those in greatest need. It is therefore paramount that services be utilized, and utilized in the most effective way.

Clinicians must encourage their patients to become informed consumers. There are many benefits to services, yet the social cost is too great if they are not used. We recognize that the elderly prefer to retain their independence. Reliance on 'others' undermines that sense of independence. We, therefore, must stress the notion of 'interdependence' rather than 'independence'. The clinician needs to encourage the use of services at all stages of the caregiving process. In this way, the caregiver will become accustomed to and comfortable with sharing the caregiving role.

Realistically, not enough services are offered to meet all the needs of the caregiver and care receiver. Social policy must address the partnership between the formal and informal systems of care with the goal of enhancing quality of life and care while meeting the goals of fiscal responsibility and restraint.

While cost containment is a major concern for today's healthcare system, quality of life and quality of care need not be sacrificed for such a large number of vulnerable citizens. It is possible to be both cost-effective and provide good care. Savings, both monetary and human, can be achieved by timely interventions in avoidable crises. Investment in a partnership between the formal and informal system will pay great dividends in prevention of caregiver burnout, improved care to the AD patient and promotion and prolongation of family life.

REFERENCES

1. Doody RS, Stevens JC, Beck C, et al. Practice parameter: management of dementia (an evidence-based review). Report of the Quality Standards Subcommittee of the American Academy of Neurology. Neurology 2001; 56:1154–1166.

2. Torti FM, Gwyther LP, Shelby DR, et al. A multinational review of the recent trends and reports in dementia caregiver burden. Alzheimer Dis Assoc Disord 2004; 18:99–109.

3. Krothe JP. Giving voice to elderly people: community-based long-term care. Pub Health Nurs 1997; 14:217–226.

4. Shapiro E, Tate RB. The use and cost of community care services by elders with unimpaired cognitive functions with cognitive impairment/no dementia and with dementia. Can J Aging 1997; 16: 665–681.

5. Zarit SH, Pearlin LI. Family caregiving: integrating informal and formal systems for care. In: Zarit SH, Pearlin LI, Schaie KW, eds. Caregiving Systems: Formal and Informal Helpers. Hillsdale: Lawrence Erlbaum Associates 1993; 303–316.

6. Bolduc M, Bélanger L, Trahan L Home care for frail elderly persons: highlights of a Quebec evaluation program. Presented at the Third Annual Conference of The Canadian Home Care Association, Fredericton 1992.

7. Brodsky J, Habib J New developments and issues in home care policies Disabil Rehab 1997; 19:150–154.

8. Levin E. Care for the carers: the role of respite services. In: Wilcock G, ed. The Management of Alzheimer's Disease. Petersfield: Wrightson Biomedical Publishing 1993.

9. Lévesque L. Québec home-care services: a program at the local community level. In: Zarit SH, Pearlin LI, Schaie KW, eds. Caregiving Systems: Formal and Informal Helpers. Hillsdale: Lawrence Erlbaum Associates 1993; 217–232.

10. National Alliance for Caregiving and AARP (2004). Caregiving in the U.S. Accessed 18 September 2005 from http://www.caregiving.org/data/04finalreport.pdf.

11. Robinson KM. The family's role in long-term care. J Gerontol Nurs 1997; 23:7–11.

12. Doty P. Family care of the elderly: the role of public policy. Milbank Quart 1986; 64:34–75.

13. Canadian Study of Health and Aging. Patterns of caring for people with dementia in Canada. Can J Aging 1994; 13:470–487.

14. Levin E. Carers: problems, strains and services. In: Jacoby R, Oppenheim C, eds. Psychiatry in the Elderly. Oxford: Oxford University Press 1991.

15. National Alliance for Caregiving and Alzheimer's Association (2004). Families care: Alzheimer's caregiving in the United States. Accessed 18 September 2005 from http://www.caregiving.org/data/alzcaregivers04.pdf.

16. Abraham IL, Onega LL, Chalifoux ZL, Maes MJ. Care environments for patients with Alzheimer's Disease. Nurs Clin North Am 1994; 29:157–172.

17. Logan JR, Spitze G. Informal support and the use of formal services. J Gerontol 1994; 49: S25–S34.

18. Silverstein NM. Informing the elderly about public services: the relationship between sources of knowledge and service utilization. Gerontologist 1984; 24:37–40.

19. Lubben JE, Damron-Rodriguez J. An international approach to community health care for older adults. Fam Commun Health 2003; 26:338–349.

20. Delgado M, Tennstedt S. Making the case for culturally appropriate community services: Puerto Rican Elders and their caregivers. Health Social Work 1997; 22:246–255.

21. Eisdorfer C. Community resources and the management of dementia patients. Med Clin North Am 1994; 78: 869–875.

22. Gaugler JE, Kane RL, Kane RA, Newcomer R. Early community-based effects on institutionalization in dementia caregiving. Gerontologist 2005; 45:177–185.

23. McPherson BD. Aging as a Social Process. Toronto: Butterworths 1990.

24. Zarit SH, Pearlin LI, Schaie KW, eds. Caregiving Systems: Formal and Informal Helpers. Hillsdale: Lawrence Erlbaum 1993; 171–173.

25. Chappell N, Blandford A. Informal and formal care: exploring the complementarity. Ageing Soc 1991; 11: 299–317.

26. Dorfman LT, Holmes CA, Berlin KL. Service utilization by wife caregivers of frail older veterans. Social Work Health Care 1997; 26:33–52.

27. Caserta MS, Lund DA, Wright SC, Redburn DE. Caregivers to dementia patients: the utilization of community services. Gerontologist 1987; 27:209–214.

28. Cox C. Findings from a state wide program of respite care: a comparison of service users, stoppers and nonusers. Gerontologist 1997; 37:511–517.

29. Mittleman MS. Community caregiving. Alzheimer's Care Quart 2003; 4:273–285.

30. Zarit SH, Leitsch SA. Developing and evaluating community-based intervention programs for Alzheimer's patients and their caregivers. Ageing Ment Health 2001; 5:S84–S98.

31. Markle-Reid M, Browne G. Explaining the use and non-use of community-based long-term care services by caregivers of persons with dementia. J Eval Clin Pract 2001; 7:271–287.

32. Conlin MM, Caranasos GJ, Davidson RA. Reduction of caregiver stress by respite care: a pilot study. South Med J 1992; 85:1096–1100.

33. Gottlieb BH. Impact of Day Programs on Family Caregivers of Persons with Dementia. Guelph: University of Guelph 1995.

34. Scharlach A, Frenzl C. An evaluation of institution-based respite care. Gerontologist 1986; 26:77–82.

35. Winslow BW. Family caregiving and the use of formal community support services: a qualitative study. Issues Ment Health Nurs 1998; 19:11–27.

36. Litwack E. Helping the Elderly: The Complementary Roles of Informal Networks and Formal Systems. New York: The Guilford Press 1985.

37. Noelker LS, Bass DM. Home care for elderly persons: linkages between formal and informal caregivers. J Gerontol 1989; 44:S63–S70.

38. Stoller EP. Formal services and informal helping: the myth of service substitution. J Appl Gerontol 1989; 8:37–52.

39. Kane RA, Penrod JD. Family caregiving policies: insights from an intensive longitudinal study. In: Zarit SH, Pearlin LI, Schaie KW, eds. Caregiving Systems: Formal and Informal Helpers. Hillsdale: Lawrence Erlbaum Associates 1993 273–292.

40. Zarit SH, Gaugler JE, Jarrot SE. Useful services for families, research findings and directions. Int J Geriat Psychiatry 1999; 14:165–181.

41. Borrayo EA, Salmon JR, Polivka L, Dunlop BD. Utilization across the continuum of long-term care services. Gerontologist 2002; 42:603–612.

42. Mullan JT. Barriers to the use of formal services among Alzheimer's caregivers. In: Zarit SH, Pearlin LI, Schaie KW, eds. Caregiving Systems: Formal and Informal Helpers. Hillsdale: Lawrence Erlbaum Associates 1993 241–259.

43. Parris Stephens MA. Understanding barriers to caregivers' use of formal services: the caregiver's perspective. In: Zarit SH, Pearlin LI, Schaie KW, eds. Caregiving Systems: Formal and Informal Helpers. Hillsdale: Lawrence Erlbaum Associates 1993 261–272.

44. Collins C. 'I don't need help!' What do dementia caregivers really mean? Home Healthcare Nurse 1992; 10: 53–56.

45. McCabe BW, Sand BJ, Yeaworth RC, Nieveen JL. Availability and utilization of services. J Gerotol Nurs 1995; 21:14–22.

46. Beisecker AE, Wright LJ, Chrisman SK, Ashworth J. Family caregiver perceptions of benefits and barriers to the use of adult day care for individuals with Alzheimer's Disease. Res Aging 1995; 18: 430–450.

47. Rands G. Working people who also care for the elderly. Int J Geriatr Psychiatry 1997; 12: 39–44.

48. Coon DW, Williams MP, Moore RJ, et al. The Northern California chronic care network for dementia. J Am Geriatr Soc 2004; 52:150–156.

49. Fox P, Newcomer R, Yordi C, Arnsberger P. Lessons learned from the medicare Alzheimer disease demonstration. Alzheim Dis Assoc Disord 2000; 14:87–93.

50. Régie Régionale de la santé et des services sociaux de Montréal Centre. Continuum de services aux personnes âgées: le CLSC: guichet unique d'accès aux services de longue durée. Montréal: Direction de la programmatioon et de la coordination 1996.

51. Renwick D. Community care and social services. BMJ 1996; 5:171–172.

52. Mahoney DF, Tarlow BJ, Jones RN. Effects of an automated telephone support system on caregiver burden and anxiety: findings from the REACH for LTC intervention study. Gerontologist 2003; 43:556–567.

53. Brennan PF, Moore SM, Smyth KA. Alzheimer's disease caregivers users of a computer network. West J Nurs Res 1992; 14:662–673.

54. Ripich S, Moore SM, Brennan PF. A new nursing medium: computer networks for group intervention. J Psychosocial Nurs 1992; 30:15–20.

55. Czaja SJ, Rupert MP. Telecommunications technology as an aid to family caregivers of persons with dementia. Psychosom Med 2002; 64:469–476.

56. The National Institute on Aging and the National Library of Medicine. Making your web site senior friendly. Available at http://www.nlm.nih.gov/pubs.checklist.pdf. [accessed on 11 August 2005].

57. Rowe WS, Dulka IM, Pepler C, Yaffe MJ. Discharge Planning Organization and Outcomes for Short Stay and Same-Day Surgery Patients Aged 55 and Over: A Descriptive Exploratory Study. Montreal: McGill University and the Centre for Applied Family Studies, School of Social Work 1997.

58. Borrayo EV, Salmon JR, Polivka L. Dunlop BD. Who is being served? Program eligibility and home- and community-based services use. Appl Gerontol 2004; 23:120–140.

59. Gaylord S, Crotty N. Enhancing function with complementary therapies in geriatric rehabilitation. Topics Geriatr Rehabil 2002; 18:63–79.

60. Coleman, LM, Fowler LB, William ME. Use of unproven therapies by people with Alzheimer's disease. J Am Geriatr Soc 1995; 43:747–750 in Gaylord S & Crotty N. Enhancing function with complementary therapies in geriatric rehabilitation. Topics in Geriatr Rehabil 2002; 18: 63–79.

61. McBee L. Mindfulness practice with the frail elderly and their caregivers: changing the practitioner–patient relationship. Topics Geriatr Rehab 2003; 19:257–264.

62. Sanders S. Is the glass half empty or half full? Reflections on strain and gain in caregivers with Alzheimer's disease. Social Work Health Care 2005; 40:57–73.

63. Stuckey JC, Post SG, Ollerton S, et al. Alzheimer's disease, religion, and the ethics of respect for spirituality: a community dialogue. Alzheimer's Care Quart 2002; 3:199–207.

64. Lenshyn J. Reaching the living echo: maintaining and promoting the spiritual in persons living with Alzheimer's disease. Alzheimer's Care Quart 2005; 1:20–28.

65. Roff LE, Parker MW. Spirituality and Alzheimer's disease care. Alzheimer's Care Quart 2003; 4:267–270.

66. Biegel D, Bass D, Schulz R, Morycz R. Predictors of in-home and out-of-home service use by family caregivers of Alzheimer's disease patients. J Aging Health 1993; 5:419–438.

67. Wallace SP, Campbell K, Lew-Ting CY. Structural barriers to the use of formal in-home services by elderly Latinos. J Gerontol Social Sci 1994; 49: S253–S263.

68. Hamilton EM, Braun JW, Kerber P, et al. Factors associated with family caregivers' choice not to use services. Am J Alzheim Dis 1996; 11: 29–38.

69. Harrison J, Neufeld A. Women's experiences of barriers to support while caregiving. Health Care Women Int 1997; 18: 591–602.

70. McCallion P, Toseland RW, Gerber T, Banks S. Increasing the use of formal services by caregivers of people with dementia. Social Work 2004; 49:441–450.

71. Collins C, Stommel M, King S, Given CW. Assessment of the attitudes of family caregivers toward community services. Gerontologist 1991; 31:756–761.

72. Smyth KA, Milidonis MK. The relationship between normative beliefs about help seeking and the experience of caregiving in Alzheimer's disease. J Appl Gerontol 1999; 18: 222–238.

73. Jette AM, Tennstedt S, Crawford S. How does formal and informal community care affect nursing home use? J Gerontol Social Sci 1995; 50B:S4–S12.

74. Brotman SL, Yaffe MJ. Expressed Needs of Family Caregivers of Frail Elderly of Montreal. Montreal: Jewish Support Services for the Elderly 1993.

75. Lawton PM, Brody EM, Saperstein AR. Respite for Caregivers of Alzheimer Patients: Research and Practice. New York: Springer 1991.

76. Innes A. The social and political context of formal dementia care provision. Ageing Soc 2002; 22:483–499.

77. Hooyman NR, Kiyak HA. Social Gerontology: A Multidisciplinary Perspective. Allyn and Bacon: Boston 1996.

78. Young HM, McCormick WM, Vitaliano PP. Attitudes towards community-based services among Japanese American families. Gerontologist 42:814–825.

79. Hong GS, Hong SY. Health care of American Indian elderly: determinants of the perceived difficulty in obtaining access to health care. J Fam Econ Issues 1997; 18:33–47.

80. Kane MN, Houston-Vega MK. Maximizing content on elders with dementia while teaching multicultural diversity. J Social Work Educ 2004; 40:285–303.

81. Roberts JC, Connell CM, Cisewski D, et al. Differences between African Americans and Whites in their perceptions of Alzheimer disease. Alzheim Dis Assoc Disord 2003; 17: 19–26.

82. Moore WR. Lesbian and gay elders: connecting care providers through a telephone support group. J Gay Lesbian Social Serv 2002; 14:23–41.

83. Newcomer RJ, Fox PJ, Harrington CA. Health and long-term care for people with Alzheimer's disease and related dementias: policy research issues. Aging Ment Health 2001; 5:S124–S137.

84. Mittelman MS, Ferris SH, Shulman E, et al. A comprehensive support program: effect on depression in spouse-caregivers of AD patients. Gerontologist 1995; 35:792–802.

85. Paun O, Farran CJ, Perraud S, Loukissa DA. Successful caregiving of persons with Alzheimer's disease: skill development over time. Alzheimer's Care Quart 2004; 5:241–251.

86. Robinson K, Yates K. Effects of two caregiver-training programs on burden and attitude toward help. Arch Psychiatri Nurs 1994; 5:312–319.

87. Biegel DE, Song LY. Facilitators and barriers to caregiver support group participation. J Case Mgmt 1995; 4:164–172.

VI Ethical and quality of life issues

25

Ethical issues

Jason Karlawish

INTRODUCTION

The goal of this chapter is to assist clinicians in addressing common and often clinically significant ethical issues they encounter in the care of persons with Alzheimer's disease (AD). The general ethical framework to organize this chapter is derived from a set of principles of bioethics: respect for autonomy (granting a competent person freedom of choice), beneficence and non-maleficence (maximizing the good and minimizing harm) and justice (treating equal people equally).

Legitimate but different conceptions of each of these principles exist and some, especially respect for autonomy, are the subject of intense meta-ethical debate based on competing theories of what it means to be autonomous.[1] In addition, some ethical schools of thought may introduce other principles, such as respect for community, or place the principles in a distinct hierarchy, such as resolving dilemmas between autonomy and beneficence in favour of respect for autonomy. However, this chapter is not organized according to a hierarchy of principles and it admits a range of reasonable conceptions of these principles.

Among the many chronic diseases medicine addresses, AD presents particularly unique and challenging ethical issues. The contours of these issues are shaped by three features. The disease is chronic and progressively disabling. Persons with the disease progressively lose their capacity to make decisions and even to express preferences and values. Finally, the disease typically involves other people in care and decision-making. These people are commonly referred to as 'carers' or 'caregivers' and are typically close family members and in some cultures, despite a balance of the population's genders, they are disproportionately female.

These three features generate a set of ethical issues listed in Table 25.1 and organized according to the

Table 25.1 The common ethical issues encountered in the care of persons with AD

Stage	Ethical issues
Very early and early stages	Identifying the 'caregivers'
	Diagnostic disclosure
	Driving
	Advance planning
	Enrolling in research
Middle stage	Advance planning
	Driving
	Enrolling in research
Severe stage	Use of treatments to slow progression
	End of life care
	Enrolling in research

stages of AD in Table 25.2. The stage based organization is intended both to highlight how some issues are stage specific, such as driving and diagnostic disclosure, while others are relevant across the stages, such as enrolling in research, although the nature of the problems and their solutions may vary across the stages.

The staging schemata to organize these issues combines the organization of the Clinical Dementia Rating Scale[2] and the standard cutpoints on the Mini-Mental State Exam.[3] Onto these we have mapped the general pattern of how persons with AD make decisions. This pattern is derived from studies of the relationship between stages of AD and patient decision-making capacity and participation in decisions.[4]

The material in the column 'decision-making' describes two components of how persons make

Table 25.2 The stages of AD

Stage	Functional abilities	Overall cognitive abilities	Decision-making
Very early (CDR 0.5)	IADL independent and assistance BADL independent	MMSE > 23 Retains all or some insight into problems	Involvement of others: collaborative/shared independent Capacity: capable to marginally impaired
Early (CDR 0.5–1)	IADL assistance and dependence BADL independent though may need reminders	MMSE 19 to 23 Retains some insight into problems	Involvement of others: collaborative/shared Capacity: capable to impaired
Middle (CDR 1–2)	IADL dependence BADL assistance	MMSE 10 to 19 Retains some insight or lacks insight into problems	Involvement of others: collaborative/shared and proxy Capacity: impaired to incapable
Late (CDR 3–5)	IADL dependence BADL dependence	MMSE < 10 Lacks insight into problems	Involvement of others: proxy Capacity: incapable

decisions: 'involvement of others' and 'capacity'. 'Involvement of others' borrows from the way clinicians assess a person's ability to perform activities of daily living (ADL). It ranges along a spectrum from independent to entirely unable. Thus, as a person looses cognitive abilities, they progress from being independent in their decision-making to needing progressively more and more assistance. Of course, just as with ADL, people have a baseline of their 'normal function' that reflects their premorbid habits, preferences and abilities. Hence, just as a person who never performed financial or household tasks is 'dependent' in these ADL, so too a person can choose to delegate much of their decision-making to other people or work in a collaborative manner to perform this task. In fact, many elderly persons who have a spouse describe a process of 'interaction with other' that involves collaboration with their spouse.[5]

The second term used in that column is 'capacity'. This term refers to a person's decision-making abilities, that is, the abilities to understand, appreciate, reason and make a choice.[6] Chapter 26 provides a detailed treatment of these abilities. Impairments in these abilities fit a person with AD into three groups – capable, marginally capable and incapable. These categories have ethical consequences on how clinicians

negotiate the balance between respect for autonomy and beneficence and non-maleficence.

The decision-making categories described in Table 25.2 are not fixed. A person with mild-to-moderate AD will likely occupy different categories depending on the complexity of the decision, how persons charged with judging capacity exercise that judgment and social and environmental factors. For example, a person with mild AD is very likely capable of voting and making that decision on his own (though a person is free to ask for assistance).[7] In contrast, that same person may not be capable of making a decision about whether to take an AD treatment and instead rely on a close relative to decide for him.[8]

The remainder of this chapter discusses each of the issues with a focus on how clinicians can address them with attention to the range of choices and approaches.

IDENTIFYING THE 'CAREGIVER(S)'

What is a caregiver? Clinicians who fail to identify this person and develop techniques to work with them face a number of potentially significant consequences for the health and well-being of their patients with AD. These include inaccurate diagnosis and staging and incomplete data to guide clinical decision-making. However, prior to labelling a person 'the caregiver' a clinician needs to understand what a 'caregiver' is.

Many persons with chronic illnesses such as emphysema and congestive heart failure develop a relationship with another person who assists them in their day-to-day ADL and thus, because they provide care, could be called a caregiver. But AD is unique among most other common and chronic diseases of adults in how it determines what the caregiver does. Caregivers have at least four roles.

The first role is that of knowledgeable informant. A critical element of the information a clinician needs in order to diagnose the cause of late-life cognitive changes is history from a collateral source. This history allows the clinician better to estimate the true nature and extent of cognitive impairments and whether they impact on the person's day-to-day function. Such data are essential to reach a diagnosis of dementia as defined by impairments in two or more cognitive domains that interfere with the ability to perform usual and everyday activities. History gained only from the person with cognitive complaints and impairment may reveal some of these problems, but the consistent tendency of persons to minimize the presence or severity of ADL impairments necessitates the role of a knowledgeable informant.[9]

A second role of a caregiver is providing assistance with ADL. By the mild stage of AD a person develops impairments in his abilities to perform instrumental ADL. While he may still do these tasks, he does not perform them as well and, as a result, someone else needs to supervise, assist or even do the task for the person.

A third role that a caregiver has is a result of the impact of the cognitive impairments on the patient's decision-making abilities. This is the role of decision-maker. Every decision involves the need to understand some body of facts, such as a medicine's risks and benefits, weigh the relative benefits and downsides of the various options, apply the facts to a person's daily life and make a choice. Deficits in short-term memory and executive function impair a person's ability to exercise these abilities independently.[10] Someone else either has to assist the person in thinking through the information or make the decision for them. In general, among persons with mild stage AD, they usually have a collaborative role with their decision-maker wherein they make decisions together and in the moderate stage of AD this transitions to a decision-maker or caregiver-dominated role, wherein that person makes the decision but checks with the person with AD.[4]

Collectively, these three roles often lead to a fourth role – that of patient. A person in a 'caregiving role' –

that is a person serving as knowledgeable informant, task doer and decision-maker – frequently reports psychiatric morbidity of depression and anxiety which can in turn lead to poor physical health.

The need for a caregiver for a person with AD is evident. Clinicians bear a beneficence based responsibility to their patient to identify a person who will serve as a knowledgeable informant, decision-maker and provide assistance with ADL. However, there may be more than one person who serves in these roles (hence the title of this section refers to 'caregiver(s)'). For example, a patient may choose to rely on his daughter to assist him with day-to-day tasks but then turn to this daughter and his son to make decisions. A clinician who fails to recognize this kind of diversity in caregivers will hazard effective communication and collaboration with the patient and their relevant caregivers.

Clinicians also have a beneficence based obligation to recognize that the caregiver may also need medical care. Short screens for burden and depression can serve as a useful way to identify these problems and then refer the person to the appropriate resources that address common causes of burden.[11]

Finally, clinicians need to recognize that the term 'caregiver' is imprecise for at least two reasons. It denotes only one of the roles that the 'caregiver' serves, and it may not be the term that the person considered a caregiver calls him- or herself. Limited data exist to describe this second reason and the kinds of persons who reject the title, but this author's clinical experience is that some family members reject the term while others wholeheartedly embrace it. Preliminary evidence from the author's lab suggests that while a term exists in Spanish for a 'caregiver' – called 'cuidadoro' – Latinos of Puerto Rican heritage do not typically use it.

DIAGNOSTIC DISCLOSURE

Diagnostic disclosure captures a classic tension between a clinician's beneficence and non-maleficence based obligations to maximize a patient's good and minimize harms, and the clinician's commitment to respect a patient's autonomous choice, which in turn requires having adequate and relevant information, such as the diagnosis and prognosis of their dementing illness. The classic case that frames this tension is the dedicated family carer who requests that the clinician should not tell the patient he or she has AD.

The common argument in support of non-disclosure is that disclosure is not in the patient's best interests. The disease is progressive and ultimately fatal. There are no treatments that slow or halt the progression. Hence, knowing one has AD will harm the person. In particular, clinicians should withhold diagnostic information, especially from patients who are depressed or prone to depression. In a phrase, ignorance is bliss.

The common argument in support of disclosure is that a clinician who chooses not to disclose a diagnosis denies the patient information that is vital to making decisions about his or her future care and plans. In addition, it leads to deception and even lying. In short, this behaviour undermines trust and honest communication between the clinician and patient which are the very foundation of human relations. There are three considerations a clinician can use to work through these two sides.

The clinician's first consideration is to identify the concerns of the person who is requesting no diagnostic disclosure. In general, a carer worries that disclosure will either worsen or precipitate patient depression or that the patient is in denial and the carer wishes to respect this denial. In response to these concerns, the clinician should learn how the carer understands their relative's mood and insight and how this understanding corresponds to the patient's actual mood and insight. The issue here is that signs and symptoms of what the carer thinks is depression may actually represent apathy, and the perceived signs or symptoms of denial may actually represent a lack of insight into the presence of cognitive and functional disorders.

How do apathy, insight and depression differ? Core features of apathy are blunted emotional response, indifference, low social engagement, diminished initiation and poor persistence.[12] These same symptoms can appear as depression, though a patient who has apathy can be entirely free of self-reported depressive symptoms. Core features of insight are awareness of problems with memory, doing tasks and concentration. These same symptoms can also appear as depression and in fact one of the strongest correlates of cognitive complaints is not performance on measures of cognition but self-reported depressive symptoms.[13] Thus, to distinguish a patient with depression from one with insight a clinician should assess for the presence of the core symptoms of depression that focus on mood: dysphoria, suicidal ideation, self-criticism, guilt, pessimism and hopelessness. For example, a patient with insight who is not depressed may very well report 'positive' responses to the two items on the 15-item geriatric depression scale that ask about 'problems with memory' and 'dropped usual activities', but otherwise deny other symptoms of depression such as not feeling satisfied with their life and feeling like something bad is going to happen to them.[14]

Insight is a multi-attribute and dimensional construct. It refers to a person's awareness of at least four attributes: cognitive problems, functional losses, diagnosis and prognosis, two of which – cognitive problems and functional losses – are dimensional. A patient may recognize some but not all of their cognitive problems and functional losses. Several studies of insight in persons with AD among persons with mild-to-moderate disease show there is a wide spectrum of awareness of the presence of problems with memory and thinking and how they impact on the person's day-to-day function. For example, Marzanski reported that nearly half (14/30) of patients with dementia were able to give a correct diagnosis or adequately describe their main symptoms,[15] and Karlawish and colleagues reported similar results with 34 per cent aware that they had memory problems that would get worse and 53 per cent that they had AD or dementia.[8]

A clinician has a clear obligation to educate the patient's family about the results of assessments of mood, apathy and insight. These data guide assessment of the value and risks of diagnostic disclosure. A patient with insight arguably knows what is going on and deserves the virtue of kind, hopeful but honest disclosure of the problem that explains their symptoms. To deny that patient this information disrespects the legitimacy of his or her suffering.

A useful clinical strategy to assess insight and a patient's desire to know their diagnosis is to assess the degree that the patient experiences symptoms: '*Do you have any problems with your memory or thinking?*' Probes may be necessary, such as whether the person has problems remembering a list of grocery items or the date, or trouble following a TV show or movie. Alternatively, ask the patient how she or he did on the cognitive testing: '*Do you think you did as well as you would have ten years ago?*'

In the case of a patient who endorses cognitive problems, the next step is to ask whether he or she wants to know the cause of those problems. If the patient answers that he does not want to know the cause, explore why. It is possible that the person has a strong view about not wanting to know certain kinds of medical information and thus a clinician may well have an obligation to respect this preference. In the case of a patient who does want to know the cause of their cognitive and functional problems, a useful follow-up question is the following: '*There any many different kinds of conditions and diseases that can cause memory and thinking problems, one of them is Alzheimer's disease. Do you want to know if you have Alzheimers disease?*' This question is another opportunity for the patient to express his preference about whether he wants to know the diagnosis.

In contrast, a patient with marked loss of insight may simply not understand or appreciate a diagnostic disclosure. Such a person simply lacks the cognitive capacity to appreciate their problem. A patient with clinically significant depression requires a clear plan to address their mood disorder. Such patients need a plan for disclosure that sensibly integrates a treatment plan for depression that includes both drug therapy and counselling.

A second consideration in addressing requests to withhold the diagnosis from the patient is to teach the family about the potential harms of non-disclosure. A well-functioning caregiver–patient dyad requires recognizing the caregiving roles and the value of intimacy between patient and caregiver. Failure to disclose the diagnosis can lead to an emotional distancing. Hence, diagnostic disclosure may actually be in the patient's *and* the caregiver's best interests.

A third consideration in the decision whether to disclose a diagnosis of AD is the claim of what is the point of disclosure because nothing can be done. In fact, a lot can be done. First, long before biomedicine took an interest in dementia as a disease, people still lived with it. Disclosure is a first step to making meaning out of the experience of an illness. Patients have kept diaries[16,17] and can participate in support groups.[18] Insight can last far into the disease. The writer Jonathan Kozol records how his father, a neurologist who diagnosed himself with AD, even at a stage when he lived in a nursing home would struggle to explain how he had selective confusion because certain neurons had degenerated.[19] Second, there is a clear need to recognize the value of non-pharmacological interventions that begin with recognizing and naming a problem. Education and skill training can improve both patient and caregiver quality of life[20] and provide an opportunity for the patient to plan future care and complete unfinished tasks.

ADVANCE PLANNING

Advance care planning describes a patient expressing how other people should manage future medical problems when the patient is no longer able to make decisions about his or her care. A patient can document these plans as witnessed legal documents. Such a document is called a living will. It describes the kinds of treatments the person would or would not want to receive. A durable power of attorney for health care describes the person who should serve as surrogate and speak on behalf of the patient. Alternatively, a patient can choose not to execute these legal documents but instead have informal guides for

care that are kept in a chart note or remembered conversation.

In general, the process of advance care planning benefits patients: decreasing depression, enhancing a sense of being in control and settling treatment preferences.[21] It may be particularly useful in the case of patients who are at risk of problems with surrogate decision-making. Specifically, the patient may be estranged from their spouse, though not divorced, and living with a partner. Or the patient may not have a partner but several children who are not in close contact with each other. There are, of course, multiple permutations upon these kinds of family situations. The general point is that they present the risk that there may be disagreements among people over who has the authority to speak on behalf of the person and what is the proper way to care for them. A useful strategy to avoid such a situation is to ask a patient *'Suppose your Alzheimer's disease gets worse so that you can't talk with me the way you are right now and instead I have to talk with someone else about how to take care of you. Who should I talk to? Who do you trust? Is there anyone in the family I should not talk to?'* However, as potentially valuable as advance care planning is, clinicians need to address three limitations to assure that advance care plans create an understanding and appreciation of the patient's future, and identify values that should help to shape that future.

The first limitation is the nature of the specificity of the directive. Living wills may seem to assure the strictest adherence to a patient's self-determination, for example, *'I do not want a feeding tube'*. However, a directive applies to specific conditions, the most common of which is the condition of a terminal illness. In other words, the directive to withhold an enteral feeding tube would only apply in the event the person is not competent and also in a terminal state. Such conditions limit the scope of the directive. And yet, the future health states that typically motivate people to make a living will are cases of a persistent vegetative state or severe dementia, both of which do not clearly describe a person who is terminal and may in fact live for at least a year or more. A clinician can address this limitation by fostering advance care planning conversations that focus on the patient's goals, values and personal concepts of best interests, and are amended to include conditions such as persistent vegetative state or severe dementia.

A second limitation of advance directives is that many people do not see them as a means to determine precisely the course of future events. Specifically, people may not want to make specific plans for their future care in the same manner that they use a will to instruct people to manage their property. Instead, people may use an advance directive to entrust others to act in their best interests.[22] Whereas a will for property typically states instructions such as 'My sister gets the car and my son gets the boat', a person may not want their living will to have the same degree of specificity. Instead of stating the decision specific 'In the event I have severe stage dementia, I do not want an enteral feeding tube', their directive would state 'In the event I have severe stage dementia, I leave it to my trusted husband to decide whether I should have an enteral feeding tube'. The clinician or whoever is helping the person complete their advance care plan then needs to ask the person what kinds of factors the trusted husband should or should not think about.

To guide this discussion of factors, a clinician should assess how much freedom or leeway a person would grant their trusted proxy over their advance care preferences and if they would grant them freedom, what factors should guide it. For example, a patient may say 'If I reach the point where I cannot recognize my family, then I don't want to be kept alive. If I get pneumonia or something, let me go. Period'. A useful probe to this statement is how much leeway or freedom the patient would give to their proxy over this decision to do the opposite. For example, this same patient may say 'Well, if I'm happy and laughing and enjoying life, it's worth taking some chances, but that's really the key – how much I am enjoying life'. This example illustrates how the person modified their initial strong preference against treatment under certain clinical circumstances to include factors that their proxy should take into consideration.

A third limitation is that a dementia patient's impairments in abstract reasoning, planning and insight may hinder their decision-making abilities to the degree that they lack the capacity to execute an advance directive.[23] A useful strategy for the clinician is to present a patient with a description of a person in the profound stage of dementia and ask the patient 'Suppose that you were in this condition. How would you want to be cared for?'.[24] The patient's answer is then a starting point both to assess their ability to make decisions about their future care and for a discussion about their goals and values of care.

USE OF TREATMENTS TO SLOW PROGRESSION

The standard model of ethics largely situates decisions about treatment as a matter of informed consent. In the case of an AD slowing treatment, a physician would disclose the treatment options and their risks and benefits. A competent patient makes a choice based on, among other considerations, his perception of his quality of life. In the care of a patient who is not competent, their proxy should make a substituted judgment, that is, they should choose as the person would have chosen if they were capable.[25] In the event the carer cannot make a substituted judgment, they should decide based on what is in the patient's best interests. This judgment will rely on how the carer perceives that patient's quality of life. This makes sense, as a maxim in the care of any progressive and incurable illness is that quality of life needs to be a focus of care.

This model likely does not reflect how decisions about an AD treatment are in fact made. In general, patients and family members describe a collaborative model of decision-making. In this process, female carers are more likely to report that the patient has the final say over whether to take a treatment.[26] In the event the carer does make the decision, his choice whether to use a treatment is largely determined by the carer's perception of the patient's quality of life.[27] Quality of life is especially important in the case of choosing whether to use a treatment that presents risk to the patient. As important as quality of life is in the care of persons with AD, clinicians need to recognize sharp differences may exist between carer and patient perspectives on the patient's quality of life.[28]

Chapter 28 addresses quality of life in greater detail. The ethical issues at stake are as follows. Patients typically rate their quality of life better than their carers rate the patients' quality of life. This applies to studies that examine satisfaction as well as measures of ADL. In the assessment of ADL, the carer's perspective is typically regarded as 'correct'. Thus, they complete assessments of function in clinical trials. But in the case of measures of satisfaction or preference, a useful strategy recognizes the value of the patient's perspective. The clinician should elicit both the caregiver's and patient's assessments.

A useful question to inaugurate a discussion of quality of life is a global rating: 'How would you rate your overall quality of life? Would you say poor, fair, good, very good or excellent?'. The advantage of a global rating is that it allows a person to integrate whatever factors they choose into this assessment. Whereas one person may value the pleasure for activities, another may value their relationships with family. In either case, a global rating allows the person to incorporate what matters to him. A clinically useful finding is that among patients who answer that their overall quality of life is less than 'good' generally often report significant depressive symptoms.[29,30] This suggests that self-reported mood is a common filter for the variety of experiences that constitute a person's quality of life. Thus, clinical interventions to improve patient quality of life ought to target patient mood. Caregivers who answer that the patient's quality of life is less than 'good' may be experiencing significant distress, depression or simply perceiving the severity of the patient's functional losses.[31] Hence, a treatment plan may need to focus on the caregiver's mood and skills in caregiving. In summary, decisions about whether to use AD treatments need to focus on the quality of *lives* – the patient's and the caregiver's.

END-OF-LIFE CARE

As dementia progresses into moderate and severe stages, the physician should discuss the options for palliative care. The term describes 'the management of patients with active, progressive, far-advanced disease for whom prognosis is limited and the focus of care is the quality of life'.[32] In the setting of full palliative care, treatments that slow the dementia are typically withdrawn. The focus is on the relief of symptoms.

Two of the most vexing issues in discussion of palliative care are effectively communicating prognosis and having a means for families to begin to plan for how the person will die with AD.[33] A useful clinical heuristic to decide whether a patient is terminal is to ask yourself the question *'Would you be surprised if you received a call that your patient had died or suffered a terminal event?'*. If the clinician's answer to this question is 'no', that suggests that patient is very well near or in the terminal stages of their illness. A useful means then to convey this to the family together with a prompt to make plans for end-of-life care is the following: *'I don't know precisely when your relative is going to die but I do know that I will not be surprised when this happens. Recognizing this, I think we need to begin to plan on how we can take care of him in a way that lets you look back after he's gone and say he was treated with dignity and quality of life'.*

Among the most difficult symptoms are dysphagia and aspiration pneumonia as a result of progressive loss of the ability to chew and swallow. A usual approach has been to recommend a percutaneous enterogastrostomy tube, a so-called PEG tube. The logic of this intervention is that bypassing the usual oropharyngeal route of eating will limit aspiration episodes. However, the practice developed largely without clear evidence that it benefits clinical outcomes. Specifically, the available data do not support that PEG tubes extend life, reduce episodes of aspiration or improve nutritional parameters.[34] Moreover, survival after placement is poor, suggesting that aspi-

ration marks a terminal event.[35] Finally, maintaining a PEG tube includes risks and indignities such as restraining the patient, stool production that can lead to skin breakdown and a loss of the intimacy from oral feeding. A reasonable approach to the management of neurogenic dysphagia is to offer a clear plan for careful oral feeding, and candidly discuss how this is a common event in the terminal phase of dementia. In cases where the family strongly wishes to use enteral feeding, a clinician should propose clear endpoints in order to reassess its efficacy.

DRIVING

The ability to drive is an expression of liberty and independence. It provides a sense of self-esteem and control of one's everyday life. Driving cessation often leads to decreased quality of life, loss of control, increased loneliness and isolation, and depression.[36] But the law recognizes driving as a privilege and not a right. In many states, physicians have a duty to protect their patient's lives and also maintain public safety. A physician must balance the autonomy and quality of life of their patient with the safety of their patient and society.

Drivers with moderate-to-severe stages of AD pose a significant safety problem.[37] They clearly should not drive. But a proportion of drivers with very-mild-to-mild dementia display driving impairment comparable to that tolerated in other segments of the driving population.[38–40] Hence, a clinician cannot infer automatically from a diagnosis of dementia in persons at this stage that a patient cannot drive.[40–44] For these kinds of patients, a recommendation to limit or cease driving should be based on relevant criteria such as tests of functional competency.

A useful strategy will focus on assessing the patient's capacity to drive. A useful question to families is *'Would you allow your relative to drive your children (or grandchildren)?'*. A negative answer to this strongly supports the need for a driving skills assessment or even simply disabling the car. Occupational therapists can perform formal driving screens that include tests of perception, cognition, reaction time and on-the-road evaluation.[42,45,46] Sometimes a patient or family will resist a driving evaluation because they report it is too expensive. A useful strategy to address this is to ask if they would pay the same amount of money to repair the car. The implication here is that if a person is willing to pay that much to repair the car, then they should similarly be willing to pay that much to assure the driver can properly operate it.

Clinicians should recognize that some states expect them to serve a public health role as well. Many states have laws requiring physicians to report patients with certain medical conditions that can impair driving ability to the Department of Transportation.[45] For example, California requires physicians to report all cases of dementia to the motor vehicle licensing administration.[47]

ENROLLING IN RESEARCH

Ethical dilemmas in clinical care typically centre on competing claims of what will benefit a patient. But research raises a unique set of dilemmas. Unlike clinical care, research is an activity that is designed to generate generalizable knowledge, not to benefit the patient. Research exposes patients to risks that are justified by the pursuit of benefit to others. Hence, it creates a dilemma between the good of the patient and the good of society.[48] This dilemma is especially vexing when the patients cannot themselves volunteer. On what grounds can another person enrol someone in an activity that benefits others, but not the person?

The general model of policies and guidelines is that it is permissible to expose a non-competent subject to research risks provided (1) the research presents a reasonable prospect of benefit to the subjects or (2) the research is not potentially beneficial but its risks are either minimal or the research promises to yield vitally important knowledge to the class of subjects under study and the subject has indicated in advance a willingness to participate in this kind of research.[49–51] In all of these cases, there is general consensus that the subject should be able to assent to enrol. Unlike consent, assent describes a lesser standard of understanding.

This model – with the exception of advance consent – is largely based on the United States regulations for research that involves children.[52] While federal research regulations only carry authority at United States institutions that accept federal monies, they are widely regarded as an ethical framework. The core of this model is the idea that research risks can be balanced against two kinds of benefits: the potential benefits to the subjects, if any, and the importance of the knowledge that can reasonably be expected to result.[52] This model is a useful starting point for investigators and institutional review boards, but two issues need further detail.

First, some patients with dementia are competent to consent to enrol in research. Studies that measure the decision-making abilities of patients with dementia with Mini-mental State Exam scores of at least 19 show that a portion of patients do have adequate abilities to be competent to provide an informed consent.[53,54]

Second, as important as the term 'minimal risk' is, it has two ambiguities. The term is defined as 'the probability and magnitude of physical or psychological harm or discomfort anticipated in the research are not greater in and of themselves than those ordinarily encountered in daily life, or during the performance of routine physical or psychological examinations or tests'.[52] While this definition details the breadth of what risks should be assessed, it lacks a subject to compare these risks to.[55] A second ambiguity is how to assess minimal risk.[56] Specifically, does minimal risk cover all of the risks encountered in a research project, or only the research risks that are not balanced by potential benefits? The following case works through a solution to these ambiguities. A 12-month-long trial will randomize subjects to one of two potential treatments for Alzheimer's disease: drug A is standard of care, drug B is a new drug – evidence suggests that it may be superior to A. A clinical trial is needed to prove this. Subjects receive periodical physical exams, cognitive testing and blood tests.

At first glance, this clinical trial seems greater than minimal risk. The subjects will receive a host of tests for one and a half years. They receive drugs that have risks. But if legitimate uncertainty exists whether B is better than A, the potential risks of each intervention are balanced by the potential benefits. The issue in assessing whether a study presents research risks that are minimal is the nature of the risks that are not balanced by potential benefits to the subjects. For example, if this clinical trial included more blood tests than are routinely part of treatment with standard of care drug A and with drug B, the risks of the additional blood tests are research risks. Another example is if the trial includes additional cognitive testing over and above that done by expert clinicians. The risks of those additional tests are research risks.

The general issue then is how the risks of research procedures whose purpose is to generate generalizable knowledge compare to the risks routinely encountered in clinical care of the patients eligible for the trial. Most reasonable people would agree that a blood draw and cognitive testing are among routine tests encountered in the care of persons with dementia. Hence, it is reasonable to conclude that the study presents minimal risks from the procedures that are done solely to generate generalizable knowledge.

In summary, the assessment of research risks relies on a two step process: (1) demarcate the risks of procedures that are done solely as part of research interventions to produce generalizable knowledge from the risks of procedures that are part of therapeutic interventions, and (2) compare research risks that are done solely as part of research interventions to produce generalizable knowledge to the risks the patients encounter in their everyday lives. If those research risks have a reasonable equivalence to daily life, the protocol likely presents minimal risk and can enrol subjects with proxy informed consent. In the event those risks are greater than minimal, proxy consent may not be appropriate.

CONCLUSION

Ethics is about choice. It is all very well for each actor to have a coherent concept of the principles of ethics and principles to balance among them. These principles will assure that choices do not offend core values and they are not irrational or even deranged. But fundamental to making a good choice is that the actors who face the decision communicate effectively. Hence, clinicians need to have standard approaches to think through and communicate about the common ethical issues encountered in the care of persons with AD. This is all the more important in AD because the patient with AD may not be capable of communicating. The clinician needs to have skills in assessing whether this is in fact true and, if it is, in how to effectively work with proxies to make decisions on behalf of the person with AD. This chapter has emphasized how standard lines akin to the way a clinician assesses a chief complaint of memory loss can be useful to assure that communication is effective and coherent.

REFERENCES

1. Beauchamp TL, Childress JF. The Concept of Autonomy. In: Beauchamp TL, Childress JF. Principles of Biomedical Ethics. New York, Oxford: Oxford University Press 1994:120–128.
2. Berg L. Clinical dementia rating (CDR). Psychopharmacol Bull. 1988; 24:637–639.
3. Folstein M, Folstein S, McHugh P. Mini-mental state: a practical method for grading the cognitive state of patients for the clinician. J Psych Res 1975; 12:189–198.
4. Hirschman KB, Xie SX, Feudtner C, Karlawish JHT. How does an Alzheimer's disease patient's role in medical decision-making change over time? J Geriatr Psych Neurol 2004; 75:55–60.
5. Padula C. Older couples' decision making on health issues. West J Nurs Res 1996; 18:675–687.
6. Grisso T, Appelbaum PS. Abilities Related to Competence. In: Grisso T, Appelbaum PS. Assessing Competence To Consent To Treatment. A guide for physicians and other health professionals. New York: Oxford University Press 1998:31–60.
7. Appelbaum PS, Bonnie RJ, Karlawish JHT. The capacity to vote of persons with Alzheimers disease. Am J Psychiatry 2005; 162:2094–2100.
8. Karlawish JHT, Casarett DJ, James BD, Xie SX, Kim SYK. The ability of persons with Alzheimers disease to make a decision about taking an AD treatment. Neurology 2005; 64:1514–1519.
9. Kiyak HA, Teri L, Borson S. Physical and functional health assessment in normal aging and in Alzheimer's disease: self-reports vs family reports. Gerontologist 1994; 34:324–330.
10. Marson D, Harrell L. Executive dysfunction and loss of capacity to consent to medical treatment in patients with Alzheimer's disease. Semin Clin Neuropsych 1999; 4:41–49.
11. Hirschman KB, Shea J, Xie SX, Karlawish JH. The development of a rapid screen for caregiver burden. J Am Geriatr Soc 2004; 52:1724–1729.
12. Landes AM, Sperry SD, Strauss ME. Apathy in Alzheimer's disease. J Am Geriatr Soc 2001; 49:1700–1707.
13. Bassett SS, Folstein MF. Memory complaint, memory performance, and psychiatric diagnosis: a community study. J Geriatr Psych Neurol 1993; 6:105–111.
14. Yesavage JA, Brink TL, Rose TL, et al. Development and validation of a geriatric depression screening scale: a preliminary report. J Psych Res 1983; 17:37–49.
15. Marzanski M. Would you like to know what is wrong with you? On telling the truth to patients with dementia. J Med Ethics 2000; 26:108–113.
16. McGowin DF. Living the Labyrinth: A Personal Journey through the Maze of Alzheimer's. New York: Dell Publishing 1993.
17. Thomas H, Thomas N. How can my mind go AWOL? Lancet 2001; 358:S2.
18. Snyder L, Quayhagen MP, Shepard S, Bower D. Supportive seminar groups: an intervention for early stage dementia patients. Gerontologist 1995; 35:691–695.
19. Kozol J. Losing my father one day at a time. The New York Times 2000 Aug 22; A21.
20. Mittelman M, Ferris S, Shulman E, Steinberg G, Levin B. A family intervention to delay nursing home placement of patients with Alzheimer's disease: a randomized controlled trial. JAMA 1996; 276:1725–1731.
21. Miles SH, Koepp R, Weber EP. Advance end-of-life treatment planning: a research review. Arch Intern Med 1996; 156:1062–1068.
22. Sehgal A, Galbraith A, Chesney M, et al. How strictly do dialysis patients want their advance directive followed? JAMA 1992; 267:59–63.
23. Fazel S, Hope T, Jacoby R. Dementia, intelligence, and the competence to complete advance directives [research letter]. Lancet 1999; 354:48.
24. Fazel S, Hope T, Jacoby R. Assessment of competence to complete advance directives: validation of a patient centred approach. BMJ 1999; 318:493–497.
25. Beauchamp TL, Childress JF. A framework of standards for surrogate decisionmaking. In: Beauchamp TL, Childress JF. Principles of Biomedical Ethics. New York, Oxford: Oxford University Press 1994:170–181.
26. Hirschman KB, Joyce CM, James B, et al. Would caregivers of Alzheimer's disease (AD) patients involve their relative in a decision to use an AD slowing medication? Am J Geriatr Psychiatry 2005; 13:1014–1021.
27. Karlawish JH, Casarett DJ, James BD, et al. Why would caregivers not want to treat their relative's Alzheimer's disease? J Am Geriatr Soc 2003; 51:1391–1397.

28. Logsdon RG, Gibbons LE, McCurry SM, Teri L. Quality of life in Alzheimer's Disease: patient and caregiver reports. J Ment Health Aging 1999; 5:21–32.

29. James BD, Xie SX, Karlawish JH. How do patients with Alzheimer disease rate their overall quality of life? Am J Geriatr Psychiatry 2005; 13:484–490.

30. Logsdon RG, Albert SM. Assessing quality of life in Alzheimer's disease: conceptual and methodological issues. J Men Health Aging 1999; 5:3–6.

31. Karlawish JHT, Casarett D, Klocinski J, Clark CM. The relationship between caregivers' global ratings of Alzheimers disease patients' quality of life, disease severity and the caregiving experience. J Am Geriatr Soc 2001; 49: 1066–1070.

32. Doyle D, Hanks GWC, MacDonald N. Oxford Textbook of Palliative Medicine, 2nd edn. New York: Oxford University Press 1998.

33. Karlawish JHT, Quill T, Meier DE. A consensus-based approach to providing palliative care for patients who lack decision-making capacity. Ann Intern Med 1999; 130: 835–840.

34. Finucane TE, Christmas C, Travis K. Tube feeding in patients with advanced dementia. A review of the evidence. JAMA 1999; 282:1365–1370.

35. Grant M, Rudberg M, Brody J. Gastrostomy placement and mortality among hospitalized Medicare beneficiaries. JAMA 1998; 279:1973–1976.

36. Marattoli RA, Meandes de Leon CF, Glass TA, et al. Driving cessation and increased depressive symptoms: prospective evidence from the New Haven EPESE. J Am Geriatr Soc 1997; 45:202–206.

37. Lucas-Blaustein MJ, Filipp L, Dungan C, Tune L. Driving in patients with dementia. J Am Geriatr Soc 1988; 36: 1087–1091.

38. Dubinsky RM, Stein AC, Lyons K. Practice parameter: risk of driving and Alzheimer's disease (an evidence-based review). Neurology 2000; 54:2205–2211.

39. Hunt L, Morris JC, Edwards D, Wilson BS. Driving performance in persons with mild senile dementia of the Alzheimer type. J Am Geriatr Soc 1993; 41:747–753.

40. Drachman DA, Swearer JM. Driving and Alzheimer's disease: the risk of crashes. Neurology 1993; 43:2448–2456.

41. Donnelly RE, Karlinsky H. The impact of Alzheimer's disease on driving ability: a review. J Geriatr Psych Neurol 1990; 3:1990.

42. Odenheimer GL. Dementia and the older driver. Clin Geriatr Med 1993; 9:349–364.

43. Trobe JD, Waller PF, Cook-Flannagan CA, Teshima SM, Bieliauskas LA. Crashes and violations among drivers with Alzheimer disease. Arch Neurol 1996; 53:411–416.

44. Fitten LJ, Perryman KM, Wilkinson CJ, et al. Alzheimer and vascular dementias and driving. JAMA 1995; 273: 1360–1365.

45. Pasupathy S, Lavizzo-Mourey R. The older driver. In: Forciea MA, Lavizzo-Mourey R, Schwab EP, eds. Geriatric Secrets, 2nd edn. Philadelphia: Hanley and Belfus 2000: 115–120.

46. Carr D, Schmader K, Bergman C, et al. A multidisciplinary approach in the evaluation of demented drivers referred to geriatric assessment centers. J Am Geriatr Soc 1991; 39: 1132–1136.

47. California Health And Safety Code 103900. Available at http://www.aroundthecapitol.com/code/code.html?sec=hsc &codesection=103900, 2000 [accessed 10 April, 2006].

48. Jonas H. Philosophical reflections on experimenting with human subjects. In: Freund PA, ed. Experimentation with Human Subjects. New York: George Braziller, 1969:1–31.

49. National Bioethics Advisory Commission. Research involving Persons with Mental Disorders that may affect their Decisionmaking Capacity. Vol I: Report and Recommendations. Rockville, MD: US Government Printing Office 1998.

50. New York State Advisory Work Group on Human Subjects Research Involving the Protected Classes. Recommendations on the Oversight of Human Subject Research Involving the Protected Classes. Albany, NY: State of New York Department of Health 1998.

51. Attorney General's Working Group. Office of the Maryland Attorney General. Third report of the attorney general's research working group. Consent to research – Protection of Decisionally Incapacitated Individuals. Baltimore, 1998.

52. Department of Health and Human Services. Common Rule, 45 CFR 46. Federal policy for the protection of human subjects; Notices and rules. Fed Reg 1991; 56:28003–28032.

53. Kim SYH, Caine ED, Currier GW, Leibovici A, Ryan JM. Assessing the competence of persons with Alzheimer's disease in providing informed consent for participation in research. Am J Psychiatry 2001; 158:710–717.

54. Karlawish JHT, Casarett DJ, James BD. Alzheimers disease patients' and caregivers' capacity, competency and reasons to enroll in an early phase Alzheimers disease clinical trial. J Am Geriatr Soc 2002; 50:2019–2024.

55. Karlawish JHT, Hall JB. The controversy over emergency research: a review of the issues and suggestions for a resolution. Am J Respir Crit Care Med 1996; 153:499–506.

56. Weijer C. The ethical analysis of risk. J Law Med Ethics 2000; 28:344–361.

26

Competency

Daniel C Marson and Laura E Dreer

INTRODUCTION

Impairments of decisional capacities and higher order functions are inevitable consequences of Alzheimer's disease (AD) and related disorders.[1,2] As persons with AD experience progressive declines in memory, judgment, reasoning, communication and attention over the course of the disease process, such cognitive changes affect abilities to participate in and perform various higher order capacities (competencies) associated with everyday living.[3] Specific capacities which become impaired over time in persons with AD include the capacity to make medical decisions (consent to treatment),[1,4,5] consent to research,[6] manage finances,[7] drive,[8,9] make a will[10,11] and vote.[12,13] Impairment and loss of these capacities significantly reduce patients' autonomy and psychological well-being,[14] cause substantial patient disability and caregiving burden for families and give rise to clinical and legal challenges for clinicians and legal professionals. Thus, loss of competency in AD has important psychological, ethical, clinical and legal implications.[3]

Over the past 20 years, competency research has begun to emerge as a recognized field of study in the literature.[15,16] Dementia related studies, and in particular those focusing on AD, form a substantial part of this emerging field. For example, prior investigations have shown that important capacities such as medical decision-making, financial management skills and research consent are impaired in patients with mild and moderate AD.[6,7,12,17,18] This line of empirical research has been based upon the recent development of conceptually grounded, empirically-based competency assessment instruments such as the McArthur Competency Assessment Instruments[19,20] and the Financial Capacity Instrument.[7] Other research studies have sought to use neurocognitive test batteries to identify cognitive functions and possible neurological substrates associated with competency impairment and loss.[5,21,22]

As discussed further below, however, the field of empirical competency research is still emerging and many knowledge gaps exist. For example, there is a significant need currently for longitudinal studies of competency to better understand clinical trajectories of impairment in various capacities across time in persons with AD and other disorders affecting cognition.

In this chapter, we present conceptual, clinical and research approaches to assessing different competencies in patients with AD. We begin by outlining basic theoretical concepts and principles related to competency evaluations, in an effort to provide a general context for understanding competency assessment and research in dementia. We then discuss AD as a paradigmatic disease for understanding competency loss, identifying specific core cognitive deficits in AD and how they can affect competency. The next section, which comprises the largest portion of the chapter, discusses conceptual and, where available, empirical aspects of five specific competencies in dementia: medical decision-making capacity (treatment consent capacity), financial capacity, testamentary capacity (capacity to execute a will), driving capacity and voting capacity. We conclude by summarizing the current state of competency research in AD, and by highlighting directions for future research.

KEY PRINCIPLES IN COMPETENCY ASSESSMENT

Competency is an elusive and at times misunderstood medical-legal construct.[3] Sound clinical assessment and empirical research in the area of competency requires identification and clarification of terminology and basic concepts.[1] In this section, we highlight a number of key points and principles.

What is 'competency'?

In general, the terms 'competency' and more recently 'capacity' relate to a person's legal status in our society to participate in certain decisions and to perform certain acts.[23,24] (These same terms are often also used in the clinical context to refer to a patient's capacity to carry out various higher order activities of daily life.) In our society, the law presumes that adults have the capacity to exercise choices and make decisions for themselves, until proven otherwise.[25] However, organic and psychiatric illnesses may cause some adults to lose the ability to make such decisions in a rational manner. In addition, some individuals with developmental or acquired disabilities in childhood will never, even as adults, possess the capacities necessary to make such decisions. In these circumstances, the state, through exercise of its protective 'parens patriae' power, may deem these persons incompetent and appoint substitute decision-makers (guardians and conservators).[26] Accordingly, while there is no single agreed upon definition of competence,[27] competency may be usefully defined as 'a threshold requirement for an individual to retain the power to make decisions for themselves'[23] (p. 218). Since a finding of incompetency may entail a significant deprivation of rights and autonomy, competency evaluations and determinations are serious matters.[1,3,23]

Capacity versus competency

The terms 'capacity' and 'competency' are often used interchangeably.[3] However, the terms are actually related but also distinct concepts.[26,28] Until recently, the term 'capacity' has denoted a clinical status as judged by a healthcare professional, whereas 'competency' has denoted a legal status as determined by a legal professional (i.e. a judge). A capacity evaluation involves a clinical assessment and judgment based on a patient's history, presentation and test performance. A clinical judgment of incapacity, however, does not permit the formal transfer of decisional authority to another (with the exception of 'springing' durable power of attorneys, which are designed to go into effect upon such a clinical judgment). At the same time, patients and families will often adhere to a clinician's capacity judgments, conferring upon them a quasi-adjudicative status.

In contrast, a legal judgment of incompetency will lead to a formal change in an individual's legal status, whether with respect to a specific transaction (e.g. making a will) or globally (guardianship). In the legal arena, a clinical judgment of capacity is simply one (albeit important) kind of evidence supporting a legal judgment of competency. A judge may consider such clinical capacity findings as part of his/her competency decision-making process, but will also consider other sources of authority, such as statutes, case law precedent and principles of equity and justice.[3] It is important and useful to be mindful of the capacity/competency distinction in approaching competency issues, even when for reasons of convenience the terms have often been used interchangeably.[3]

To make matters more complicated, in recent years the legal field (in particular the area of guardianship law), has begun to use the term 'capacity' as a replacement term for the older term 'competency' (which has fallen into disfavour).[24] Unfortunately, this new usage tends to undermine the valuable distinctions drawn above. In order to preserve clarity of usage, it may be best currently to use the terms 'clinical capacity judgment' and 'legal capacity judgment' to distinguish the contexts and status of the decisions made.

Multiple competencies: competency to do what?

The term 'competency' is often used in an undifferentiated way to describe a variety of capacities.[1,3] Competency, however, is not a unitary concept or construct: there is not simply 'one' competency. The normal adult has distinct and multiple competencies, including the capacity to make a will, to drive, to consent to medical treatment, to manage his or her financial affairs and, ultimately, to manage all of his or her personal affairs. Each capacity involves a distinct combination of functional abilities and skills that sets it apart from other competencies.[29] For example, the cognitive and physical capacities requisite for driving are arguably quite distinct from those for making a will. In addition, each competency tends to operate in a context specific to itself.[30] For instance, the capacity to consent to treatment almost always arises in a medical setting. The reality of multiple competencies indicates that the operative question should not be 'Is he/she competent?', but rather, 'Is he/she competent to do X in Y context?'.[1,3]

Specific versus general competency

One useful distinction for analysing different competencies is that of 'specific' versus 'general' competency.[1,23] General competence is defined as the capacity to manage 'all one's affairs in an adequate manner',[23] and is the focus of most state statutes in the US governing guardianship. Specific competency, in contrast, concerns the capacity to perform a specific act or set of specific actions.[1] As suggested above, there are many specific civil and criminal competencies recognized by the law, including the capacity to manage financial affairs, make a will, be a parent (adoption and custody), consent to medical treatment and stand trial. In the authors' experience, each specific competency must be approached and analysed discretely, as each has distinct functional abilities underlying it.[3]

Limited competency

Because competency determination by its nature results in a categorical assignment (e.g. competent vs incompetent), outcomes in the past have generally been dichotomous, 'all or nothing' propositions.[3,23] Limited competency refers to the fact that, within a general or specific competency, an individual may have the capacity to perform some actions but not others. For example, a mildly demented AD patient may no longer be able to handle more complex investment and financial decisions, but might still be able to write cheques and handle small daily sums of money.[3] Such an individual could be characterized, therefore, as having limited competency to manage his or her financial affairs. The legal system has recognized the importance of limited competency through its increasing use of limited guardianships and conservatorships.[3]

Intermittent competency and restoration of competency

It is important to realize that competency status may change over time.[3] For example, fluctuations in chronic psychiatric illness may periodically compromise an individual's capacity to give consent to medications or to manage his or her personal affairs. The competency of a patient with AD or related dementia, in contrast, is usually more stable over time, although over time the capacity will be lost forever. In situations of intermittent competency, periodic re-evaluations are indicated. In some cases, the underlying organic or psychiatric condition compromising an individual's competency may resolve, resulting in the individual regaining decision-making abilities. In such cases, legal competency may be restored through a formal court hearing and decision.[3]

Dementia diagnosis does not constitute incompetency

A diagnosis of dementia is not synonymous with incompetency.[3] A patient who meets the NINCDS-ADRDA criteria for probable AD[31] may, nonetheless, be competent to consent to medical treatment or research, or other activities such as driving or managing financial affairs. A determination of competency should always involve a 'functional' analysis: does the person possess the skills and abilities integral to performing a specific act in its context?[32] Dementia diagnosis is certainly a relevant factor in evaluating competency. However, because diagnosis conveys no specific functional information, it cannot by itself be dispositive of the competency question.[1,3]

Cognitive impairment does not constitute incompetency

For similar reasons, neuropsychological and mental status test measures by themselves cannot, and should not, decide issues of capacity.[3] Such test results are important for diagnosing AD and for measuring level of cognitive impairment, and they certainly are relevant to a competency evaluation. However, again, they cannot by themselves be dispositive of the competency issue.[30,33] As noted by Grisso, decision-makers must go further and 'present the logic that links these clinical observations [i.e. test results] to the capacities with which the law is concerned'.[29] For example, neuropsychological impairments in attention, auditory verbal comprehension and abstractive capacity become relevant to a competency determination only when they are meaningfully related to competency-specific functional impairments – for instance, the inability to express a treatment preference, to understand what a will is or to operate a motor vehicle.

ALZHEIMER'S DISEASE AND COMPETENCY

Cognition and with it higher and basic functional abilities are progressively and relentlessly eroded in AD and related dementias.[3] As a result, AD is a paradigmatic disease through which to understand competency impairment and loss. It is therefore instructive to consider, from a conceptual and neuropsychological standpoint, how AD affects core cognitive abilities relevant to a range of different capacities.

The first area to consider is that of short-term memory and new learning. Anterograde amnesia is the hallmark clinical feature of early AD and substantially impairs patients' capacity to encode and consolidate new verbal and visual information.[34] Such a deficit has enormous ramifications for competency. For example, verbal memory impairment will substantially limit a patient's capacity to retain information relating to his/her medical condition (e.g. as related by his/her physician) and thus will affect the patient's capacity to make medical treatment decisions. The same verbal memory deficit can make highly problematic a patient's participation in a contract or other financial transaction, as the patient will be unable to recall and draw upon key factual aspects of the deal.

A second and perhaps less appreciated area of cognitive deficit involves access to historical memory. As AD progresses, patients' access to their own personal historical archive of episodic memories is also increasingly reduced. As a result, patients with AD may not have immediate recourse to episodic memories, template experiences and personal values that have guided their decision-making in the past.[35] This deficit, in turn, can lead to uncharacteristic and unreflective medical treatment choices, or may cause the individual to make fundamental or naïve mistakes in a business transaction that would have been unheard of a decade previously.

A third area of cognitive deficit in AD affecting capacity is semantic knowledge. Disruption and progressive loss of semantic knowledge networks is another characteristic of cognitive change in AD.[36] As a result, patients with AD over time begin to lose their established fund of conceptual knowledge, in addition to experiencing substantial difficulty learning new concepts as well. Such loss of conceptual knowledge is arguably as great a threat to competency as short-term memory loss. When an individual no longer fully appreciates concepts such as 'side effect', their ability to engage in a meaningful treatment consent dialogue with their physician, and in medical treatment decision-making generally, becomes highly questionable. Similarly, if an individual no longer understands terms such as 'interest rate' or 'escrow', their ability to participate in a financial transaction becomes problematic. Such frank losses in semantic knowledge can particularly occur in the mild to moderate stages of AD and are reflected in the often palpable confusion of the patient as he/she struggles to follow conversations relevant to a medical or financial transaction.

Executive function and judgment comprise a fourth cognitive domain closely implicated in competency loss.[37] Executive functions concern those frontally mediated cognitive abilities that permit us to engage in goal oriented activity serving our self-interest and that of others. These abilities include mental sequencing, mental flexibility and self-monitoring and correcting functions, and the capacity to integrate emotional/affective input into decisional processes.[38,39] The value of such executive abilities to decision-making is apparent, as they permit flexible approaches to decision-making and the exercise of judgment based upon both informational and emotional sources. Executive dysfunction is a characteristic cognitive deficit that occurs

early in AD,[40–42] sometimes emerging concurrently or shortly after pronounced short-term memory loss. As a result, patients with AD early on begin to lose the ability to consider a range of alternatives in their decision-making, and to examine and weigh the respective merits of different decisional paths. They are more likely to become 'fixed' upon one approach to a medical or financial decision, even if the evidence suggests that it may not be the most promising. Patients also lose the ability to exercise judgment and to detect issues of personal risk and exploitation represented by lotteries, magazine subscriptions and related money scams.[7,43]

A fifth area of cognitive deficit in AD involves communication abilities and their relevance to competency. Towards the moderate stage of the disease, patients' expressive ability to speak and to express choices and preferences can become substantially impaired, and their receptive abilities to understand spoken language start to become affected.[2,5] Thus, apart from the core deficits in memory, understanding and mental flexibility/judgment described above, AD patients' basic abilities to express simple choices and to process spoken (and usually written) language become impaired. Loss of these fundamental verbal abilities obviously has a devastating impact on those residual capacities and everyday functions the patient can still engage in. For example, such loss threatens a patient's capacity simply to register a medical treatment choice, or even to assent to a medical choice made by a duly authorized proxy decision-maker.

SPECIFIC COMPETENCIES AFFECTED IN PERSONS WITH AD

Medical decision-making capacity

The capacity to make medical treatment decisions about the care of one's body and mind is a higher order ability and fundamental aspect of personal autonomy.[44] Treatment consent capacity, or medical decision-making capacity (MDC), refers to a patient's cognitive and emotional capacity to accept a proposed treatment to refuse treatment, or to select among treatment alternatives.[28,29] Treatment consent capacity is an integral element of the legal doctrine of informed consent, which requires that a person's consent be informed, voluntary and *competent*.[26] From a functional standpoint, consent capacity may be viewed as an 'advanced activity of daily life'[30] and an important aspect of functional health and independent living skills in both younger and older adults.[37]

MDC is distinctive in that it is a 'generic' instrumental activity of daily life (IADL) common to all independent, community-dwelling older adults. In our society, all independently functioning adults are presumed to possess MDC and are expected to exercise this capacity in encounters and treatment decisions with physicians and other healthcare providers.[45] Due to the heightened incidence and prevalence of medical illnesses that come with ageing, older adults must make a disproportionately higher number of personal medical decisions relative to other age groups.[45] In this regard, patients with AD are increasingly called upon to make medical treatment decisions, as new therapeutics designed at prevention or symptomatic relief are introduced.[46] Consent capacity is also an ethical issue in the research sphere, as patients with AD increasingly must choose whether to participate in clinical research trials aimed at developing new treatments.[6]

Conceptually, MDC consists of four core consent abilities: the ability to communicate a treatment choice (*evidencing choice*); the ability to appreciate the consequences of a treatment choice (*appreciation*); the ability to reason about different treatment choices (*reasoning*) and the ability to understand the treatment situation and choices (*understanding*).[2,20,31] Prior research in older adult and dementia populations has suggested that MDC draws upon a number of neurocognitive functions including verbal conceptualization, verbal memory, executive functioning, language, and attention.[4,5,21,22]

Over the past decade, a number of investigators have developed instruments for the assessment of decisional capacity in different patient populations.[2,19,20,47,48] Our own research group sought to develop a reliable and valid instrument for assessment of treatment consent capacity in patients with AD. Using the above conceptual model, we developed a psychometric instrument consisting of two specialized clinical vignettes (vignette A: neoplasm; vignette B: cardiac) that tested MDC using the consent abilities detailed above (*Capacity to Consent to Treatment Instrument*, CCTI).[2]

Each CCTI vignette presents a hypothetical medical problem and symptoms, and two treatment alternatives with associated risks and benefits. The medical content of each vignette was reviewed by a neurologist with expertise with the elderly and dementia. The vignettes, which are presented orally and in writing to participants in an uninterrupted disclosure format,[49] are written at a 5th to 6th grade reading level[50] with low syntactic complexity and a moderate information load. The administration format approximates an informed consent dialogue and requires the subject to consider two different treatment options with associated risks and benefits. Vignettes are administered by having subjects simultaneously read and listen to an oral presentation of the vignette information. Participants then answer standardized questions designed to test consent capacity under the four standards set forth above. The CCTI has a detailed and well-operationalized scoring system for each vignette standard and good psychometric properties in patients with AD.[2,4,5,51]

Prior work with the CCTI has shown that treatment consent capacity is significantly impaired in patients with mild and moderate Alzheimer's disease.[2,17,18] In a cross-sectional study, our group found that patients with mild AD demonstrated significant impairments in treatment consent abilities of *understanding treatment* and *reasoning about treatment*,[2,18] and were at risk for competency loss in certain medical situations.[17,18] Patients with moderate AD demonstrated deficits in *understanding treatment*, *reasoning* and *appreciation*, as well as some initial problems with the basic consent abilities of *evidencing a choice* and *making the reasonable choice*.

Cognitive studies with the CCTI have shown that measures of semantic knowledge, executive function and verbal memory are key predictors of consent ability performance and outcome in AD patients.[4,5] Specifically, deficits in conceptualization, semantic memory and probably verbal recall appear to be associated with the significantly impaired capacity of both mild and moderate AD patients to *understand* a treatment situation and choices. Deficits in simple executive dysfunction (word fluency) appear linked to the impaired capacity of both mild and moderate AD patients to provide *reasoning* for a treatment choice, and to the impaired capacity of moderate AD patients to *appreciate* the personal consequences of a treatment choice. Finally, receptive aphasia and advanced semantic memory loss (severe dysnomia) may be associated with the impaired ability of moderate AD patients to *evidence* a simple treatment choice. Results from these studies offer insight into the relationship between different consent abilities and the progressive cognitive changes characteristic of AD, and represent an initial step toward a neurological model of competency.[4,5]

Factor analysis of the CCTI has also provided a valuable glimpse into the neurocognitive basis of MDC as a construct in patients with AD.[21] We investigated the competency construct through a series of exploratory and validation factor analyses of the CCTI consent items in a sample of 82 patients with mild and moderate AD. In the exploratory phase, principal components analyses revealed that the CCTI is composed of two orthogonal factors: verbal conceptualization/reasoning and verbal memory. In the validation phase, principal components analysis of individual factor scores and neuropsychological test performance supported and further elaborated the two-factor structure. The neuropsychological test measures differentially loaded on the different validation factors in a manner reflecting their neurocognitive basis and relationship to the exploratory factor scores. Measures of conceptualization, executive function, language/semantic memory and attention loaded heavily on the first factor corresponding to verbal conceptualization/reasoning. In addition, five measures of immediate and delayed verbal recall and memory loaded heavily on the second factor corresponding to verbal memory. The findings provided strong evidence that treatment consent capacity in an AD population is a multidimensional construct represented by neurocognitive factors of verbal reasoning and verbal memory. From a clinical standpoint, neuropsychological measures of verbal conceptualization/reasoning and verbal memory are likely to be quite sensitive to declining treatment consent capacity in older adults with AD.

Financial capacity

Financial capacity (FC) is a second important IADL and competency that is usually compromised in persons with AD.[3,7,52] FC consists of a broad range of conceptual, pragmatic and judgment abilities, ranging from basic skills of identifying and counting coins and currency to paying bills, managing a bank statement and exercising financial judgment. FC is a core aspect of individual autonomy in older adults.[3,53] It has been suggested that 'everyday use of money will be highly correlated with general success in independent living',[54] and it is possible that loss of financial skills is the primary litmus for declining capacity to live independently.[7]

Epidemiological ageing research has confirmed the special character of financial capacity as an IADL.[7] Financial capacity has been found to be an 'advanced ADL' (along with using the telephone and eating), conceptually and statistically distinct from 'household' ADLs (meal preparation, shopping, light and heavy housework) and 'basic' ADLs (bathing, dressing, walking, toileting).[30] The advanced ADLs are specifically associated with cognitive function[55] and their loss differentially predicts hospital contact and mortality.[30] Thus, FC represents a cognitively complex set of knowledge and skills which is particularly vulnerable to cognitive ageing, dementia and other neurocognitive disorders.[7,56]

Financial capacity also has clinical relevance to healthcare professionals who assess and treat AD patients.[7] Impairments in financial skills and judgment are often the first functional changes demonstrated by patients with early dementia.[7,56] In our clinical experience, family complaints of financial declines in patients with early AD (neglecting bills, repetitively paying bills, problems balancing a chequebook, poor financial judgment) may sometimes be concurrent with characteristic complaints of significant short-term memory loss.

Like medical decision-making capacity, financial capacity is also a 'generic' IADL common to virtually all community-dwelling older adults. Unlike gender-based activities like cooking, laundry or car repair, and unlike individual specific hobbies like playing bridge or tennis, almost all adults have developed a set of financial skills during their lifetime which can be evaluated in later life. It is true that such financial experience varies across individuals, and in some households many or most financial tasks may be delegated to one spouse. But nonetheless there are core financial skills (basic monetary skills, financial conceptual knowledge, cash transaction abilities, judgment of fraud risk, bill payment, knowledge of personal assets/estate arrangements) that are common to all independently functioning adults.[7] There are also more specialized financial skills (chequebook management, bank statement management, investment decision-making) which many individuals may have used during their lifetime and continue to possess, even if another member of the household is currently responsible for them.

Despite its clear importance to everyday living and independence, there has been a surprising lack of conceptual and empirical study of financial capacity.[7] Our own conceptual model of financial capacity views financial capacity as comprising three levels:[57]

(1) specific financial abilities or tasks, each of which is relevant to a particular domain of financial activity;
(2) general domains of financial activity, which are clinically relevant to the independent functioning of community-dwelling older adults and
(3) overall financial capacity, which reflects a global assessment of financial capacity based on domain- and task-level performance.

As part of the model, we currently have identified nine domains of financial activity: 1 – Basic Monetary Skills; 2 – Conceptual Knowledge; 3 – Cash Transactions; 4 – Chequebook Management; 5 – Bank Statement Management; 6 – Financial Judgment; 7 –

Bill Payment; 8 – Knowledge of Personal Assets/Estate Arrangements; 9 – Investment Decision-Making. A schema of the model is set forth in Table 26.1. This model has been the basis for instrument development and for ongoing studies of financial capacity in AD discussed below. The model is discussed in detail elsewhere.[3,7,52]

Studies of financial capacity

Using this model, and a psychometric assessment instrument based upon the model (Financial Capacity Instrument, FCI), our group has conducted several studies of financial capacity in patients with AD and mild cognitive impairment (MCI).[3,7,57] In an initial study, a sample of 23 older controls and 50 AD patients (30 with mild dementia and 23 with moderate dementia) were administered the FCI-6 (initial six-domain version of FCI).[7] We found that mild AD patients performed equivalently with control subjects on the domain of basic monetary skills, but significantly below controls on the domains of conceptual knowledge, cash transactions, chequebook management, bank statement management and financial judgment. Moderate AD patients performed significantly below controls and mild AD patients on all domains. At the task level, mild AD patients performed equivalently with controls on simple tasks such as naming and counting coins/currency, understanding parts of a chequebook and detecting risk of mail fraud, but significantly below controls on more complex tasks such as applying financial concepts, obtaining change for vending machine use, understanding and using a bank statement and making an investment decision. Moderate AD patients performed significantly below controls and mild AD patients on all tasks.

Findings from this study represented perhaps the first effort to investigate, empirically, loss of financial capacity in patients with AD. The findings suggested that, early on in AD, there is significant impairment of financial capacity. Mild AD patients appear to experience deficits in complex financial abilities (tasks) and some level of impairment in almost all financial activities (domains). Moderate AD patients appear to experience loss of both simple and complex financial abilities, and severe impairment across all financial activities. Accordingly, we have proposed two preliminary clinical guidelines for assessment of financial capacity in AD patients:

(1) Mild AD patients are at significant risk for impairment in most financial activities, in particular complex activities like chequebook and bank statement management. Areas of preserved autonomous financial activity should be carefully evaluated and monitored.

(2) Moderate AD patients are at great risk for loss of all financial activities. Although each AD patient must be considered individually, it is likely that most moderate AD patients will be unable to manage their financial affairs.

In a subsequent study using a revised and expanded assessment measure (FCI-9), our group examined financial capacity in patients with mild cognitive impairment (MCI).[57] The FCI-9 was administered to groups of older controls, patients with amnestic MCI and patients with mild AD. The groups were well matched on demographic variables of education, gender, race and socio-economic status. At the domain level, controls performed significantly better than mild AD subjects on all domains with the exception of Domain 8 (Knowledge of Assets/Estate).[57] Controls performed significantly better than the MCI group on Domains 2 (Financial Concepts), 4 (Chequebook Management), 5 (Bank Statement Management), 6 (Financial Judgment) and 7 (Bill Payment). In turn, the MCI group performed significantly better than mild AD patients on Domains 1 (Basic Monetary Skills), 2, 3 (Cash Transactions), 4, 5, 7 and 9 (Investment Decision-Making). There were no domains on which the MCI group performed better than controls.

For overall financial capacity (Domains 1–7), control participants performed significantly better than MCI and AD participants, and MCI participants performed significantly better than AD participants. On an experimental measure of overall financial capacity that included knowledge of assets and estate arrangements (Domains 1–8), smaller samples of control and MCI subjects performed significantly better than AD patients ($p < 0.001$) but did not differ significantly from each other.

This study is one of the first published reports of direct assessment evidence for higher order functional decline and capacity loss in MCI.[57] We found that patients with amnestic MCI demonstrated significant, albeit mild, declines on some (but not all) financial abilities compared to age, education, gender and racially matched normal controls. MCI patients showed a decline in overall financial capacity (Domains 1–7) of 1.74 SD units compared to control subjects. These results strongly suggested that decline in financial abilities is an aspect of functional change in MCI.[57]

In summary, these two studies support the value of the conceptual model and the FCI as new approaches for assessing financial capacity across the spectrum of patients with both preclinical and clinical AD. The

Table 26.1 Financial conceptual model: tasks, domain and global levels

Task description		Difficulty
Domain 1	**Basic Monetary Skills**	
Task 1a	Naming coins/currency Simple	Identify specific coins and currency
Task 1b	Coin/currency relationships Simple	Indicate relative monetary values of coins/currency
Task 1c	Counting coins/currency Simple	Accurately count groups of coins and currency
Domain 2	**Financial Conceptual Knowledge**	
Task 2a	Define financial concepts Complex	Define a variety of simple financial concepts
Task 2b	Apply financial concepts Complex	Practical application/computation using concepts
Domain 3	**Cash Transactions**	
Task 3a	1 item grocery purchase Simple	Enter into simulated 1 item transaction; verify change
Task 3b	3 item grocery purchase Complex	Enter into simulated 3 item transaction; verify change
Task 3c	Change/vending machine Complex	Obtain change for vending machine use; verify change
Task 3d	Tipping Complex	Understand tipping convention; calculate/identify tips
Domain 4	**Chequebook Management**	
Task 4a	Understand chequebook Simple	Identify and explain parts of cheque and cheque register
Task 4b	Use chequebook/register Complex	Enter into simulated transaction; pay by cheque
Domain 5	**Bank Statement Management**	
Task 5a	Understand bank statement Complex	Identify and explain parts of a bank statement
Task 5b	Use bank statement Complex	Identify specific transactions on bank statement
Domain 6	**Financial Judgment**	
Task 6a	Detect mail fraud risk Simple	Detect and explain risks in mail fraud solicitation
Task 6c	Detect telephone fraud risk Simple	Detect and explain risks in telephone fraud solicitation
Domain 7	**Bill Payment**	
Task 7a	Understand bills Simple	Explain meaning and purpose of bills
Task 7b	Prioritize bills Simple	Identify bills; identify overdue utility bill
Task 7c	Prepare bills for mailing Complex	Prepare simulated bills, cheques, envelopes for mailing
Domain 8	**Knowledge Assets/Estate** Simple	Indicate knowledge of asset ownership, estate arrangements
Domain 9	**Investment Decision Making** Complex	Understand investment options; determine returns; make decision
Overall Financial Capacity	Complex	Overall functioning across tasks and domains

FCI represents a potential advance in functional assessment in dementia. It is specific to the construct of financial capacity and is based on a model conceptualizing financial capacity as a series of discrete spheres of activity (domains) linked to independent community function. The FCI operationalizes domains with actual tests of specific financial abilities (tasks), which are objective and behaviourally anchored. Finally, the FCI has demonstrated initial construct validity by discriminating financial performance and capacity outcomes of controls, mild AD and moderate AD patients, and of controls, MCI and mild AD patients.

TESTAMENTARY CAPACITY

An important civil competency related to, but also distinct from, financial competency is the capacity to make a will (testamentary capacity).[11] The freedom to choose how one's property and other possessions will be disposed of following death – known as the right of *testation* – is a fundamental right under Anglo-American law.[11,58] A key requirement of the law of testation is that a testator (person making the will) has *testamentary capacity* or *competency* (TC): 'that measure of mental ability recognized in law as sufficient for the making of a will'.[59] If testamentary capacity is lacking at the time of execution of the will, the will is invalid and void in effect.[60] The legal requirement of testamentary capacity exists across all state jurisdictions. In order to make a valid will, the law also requires that the testator be free from *undue influence* by another individual who may profit from a new will or a legal amendment of an existing will (codicil).[61] Thus a validly executed will may be voided by the court if the court deems that the volition of the testator was in effect supplanted by an individual exercising undue influence over him/her. The doctrine of undue influence, which also exists across state jurisdictions, is analytically distinct from testamentary capacity insofar as it applies in cases in which the testator possesses testamentary capacity.[58] Nonetheless, in the case of a will contest, these two legal issues often co-occur and intertwine.[11]

Anglo-American law has strongly supported testation over intestacy.[11,58] Public policy and legal precedent have clearly favoured allowing individuals to choose how their property will be distributed after death rather than leaving such decisions to state laws governing intestacy.[11] However, despite the legal system's tendency to favour the rights of the testator, cases challenging the validity of wills and specifically the testamentary capacity and/or independent volition of testators are common and in fact appear to be increasing in number.[62] This increase in will contest litigation reflects a number of factors, in particular our ageing society and increasing numbers of older adults with neurological, psychiatric and medical impairments that adversely affect their mental capacities.[11] Other factors include the breakdown of the nuclear family and increase in blended families with conflicting agendas, and the enormous transfer of wealth currently ongoing between the World War II and baby boomer generations.[62]

The current legal requirements for testamentary capacity in the United States vary to some degree from state to state, but in many states (although not all) four specific criteria or elements are recognized.[11] A testator must:

(1) understand the nature of the testamentary act (i.e. know what a will is);
(2) understand and recollect the nature and situation of his or her property;
(3) have knowledge of the persons who are the natural objects of his or her bounty and
(4) know the manner in which the disposition of the property is to occur.[10,11]

The way in which these elements are weighed by courts in determining the validity of a will varies across states.[58,61] Some states require that the testator meet only one of the criteria for a will to be valid, while others require that the testator understand a will and demonstrate memory of all property and potential heirs and hold this information in mind while developing a plan for disposition of assets.[10,63]

In addition to the four elements mentioned above, many states also require that the testator at the time the will is executed does not exhibit delusions and/or hallucinations which result in a will that excludes or favours potential heirs based on false beliefs and/or is uncharacteristic of the testator's preferences in the absence of delusions and hallucinations.[10,63] However, a will may be ruled valid if delusions and hallucinations are discrete, unassociated with the testator's property and potential heirs and/or have seemingly little or no impact on testator's plan for the disposition of assets.[11,63]

Currently there is little or no published research investigating the conceptual or empirical bases of testamentary capacity,[11] and there are no published studies of testamentary capacity in dementia populations. In part this reflects the still early developmental stage of the field of capacity assessment generally. With the exception of treatment consent capacity, for which there is now a reasonable body of research,[2,6,19,20,64] relatively little conceptual and empirical research has been conducted thus far regarding other important civil competencies.[3,7] However, this point notwithstanding, the area of testamentary capacity has been neglected. The authors have identified no cognitive or neuropsychological models, direct assessment instruments or published empirical research regarding either testamentary capacity or undue influence in the psychological literature. Given the prevalence and importance of inheritance by will, this represents a key knowledge gap in the competency literature.

A starting point for addressing this knowledge is to develop a cognitive model for the legal elements of testamentary capacity, particularly in the context of dementia.[11] Our capacity research group has begun work in this area and offers the following preliminary discussion concerning hypothesized cognitive components for each of the four legal elements of testamentary capacity. These are outlined below:

1. *Cognitive Functions Related to Understanding the Nature of a Will:* This element requires a testator to understand the purposes and consequences of a will, and to express these verbally or in some other adequate form to an attorney or judge.[11] Possible cognitive functions involved may include semantic memory regarding terms such as death, property and inheritance, verbal abstraction abilities permitting basic understanding that a will permits designated disposal of property to loved ones after one's own death and sufficient language abilities to express the testator's understanding. All of these are abilities that are affected in mild to moderate AD.

An AD patient's reply of '*yes*' or '*no*' to an attorney's queries regarding the nature of a will is unlikely to be satisfactory in this regard, as such responses do not clearly support the patient's independent understanding of the will element. Similarly, a testator's signature on a legal document by itself does not demonstrate understanding, as a signature is an automatic procedural behaviour not dependent upon higher level cognition.[65] Many patients with AD can still sign their names but would lack understanding of the testamentary documents they are signing.

2. *Cognitive Functions Related to Knowing the Nature and Extent of Property:* The second legal element of testamentary capacity requires that the testator remember the nature and extent of his or her property to be disposed.[11] As reported earlier, some states differ in their interpretation of this (§2.04 Variation in Requirements, 2–13).[63] Possible cognitive functions involved here would include semantic memory concerning assets and ownership, historical memory and short-term memory enabling recall of long-term and more recently acquired assets and property, and comprehension of the value attached to different assets and property. In most cases, patients with mild AD can identify major assets, although some may be overlooked without specific prompting. However, if the patient with AD has recently purchased new possessions prior to his or her execution of a will, then impairment in short-term memory (the hallmark sign of early AD) can significantly impact his or her recall of these items. Testators must also be able to form working estimates of value for key pieces of property that reasonably approximate their true value. It is likely that executive function abilities play a key role here, and in the first author's experience AD patients are prone to misestimations of previously known property values.

3. *Cognitive Functions Related to Knowing the Objects of One's Bounty:* This legal element requires that the testator be cognizant of those individuals who represent his natural heirs, or other heirs who can place a reasonable claim on the estate.[11] Historical and also short-term episodic personal memory of these individuals, and of the nature of their relationships with the testator, would appear to be prominent cognitive abilities associated with this element. As dementias like AD progress to the moderate and severe stages, potential testators will be increasingly unable even to recall family members and acquaintances, leading ultimately to failure to recognize these individuals in photographs or even when presenting in person.

4. *Cognitive Functions Related to a Plan for Distribution of Assets:* This final legal element of testamentary capacity requires that the testator be able to express a basic plan for distributing his assets to his intended heirs.[11] Insofar as this element integrates the first three elements in a supraordinate fashion, the proposed cognitive basis for this element arguably represents an integration of the cognitive abilities underlying the other three elements. Accordingly, higher order executive function abilities are implied as the testator must demonstrate a projective understanding of how future dispositions of specific property to specific heirs will occur.

The preliminary cognitive psychological model of testamentary capacity proposed above represents a first step towards model building in this area. Such a model awaits empirical verification in older control and dementia patient samples through use of a testamentary capacity instrument and neuropsychological test measures.

DRIVING CAPACITY

Driving is an advanced IADL that, like financial capacity, is integral to the independence of community-dwelling older adults.[66] Driving is a distinct capacity insofar as it comprises a set of overlearned and automatic motor, visuospatial and procedural skills with simultaneous, intermittent demands on controlled processing abilities, including higher order attention, judgment and decision-making skills. As discussed below, it is probably the least verbally mediated of the five specific capacities presented here and accordingly it may be the least amenable to cognitive modelling.

The capacity of older adults to drive is a clinical and public policy issue of substantial and growing importance.[66] Older adults represent the fastest growing segment of the driving population.[67] In the United States, the number of older drivers is projected to increase from 13 million in 1994 to 30 million by 2020.[68] Research suggests that older adults, particularly those over the age of 85, are at higher risk for automobile accidents than any other age group.[69] This finding is particularly concerning as increased risk associated with driving persists, even in the light of self-limiting behaviour typical among older adult drivers such as driving fewer miles and avoiding driving at night or in bad weather.[69–71] Elderly drivers over the age of 65 are one to three times more likely to be injured in a motor vehicle accident than drivers between the ages of 25 and 64 years, and have more fatal crashes per mile driven than any other age group except teenage males.[70–74] Furthermore, nearly one-third of all deaths occurring at intersections involve older adults and, interestingly, 50 per cent of these elders died while attempting left turns.[70]

Medical conditions that compromise driving can occur at any age, but they are more likely to occur with advancing age.[66,75] In particular, AD and related dementias represent a direct challenge to driving capacity. Individuals with AD typically demonstrate progressive deficits in memory, executive functioning, visuospatial ability and judgment that, over time, severely impair their ability to operate a motor vehicle.[69,76] Studies of driving in AD have examined issues such as the prevalence of automobile accidents or 'near accidents' relative to other groups of drivers, causes of and factors contributing to automobile accidents and the reliability and validity of neuropsychological tests or simulator performance in predicting driving aptitude.[8,9,77,78]

AD patients as a group drive more poorly and have a higher crash risk than their normal older peers.[66,69,71,79,80] Dubinsky et al[69] conducted a systematic review of the literature to develop practice parameters for neurologists specific to driving and AD. Individuals with AD were found to demonstrate significantly poorer driving performance than controls for both on-the-road and simulator assessments as well as higher error rates on a simple traffic sign recognition task. Only one study failed to find increased risk of motor vehicle accidents and violations among individuals with AD relative to cognitively intact older drivers.[81] Friedland and colleagues[80] found that a sample of AD drivers were 4.7 times more likely than controls to have had at least one crash in the past five years, and these accidents were associated with errors related to manoeuvring intersections, obeying traffic lights and making lane changes. Moreover, individuals with AD are more likely than cognitively intact older drivers to experience disorientation in familiar as well as unfamiliar areas and a decrease in both comprehension of traffic signs and general driving performance relative to other groups of drivers.[69,78,82] Increased risk in the AD group persists even though AD patients reported driving less at night, on freeways and in unfamiliar places.[76] In fact, research has shown that individuals with AD report driving one-quarter as many kilometres as age-matched controls.[69,81]

Some studies suggest that drivers in the early stages of AD have no more crashes than matched controls or drivers of all ages.[8,81] Trobe and colleagues[81] compared Michigan State driving records from 1986 to 1993 for 143 individuals with AD and 715 controls matched for age, sex and county of residence. Crash rates were nearly identical between the two groups, with 77 to 78 per cent of subjects in both groups having no crashes, 17 to 20 per cent having one crash and 3 to 5 per cent having more than one crash. Several limitations of this study which may have resulted in equivalent crash and violation rates for AD drivers and controls include (1) the absence of cognitive status testing for control subjects who were presumed not to be demented, thereby potentially inflating cognitive deficits in the control group, (2) failure to include minor collisions that may not be reported to the police and (3) confounding of reduced driving exposure among subjects with AD relative to controls.

As is true with other higher functional abilities like financial capacity,[83] AD patients as a group appear to demonstrate anosognosia and denial with respect to their driving deficits.[66] Research has found that AD drivers are no more likely than cognitively-intact older adults to have discussed or made plans for driving cessation.[76,84] In fact, Adler and colleagues[76,85] found that 59 to 63 per cent of AD drivers in each sample ($N = 54$ and 75) felt that their memory problems would not cause them to stop driving. Furthermore, 43 per cent of collaterals (i.e. spouse or other individual familiar with the subject's driving habits) believed that subjects with AD would be able to continue driving throughout the disease course.[85] Additional research has shown that individuals with AD continue to drive after both onset of clinical symptoms and diagnosis of dementia.[71,84] Thus, the lack of awareness of impaired abilities among older drivers with dementia and their family members raises clear issues for public policymakers as they seek to protect both individual rights and public safety.

In summary, research supports that neurocognitive decline associated with AD results in impaired driving performance over time. Increased crash rate, significant impairment in driving ability and significant deficits in visual processing have been found in drivers with AD, and these impairments may be evident even in the early stages of the disease process.[67,69] However, the negative impact of dementia on driving performance is poorly understood by patients and their caregivers. As such, many individuals with AD continue driving for many months or even years following diagnosis, thereby posing challenges to public safety.[76,84] Matters are further complicated in that some patients with mild AD retain good driving skills, suggesting that many basic skills involved in driving are automatized and reflective of procedural knowledge which is relatively spared in early AD.[67,71,81] Although data on crash rates during the first few years after symptom onset and diagnosis of AD do not pose a significant problem, the precise point in time at which risk becomes unacceptable remains to be determined, and almost certainly varies across individuals and contexts.[71] Unfortunately, tests of mental status, neuropsychological measures and rating scales of functional performance administered within a clinical setting are limited in their ability to predict driving performance.[71,81] As with other capacities, *direct assessment* of driving capacity, via simulator or on the road testing, remains the gold standard. However, although driving simulators are valid measures of driving aptitude, they are more costly, less accessible and more difficult to administer than mental status tests, neuropsychological assessment or state road tests.[69,86]

The issue of driving capacity among older adults, and older adults with dementia, will become increasingly prominent over the next several decades as our ageing society struggles to balance the individual rights of our older adult population with the demands of public safety. Current needs at the present time include conceptual models of driving capacity, better assessment tools to identify individuals at high risk for crashes and violations and the creation of alternatives to driving which are both appropriate and acceptable to high-risk older drivers.[76]

VOTING CAPACITY

Voting capacity has recently received attention in the context of patients with cognitive impairment and dementia.[12,13,87] Voting is considered an integral aspect of participation within democratic societies, and represents an individual's ability to express his or her political will, values and ideals.[88] Exercising the right to vote is considered an important freedom, and limitations and infringements on this freedom have significant implications for public policy, the political system and society.

In the United States, the right to vote is defined and regulated by federal, state and local laws, and by relevant court decisions. Federal law acknowledges the state's authority to define and regulate voter qualifications relating to a person's residency, citizenship, criminal record and mental capacity.[89] State laws, however, vary substantially across jurisdictions.[13]

There is currently not an accepted conceptual model for voting capacity. It would appear that basic understanding and reasoning standards would apply, as drawn from the treatment consent and research consent literature. However, voting competency also has features which set it apart from other decisional capacities. For example, in contrast to other decisional capacities such as medical decision-making capacity, research consent capacity or financial capacity, the voting process and outcome do not place a patient (or other third parties) at risk or in harm's way. In addition, a person's voting choice is difficult to evaluate or critique as an outcome, since no clear consensus exists on what constitutes an inappropriate voting decision.[12]

Inquiries have been raised recently as to whether an individual with dementia is competent to vote.[90] Reasons underlying this interest include the growth of the oldest-old segment of our population, the corresponding increase in dementing disorders and not least of all the fact that national as well as local elections can sometimes be decided by narrow vote margins. To date, however, no practice guidelines or recommendations currently exist regarding voting among persons with AD or other dementias.[90] Little attention has been paid to voting competency, and currently there are no accepted conceptual models or methods for evaluating voting competency in patients with dementia.

As a result, there are a large number of unresolved assessment and related ethical, legal and social issues regarding voting competency, and that make voting integrity in the elderly an emerging public policy problem.[91] First, there is enormous variability and presumably unreliability in the assessment of voting competency among cognitively impaired elderly. On the one hand, individuals with dementia who remain capable of engaging in the voting process, and who wish to do so, are sometimes mistakenly denied this right based solely on their diagnosis. Caregivers and institutional administrators may incorrectly assume that persons with dementia lack voting capacity, or the person with dementia may lack access to voting technologies tailored to cognitive disabilities.[13] Related to this issue, supervisory personnel in long-term care facilities may not always inform residents of their right to vote, or choose to assist them in registering or voting.[13] A person may also be denied the right to vote due to a voting official doubting his or her capacity and refusing to supply a registration form or ballot.

When a person is disqualified from voting – regardless of the reason – that person and his/her ballot are excluded from the democratic process, as no proxy vote can be substituted. Voting is one capacity in particular in which a proxy is legally not authorized to vote on behalf of another person.[13]

On the other hand, voting integrity can also be jeopardized by patients with AD who cognitively have lost the capacity to vote, but still engage in such activity. Alternatively, as Karlawish et al note, caregivers may themselves cast votes on behalf of persons with AD, thereby substituting their voting preference for patients whose own voting capacity is undetermined and possibly impaired.[13]

There is a clear need currently for development of methods to assess the capacity to vote. Karlawish and colleagues are currently in the process of developing a measure to evaluate whether an individual understands the act of voting.[13] For example, with their measure individuals are asked to imagine that it is election day for the governor of his or her state and are then asked how people of the state will pick the next governor (correct answer is that people will vote). To assess whether the individual understands the effects of voting, the individual is asked how it will be decided who won the election (the correct answer is that whoever gets the majority of votes wins). Lastly, to evaluate the individual's ability to make a choice, the person is presented with a short description of two candidates and is asked to choose one of them. This method offers an initial step toward evaluating voting capacity.

Empirical investigations examining voting capacity and dementia have just begun to emerge in the literature. In a descriptive investigation surveying 75 caregivers of patients with dementia, Karlawish and colleagues[12] found that a substantial number of community-dwelling persons with dementia participating in the Alzheimer's Disease Center at a major academic medical centre had cast ballots in the 2000 US presidential election. While their particular sample consisted of research clinic patients (which may be a highly motivated group), the proportion of voters with AD (69 per cent) actually exceeded the proportion of registered voters nationwide who voted in that election.[12] This suggests that a large proportion of patients with dementia may continue to vote.[12] Interestingly, patients cared for by spouses were more likely to vote than patients cared for by adult children. The authors also found that patients with relatively mild dementia were more likely to vote than those with more advanced dementia. However, a quarter of those who voted had moderate to severe dementia.[12]

Other research has also found that a significant number of cognitively impaired older adults, some with severe dementia, continue to vote. Ott and colleagues[91] surveyed 100 outpatients with dementia during two months following the November 2000 US presidential election. Results revealed that a majority of the outpatient respondents had voted in the election (60 per cent). Increasing severity of dementia was associated with reduced knowledge about the election, along with reduced voting participation by patients and caregivers. Those individuals who voted possessed knowledge about the election, as evidenced by their matching candidate photographs with names and party labels. However, patients were most impaired on free recall of information about the candidates.[91]

Given the importance of the topic and the current paucity of studies, further research into the voting competency of older adults is clearly needed. Investigations examining the complexity of ballot designs for older adults (i.e. butterfly ballot) and potential modification of such ballots represent one area of interest.[91] Other issues warranting attention include methods to support voting capacity in cognitively impaired elderly, development of voting capacity assessment measures, the use and misuse of absentee voting from long-term care facilities and the influence of caregivers on voting patterns of cognitively impaired older adults. These research efforts can lead to improved voter guidelines and electoral processes regarding the elderly, and can minimize opportunities for voter fraud and inappropriate participation by patients with dementia who lack capacity.[13]

SUMMARY AND FUTURE DIRECTIONS

In this chapter, we have discussed conceptual, clinical and empirical aspects of competency loss in AD and related dementias. We have presented key conceptual principles of capacity assessment and also examined how dementia causes capacity impairment and loss. We then discussed five specific civil competencies: treatment consent capacity, financial capacity, testamentary capacity, driving capacity and voting capacity. Each of these capacities requires discrete study, as each draws upon different constituent functional abilities, and the legal and environmental context for each differs as well.

By virtue of its relentless progressive nature, AD is perhaps the most useful disease through which to begin to understand relationships between abnormal cognition and loss of decisional capacity. Future studies, however, should examine how cognitive changes in other neurodegenerative diseases, such as Huntington's disease, ALS or MS, other dementing processes such as vascular dementia and acquired disorders such as severe traumatic brain injury or cerebrovascular accident, may also affect different competencies.[51] In addition, normal age-related cognitive changes may affect higher order functional capacities like consent capacity and financial capacity.[56,92,93] Little is known about whether and to what extent such normative age-related changes may affect the competency of non-demented older adults. Thus studies using different age cohorts of normal adults, as well as patient groups with neurodegenerative diseases and dementias other than AD, are necessary to expand our understanding of competency in dementia and in normal ageing.

Finally, there is an increasing need for longitudinal studies of competency impairment and loss in dementia populations. Such studies can reveal the natural history of competency loss in conditions like AD, and can establish neuropsychological and other behavioural markers demarcating impairment and loss of specific functional abilities.

ACKNOWLEDGEMENTS

This work was supported in part by grant 1 R01 AG021927 (Marson, PI) and an Alzheimer's Disease Research Center grant (NIH, NIA 1P50 AG16582) (Marson, PI) from the National Institute on Aging, a grant from the National Institute of Mental Health (NIH, NIMH 1 R01 MH55427) and grants from the Alzheimer's Association (IIRG 93-051 and PRG-91-122) (Marson, PI), the Alzheimer's Disease Cooperative Study (NIH, NIA AG 10483-12) (Thal, PI) and the National Institute on Child Health and Human Development (Grant #T32-HD07420).

REFERENCES

1. Marson DC, Schmitt F, Ingram KK, Harrell LE. Determining the competency of Alzheimer's patients to consent to treatment and research. Alzheimer Dis Assoc Disord 1994; 8(suppl 4):5–18.
2. Marson DC, Ingram KK, Cody HA, Harrell LE. Assessing the competency of patients with Alzheimer's disease under different legal standards. Arch Neurol 1995; 52:949–954.
3. Marson D, Briggs S. Assessing competency in Alzheimer's disease: Treatment consent capacity and financial capacity. In: Gauthier S, Cummings JL, eds. Alzheimer's Disease and Related Disorders Annual 2001. London: Martin Dunitz 2001.
4. Marson DC, Cody HA, Ingram KK, Harrell LE. Neuropsychologic predictors of competency in Alzheimer's disease using a rational reasons legal standard. Arch Neurol. 1995; 52:955–959.
5. Marson DC, Chatterjee A, Ingram KK, Harrell LE. Toward a neurologic model of competency: cognitive predictors of capacity to consent in Alzheimer's disease using three different legal standards. Neurology 1996; 46:666–672.
6. Kim S, Caine E, Currier G, Leibovici A, Ryan M. Assessing the competence of persons with Alzheimer's disease in providing informed consent for participation in research. Am J Psychiatry 2001; 158:712–717.
7. Marson D, Sawrie S, Snyder S, et al. Assessing financial capacity in patients with Alzheimer Disease. Arch Neurol 2000; 57:877–884.
8. Drachman D, Swearer J, Group CS. Driving and Alzheimer's disease: the risk of crashes. Neurology 1993; 43:2448–2456.
9. Hunt L, Murphy C, Carr D, et al. Reliability of the Washington University Road Test: a performance-based assessment for drivers with dementia of the Alzheimer type. Arch Neurol 1997; 54:707–712.
10. Spar J, Garb A. Assessing competency to make a will. Am J Psychiatry 1992; 149:169–174.
11. Marson D, Huthwaite J, Hebert T. Testamentary capacity and undue influence in the elderly: a jurisprudent therapy perspective. Law Psychol 2004; 28:71–96.
12. Karlawish J, Casarett M, James B, Propert K, Asch D. Do persons with dementia vote? Neurology 2002; 58: 1100–1102.
13. Karlawish J, Bonnie R, Appelbaum P, et al. Addressing the ethical, legal, and social issues raised by voting by persons with dementia. JAMA 2004; 292:1345–1350.
14. Moye J. Theoretical frameworks for competency in cognitively impaired elderly adults. J Aging Studies 1996; 10:27–42.
15. Marson D, Ingram K. Competency to consent to treatment: a growing field of research. J Ethics Law Aging 1996; 2:59–63.
16. Marson D. Competency assessment and research in an aging society. Generations 2002; 26:99–103.
17. Marson D, McInturff B, Hawkins L, Bartolucci A, Harrell L. Consistency of physician judgments of capacity to consent in mild Alzheimer's disease. J Am Geriatr Soc 1997; 45:453–457.
18. Marson D, Earnst K, Jamil F, Bartolucci A, Harrell L. Consistency of physicians' legal standard and personal judgments of competency in patients with Alzheimer's disease. J Am Geriatr Soc 2000; 48:911–918.
19. Grisso T, Appelbaum P. The MacArthur Treatment Competence Study. III: Abilities of patients to consent to psychiatric and medical treatments. Law Hum Behav 1995; 19:149–169.

20. Grisso T, Appelbaum P, Mulvey E, Fletcher K. The MacArthur Treatment Competence Study. II: Measures of abilities related to competence to consent to treatment. Law Hum Behav 1995; 19:127–148.

21. MP, Marson DC, Harrell L. Factor structure of capacity to consent to medical treatment in patients with Alzheimer's disease: an exploratory study. J Foren Neuropsychol 1999; 1: 27–48.

22. Earnst K, Marson D, Harrell L. Cognitive models of physicians' legal standard and personal judgments of competency in patients with Alzheimer's disease. J Am Geriatr Soc 2000; 48:919–927.

23. Appelbaum P, Gutheil T. Clinical Handbook of Psychiatry and the Law, 2nd edn. Baltimore, MD: Williams & Wilkins 1991.

24. American Bar Association Commission on Law and Aging, Association AP. Assessment of Older Adults with Diminished Capacity: A Handbook for Lawyers. Washington, DC: American Bar Association and American Psychological Association 2005.

25. Appelbaum P, Roth L. Clinical issues in the assessment of competence. Am J Psychiatry 1981; 138:1462–1467.

26. Kapp M. Geriatrics and the Law: Patient Rights and Professional Responsibilities. New York: Springer 1992.

27. Glass K, Silberfeld M. Determination of competence. In: Gauthier S, ed. Clinical Diagnosis and Management of Alzheimer's Disease, 2nd edn. London: Martin Dunitz 1999.

28. Tepper A, Elwork A. Competency to consent to treatment as a psychological construct. Law Hum Behav 1984; 8:205–223.

29. Grisso T. Evaluating Competencies: Forensic Assessments and Instruments. New York, NY: Plenum Press 1986.

30. Wolinsky F, Johnson R. The use of health services by older adults. J Gerontol Social Sci 1991; 46:345–357.

31. Appelbaum P, Grisso T. Assessing patients' capacities to consent to treatment. N Engl J Med 1988; 319:1635–1638.

32. Grisso T. Evaluating competencies: Forensic Assessments and Instruments. 2nd edn. New York, NY: Plenum Press 2003.

33. Grisso T. Clinical assessments for legal competence of older adults. In: Storandt M, VandenBos G, eds. Neuropsychological Assessment of Dementia and Depression in Older Adults: A Clinician's Guide. Washington, DC: American Psychological Association 1995.

34. Welsh K, Butters N, Mohs R, et al. The Consortium to establish a registry for Alzheimer's disease (CERAD): Part V. A normative study of the neuropsychological battery. Neurology 1994; 44:609–614.

35. Moye J. Mr. Franks refuses surgery: cognition and values in competency determination in complex cases. J Aging Stud 2000; 14:385–401.

36. Butters M, Salmon D, Butters N. Neuropsychological assessment of dementia. In: Storandt M, VandenBos G, eds. Neuropsychological Assessment of Dementia and Depression in Older Adults: A Clinician's Guide. Washington, DC: American Psychological Association 1994: 33–59.

37. Marson D, Harrell L. Executive dysfunction and loss of capacity to consent to medical treatment in patients with Alzheimer's disease. Semin Clin Neuropsychiatry 1999; 4: 41–49.

38. Litvan I, Mohr E, Williams J, Gomez C, Chase T. Differential memory and executive functions in demented patients with Parkinson's and Alzheimer's disease. J Neurol Neurosurg Psychiatry 1991; 54:25–29.

39. Damasio A. Concluding comments. In: Levin H, Eisenberg H, Benton AL, eds. Frontal Lobe Function and Dysfunction. New York, NY: Oxford University Press 1991: 401–407.

40. Swanberg M, Tractenberg R, Mohs R, Thal L, Cummings J. Executive dysfunction in Alzheimer Disease. Arch Neurol 2004; 61:556–560.

41. Sgaramella T, Borgo F, Mondini S, et al. Executive deficits appearing in the initial stage of Alzheimer's disease. Brain Cogn 2001; 46:264–268.

42. Binetti G, Magni E, Padovani A, et al. Executive dysfunction in early Alzheimer's disease. J Neurol Neurosurg Psychiatry 1996; 60:91–93.

43. Marson D. Cognitive models of financial capacity in MCI. Paper presented at Gerontological Society of America, 2002; Boston, MA.

44. Marson D. Loss of competency in Alzheimer's disease: conceptual and psychometric approaches. Int J Law Psychiatry 2001; 8:109–119.

45. Marson D, Annis S, McInturff B, Bartolucci A, Harrell L. Error behaviors associated with loss of competency in Alzheimer's disease. Neurology 1999; 53:1983–1992.

46. Morris J. Challenging assumptions about Alzheimer's disease: mild cognitive impairment and the cholinergic hypothesis. Ann Neurol 2002; 51:143–144.

47. Janofsky J, McCarthy R, Folstein M. The Hopkins Competency Assessment Test: a brief method for evaluating patients' capacity to give informed consent. Hosp Commun Psychiatry 1992; 43:132–136.

48. Edelstein B, Nygren M, Northrop L, Staats N, Pool D. Assessment of capacity to make medical and financial decisions. Paper presented at 101st Annual Convention of the American Psychological Association, 1993; Toronto, Canada.

49. Grisso T, Appelbaum P. Mentally ill and non-mentally ill patients' abilities to understand informed consent disclosure for medication. Law Hum Behav 1991; 15:377–388.

50. Flesch R. The Art of Readable Writing. New York: Harper & Row 1974.

51. Dymek M, Atchison P, Harrell L, Marson D. Competency to consent to treatment in cognitively impaired patients with Parkinson's disease. Neurology 2001; 56:17–24.

52. Earnst K, Wadley V, Aldridge T, et al. Loss of financial capacity in Alzheimer's disease: the role of working memory. Aging Neuropsychol Cogn 2001; 8:109–119.

53. Kane R, Kane R. Assessing the elderly: A Practical Guide to Measurement. Lexington, MA: Lexington Books 1981.

54. Melton G, Petrila J, Poythress N, Slobogin C. Psychological Evaluations for the Courts. New York: Guilford Press 1987.

55. Fitzgerald J, Smith D, Martin D, Freedman J, Wolinsky F. Replication of the multidimensionality of the activities of daily living. J Gerontol Social Sci 1993; 48:S28–S31.

56. Willis S. Everyday cognitive competence in elderly persons: conceptual issues and empirical findings. Gerontologist 1996; 36:595–601.

57. Griffith H, Belue K, Sicola A, et al. Impaired financial abilities in mild cognitive impairment: a direct assessment approach. Neurology 2003; 60:449–457.

58. Frolik L. The strange interplay of testamentary capacity and the doctrine of undue influence. Are we protecting older testators or overriding individual preferences? Int J Law Psychiatry 2001; 24:253–266.

59. Black HC. Black's Law Dictionary 1644, 4th edn. Minnesota, West Publishing Company 1968.

60. Perr I. Wills, testamentary capacity, and undue influence. Bull Am Assoc Psychiatry Law 1981; 9:15–22.

61. Spar J, Hankin M, Stodden A. Assessing mental capacity and susceptibility to undue influence. Behav Sci Law 1995; 13:391–403.

62. Nedd H. Fighting over the care of aging parents: more siblings clashing over money and control. USA Today 30 July 1998 1A.

63. Walsh AC, Brown BB, Kaye K, Grigsby J. Mental Capacity: Legal and Medical Aspects of Assessment and Treatment, 2nd edn. Deerfield: Clark, Boardman, and Callaghan 1997.

64. Appelbaum P, Grisso T. The MacArthur Treatment Competence Study. I: Mental illness and competence to consent to treatment. Law Hum Behav 1995; 19:105–126.

65. Greiffenstein M. The neuropsychological autopsy. Michigan Bar J 1996; May:424–425.

66. Marson D, Hebert K. Functional assessment. In: Attix D, Welsh-Bohmer K, eds. Geriatric Neuropsychology: Assessment and Intervention. New York: Guilford Press 2005: 166–205.

67. Duchek J, Hunt L, Ball K, Buckles V, Morris JC. The role of selective attention in driving and dementia of the Alzheimer type. Alzheimer Dis Assoc Disord 1997; 11(suppl 1):48–56.

68. Eberhard J. Mobility and safety: the mature driver's challenge. Paper presented at Fourteenth International Technical Conference on the Enhanced Safety of Vehicles, 1994; Munich, Germany.

69. Dubinsky R, Stein A, Lyons K. Practice parameter: risk of driving and Alzheimer's disease (an evidence-based review). Am J Neurol 2000; 54:2205–2211.

70. Fitten L. Driver screening for older adults [comment]. Arch Intern Med 2003; 163:2126–2128.

71. Lundberg C, Johansson K, Ball K, et al. Dementia and driving: an attempt at consensus. Alzheimer Dis Assoc Disord 1997; 11:28–37.

72. Grabowski D, Campbell C, Morrisey M. Elderly licensure laws and motor vehicle fatalities. JAMA 2004; 291: 2840–2846.

73. Levy D, Wernick J, Howard K. Relationship between driver's license renewal policies and fatal car crashes involving drivers 70 years or older. JAMA 1995; 274:1026–1030.

74. Lyman S, Ferguson S, Braver E, Williams A. Older driver involvement in police reported crashes and fatal crashes: trends and projections. Injury Prev 2002; 8:116–120.

75. Dobbs B, Carr D, Morris J. Evaluation and management of the driver with dementia. Neurologist 2002; 8:61–70.

76. Adler G, Rottunda S, Bauer M, Kuskowski M. The older driver with Parkinson's disease. J Gerontol Social Work 2000; 342:39–49.

77. Fitten L, Colemen L, Siembieda D, Yu M, Ganzell S. Assessment of capacity to comply with medication regimens in older patients. J Am Geriatr Soc 1995; 43:361–367.

78. Rizzo M, McGehee D, Petersen, AD, Dingus T. Development of an unobtrusively instrumented field research vehicle for objective assessments of driving performance. In: Rothengatter T, Carbonnel V, eds. Traffic and Transport Psychology: Theory and Application. New York: Pergamon 1997: 203–208.

79. Ball K, Owsley C. Driving competence: it's not a matter of age. J Am Geriatr Soc 2003; 51:1499–1501.

80. Friedland R, Koss E, Kumar A, et al. Motor vehicle crashes in dementia of the Alzheimer type. Ann Neurol 1989; 24: 415–416.

81. Trobe J, Waller P, Cook-Flannagan C, Teshima S, Bieliauskas L. Crashes and violations among drivers with Alzheimer disease. Arch Neurol 1996; 53:411–416.

82. Carr D, LaBarge E, Dunnigan K, Storandt M. Differentiating drivers with dementia of the Alzheimer type from healthy older persons with a traffic sign naming test. J Gerontol Series A Biol Sci Med Sci 1998; 53A: M135–M139.

83. Wadley V, Harrell M, Marson D. Self and informant report of premorbid and current financial abilities in patients with Alzheimer's disease: how reliable and valid? J Am Geriatr Soc 2003; 51:1621–1626.

84. Hebert K, Martin-Cook K, Svetlik D, Weiner M. Caregiver decision-making and driving: what we say versus what we do. Clin Gerontol 2002; 26:17–29.

85. Adler G, Rottunda S, Kuskowski M. Dementia and driving: perceptions and changing habits. Clin Gerontol 1999; 20: 23–34.

86. Odenheimer G. Dementia and the older driver. Clin Geriatr Med 1993; 9:349–364.

87. Karlawish J, Casarett D. Addressing the ethical challenges of clinical trials that involve patients with dementia. J Am Geriatr Soc 2001; 14:222–228.

88. Nash M. Voting as a means of social inclusion for people with a mental illness. J Psychiatr Ment Health Nurs 2002; 9: 697–703.

89. Issacharoff S, Karlan P, Pildes R. The Law of Democracy: Legal Structure of the Political Process, 2nd edn. New York: Foundation Press 2001.

90. Henderson V, Drachman D. Dementia, butterfly ballots, and voter competence. Neurology 2002; 58:995–996.

91. Ott B, Heindel W, Papandonatos G. A survey of voter participaton by cognitively impaired elderly patients. Neurology 2003; 60:1546–1548.

92. Park D. Applied cognitive aging research. In: Craik F, Salthouse T, eds. Handbook of Aging and Cognition. Hillsdale, NJ: Erlbaum 1992:449–493.

93. Diehl M, Willis S, Schaie K. Everyday problem solving in older adults: observational assessment and cognitive correlates. Psychol Aging 1995; 10:478–491.

27

Genetic counselling

Simon Lovestone and A Dessa Sadovnick

INTRODUCTION TO GENETIC COUNSELLING AND MOLECULAR GENETIC TESTING

The role of genetic factors in disease is increasingly recognized. This role ranges from causation of disease through to relatively minor alterations in susceptibility to disease and possibly, although there is not much evidence for this yet, to response to treatment. The diseases concerned range from those present at birth, to disorders manifesting themselves later in life from childhood through early to middle adulthood right through to late life conditions. This trend of identifying genetic components for an increasing number of relatively common complex disorders (e.g. multiple sclerosis, breast cancer, heart disease) is expected to continue given progressively sophisticated uses of new genetic technology. The purpose of the research that leads to the identification of genes interacting with disease is primarily to understand molecular pathogenesis in the hope that this will yield disease-modifying treatment. However, the lag between identification of a gene and the introduction of therapies based upon that identification is measured in decades. The very first consequences of gene identification might therefore be genetic testing in all its variants and, at least until the present time, this is always accompanied by genetic counselling.

It is difficult to define genetic counselling in a way that encompasses all its aspects. The following, although published more than 30 years ago, is probably still one of the best available descriptions: 'A communication process which deals with human problems associated with the occurrence, or risk of occurrence, of a genetic disorder in a family. This process involves an attempt by one or more appropriately trained persons to help the individual or the family to: (1) comprehend the medical facts including the diagnosis, the probable cause of the disorder and the available

management; (2) appreciate the way heredity contributes to the disorder and the risk of recurrence in specified relatives; (3) understand the options for dealing with the risk of recurrence; (4) choose the course of action which seems appropriate to them in view of their risks and their family goals and act in accordance with that decision; and (5) make the best possible adjustment to the disorder in an affected family member and/or to the risk of recurrence of that disorder'.[1]

The documentation and interpretation of family history information and molecular genetic data is not straightforward for the majority of disorders including the dementias. Clinical genetics is now a recognized medical speciality, which generally uses a team approach including both the clinician geneticist and a counsellor who often has a nursing background and may have a master's degree in genetic counselling. In many instances the genetics team will work closely with a disease-specific team, often holding joint clinics.

Historically medical genetics and genetic counselling services developed within paediatrics. Clinical geneticists were initially paediatricians, but now also include other medical specialists, such as neurologists and obstetricians, general physicians and in some instances psychiatrists. This early association of genetics with paediatrics is reflected today in the organization of clinical genetics and the perceived need for clinical genetic counselling. For example, the British Department of Health, in a paper exploring the needs for genetic services, noted that the reasons for seeking counselling are to make informed decisions regarding parenthood and pregnancy as well as to aid in the diagnosis of congenital disorders and to facilitate life planning decisions.[2] Historically, the vast bulk of the work of a department of medical genetics has been concerned with classical autosomal dominant, sex-linked or recessive Mendelian disorders. However, the challenge for the future is the provision of genetic counselling and information for complex multifactorial diseases with non-determinative genetics and increasingly for late life conditions. Alzheimer's disease (AD) and the other dementias thus provide something of a test case for the future of medical genetics.

Up to very recent times though, the focus of a genetics department has been to a large degree that of congenital malformations and birth defects. The clinician would make a diagnosis, where possible, by putting together various symptoms into syndromes, and then would provide the best available recurrence risk data to families. For disorders where the mode of inheritance was relatively clear-cut, risk counselling would follow Mendelian rules of inheritance. For example, a couple having a child with an autosomal recessive condition would be counselled that a subsequent pregnancy would carry a 25 per cent recurrence risk. For more complex multifactorial (genetic and environmental causes) disorders such as neural tube defects, risks were based on empirical or observed data rather than theoretical models. Since the early 1970s, prenatal monitoring and diagnosis have evolved to include various techniques such as foetal scans, maternal serum screening, chorionic villi sampling, etc., thus raising awareness about the resultant legal, ethical, psychological, moral and social issues. For example, in the 1970s, prenatal diagnosis by amniocentesis could only identify whether a foetus at risk for an X-linked recessive condition was a male (50 per cent risk of being affected) or female (virtually 0 per cent risk of being affected). Parents who terminated a pregnancy with a high probability of an affected foetus, i.e. a male, have had to deal with the realization that the aborted male foetus had a 50 per cent chance of being unaffected. Today, we are struggling with molecular genetic advances that have the potential of predictive testing in clinically asymptomatic individuals. The need to assess the legal, ethical, psychological, moral and social implications of such testing remains a critical issue to those practising medical genetics and genetic counselling.

These wider issues become even more difficult when considering complex multifactorial disorders. Thus, in addition to the complex ethical issues that apply to single-gene determinative disorders, for late-onset complex disorders one has additional complexities introduced by molecular complexities and often environmental influences. The nature of genetic risk in late-onset complex disorders is itself complex and consequently harder to convey to families. The relationship between gene and disease is not straightforward and other non-genetic factors may also be involved. The value and the purpose of providing genetic information to these families is largely at present unexplored. This is illustrated, for example, by one of the genes associated with AD (discussed below), apolipoprotein E (apoE). The risk that the gene conveys in relation to AD is age specific[3] and knowledge about apoE provides information regarding risk not only of AD, but also of coronary heart disease, which brings additional ethical complexity.[4] However, a risk factor, even if genetic in origin such as apoE, does not allow one to predict specifically which unaffected individual will become affected (or remain unaffected) in the future.

THE ROLE OF GENETIC FACTORS IN THE CAUSE OF OR SUSCEPTIBILITY TO ALZHEIMER'S DISEASE

It is now well recognized that the aetiology of AD, and other dementias, is highly heterogeneous. Broadly speaking, the dementia disorders can be divided into common late-onset syndromes, where genetic variants alter susceptibility to but do not cause disease, and a considerably smaller number of early-onset highly familial and usually autosomal dominant disorders, where genetic variants in effect are the primary cause of the disorder.

Early-onset familial dementias include AD (mutations in the APP, PS-1 and PS-2 genes), some cases of frontotemporal dementias (mutations in the gene encoding tau; MAPT), familial spongiform encephalopathies including Creutzfeld–Jakob disease (CJD; mutations in the PrP gene) and other disorders including familial British and Danish dementia, common CADASIL and Huntington's disease.

In contrast for example with Huntington's disease, where the mutation is a single locus, there are many mutations in the genes related to dementia (APP, MAPT, PS-1, PS-2). This adds to the complexity of genetic testing and counselling as discussed below. A central publication forum for mutations in the dementia genes is held on the Alzheimer Research Forum (www.alzforum.org>mutations).

Familial AD is, however, a very rare disorder. Liddell et al[5] calculated from published epidemiological studies that in the United Kingdom, with a population of some 60 million people, there are approximately 600 individuals likely to be affected by early-onset autosomal dominant or familial AD, in contrast to the 750 000 estimated people with dementia. Although small in number, these individuals require considerable attention through clinical genetic services as predictive testing for family members is possible. The decision to take a predictive test by an unaffected individual is a personal choice, which must be made in a setting that allows for informed consent, genetic and psychological counselling and confidentiality. The issue of disclosure of familial genetic information to 'at risk' family members is the subject of much discussion.[6]

For the vast majority of dementias in general, and for late-onset AD in particular, there are no known determinative (causal) genes. However, the apoε4 allele, particularly in its homozygous state, is at present the only confirmed genetic risk (susceptibility) factor for AD, although it is estimated that five to seven as yet unknown genetic variants exist in other genes.[7] There are a number of genomic regions that have been linked to AD in a series of family-based studies and a very large number of genes associated with AD, although none of these unequivocally replicated. Following this complex literature is exceedingly difficult and we would recommend the AlzGene database maintained on the Alzheimer Research Forum (www.alzforum.org>genes[8]). Here one can search for genes associated with AD by gene, by chromosome or by a number of other parameters, find the latest published data on the association and perform a meta-analysis for all published studies for that particular gene.

Given recent advances, any discussion of genetic counselling for AD must include the issues related to genetic screening for AD. For the purpose of this discussion, genetic screening is defined as the identification of an asymptomatic individual in a general population or within a specific family who possesses a certain genotype(s) which is/are associated with or is a risk factor predisposing to AD. For a more detailed and generalized discussion of genetic screening, see Holtzman and Andrews.[9]

GENETIC TESTING IN DIAGNOSIS AND SCREENING

Molecular genetic information can be used in diagnosis and screening, the former being relevant to symptomatic individuals and the latter to those currently unaffected but 'at risk'. This statement raises the question 'What does it mean to be at risk for AD?'. For the purposes of this chapter, we will concentrate upon individuals who are 'at risk' because of a particularly strong family history of reported dementia. To date, such families constituted virtually all recipients of genetic counselling. However, as late-onset common complex disorders such as AD are increasingly recognized to have genetic components, the definition of 'at risk' individuals could be said to include the entire population. As a result, the popular media has given a high profile to this area of genetics, particularly the genetics of AD. While we recognize the concern of many individuals, we expect genetic testing for AD to be limited to those with a strong family history for practical reasons in the foreseeable future. However, increasing research attention is being paid to people who consider themselves at risk of AD despite having only one affected family member, usually a parent or sibling.

GENETIC TESTING AND DIAGNOSIS

Genetic testing for early-onset familial dementia may contribute towards making the differential diagnosis, although not to the diagnosis itself, which remains a clinical process. Confronted with a patient with a family history of early-onset dementia and complaints of memory impairment, the clinician must first make a definitive diagnosis of a dementia syndrome and the molecular testing can only contribute towards deciding which of the dementia diseases is likely to be causing the syndrome. This is a particularly important distinction early in the disease when the presenting symptoms can easily be confused with anxiety or mood disturbance, both of which may be understandable in members of kindreds with a very high frequency of an early-onset neurodegenerative disorder.

Molecular genetic testing for diagnosis may appear to be less problematic than testing for screening purposes. However, although diagnostic testing requires considerably less 'counselling work-up' with respect to the symptomatic individual, one must not ignore potential indications for other family members. Before any genetic testing for a diagnosis of AD, informed consent must be received from the patient or proxy, as appropriate. It must be clearly explained that the likelihood of identifying a known mutation is relatively small and that the failure to identify a known mutation does not add further clinical information.

Molecular genetic testing for diagnostic purposes in late-onset AD remains highly contentious. Considerable energies continue to be expended to find molecular and biochemical markers for AD, but none are currently accepted for widespread use.[10,11] This search becomes more important as results of clinical treatment trials become available and treatments are approved for disease modification in AD and other dementias.

MOLECULAR TESTING IN SCREENING

Genetic screening for AD and other dementias falls into the category of 'late-onset screening'. Late-onset screening refers to genetic screening in children or adults with genotypes known to be the cause of disease which has its onset later in life (e.g. Huntington's disease) or to be a risk factor for a late-onset condition (e.g. hyperlipidaemia). Ideally, late-onset screening would lead to early intervention, which could prevent or delay the eventual onset of symptoms and/or effectively treat the disease. However, for many complex diseases such as AD, definitive effective intervention is not yet at hand.

Before continuing a discussion of 'late-onset screening' in AD, it must be recognized that in some rare families with an identified family-specific mutation, molecular genetic prenatal diagnosis is an option for an autosomal dominant dementia. However, although technically possible, prenatal diagnosis for familial dementias in these situations is not considered appropriate by the majority of clinical geneticists. While there is agreement that a young person carrying a family-specific genetic mutation needs genetic counselling about the risks of passing that mutation to a child, there is great concern among much of the genetics community about terminating a pregnancy when the disease onset will probably not occur for several decades. It is to be hoped that the progress in understanding the molecular pathogenesis of dementias may realistically be expected to lead to effective treatment or ideally prevention within the next few decades. For this reason, the present discussion will be limited to 'late-onset screening', rather than also including 'prenatal screening'.

When discussing genetic screening for AD and other autosomal dominant dementias, one must clearly understand the differences between the following two types of genetic screening: (1) predictive genetic testing and (2) genetic risk assessment or screening.

Predictive genetic testing

Predictive genetic testing (PGT) refers to testing for an inherited (genetic) material in an asymptomatic individual which, with a high degree of certainty, 'predicts whether or not the individual will develop AD or another dementia in the future'. At present, PGT can only be offered to individuals from a very few families characterized by an early-onset dementia (usually under the age of 60) and in which the disease can be traced from generation to generation, with affected individuals passing the disease to approximately 50 per cent of their male and female offspring, i.e. following an autosomal dominant mode of inheritance. In these very rare families (constituting only a few per cent of all dementia and a small proportion of all early-onset dementia), a specific genetic change (mutation) travels through the family with the disease. Disease where this occurs includes familial AD with mutations on the amyloid precursor protein (APP), presenilin 1 (PS-1) and presenilin 2 (PS-2) genes, frontotemporal dementias with mutations in MAPT (the gene for tau), spongiform encephalopathies such as CJD with mutations in the PrP gene and some as yet unidentified families.

These genetic changes can be shared by more than one family or can be specific to one family. PGT is presently possible if a family-specific mutation is identified in at least one affected family member. Usually there will in addition be postmortem confirmation of the pathology in an affected family member. An asymptomatic family member, usually a first-degree relative (sibling, child) of the affected individual with the mutation, may then be offered PGT for the presence of absence of the specific mutations. In this asymptomatic family member, the presence of the mutation increases the likelihood that he or she will develop the dementia being tested for from the 25 to 50 per cent risk predicted by the autosomal dominant model to almost 100 per cent. Conversely, the absence of such a mutation in the family member would decrease the likelihood that he or she would develop the specific dementia being tested for from the 25 to 50 per cent a priori risk predicted by the autosomal dominant transmission to virtually the risk for the general population.

It must, however, be mentioned that the penetrance of identifying mutations for AD is still not completely understood. Occasional families have been reported in which an individual carries the pathogenic mutation and yet remains unaffected, despite being more than two standard deviations above the average age of onset within that family. Whether there is interaction of genetic and non-genetic factors is still unclear, for example does the presence or absence of an apoEε4 allele in addition to a family-specific mutation influence penetrance and age of onset? In contrast to the situation for Huntington's disease,[12] but similar to that for breast cancer,[13] an individual for whom PGT for familial dementia is an option must fully understand that the absence of a family-specific mutation does not protect that individual from AD or another dementia due to causes other than the family-specific mutation. In other words, the absence of the mutation simply restores the level of risk to that of the general population, which for a common disorder such as AD is intrinsically high.

Genetic risk assessment or screening

Genetic risk assessment or screening (GRA/S) is the identification of a risk factor(s) which could potentially increase an asymptomatic individual's chance to develop AD or another dementia. In contrast to the situation for PGT, the presence of a genetic risk factor does not increase the risk for AD to almost 100 per cent. Similarly, its absence does not dramatically reduce the risk for the age and gender matched population. AD can occur in an individual whether or not a genetic risk factor has been identified.[3,6]

The best documented genetic risk or susceptibility factor for AD is the apolipoprotein ε4 (apoE ε4) allele located on chromosome 19. The apoE gene has three alleles (ε2, ε3, ε4) with six possible genotypes ε2/ε2, ε2/ε3, ε2/ε4, ε3/ε3, ε3/ε4, ε4/ε4. The protein products differ with respect to two amino acid substitutions, but the role of these in mediating AD remains a subject of some contention. The association between apoE and AD remains at the current time the only unequivocally replicated association study in AD and indeed one of the very few confirmed associations of a susceptibility gene with a complex disorder. Currently, apoE genotyping has no clinical utility, although a possible role of apoE genotyping in diagnosis, in clinical management and in GRA/S has been suggested.[14]

With respect to diagnosis, one must remember that the apoEε4 allele is carried by many elderly people without dementia and, conversely, a large proportion if not the majority of people with AD do not carry an apoEε4 allele. Thus, its role in the differential diagnosis is at best limited. This is complicated by the fact that apoE alleles have been associated with other non-AD dementias. Large studies have demonstrated that apoEε4 genotyping contributes relatively little to diagnostic certainty.[15] The role of apoE genotyping for clinical management is equally limited. Early studies suggested that there was a differential response to cholinesterase inhibitors based upon apoE genotype, but these findings have not been unequivocally replicated in subsequent studies.[16–19] Finally, apoE genotyping for genetic risk assessment or screening is not currently recommended by a number of consensus groupings,[20–26] although research in this area is continuing (see below).

CLINICAL APPLICATIONS

The discussion in this chapter focuses on genetic counselling, including screening, for asymptomatic first-degree relatives of individuals with dementia, who can be subgrouped as follows: (1) early-onset autosomal dominant dementia – family-specific mutation identified; (2) early-onset autosomal dominant dementia – no family-specific mutation identified to date; (3) late-onset autosomal dominant AD; (4) family aggregates (two or more relatives with AD, but the pedigree is not consistent with autosomal dominant inheritance and (5) apparently sporadic AD (only one affected family member). The statements listed below are applicable for the majority of individuals in each category but there are always exceptions to the rules.

Early-autosomal dominant dementia – family-specific mutation identified

PGT can be an option for asymptomatic relatives, usually first-degree, of a person with AD, FTD or one of the rarer autosomal dominant dementias where a mutation has been identified in that family. One-on-one counselling (genetic, psychological) by trained health professionals is mandatory if PGT is to be considered. If PGT is not being considered, genetic counselling is still recommended, based on the predictions of the autosomal dominant inheritance. Figure 27.1 illustrates a family in which PGT can be offered.

The situation is more complex for individuals II-5 and III-5 in the pedigree shown in Figure 27.1. II-5 is 38 years of age and is asymptomatic. She knows that she has a 50 per cent risk of being M+, based on her family history, and is also very aware that the next few years will be critical in determining whether or not she will express AD because of the family-specific mutation. Nevertheless, II-5 does not want PGT. III-5 is the 20-year-old daughter of II-5. She is adamant that she wants PGT so that her risk for AD, because of the family-specific mutation, can be changed to either the general population age-specific risk or almost 100 per cent from her prior empirical risk of 25 per cent. III-5 feels that she has a right to PGT, yet II-5 has a right not to know whether or not she has the family-specific mutation. However, if III-5 has PGT, there are definite implications for II-5. If III-5 is M−, this could be either because she did not inherit the chromosome with the M+ from her mother or because her mother did not have the M+ to pass on. These results would not realistically change the situation for II-5. However, if III-5 has the family-specific mutation, II-5 would learn that she will develop AD with almost 100 per cent certainty in the very near future. What are the ethical, legal, moral, social and psychological implications of this situation? In this situation, it would be important to include others such as an experienced genetic ethicist or psychiatrist/psychologist as well as a clinical geneticist and genetic counsellor in

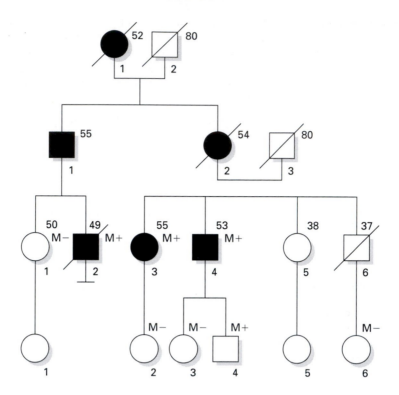

Figure 27.1 Pedigree of a family for whom PGT is an option. M+, family-specific mutation identified; M−, family-specific mutation not identified.

the multidisciplinary team discussions. These are difficult issues, but issues that have been explored most thoroughly in Huntington's disease and other autosomal dominant disorders. A comprehensive consideration of these and other issues together with the viewpoint of the recipient of counselling can be found in Marteau and Richards.[27]

With comprehensive counselling most people undergoing PGT do well. For example, in Huntington's disease, there was a significant reduction in psychological distress in those undergoing PGT although a significant number of counsellees experienced an adverse event.[28] Although more frequent in people having an adverse test result, adverse psychological events as a consequence of PGT also include those people who have reduced or no risk at the end of the counselling process.[29] This, initially counterintuitive, result is most likely due to a combination of survivor guilt and the extensive re-evaluation that occurs in someone who has lived for some considerable time with a concept of a 50 per cent risk of an inevitably

fatal disease being told that they now carry little or even no risk at all.

Early-onset autosomal dominant AD – no family-specific mutation identified to date

PGT is not possible for asymptomatic relatives of a person with AD or another autosomal dominant dementia unless a family-specific mutation is identified. Nevertheless, one-on-one counselling by trained health professionals is strongly suggested to ensure that the asymptomatic individual (1) understands his or her risk based on the autosomal dominant model and (2) has the option of DNA banking, which is important as genetic advances continue and could result in the identification of new mutations in the future. It is likely that the majority of autosomal dominant families with dementia have already been identified and mutations ascertained in one or another members of these families. However, it is known that there are some chromosome 3 and chromosome 9 linked families where the mutations have not yet been discovered and some families where no mutation or linkage is currently known. At present, we are unable to alter risks predicted by the autosomal dominant model with any degree of certainty, even if other genetic risk factors such as apoE genotype are identified. This situation may, of course, change in the future.

Late-onset familial autosomal dominant AD

PGT is not available for asymptomatic first-degree relatives of a person with late-onset autosomal dominant dementia and will not be available until a family-specific mutation can be identified. To date research continues, but no causal (deterministic) mutation has yet been identified for this group of individuals.

One-on-one counselling by trained health professionals is strongly suggested to ensure that the asymptomatic individual (1) understands his or her risk based on the autosomal dominant model and (2) has the option of DNA banking for the future. At present, we are unable to alter risks predicted by the autosomal dominant model and as before this situation may change in the future.

Family aggregates (two or more relatives with AD, but the pedigree is not consistent with autosomal inheritance) and sporadic AD

In the majority of families, there is no evidence for autosomal dominant inheritance of AD or another dementia. However, a series of family-based studies has indicated that risk is altered by the presence or absence of a family history, even in one family member. Recently survival data from a longitudinal study and apoE odds ratios have been used to estimate risk curves for first-degree family members that might be utilized in genetic counselling.[3] Thus at age 80 the risk for an individual with a first-degree relative affected by AD is roughly twice that of the population and this risk is increased considerably by possession of an apoEε4 allele. A male aged 65 has a risk of a little over 13 per cent in developing AD at the age of 80, a risk that increases to 28 per cent if he is apoEε3/ε4.

Familial risk counselling for asymptomatic first-degree relatives of an affected individual must be based on empirical data such as that reported in,[3] rather than theoretical genetic models. PGT is not an option, but may be considered in special circumstances where the affected relative is or was very young and the family history is non-contributory, e.g. no

other first-degree relative survived the age at which the AD would be expected to appear in the family. However, as previously stated, GRA/S, specifically with reference to the apoE genotype, is not recommended for asymptomatic individuals at this time.

It is an open question at the current time as to whether people would find the age and family-specific risk information as produced by Cupples et al[3] useful. Neumann et al[30] suggested that up to 80 per cent of respondents in a study in the general population might be interested in such information. However, the actual uptake of such tests is likely to be considerably less than this. A similar situation was found for Huntington's disease, where nearly 60 per cent of family members suggested they might want to take a test,[31] but only a little over 10 per cent proceeded to testing.[32] Our own personal experience in genetic counselling for dementia is that there is a degree of unmet need. For example, one of us (SL) has run a specific Alzheimer's disease genetic counselling unit for more than 10 years. Initially this clinic was planned as a joint clinic with the medical genetics department to identify early-onset autosomal dominant families and provide them with PGT. Although this was the target population, an audit of the clinic activity suggested that the majority of those being counselled had small numbers (one or two only) of affected family members and that the age of the affected family members was clearly late-onset. Those receiving counselling had high rates of clinically relevant anxiety or depression. The experience in another clinic for AD and related disorders where one of us (ADS) has worked since 1984 has been similar.

This clinical experience is matched in the first report from the REVEAL study.[33] This is a large, randomized control trial of susceptibility testing in AD. Participants were recruited from two sources – those who self-referred after public appeal through various sources of media and those contacted by the research team as having previously been identified as a first-degree relative of an Alzheimer patient known to Alzheimer centres participating in the REVEAL study. After a process of explanation of the study, individualized genetic counselling and consent for apoE testing, subjects were randomized into two arms of the study as follows:

(1) Risk to develop AD is given, controlling for gender, race and family history of AD.
(2) Risk to develop AD is given as in (1), but the additional factor of apoE genotype is included in the risk calculation.[3] A relatively small proportion of those who were systematically collected as family

members of people with AD proceeded to randomization and only a little over 60 per cent of those who referred themselves proceeded. When comparing those who progressed to randomization to those who did not, participants who were systematically collected were more likely to progress to randomization if they were highly educated and young, whereas those progressed to randomization who referred themselves were more likely to be very worried about inheriting dementia.[33] These research findings and findings from our clinical experience suggest that the introduction of GRA/S for late-onset dementia needs to be accompanied by counselling, not least because those who volunteer for such information disclosure are likely to have serious concerns and perhaps even psychiatric symptoms that need addressing individually. REVEAL II is in progress to study further these issues of disclosure and its impact.

SUMMARY

In summary, advances in understanding the role of genetic factors in the causation of (or susceptibility to) common complex disorders such as AD have been rapid. Caution must be exhibited when providing genetic counselling, which may include genetic testing where appropriate. Such counselling must be family structure specific. While there is understandably much pressure from the community to offer molecular genetic testing, and to some extent diagnostic testing, in most situations we cannot at present do this with sufficient accuracy and understanding to justify the potential social, legal, psychological, ethical and moral implication. To a large extent, this perceived pressure for molecular genetic testing is from relatives of patients with dementia who state that they want PGT but fail to understand that this is only possible for the very few families with an identified specific genetic mutation. Other relatives of people with AD have concerns and anxieties about dementia that must be addressed separately from any concerns regarding inheritance for themselves. If and when an effective diagnosis-specific treatment for dementia is proven, these same individuals will be expected to lobby for molecular genetic testing which is not causal but is more GRA/S diagnostic testing.

Although it is our opinion, as discussed previously, that the time for PGT has not yet arrived for the majority of families, this opinion does not hold true for genetic counselling. We emphasize the view of Professor Clarke Fraser[1] as cited in the introduction that genetic counselling consists of more than testing. Family members deserve an opportunity to discuss their concerns about inheriting AD and related dementias and should be able to insist upon the best and most current advice related to their own situation. This process has in fact begun in many centres.

The experience with Huntington's disease cannot be used uncritically as a paradigm for AD. However, the Huntington's disease experience did clearly show that the unexpected can occur and also demonstrated the need for well-designed longitudinal studies to assess the process and impact of counselling and testing. Clinical practice and research in this area provides an ideal opportunity for collaboration between clinicians with experience in genetics and those with experience in dementia.

The research continues to progress at times rapidly, at other times frustratingly slowly. Nonetheless, progress is being made and it is likely that DNA-based diagnosis prediction and influence on clinical management will become increasingly a part of dementia medicine as in most other areas of medicine. For that reason, DNA banking for affected individuals should be encouraged. Similarly, because of the possible error in the clinical diagnosis, neuropathological diagnosis continues to be the gold standard and should be encouraged wherever possible. DNA banking and neuropathological diagnosis may not benefit the affected individual or at risk individuals today, but it certainly appears that having this information available or accessible will certainly help those affected and at risk in the near future.

For these reasons, we recommend that during this period of ever-accumulating data, genetic assessment should be performed in close collaboration with geneticists, genetic counsellors and clinicians in specialized dementia clinics. It is unrealistic to expect non-genetic clinicians to be always abreast of developments in this fast-changing field.[34] Provision of assessment, testing and counselling in the future for this relatively common disorder will have to be very carefully planned.

REFERENCES

1. Fraser FC. Genetic counseling. Am J Hum Genet (1974) 26: 636–661.
2. Department of Health Population Needs and Genetic Services. London: HMSO 1993.
3. Cupples LA, Farrer LA, Sadovnick AD, et al. Estimating risk curves for first-degree relatives of patients with Alzheimer's disease: the REVEAL study. Genet Med 2004; 6:192–196.
4. Wachbroit R. The question not asked: the challenge of pleiotropic genetic tests. Kennedy Inst Ethics J 1998; 8: 131–144.

5. Liddell MB, Lovestone S, Owen MJ. Genetic risk of Alzheimer's disease: advising relatives, Br J Psychiatry 2001; 178:7–11.

6. The American Society of Human Genetics Social Issues Subcommittee on Familial Disclosure. ASHG statement. Professional disclosure of familial genetic information. Am J Hum Genet 1998; 62:474–483.

7. Owen M, Liddell M, McGuffin P. Alzheimer's disease. BMJ 1994; 308:672–673.

8. Bertram L, McQueen M, Mullin K, Blacker D, Tanzi R. The AlzGene Database. Alzheimer Research Forum. Available at http://www.alzforum.org. 1996 [accessed 10 October 2005].

9. Holtzman NA, Andrews LB. Ethical and legal issues in genetic epidemiology. Epidemiol Rev 1997; 19:163–174.

10. De Leon MJ, Desanti S, Zinkowski R, et al. MRI and CSF studies in the early diagnosis of Alzheimer's disease. J Intern Med 2004; 256:205–223.

11. Sunderland T, Gur RE, Arnold SE. The use of biomarkers in the elderly: current and future challenges. Biol Psychiatry 2005; 58:272–276.

12. Wiggins S, Whyte P, Huggins M, et al. The psychological consequences of predictive testing for Huntington's disease. Canadian Collaborative Study of Predictive Testing [see comments]. N Engl J Med 1992; 327:1401–1405.

13. Claus EB, Schildkraut JM, Thompson WD, Risch NJ. The genetic attributable risk of breast and ovarian cancer. Cancer 1996; 77:2318–2324.

14. Roses AD. Apolipoprotein E genotyping in the differential diagnosis, not prediction, of Alzheimer's disease. Ann Neurol 1995; 38:6–14.

15. Mayeux R, Saunders AM, Shea S, et al. Alzheimer's Dis Ctr Consortium Apolipo. Utility of the apolipoprotein E genotype in the diagnosis of Alzheimer's disease. N Engl J Med 1998; 338:506–511.

16. Poirier J, Delisle MC, Quirion R, et al. Apolipoprotein E4 allele as a predictor of cholinergic deficits and treatment outcome in Alzheimer disease. Proc Natl Acad Sci USA 1995; 92:12260–12264.

17. Rigaud AS, Traykov L, Caputo L, et al. The apolipoprotein E epsilon4 allele and the response to tacrine therapy in Alzheimer's disease. Eur J Neurol 2000; 7:255–258.

18. Aerssens J, Raeymaekers P, Lilienfeld S, et al. APOE genotype: no influence on galantamine treatment efficacy nor on rate of decline in Alzheimer's disease. Dement Geriatr Cogn Disord 2001; 12:69–77.

19. Farlow M, Lane R, Kudaravalli S, He Y. Differential qualitative responses to rivastigmine in APOE epsilon4 carriers and noncarriers. Pharmacogenom J 2004; 4:332–335.

20. American College of Medical Genetics/American Society of Human Genetics Working Group on ApoE and Alzheimer disease. Statement on use of apolipoprotein E testing for Alzheimer disease. JAMA 1995; 274:1627–1629.

21. Fisk JD, Sadovnick AD, Cohen CA, et al. Ethical guidelines of the Alzheimer Society of Canada. Can J Neurol Sci 1998; 25:242–248.

22. Alzheimers Assoc, Natl Inst Aging. Consensus report of the Working Group on: 'Molecular and Biochemical Markers of Alzheimer's Disease'. Neurobiol Aging 1998; 19:109–116.

23. Farrer LA, Brin MF, ELsas L, et al. Statement on use of apolipoprotein E testing for Alzheimer disease. JAMA 1995; 274:1627–1629.

24. Relkin NR, Kwon YJ, Tsai J, Gandy S. The National Institute on Aging/Alzheimer's Association recommendations on the application of apolipoprotein E genotyping to Alzheimer's disease. Ann NY Acad Sci 1996; 802:149–176.

25. Lovestone S, Wilcock G, Rossor M, Cayton H, Ragan I. Apolipoprotein E genotyping in Alzheimer's disease. Lancet 1996; 347:1775–1776.

26. Medical and scientific committee, ADI, Brodaty H, Conneally M, Gauthier S, et al. Consensus statement on predictive testing. Alzheimer Dis Assoc Disord 1996; 9: 182–187.

27. Marteau T, Richards M. The Troubled Helix. Cambridge: Cambridge University Press 1996.

28. Almqvist EW, Brinkman RR, Wiggins S, Hayden MR. Psychological consequences and predictors of adverse events in the first 5 years after predictive testing for Huntington's disease. Clin Genet 2003; 64:300–309.

29. Lawson K, Wiggins S, Green T, et al. Adverse psychological events occurring in the first year after predictive testing for Huntington's disease. The Canadian Collaborative Study Predictive Testing. J Med Genet 1999; 33:856–862.

30. Neumann PJ, Hammitt JK, Mueller C, et al. Public attitudes about genetic testing for Alzheimer's disease. Health Aff (Millwood) 2001; 20:252–264.

31. Tyler A, Harper PS. Attitudes of subjects at risk and their relatives towards genetic counselling in Huntington's chorea. J Med Genet 1983; 20:179–188.

32. Bloch M, Adam S, Wiggins S, Huggins M, Hayden MR. Predictive testing for Huntington disease in Canada: the experience of those receiving an increased risk. Am J Med Genet 1992; 42:499–507.

33. Roberts JS, Barber M, Brown TM, et al. Who seeks genetic susceptibility testing for Alzheimer's disease? Findings from a multisite, randomized clinical trial. Genet Med 2004; 6:197–203.

34. Suchard MA, Yudkin P, Sinsheimer JS, Fowler GH. General practitioners' views on genetic screening for common diseases. Br J Gen Pract 1999; 49:45–46.

28

Health-related quality of life measurement techniques in the management of dementia

Sam Salek and Mel Walker

INTRODUCTION

The focus of healthcare provision in the Western world has shifted over time due to a significant increase in the average life span. This increase is as a result of a number of factors including environmental improvements, provision of social services, effective health promotion and improved diet. Significant advances in modern medicine have resulted in the cure or prevention of many life-threatening infectious diseases as well as the development of numerous treatments that can control or alleviate the symptoms of chronic disease. This longer life expectancy has resulted in the expansion of the elderly sector of the population and an increase in illness associated with ageing. Consequently, dementia sufferers, being predominantly elderly people, have become an increasingly important subgroup of the population, with recent estimates suggesting that there are currently 20 million dementia sufferers worldwide, a figure that is expected to double by the year 2025.[1] Of these 40 million, 56 per cent will be suffering from Alzheimer's disease (AD), which is the fourth most common cause of death in the Western world after heart disease, cancer and strokes. It is not surprising, therefore, that dementia is considered to be a major public health problem and is an increasingly important target area for medical and pharmaceutical research.

Research into any therapeutic area aims to develop an understanding of the various aspects of the disease and its impact. Investigating the psychological, social and economic impact of a disease is as important as developing a greater knowledge of the underlying biological and physiological mechanisms. Understanding these aspects is facilitated by the use of various approaches that include traditional biomedical assessments as well as newer techniques such as quality of life measurement. Various scales have been developed for use in dementia, and especially AD, to measure different aspects of the condition.[2,3] These include performance-based cognitive measures,[4,5] neuropsychiatric evaluations,[6–8] activities of daily living (ADL) scales,[9] assessments of clinical global change[10] and quality of life measures.[11–13] Of these scales, quality of life measures offer a more holistic and patient-centred approach to assessing patients with dementia.

'Quality of life' is used to describe how a person feels and functions in their everyday life.[14] The components that make up a good quality of life vary from person to person as well as the emphasis placed on each of these components. Quality of life is affected by many factors including education and environment as well as cultural, political and religious beliefs, but one of the most important influences is an individual's state of health. When a person's health is affected by disease, there is a resulting impact on a number of aspects of everyday life including physical functioning, self-care, psychological well-being, social interaction and overall life satisfaction. Those aspects of a person's life which are affected by their health are collectively used to describe an individual's health-related quality of life (HRQOL).[15]

Improvement in HRQOL is the ultimate goal of healthcare and measuring the impact of disease and drug treatment on this outcome is an important component in the effective and efficient treatment of patients. HRQOL assessments can be used to make comparisons across disease states, evaluate drug performance, predict outcomes and assess healthcare provision. Additionally, they can be used as a final health outcome for monitoring a patient with respect to disease progression and response to therapy and are also useful for estimating disease costs in pharmacoeconomic studies.

There are many differing opinions on what HRQOL actually is and the problem of developing a suitable definition for use in dementia is made more difficult as HRQOL for a demented person may be influenced by factors that are very different to those which determine the HRQOL of an individual who is not cognitively impaired. It has been proposed that the following domains should be covered in outcome measures for patients with dementia: personal self-care, ADL, physical health, psychological well-being, cognitive decline, inappropriate behaviour, social functioning and satisfaction.[16] Of these aspects, it is psychological well-being that is the crucial component of HRQOL measurement. The International Working Group on Harmonisation of Dementia Drug Guidelines has produced the following definition of HRQOL in the context of dementia: 'Quality of life is the integration of cognitive functioning, activities of daily living, social interactions, and psychological well-being'.[17]

The subjective nature of psychological well-being presents difficulties in patients suffering from cognitive impairment, loss of insight and decreased ability to make judgments. In such cases, patients may not be a reliable source of HRQOL data.[18] Thus, the majority of approaches to HRQOL assessment in dementia make use of proxies and there are a number of issues to be considered when utilising informant reports.[19] Research has shown that carers may be more accurate in assessing patients' psychological and social health,[20] but careful documentation of the potential error introduced by the use of proxies has been suggested.[21] Carers also play an important role in providing a complete picture of HRQOL by supplying a self-assessment of their own HRQOL. Such assessments are important because informal care for patients suffering from dementia is provided at a great cost to the carer in a variety of ways and a number of studies have documented the deleterious impact of dementia on families.[22,23]

A number of instruments have been used to assess HRQOL in dementia and others are in development. Some instruments claim to measure HRQOL but are actually measuring different, although related, concepts. Other instruments are only measuring one or two of the domains necessary for a comprehensive picture of HRQOL, while some instruments have not undergone adequate psychometric testing. Recent reviews of the literature included many of these instruments[12,13] and therefore it was decided to evaluate a selection of these along with some recent additions based on certain criteria. Instruments were chosen if they were considered actually to measure or be very close to measuring HRQOL. Measures that

have been extensively used in the literature to assess HRQOL were also selected for evaluation. The resulting instruments represent a selection of the most theoretically accurate or the most often used measures available and therefore provide a good starting point for developing an understanding of various approaches to assessing HRQOL in dementia. Critical evaluation of these measures will provide the reader with insight into how appropriate instruments can be selected for use in dementia research. Instruments have been divided into generic, utility and disease-specific measures.

GENERIC MEASURES

The measures described here were designed to assess HRQOL in a broad range of populations and are useful for comparisons between different disease areas. Each instrument's attributes are described in Table 28.1 while their application, strengths and weaknesses are described in the text.

Blau's QOL Scale

Application
This scale was developed for use in psychotherapy[24] and has been used in a number of clinical trials of donepezil.[25–27]

Strengths
This scale is short and easy to complete with a simple scoring method and the patient-rated version has demonstrated some evidence of sensitivity.

Weaknesses
Blau's research refers to a 10-item scale assessed by patients or external judges, but the trials of donepezil documented the use of a 7-item scale completed by the patient and the carer. These studies offer little evidence in support of the validity of this scale or even how the scale has been adapted to include only seven items. Mention of inter- and intrapatient variability suggests that reliability may have been looked at, but no explicit evidence is available. The carer-rated version was not able to demonstrate any significant difference from placebo.

Medical Outcomes Study 36-Item Short Form Health Survey (SF-36)

Application
The SF-36[28,29] is a health status measure that has been validated for use in the UK.[30,31] It has been

Table 28.1 Generic measures

Instrument	Areas covered (No. items)	Total items	Largest sample	Population	Administration	Rater	Scaling	Scoring
Blau's QOL Scale	Working (1) Leisure (1) Eating (1) Sleeping (1) Social contact (1) Earning (1) Parenting (1) Loving (1) Environment (1) Self-acceptance (1)	10 (9 if no children as parenting item omitted)	473	Mild-to-moderate AD	Self	Patient (QOL-P) Informal carer as a proxy (QOL-C)	VAS marked With 0 to 50 in increments of 10 with descriptors provided for 0, 10, 30 and 50 (0 representing 'non-existent or no opportunity' and 50 being 'best possible')	QOL scores are calculated by summing the scores for each QOL variable giving an index score ranging from 0 to 500 (or 0 to 450 if no children)
Medical Outcomes Study short form 36-item health status measure (SF-36)	Physical functioning (10) Role – physical (4) Bodily pain (2) General health (5) Vitality (4) Social functioning (2) Role – emotional (3) Mental health (5) Self-evaluation of change (1)	36	1014	Mild-to-severe cognitive dysfunction	Interviewer Self	Patient Patient	A series of scales ranging from yes/no answers up to 6-point multiple response scales	Responses to each item within a dimension are summated to give a score from 0 (worst health) to 100 (best health)
QOL Assessment Schedule (QOLAS)	Physical (2) Psychological (2) Social/family (2) Daily activities (2) Cognitive (2)	10	37	Mild-to-moderate dementia	Interviewer Interviewer	Patient Informal carer as a proxy	Two constructs are elicited for each domain and then scored on a 6-point scale rating how much of a problem the construct is from no problem (0) to it could not be worse (5)	Scores for the 2 constructs are summated to give a domain score out of 10 and the total of each domain is then summated to give an overall QOLAS score out of 50

Table 28.1 Generic measures (cont.)

Instrument	Areas covered (No. items)	Total items	Largest sample	Population	Administration	Rater	Scaling	Scoring
Schedule for the Evaluation of Individual Quality of Life (SEIQOL)	Five areas of life considered to be important determinants of QOL are nominated by the patient (5) / Overall QOL (1) / Randomly-generated hypothetical life profiles based on the patient-nominated cues (30)	36	20	Mild-to-moderate dementia	Interviewer	Patient	VAS (Vertical & Horizontal) each with 5 intervening descriptors / Hypothetical Life Profiles possess endpoint labels only	Policy PC Software assigns relative weights for each cue and calculates an overall QOL score
Sickness Impact Profile (SIP)	Body care & movement (23) / Mobility (10) / Ambulation (12) / Emotional behaviour (9) / Social interaction (20) / Alertness behaviour (10) / Communication (9) / Sleep & rest (7) / Eating (9) / Work (9) / Recreation & pastimes (8) / Home management (10)	136	30	Mild-to-moderate AD	Self	Informal carer as a proxy	Tick placed adjacent to statements applicable to the patient	Percentage scores may be calculated for each domain, for two dimensions (Physical and Psychosocial) and for the overall instrument (index)

Instrument	Areas covered (No. items)	Total items	Largest sample	Population	Administration	Rater	Scaling	Scoring
Sickness Impact Profile (SIP) (Work subscale excluded)	Body care & movement (23) Mobility (10) Ambulation (12) Emotional behaviour (9) Social interaction (20) Alertness behaviour (10) Communication (9) Sleep & rest (7) Eating (9) (Work subscale excluded) Recreation & pastimes (8) Home management (10)	127	105	Mild AD	Interviewer (trained research nurse)	Patient Informal carer as a proxy	Tick placed adjacent to statements applicable to the patient	As for original SIP but final percentage scores did not incorporate work subscale as this was excluded due to perceived inappropriateness for geriatric patients
Sickness Impact Profile-Nursing Home (SIP-NH)	Body care & movement (11) Mobility (6) Ambulation (8) Emotional behaviour (6) Social interaction (9) Alertness behaviour (5) Communication (5) Sleep & rest (4) Eating (5) Work (0) Recreation & pastimes (7) Home management (0)	66	231	Mild-to-moderate cognitive impairment	Interviewer	Nursing home residents	Tick placed adjacent to statements applicable to the patient	As for original SIP but each category total weight equals the sum of the item weights remaining after the reduction process
UK Sickness Impact Profile (UKSIP)	Body care & movement (23) Mobility (10) Ambulation (12) Emotional behaviour (9) Social interaction (20) Alertness behaviour (10) Communication (9) Sleep & rest (7) Eating (9) Work (9) Recreation & pastimes (8) Home management (10)	136	106	Mild-to-severe dementia	Self	Informal carer as a proxy	Tick placed adjacent to statements applicable to the patient	As for original SIP

Table 28.1 Generic measures (cont.)

Instrument	Areas covered (No. items)	Total items	Largest sample	Population	Administration	Rater	Scaling	Scoring
Summary UK Sickness Impact Profile (S-UKSIP)	Body care & movement (1) Mobility (1) Ambulation (1) Emotional behaviour (1) Social interaction (1) Alertness behaviour (1) Communication (1) Sleep & rest (1) Eating (1) Work (1 Recreation & pastimes (1) Home management (1) Overall QOL (1)	13	106	Mild-to-severe dementia	Self	Informal carer as a proxy	VAS numbered from 0–10 at equal intervals Ends anchored by 'best possible' and 'worst possible' scenarios	Scores from 0–10 possible for each scale Converted into a percentage and given as total or separate dimension scores
World Health Organization Quality of Life Assessment (WHOQOL 100)	Physical health (12) Psychological (20) Level of independence (16) Social relationships (12) Environment (32) Spirituality/religion/personal beliefs (4) Overall QOL and health (4)	100	57	Moderate dementia	Interviewer-assisted	Patient	Uses a 5-point rating scale for each item with higher score indicating better HRQOL	24 facet and 6 domain scores can be calculated by summation A profile of domain scores is generated along with a score for overall QOL and health based on four general questions

subsequently used in studies that have included patients with some degree of cognitive impairment.[32-34]

Strengths

The SF-36 has been evaluated, validated and recommended for use in a variety of populations and evidence supporting its validity and reliability in non-cognitively impaired elderly populations has been demonstrated.

Weaknesses

Evidence from a study in older physically disabled patients found that previously reported levels of reliability and validity for the SF-36 in younger patients were not attained. In addition, patients with coexistent cognitive impairment performed worse than those who were cognitively normal.[35] Response rates to the SF-36 are negatively affected by cognitive impairment and, although interviewer administration improved response rates, patients with even mild cognitive impairment were significantly less likely to return the SF-36. The SF-36 was considered to be insensitive to change and unsuitable for use in community-based healthcare settings.[33]

Quality of Life Assessment Schedule (QOLAS)

Application

The Repertory Grid Technique, used for patients with neurological disorders,[36] was streamlined to produce the QOLAS.[37] This instrument was then modified and used to generate proxy-rated and patient-rated HRQOL data for patients with dementia during its psychometric evaluation.[38,39]

Strengths

The QOLAS uses an individualised approach that allows respondents to choose items of importance to their own quality of life which may be particularly useful in exploratory research. The QOLAS has demonstrated that it can elicit quality of life information from patients with mild-to-moderate dementia and evidence has been provided that supports its validity and internal consistency reliability.

Weaknesses

The QOLAS may be limited in terms of direct patient assessment as about a third of patients, all with scores on the Mini-Mental State Examination (MMSE)[40] less than 10, could not be interviewed. In addition, the discrepancy between carer and proxy ratings using this measure needs to be investigated. Test-retest reliability

was not evaluated for the QOLAS and its sensitivity to clinically important change has yet to be determined.

Schedule for the Evaluation of Individual QOL (SEIQOL)

Application

The SEIQOL[41,42] has been used to measure HRQOL in small populations of patients with dementia.[43-45]

Strengths

Reliability and validity were acceptable for patients who managed to complete the instrument, but this constituted under a third of respondents in the largest study ($N = 20$) and should therefore be regarded as questionable.

Weaknesses

All studies using this instrument were carried out in very small populations (between 5 and 20 patients). Patients able to complete the SEIQOL were generally less cognitively impaired as measured by the CAMCOG, the cognitive section of the Cambridge Examination for Mental Disorders in the Elderly (CAMDEX),[46] and this indicates that the SEIQOL is only of use in very mild cognitive impairment.

Modifications

The SEIQOL-Direct Weighting (SEIQOL-DW)[47] is a simplified version of the SEIQOL that has been used to elicit HRQOL information in a sample of 35 cognitively impaired subjects with serious mental illness.[48] The SEIQOL-DW's global index was correlated with the Satisfaction With Life Scale (SWLS)[49] and the Quality Of Life Inventory (QOLI),[50] providing some evidence for the SEIQOL-DW's validity.

Sickness Impact Profile (SIP)

Application

The SIP[51,52] has been used in AD as a measure of functional health status[53,54] and as an HRQOL measure in a clinical trial of levocarnitine.[55] It has been used to compare family member assessments with patient's own self-assessment. It has also been used in a number of studies to measure general health status in people with cognitive impairment due to brain injury, cerebrovascular accident, multiple sclerosis and learning disability.[34]

Strengths

The SIP has demonstrated good psychometric properties in a number of disease areas and some supporting evidence for some of these properties in cognitively impaired populations has been provided by the studies mentioned here. Evidence of reliability and validity has been shown for the SIP and completions of this measure by family members were found to correlate with the modified Dementia Rating Scale (mDRS)[56] and the MMSE.[40]

Weaknesses

Removal of the work subscale from the SIP in one study[53] due to its perceived inappropriateness may invalidate data produced by the modified instrument. Additionally, patient-completed SIPs were found to be invalid. The SIP failed to demonstrate sensitivity in the clinical trial of levocarnitine, but this may have been due to a lack of clinical change during the trial.

Modifications

Modifications of the SIP have also been used in cognitively impaired populations including the SIP for nursing homes,[57,58] the United Kingdom SIP (UKSIP)[59,60] and the Summary United Kingdom SIP (S-UKSIP).[61] Evidence of reliability and validity has been shown for the SIP-NH, which demonstrated good correlation with the original SIP and significant correlation with the Geriatric Depression Scale (15-item version),[62] MMSE, Physical Disability Index (PDI)[63] and Katz Activities of Daily Living (Katz ADL).[64] The UKSIP has shown reasonable validity as demonstrated by correlation with the MMSE and a degree of sensitivity by detection of changes as a result of memory clinic intervention, but reliability for this version of the SIP in cognitively impaired individuals has not been explored. The S-UKSIP has only demonstrated minimal evidence of validity in populations with dementia.

World Health Organization Quality of Life Assessment (WHOQOL)

Application

The WHOQOL or WHOQOL 100[65] has been used to explore the differences in HRQOL between patients with moderate dementia and patients with cancer.[66]

Strengths

The reliability of the responses was tested in this study and clear and significant differences between the patient groups were identified. This research therefore provided some evidence of discriminative validity for the WHOQOL.

Weaknesses

The WHOQOL is a relatively lengthy instrument and may be too burdensome for use in dementia. Construct validity has not been evaluated for the WHOQOL in this disease area and its sensitivity to clinically important change has yet to be explored.

UTILITY MEASURES

The measures described here can be used to provide an estimate of patients' overall preferences for different health states. They have been included as a separate category of instrument because they represent a distinct group of instruments that use a preference-based approach to HRQOL assessment, but they can also be considered as generic measures that allow the valuation of health states. Such instruments are particularly useful in economic analyses. Each instrument's attributes are described in Table 28.2 while their application, strengths and weaknesses are described in the text.

EuroQOL-5D (EQ-5D)

Application

The EQ-5D[67] is an established generic HRQOL instrument that has been used in a range of patient groups.[68–70] In dementia, it has been used in a study of inter-rater agreement between patients and proxies (carer and physician)[71] and in patients with young-onset dementia.[72] Other research has used the EQ-5D in a psychometric evaluation of the Quality of Life Assessment Schedule (QOLAS) in dementia.[38,39]

Strengths

The EQ-5D is short and simple to administer. The validity and reliability of the EQ-5D have been demonstrated in other disease areas,[73–75] although these criteria still need to be evaluated in dementia. It has potential use in cognitively impaired individuals when completed by a proxy and unpublished research has demonstrated its discriminative validity. The EQ-5D can be used to generate utility scores that make it a useful instrument for use in economic analyses.

Weaknesses

Research has raised concerns regarding the validity of patient self-ratings using the EQ-5D. Only poor to fair agreement between patient self-rating and carer proxy ratings has been demonstrated and it is unclear as yet whether carers or physicians represent better proxies. Proxy-rated versions of the EQ-5D must be used with

Table 28.2 Utility measures

Instrument	Areas covered (No. items)	Total items	Largest sample	Population	Administration	Rater	Scaling	Scoring
EuroQOL-5D (EQ-5D)	Mobility (1) Self-care (1) Usual activities (1) Pain/discomfort (1) Anxiety/depression (1) Current health state (1)	6	64	Mild-to-moderate dementia	Interviewer-assisted Self	Patient Informal carer as a proxy Physician as a proxy	A 3-level scaling system for each of five domains plus a vertical visual analogue scale for current health state – 243 unique health states possible	Responses converted to 5 digit number representing health state across 5 domains, can convert into utility scores ranging from 1 (full health) to less than 0 (worse than death) Response to overall health state converted to a figure between 0 and 100
Health Utilities Index Mark II (HUI:2)	Sensation (1) Mobility (1) Emotion (1) Cognition (1) Self-care (1) Pain (1) Fertility (1)	7	679	Mild-to-severe AD	Interviewer	Informal carer as a proxy Formal carer as a proxy	Multi-attribute preference-based system with three to five levels of severity within each domain – 24 000 unique health states possible	Responses converted to single and multi-attribute utility scores between 0 and 1 reflecting desirability for levels of function within each attribute
Health Utilities Index Mark III (HUI:3)	Vision (1) Hearing (1) Speech (1) Ambulation (1) Dexterity (1) Emotion (1) Cognition (1) Pain (1)	8	679	Mild-to-severe AD	Interviewer	Informal carer as a proxy Formal carer as a proxy	Multi-attribute preference-based system with five or six levels of severity within each domain – 972 000 unique health states possible	Responses converted to single and multi-attribute utility scores between 0 and 1 reflecting desirability for levels of function within each attribute

Table 28.2 Utility measures (cont.)

Instrument	Areas covered (No. items)	Total items	Largest sample	Population	Administration	Rater	Scaling	Scoring
Quality of Well-Being Scale (QWB) aka Index of Well-Being (IWB) aka Health Status Index (HSI)	Self-care (1) Mobility (3) Travel (2) Body movement (4) Medical condition (4) Work (4) (main areas are mobility, physical and social activity having 5, 4 and 5 function levels respectively)	18 items (minimum)	211	Mild-to-severe dementia	Interviewer	Patient	43 possible combinations of function levels each having an established preference weight from 0 (death) to 1 (complete well-being)	Preference weight is assigned to functional level giving QWB score – adjusted to incorporate prognoses – weighted using list of 36 problems & symptoms

caution until further research has established their validity. The EQ-5D may be limited in populations with dementia by the lack of a cognitive domain and sensitivity has not yet been investigated in this patient group.

Health Utilities Index (HUI)

Application

Two versions of the HUI systems[76] have been used in AD. These are the HUI Mark II (HUI:2)[77] and the HUI Mark III (HUI:3).[78] The HUI:2 has been used in a cross-sectional study of patients and carers in AD.[79] The carers in this study responded as proxies for patients as well as for themselves. The Health Utilities Index Mark III (HUI:3) was used in a Japanese cross-sectional study of patients with AD.[80] There has also been a paper documenting the use of proxy-rated HUI:2 and HUI:3 utility scores in AD.[81]

Strengths

Both the HUI:2 and the HUI:3 have demonstrated the ability to discriminate between stages of AD as measured by the Clinical Dementia Rating (CDR) scale.[82] Compared with other utility measures, the HUI may be more useful in dementia due to the inclusion of a separate cognition domain. Both versions of the HUI appeared to reflect appropriately patient HRQOL, but the HUI:3 may allow a more comprehensive assessment due to the larger number of domains and severity levels for each attribute.

Weaknesses

Inter-rater agreement between patients and proxies has not been investigated for the HUI:2 or the HUI:3 in populations with dementia. The scoring methods for these instruments are complex and neither version has been tested for reliability or sensitivity in dementia populations.

Quality of Well-Being Scale (QWB)

Application

The QWB[83] has also been known as the Index of Well-Being (IWB)[84] and originally as the Health Status Index (HSI).[85] The QWB has been used in a cost utility analysis (CUA) of group living in dementia care[86] using data from the Global Deterioration Scale (GDS)[87] and its validity has been explored in AD.[88]

Strengths

The QWB, like other utility measures, is useful in economic analyses. Some evidence supporting the validity

of this measure has been provided because scores on the QWB have been shown to be significantly associated with dementia ratings, behavioural problems and carer use of respite time.

Weaknesses

The QWB is more complex and burdensome to use in comparison to other utility measures while incorporating minimal detail relating to cognition. There is also little evidence to support its reliability and sensitivity to change in populations with dementia.

DISEASE-SPECIFIC HRQOL MEASURES

The measures described here were developed especially to assess HRQOL in cognitively impaired populations and cannot be used for comparisons between different disease areas. However, disease-specific instruments are more likely to be of use in clinical trials as they may be more sensitive to changes in a patient's disease-related HRQOL. Each instrument's attributes are described in Table 28.3 while their application, strengths and weaknesses are described in the text.

Alzheimer's Disease-Related QOL (ADRQL)

Application

The ADRQL was specifically developed to assess HRQOL in AD and its conceptual development has been well documented.[89] The ADRQL has been used to evaluate the HRQOL of patients with dementia in long-term care.[90]

Strengths

The ADRQL has been developed using sound conceptual development methodology and includes domains and indicators that relate to psychological well-being, perceived quality of life and the social component of behavioural competence. Items were weighted on the basis of carer rankings, which may increase the overall sensitivity of the measure and reduce the undue influence that more commonly observed items might have on overall HRQOL scores.

Weaknesses

Although the ADRQL was validated for proxy completion by family carers, the study of patients with dementia in long-term care used 32 facility staff members to assess the HRQOL of 120 residents and this method had not been previously validated. Also, items relating to physical and cognitive aspects of behavioural

Table 28.3 Disease-specific measures

Instrument	Areas covered (No. items)	Total items	Largest sample	Population	Administration	Rater	Scaling	Scoring
Alzheimer's Disease-Related Quality of Life Instrument (ADRQL)	Social Interaction (12) Awareness of self (8) Feelings and mood (15) Enjoyment of activities (5) Response to surroundings (7)	47	120	Mild-to-severe AD	Interviewer	Informal or formal carer as a proxy	Response choices for each item are dichotomous consisting of either agree or disagree	Responses reflecting good QOL are assigned a scale value which are summated, divided by number of items and multiplied by 100 to obtain domain scores and instrument total score
Community Dementia Quality of Life Profile (CDQLP)	Patient HRQOL: Communication, self-care & dexterity (7) Spare time & household maintenance (4) Memory & cognitive function (4) Family & community interaction (4) Irritability & insight (5) Mobility (3) Sleep & motivation (4) Self-sustenance (2) Carer HRQOL: Carer burden (4) Emotional behaviour (4) Life adjustment (5)	46	175	Mild-to-moderate dementia	Self	Informal carer as a proxy	A 4-point categorical response scale for each item with response choice ranging from 0 to 3 (0 – not at all; 1 – sometimes; 2 – often; 3 – always)	Item scores are summated and divided by the number of items and multiplied by 100 to obtain individual category scores. Overall HRQOL index scores are also calculated in a similar fashion for the patient and carer sections. Patient and carer scores are not combined
Cornell-Brown Scale for Quality of Life in Dementia (CBS)	Mood-related signs (4) Ideational disturbance (4) Behavioural disturbance (4) Physical signs (3) Cyclic functions (4)	19	50	Mild-to-moderate dementia	Interviewer	Joint interview with patient and carer	Visual analogue dysphoria scale The scale is a 100 mm vertical line anchored by happy and sad cartoon faces	The rating scale ranges from −2 to +2 with higher scores indicating a greater positive mood

Instrument	Areas covered (No. items)	Total items	Largest sample	Population	Administration	Rater	Scaling	Scoring
DEMQOL **DEMQOL-** **Proxy**	DEMQOL Health and well-being (14) Cognitive functioning (7) Social relationships (5) Daily activities (2) DEMQOL-Proxy Health and well-being (12) Cognitive functioning (9) Social relationships (2) Self-concept (1) Daily activities (7)	28 31	241 patients 225 carers	Mild-to-moderate dementia Mild-to-severe dementia	Self Proxy	Patient Carer as proxy	4-point response scale ranging from a lot to not at all	Higher = better QoL
Dementia-QOL Instrument (DQOL)	Discretionary activities (6) Social well-being (4) Interaction capacity (3) Bodily well-being (3) Psychological well-being (29) Sense of aesthetics (8) Overall global QOL (3)	56 reduced to 29	99	Mild-to-moderate dementia	Interviewer	Patient	Six multiple-response visual scales each having 5-point options with descriptors for each point tailored to the question asked	Scores ranged from 1 to 5 for each scale with higher scores indicating better QOL (range 1 to 2 for items with yes/no answer)
Modified Pleasant Events Schedule-AD (modified PES-AD)	15 activities including: Going outside Going for a ride in a car Visiting with family and friends Exercising Reading or being read a story Going to a museum Watching a movie Working on a craft (Full list not provided) Also Six Affects including: Pleasure, interest, contentment, anxiety, anger & depression	15 (and 6 affects)	196	Mild-to-severe AD	Interviewer	Informal carer as a proxy Formal carer as a proxy	A 3-point response scale for frequency of activities in previous week (frequency, opportunity and yes/no response for current enjoyment) Frequency of affects during previous week (5-point scale)	Activity measure defined as sum of frequency that activities performed in previous week Summary +ve and summary −ve scores obtained for affects by summing frequencies

Table 28.3 Disease-specific measures (cont.)

Instrument	Areas covered (No. items)	Total items	Largest sample	Population	Administration	Rater	Scaling	Scoring
Progressive Deterioration Scale (PDS)	Extent to which patient can leave immediate neighbourhood Ability to travel distances alone Confusion in familiar settings Use of familiar household implements Participation/enjoyment of leisure/cultural activities Extent to which patient does household chores Involvement in family finances, budgeting, etc. Interest in doing household tasks Travel on public transportation Self-care and routine tasks Social function/behaviour (number of items in each content area has not been stated)	27	725	Mild-to-severe AD	Self	Informal carer as a proxy	Bipolar analogue scale with endpoints anchored by statements about patients' abilities at time of evaluation	Distance along line where cross placed by carer was measured and scored on a scale of 0 to 100
QOL in AD Measure (QOL-AD)	Physical health (1) Energy (1) Mood (1) Living situation (1) Memory (1) Family (1) Marriage (1) Friends (1) Self as a whole (1) Ability to do chores (1) Ability to do things for fun (1) Money (1) Life as a whole (1)	13	177	Mild-to-moderate AD	Interviewer (for patients) Self (for carers)	Patient Informal carer as a proxy	A multiple-response visual scale having four-point options consisting of descriptors ranging from 'poor' (1) to 'excellent' (4)	Separate scores calculated for patient's and carer's ratings Can be combined together into a weighted composite QOL-AD score
Vienna List	Communication (15) Negative affect (10) Bodily contact (5) Aggression (4) Mobility (6)	65	682	Severe dementia	Interviewer	Physician/nurse as proxy	Electronic 5 point likert scale ranging from 0 = never to 4 = always	Summation – higher impairment with increased score

competence have not been included in the ADRQL, which may reduce the comprehensiveness of the measure. Currently, data demonstrating the psychometric properties of the ADRQL are not available, although future research is in progress to address these issues.

Community Dementia Quality of Life Profile (CDQLP)

Application
The CDQLP is a recently developed measure that has been designed to assess the HRQOL of both the dementia sufferer and their primary informal carer. This measure has been used in a number of developmental and psychometric studies.[91-94] It has also been used to compare statutory with non-statutory care services[95] and may be useful in assessing patient needs in dementia.[96]

Strengths
It is short, easy to complete and self-administered and uses a categorical multiple response scale that provides category scores as well as an index score resulting from summation of the individual item scores. The CDQLP is the result of sound development methodology including factor analysis. It has been shown to be a reliable and valid instrument for assessing HRQOL in dementia.

Weaknesses
Although data as yet unpublished have provided some evidence that the CDQLP is responsive to change, this measure has yet to demonstrate sensitivity to important clinical change in the context of a controlled clinical trial. Both sections of the CDQLP must possess adequate sensitivity and be capable of measuring real changes in the HRQOL of the patient and the carer.

Cornell-Brown Scale for Quality of Life in Dementia (CBS)

Application
The CBS[97] was developed as a modification of an instrument to assess negative effect: the Cornell-Brown Scale for Quality of Life in Dementa[98] and has been designed to give a global assessment of QoL of dementia patients. The scale was developed based on the conceptualisation that high QoL is indicated by the presence of positive affect, physical and psychological satisfactions, self-esteem and the relative absence of negative affect and experiences.

Strengths
The CBS incorporates patient and caregiver perspectives into one rating. The scale shows acceptable reliability and validity and thus is a promising instrument to measure QoL in patients with dementia.

Weaknesses
More work is needed to evaluate the reliability and validity of the scale in larger and more diverse patient samples, its sensitivity to change over time, and the impact of repeated assessment on patient scores. This information also would be necessary to determine whether the scale would be sensitive to changes related to pharmacologic, social, or environmental interventions. Exploration of utility of the scale in nondemented elderly individuals is also warranted.

DEMQOL and DEMQOL-Proxy

Application
The DEMQOL[99] was conceptualised on the basis that HRQOL is a multidimensional concept that reflects the individual's subjective perception of the impact of a health condition on everyday living. It includes only the aspects of quality of life that are affected by a health condition. The 28-item DEMQOL and the 31-item DEMQOL-Proxy provide a method for evaluating HRQOL in dementia as self- and proxy-report version, respectively and are appropriate for use in mild to moderate dementia (MMSE = 10) for use in the UK. As DEMQOL and DEMQOL-Proxy give different but complementary perspectives on QoL in dementia, it is recommended that both measures are used together. In severe dementia, however, only DEMQOL-Proxy should be used.

Strengths
The DEMQOL has been developed using a sound conceptual framework including both 'top-down' (existing literature and expert consensus) and 'bottom-up' (in-depth quantitative interviews) approaches. A final framework was developed that includes five domains: daily activities and looking after yourself; health and well-being; cognitive functioning; social relationships; and self-concept. Both instruments show good psychometric properties, provide both self and proxy report versions for people with dementia and their carers, are appropriate for use in mild to moderate dementia (MMSE = 10) and are suitable for use in the UK. DEMQOL-Proxy also shows promise in severe dementia.

Weaknesses

Further research with DEMQOL is needed to confirm these findings in an independent sample, evaluate responsiveness, investigate the feasibility of use in specific subgroups and in economic evaluation and develop population norms.

Dementia QOL Instrument (DQOL)

Application

The DQOL[100] has been designed for use in cognitively impaired populations. The conceptualisation and development of this instrument, which uses a direct patient interview to assess HRQOL, has been documented.[101]

Strengths

The five domains in this instrument each possess good internal consistency and test-retest reliability. Preliminary evidence of construct validity was also demonstrated by correlation with the 15-item Geriatric Depression Scale[62] and the authors conclude it is feasible to assess HRQOL using the DQOL by direct patient assessment in individuals with a score greater than 12 on the MMSE.

Weaknesses

Only some of the domains that make up HRQOL can be rated by direct patient assessment and further work needs to be carried out to confirm validity. The authors were unable to derive acceptable scales for some of the concepts requiring assessment (e.g. ADL, mobility and confusion). Sensitivity for this instrument has not yet been explored.

Pleasant Events Schedule-AD (PES-AD)

Application

The PES-AD[102] has been modified[103] and used in conjunction with Lawton's 'apparent emotion' items[104] to measure HRQOL by combining objective indicators (activity) with subjective indicators (affect).[105] Two studies have used this composite measure. One was a comparison of proxy-reported quality of life in clinical and population-based samples of AD patients[106] and the other was a longitudinal study in advanced AD.[107] Further research was carried out to compare formal and informal home healthcare for patients with AD.[108]

Strengths

The reliability of this method was adequate and evidence of validity was demonstrated by significant cor-

relation with severity of cognitive deficit as measured by the modified MMSE.[109] Results using this method of quality of life assessment supported proxy rating by family members in AD.

Weaknesses

The study of home healthcare in AD used the modified PES-AD alone to measure patient HRQOL, but the authors recognised that a simple count of activities was not a foolproof indicator of HRQOL. Sensitivity to clinically important change has not yet been explored for the PES-AD.

Progressive Deterioration Scale (PDS)

Application

The PDS[110] has been used in a number of clinical trials. Studies of tacrine[111-113] used the PDS as a measure of HRQOL, while studies of rivastigmine[114-118] used the PDS as a measure of ADL. The PDS has also been used in clinical trials of donepezil[119] and galantamine.[120]

Strengths

The PDS has been cross-validated using the Global Deterioration Scale[87] and demonstrated good internal consistency and test-retest reliability. It also achieved 80 per cent overall accuracy in discriminating non-AD elderly from patients in early, middle and late stages of AD. It demonstrated significant improvement during clinical trials of rivastigmine[121,122] and demonstrated significant advantages over placebo during trials of donepezil and galantamine, thus showing sensitivity to change.

Weaknesses

Although the PDS has good psychometric properties, its perception in earlier studies as an HRQOL instrument was inaccurate. This perception has now changed, such that in more recent studies it is referred to as a measure of ADL. This change has resulted from an increased knowledge among researchers as to the differences between ADL and HRQOL and their definitions. Although individual trials of tacrine demonstrated improvement on the PDS, a meta-analysis of 12 tacrine trials, including 1984 patients with AD, found that 'improvement on the PDS, largely an index of functional activities, was not significant'.[123] However, this may have been due to a lack of drug effect rather than a lack of sensitivity.

QOL-Alzheimer's Disease (QOL-AD)

Application

The QOL-AD[124] has been designed for use in AD and is interviewer-administered to the patient and self-administered to the carer, who fills it in as a proxy with reference to the patient's HRQOL. Research exploring the reliability and validity of this measure has been documented[125] along with a further study using this instrument in a larger population.[126]

Strengths

This instrument is short, simple and easy to complete and score. Internal consistency was good and test-retest reliability was acceptable for both patient and carer reports. These results were confirmed when the QOL-AD was tested in a larger population. The validity of the QOL-AD has been extensively explored by correlating it with a number of other measures including the Hamilton Depression Rating Scale (HDRS),[127,128] the Geriatric Depression Scale,[62] the Pleasant Events Schedule-AD (PES-AD),[102] the Physical Self Maintenance Scale (PSMS)[129] and the MMSE. The QOL-AD has been shown to be reliable and valid for use in individuals with MMSE scores between 10 and 28. Although the QOL-AD was designed for use in the US, preliminary evidence suggests it may also be of use in the UK following a full cross-cultural validation study.[130]

Weaknesses

Correlation between patient and carer reports was modest and was found to be less for patients with lower cognitive functioning. The composite score based on an arbitrary combination of carer-rated and patient-rated HRQOL weighted in the patient's favour, therefore it may require some conceptual justification as well as longitudinal validation. Evidence supporting the sensitivity of the QOL-AD has not yet been presented, although research is currently in progress to examine longitudinal data with a view to establishing this psychometric property.

Vienna List

Application

The Vienna List[131,132] is a recently developed instrument to measure clinical proxy-ratings (i.e. physicians and nurses) for old-old patients with severe dementia. Validity and reliability of this instrument is documented. The final version of the Vienna List consists of five factors: communication; negative effect; bodily contact; aggression; and mobility.

Strengths

A useful, differentiating, time-saving and practical tool for both severely demented patients and for the documentation of the outcome of old-old geriatric inpatient rehabilitation.

Weaknesses

The instrument's constructs are based on items generated by the target population but come from physicians and nurses. Responsiveness unsatisfactory.

ADDITIONAL INSTRUMENTS

In recent years, a number of existing HRQOL instruments have been tested in populations with dementia and new instruments have also been designed specifically for use in this disease area. A number of instruments used to measure quality of life in the literature did not meet the criteria set out by the authors earlier in this chapter, but have been briefly mentioned for the purposes of completeness. These measures include:

- Pearlman and Uhlmann's Patient QOL Ratings,[133,134] used in a study of elderly chronically ill patients[135] and a study looking at spousal life-sustaining treatment decisions in AD.[136]
- The Byrne–MacLean QOL Index[137] and the Cognitively Impaired Life Quality Scale (CILQ),[138] which are better defined as measuring quality of care rather than quality of life.
- The Squires Memory Questionnaire (SMQ),[139] which is actually a measure of memory function but was used, along with the SIP, to assess HRQOL in a study of levocarnitine.[55]
- The Italian Quality of Life Scale (IQLS)[140] that was used in a clinical trial of oxiracetam in dementia,[131] but was only available in Italian.
- The Guinot Behavioural Rating Scale[142] that was used in a clinical trial of *Ginkgo biloba* leaf extract preparation.[143]
- Yehuda's QOL Scale which was used in a study of the effect of an essential fatty acid preparation (SR-3) on the quality of life of patients with AD[139] with no prior or concurrent investigation of the measure's reliability, validity or sensitivity.
- The Lancashire Quality of Life Profile (Residential) (LQOLP(R)) which is an adaptation of the original LQOLP[145] that has been used in elderly cognitively impaired individuals,[146] but has not been tested psychometrically.
- The Duke health profile,[147] which has been translated into French[148] and used to measure quality of life in a sample of dementia patients.[149]

- The Physical Self Maintenance Scale (PSMS) and Instrumental Activities of Daily Living (IADL),[129] which are actually measures of ADL but have been used to measure HRQOL in clinical trials of tacrine.[111,112]

These measures have been discussed further in a review of quality of life measures used in dementia[12,13] but were not included here due to inadequate psychometric testing, limited use and experience in dementia or because they are not actually measuring quality of life. A number of different instruments and methodologies have been used to assess HRQOL in AD and, more generally, in populations suffering from dementia. The lack of consensus about how to measure HRQOL in AD has resulted in a number of questionnaires available that either do not include all the components that constitute HRQOL or are measuring a concept that is not actually HRQOL but a related notion. Methods of cost-effectiveness analysis suitable for drugs used in AD have been reviewed.[150] The authors of this paper compiled a list of those measures which seemed to be most in accordance with the HRQOL concept. Many of these instruments, including the Carer Hassles Scale,[151] the Revised Memory and Behaviour Problem Checklist,[147] the Burden Interview,[153] the OARS Multidimensional Functional Assessment Questionnaire,[154] the Barthel Index,[155] the Cleveland Scale for Activities of Daily Living[156] and the Nurses' Observation Scale for Geriatric Patients[157] have also not been reviewed here because they do not purport to measure HRQOL, although in some cases they do assess closely related ideas. It is the view of the authors that in order for an instrument to be classified as an HRQOL measure it must comprehensively assess all the components that constitute HRQOL.

INSTRUMENTS IN DEVELOPMENT

There are also some new measures being developed to assess quality of life in dementia which have not yet been fully documented in the literature. For example, the instrument being developed at the Research Institute for the Care of the Elderly in the UK that is exploring the direct assessment of patients with mild-to-moderate stage dementia. This project is using the novel approach of developing a brief screening tool to assess whether patients are capable of answering questions about their own quality of life, before developing and testing the quality of life instrument itself.

Other research in progress includes the development of a practical 'toolkit' of valid and reliable measures with which to measure outcome and evaluate clinical and psychosocial interventions for people with dementia.[158] This QOL toolkit is being developed for use with proxy informants, but will reflect the perspective of people with dementia.

HRQOL CONSIDERATIONS FOR INSTRUMENT SELECTION

When developing an instrument for dementia it is important to select items that are directly relevant to the patient and carer, and these items should be derived from information provided from these individuals. This process contributes to the instrument's content validity. Item reduction is performed by determining the frequency with which each item is identified as a problem and the relative importance of each of the items. This is often carried out by performing a factor analysis. The potential responsiveness of each item to change must also be evaluated and wording must be short, simple and unambiguous.

Reproducibility and reliability are interchangeable terms and this property must be demonstrated in order to ensure that changes in HRQOL measured are actually due to a real change and not just to random variations that occur when completing the instrument. This property may be demonstrated by administering the instrument to a group of subjects on two occasions over a short period, during which the state of the individuals must remain constant. This type of reliability is known as test-retest reliability and is only required for self-administered instruments. If the two sets of results obtained from this procedure correlate within the required parameters and discriminate consistently between individuals then it can be said that the instrument is precise in its measurement. It is also necessary to demonstrate that an instrument is internally consistent.

HRQOL measurement in dementia has only recently become a research priority and there is currently no instrument that can be considered the gold standard. It is therefore not possible to perform criterion validation and other methods of determining validity must be used. Construct validation is the most common and clinically relevant approach and involves comparing the HRQOL scores obtained with the results of other measures. In dementia this may be done by comparing the instrument with other assessment tools, e.g. measures of HRQOL, functional status or cognitive function. In order for the instrument to demonstrate construct validity, the functional component of the HRQOL measure should alter in the expected direction with changes in functional status and a shift in cognitive status should similarly affect the appropriate domains in the HRQOL measure.

In addition to the above measurement properties, an instrument designed to assess HRQOL in a chronic condition must be responsive to change, especially if it is to be used as an outcome measure in clinical trials. Such change might be due to deterioration over time or to a particular intervention. Therefore individual items should not only be relevant to the condition but also responsive to changes in that condition. Responsiveness or the power of the instrument to detect a real difference is also known as sensitivity.

HRQOL is a multidimensional concept but the use of more than one instrument in its assessment may increase the possibility of measurement errors. Therefore, incorporating these dimensions into a single instrument would appear to be the best approach to HRQOL assessment. It should also be remembered that a measure must be feasible for use as well as comprehensive and it may therefore be necessary to strike a balance between the two. Juniper and colleagues present a general approach to instrument development and testing that is robust and replicable and which, if followed, should produce satisfactory measurement properties.[159]

It should be noted that, although an instrument in developmental stages may not yet possess certain of the psychometric properties necessary for an HRQOL measure, research may be in progress that will subsequently demonstrate criteria that are not available at the present time. It should also be remembered that whenever an instrument is modified in some way, or is used in a manner that deviates from the intended methodology, then it must be revalidated.

ASSESSMENT OF CARER HRQOL IN DEMENTIA RESEARCH

The importance of considering the HRQOL of the carer as well as that of the patient in assessments of the impact of dementia and the effects of interventions must not be overlooked. Although there are numerous examples of methods used to assess carer HRQOL,[160–164] it is usually considered in isolation and not together with the HRQOL of the patient. There are also a number of other carer instruments that have been developed which are not described as HRQOL measures. Problems with definition may also lead to confusion. A number of researchers refer to 'stress', 'strain' or 'burden' as the primary outcomes to consider when assessing the impact of dementia on the carer.[165,166] A number of instruments have been developed to assess such outcomes that are often regarded

as synonymous with HRQOL.[167] Carer well-being is also a term discussed in some papers,[168,169] which is considered to be even closer to HRQOL than 'stress' or 'burden'.

It is essential to remember that the carer is integral to a demented patient's HRQOL and without the carer's input it is impossible to formulate meaningful and practical care plans. Any discussion of HRQOL and dementia must therefore include consideration of both patient and carer and the ideal assessment instrument will concurrently measure the impact of the disease on the everyday functioning and feelings of both.

FUTURE DIRECTIONS FOR HRQOL RESEARCH IN DEMENTIA

Alzheimer's disease and dementia is currently one of the most exciting areas of medical research, and the assessment of HRQOL in dementia is becoming increasingly important as drugs in development begin to reach the market place. As purchasers of healthcare becoming increasingly interested in HRQOL outcomes, healthcare providers must look more and more towards producing data that demonstrate that their products show real improvements in this area. The pharmaceutical industry needs to demonstrate a positive impact on HRQOL, not only to support licence applications to regulatory authorities, but also to facilitate marketing of new drugs and to encourage government acceptance and reimbursement of their products. However, it is not only pharmaceutical companies who wish to generate such data. HRQOL assessments are essential in providing a patient-orientated approach to evaluating healthcare services as well as demonstrating the impact of disease.

Despite the increasing emphasis on HRQOL in populations with dementia, efforts directed towards developing and using instruments in clinical trials have produced very few measures that are satisfactory in terms of validity, reliability, sensitivity and feasibility for use in this context. Some instruments are promising, based on initial results, and research should be focused on using these instruments, both cross-sectionally and longitudinally, in order to identify their strengths and weaknesses. Research efforts should concentrate on eliminating instrument weaknesses and building on the strengths identified to produce measures that are sensitive to change as well as being able to produce valid and reliable results. Head to head comparisons of HRQOL measures will help to identify the best measures for use in dementia research. Conceptual research should also be continued to explore new methods of assessing HRQOL in dementia. Extensive well-designed research efforts carried out to thoroughly establish the necessary psychometric criteria will ensure that HRQOL data can be accepted at face value, allowing comparisons between different therapeutic options to be made more easily. One must ensure that instruments chosen for use in dementia research are actually measuring HRQOL as well as possessing the necessary psychometric properties. As HRQOL instruments become established conceptually and psychometrically, new ways of collecting and presenting HRQOL data can be explored in order to facilitate its routine use in clinical research and practice.

The incorporation of HRQOL measures into routine clinical practice relies to a certain extent on the willingness of clinicians to use them. HRQOL instruments are often challenged on the grounds that they are 'soft' measures that are inferior to 'hard' physiological measures[170] and there is also a lack of familiarity on the part of physicians with these measures and their application in clinical practice. However, with systematic use of HRQOL instruments and a measure of optimism, physicians would be able to familiarise themselves with the assessment and use of HRQOL data in a similar way to new biomedical technology when it was first introduced.[171] The presentation of HRQOL data is also very important in improving acceptability of HRQOL measures to physicians. Statistical terminology may be of little meaning to physicians and HRQOL measurements must be linked to specific actions in terms of disease management where possible. If HRQOL data were converted into clinically useful indicators of improvement or deterioration that can be easily interpreted and acted upon, then it may be possible to encourage physicians to include this type of patient-based outcome which has traditionally been ignored. The interpretation of HRQOL data may be enhanced by using HRQOL profiles in the form of bar charts, separated into HRQOL domains that can be easily understood. HRQOL scores must also be easily interpreted in terms of measuring change over time for patients and carers. Research should therefore focus on evaluating and defining minimal clinically important differences. A minimal clinically important difference may be described as the smallest difference in a score in a domain of interest that is perceived as significant by the patient and that would mandate a change in the patient's clinical management. The clinical significance of a change is often evaluated by measuring the effect size, which is where the importance of a change is scaled by comparing the magnitude of the change to the variability in stable subjects, for example on

baseline or among untreated individuals. However, research looking at new ways of measuring the clinical significance of changes in HRQOL scores will help to increase the acceptability of HRQOL instruments by making them more interpretable and thus more relevant to the clinicians using them.

Resistance and attitudinal barriers to HRQOL assessment may also arise from a lack of information and education. The provision of clinician training and interpretation guides has been suggested[172] as a way of improving physicians' knowledge about this important outcome. In addition, the usefulness of HRQOL data should be demonstrated for the benefit of the patient and carer as well as for the physician. Patients and carers completing HRQOL measures must appreciate the purpose of the assessment.[173] More research demonstrating the importance of HRQOL information to patients, carers and physicians in the area of dementia is therefore indicated.

The acceptability of HRQOL measures to patients and carers should also be addressed. Instruments should also be relatively simple, of an appropriate length, completed within a reasonable time period and place minimal burden on the patient and carer. They should also be relevant to the condition and the setting in which they are to be used and user-friendly for both staff and patients.[174] The feasibility of collecting HRQOL data while waiting to see the physician has been explored[175] and is a way of increasing acceptability to patients and carers. Consideration of reading level, language barriers and illiteracy must be considered if HRQOL is to be assessed routinely for all patients and carers, and therefore interviewer-assisted methods should be made available. The exploitation of information technology in terms of touch-screen technology and the internet should also be investigated further.[176,177] With more and more people connecting to the internet every day, the development of internet versions of HRQOL instruments will become an increasingly useful approach.

This chapter would not be complete without mentioning the phenomenon of 'response shift'. This is a change in score due to a change in internal standards, in values or in conceptualisation of quality of life.[178] One can produce a response shift by facilitating coping processes which in turn leads to an improvement in quality of life.[179] This can be done by understanding the psychological, social and cultural context of an illness, ensuring effective physician–patient relationships and helping carers to cope by the provision of training by carer support groups, for example. In chronic diseases with limited treatment options, the goal of maximising HRQOL can be achieved by providing care and teaching coping strategies. This research area is still not fully understood but it has led to a new approach to HRQOL assessment with the goal of producing 'response shift' phenomena. This approach may be a future avenue of research for exploration in the context of dementia but, when evaluating the impact of treatments, it is necessary to distinguish objective change from changes in internal standards, in values or in the conceptualisation of quality of life.

CONCLUDING REMARKS

In today's climate of patient empowerment, there is an increasing focus on patient-based outcomes that will result in a greater emphasis on the assessment of HRQOL. Incorporating HRQOL measurement into routine practice will provide clinicians with a broader view of the effects of interventions while reflecting relevant outcomes. Such an outlook is especially important in dementia, where treatment options effecting a cure are non-existent and even treatments that delay the progression of the disease are still limited. The goal in such patients should be to achieve the best possible HRQOL for the remaining life they have left. Efforts to improve and maintain carer HRQOL are also necessary as in the long run this may delay institutionalization and improve HRQOL of the patient as well as saving on the costs of long-term care. HRQOL measures should strike a balance between symptoms and overall well-being and should relate to the original goal of the assessment as well as to the severity of dementia. Working partnerships should be developed between quality of life researchers, physicians, patients and carers with a view to fine tuning suitable HRQOL measures for the routine clinical assessment of patients with dementia and their carers.

In order to facilitate the integration of HRQOL data into routine clinical practice, research needs to clarify what new information is provided by HRQOL data and for which patients it is most useful. Physicians need to be informed how often HRQOL assessment results in a change in the management of the condition and whether such changes result in improved control or decreased adverse effects and whether an overall improvement in quality of life and an increased satisfaction with care are observed. In practice, those patients and carers with the worst HRQOL should be identified and more closely monitored. Support should be provided before carers reach the point of emotional breakdown. HRQOL assessment should be viewed by patients, carers and physicians as an opportunity to enhance communication by stimulating dialogue and improving the quality of interaction, with the ultimate aim of promoting a 'partnership culture' in the management of dementia.

REFERENCES

1. The Wellcome Trust Research directions in Alzheimer's disease. Wellcome News Suppl 1998; Q3(S):4.
2. Kluger A, Ferris SH. Scales for the assessment of Alzheimer's disease. Psychiatr Clin North Am 1991; 14:309–326.
3. Morgan CD, Baade LE. Neuropsychological testing and assessment scales for dementia of the Alzheimer's type. Psychiatr Clin North Am 1997; 20:25–43.
4. Ferris SH, Kluger A. Assessing cognition in Alzheimer's disease research. Alzheimer Dis Assoc Disord 1997; 11(suppl 6):45–49.
5. Ferris SH, Lucca U, Mohs R, et al. Objective psychometric tests in clinical trials of dementia drugs. Alzheimer Dis Assoc Disord 1997; 11(suppl 3):34–38.
6. Weiner MF, Koss E, Wild KV, et al. Measures of psychiatric symptoms in Alzheimer patients: a review. Alzheimer Dis Assoc Disord 1996; 10:20–30.
7. Ferris SH, Mackell JA. Behavioural outcomes in clinical trials for Alzheimer disease. Alzheimer Dis Assoc Disord 1997; 11(suppl 4):S10–S15.
8. Cummings JL. Changes in neuropsychiatric symptoms as outcome measures in clinical trials with cholinergic therapies for Alzheimer disease. Alzheimer Dis Assoc Disord 1997; 11(suppl 4):S1–S9.
9. Teunisse S. Activities of daily living scales in dementia: their development and future. In: Levy R, Howard R, eds. Developments in Dementia and Functional Disorders in the Elderly. Petersfield: Wrightson Biomedical Publishing 1995.
10. Reisberg B, Schneider L, Doody R, et al. Clinical global measures of dementia. Alzheimer Dis Assoc Disord 1997; 11(suppl 3):8–18.
11. Howard K, Rockwood K. Quality of life in Alzheimer's disease. Dementia 1995; 6:113–116.
12. Walker MD, Salek SS, Bayer AJ. A review of quality of life in Alzheimer's disease. Part 1: Issues in assessing disease impact. Pharmacoeconomics 1998; 14:499–530.
13. Salek SS, Walker MD, Bayer AJ. A review of quality of life in Alzheimer's disease. Part 2: Issues in assessing drug effects. Pharmacoeconomics 1998; 14:613–627.
14. Walker SR. Industry perspectives on quality of life. In: Walker SR, Rossor RM, eds. Quality of Life Assessment: Key Issues in the 1990s. London: Kluwer Academic Publishers, 1993; 383–392.
15. Coons SJ, Kaplan RM. Assessing health-related quality of life: application to drug therapy. Clin Therapeut 1992; 14:850–858.
16. Ramsay M, Winget C, Higginson I. Review: measures to determine the outcome of community services for people with dementia. Age Ageing 1995; 24:73–83.
17. Whitehouse PJ, Orgogozo JM, Becker RE, et al. Quality-of-life assessment in dementia drug development. Alzheimer Dis Assoc Disord 1997; 11(suppl 3):56–60.
18. Logsdon RG, Albert SM. Assessing quality of life in Alzheimer's disease: conceptual and methodological issues. J Ment Health Aging 1999; 5:3–6.
19. Zimmerman SI, Magaziner J. Methodological issues in measuring the functional status of cognitively impaired nursing home residents: the use of proxies and performance-based measures. Alzheimer Dis Assoc Disord 1994; 8(suppl 1): S281–S290.

20. Sprangers MAG, Aaronson NK. The role of health care providers and significant others in evaluating the quality of life of patients with chronic disease: a review. J Clin Epidemiol 1992; 45:743–760.

21. Magaziner J. Use of proxies to measure health and functional outcomes in effectiveness research in persons with Alzheimer's disease and related disorders. Alzheimer Dis Assoc Disord 1997; 77(suppl 6):168–174.

22. Rabins PV, Mace HL, Lucas MJ. The impact of dementia on the family. JAMA 1982; 248:333–335.

23. Levin E, Sinclair I, Gorbach P. Families, Services and Confusion in Old Age. Aldershot: Gower Publishing Group, 1989; 1–328.

24. Blau TH. Quality of Life, social indicators and criteria of change. Prof Psycho 1977; 8:464–473.

25. Rogers SL, Friedhoff LT, Apter JT, et al. The efficacy and safety of donepezil in patients with Alzheimer's disease: results of a US multicentre, randomized, double-blind, placebo-controlled trial. Dementia 1996; 7:293–303.

26. Rogers SL, Farlow MR, Doody RS, et al. A 24-week, double-blind, placebo-controlled trial of donepezil in patients with Alzheimer's disease. Neurology 1998; 50:136–145.

27. Burns A, Rossor M, Hecker J, et al. The effects of donepezil in Alzheimer's disease – results from a multinational trial. Dementia Geriatr Cogn Disord 1999; 10:237–244.

28. Ware JE, Sherbourne CD. The MOS 36-item Short-Form health status survey 1: Conceptual framework and item selection. Med Care 1992; 30:473–483.

29. Ware JE, Snow KK, Kosinski M, et al. SF-36 Health Survey Manual and Interpretation Guide. Boston: New England Medical Center, The Health Institute, 1993.

30. Brazier JE, Harper R, Jones NMB, et al. Validating the SF-36 health survey questionnaire: new outcome measure for primary care. BMJ 1992; 205:160–164.

31. Jenkinson C, Wright L, Coulter A. Quality of Life Measurement in Health Care: A Review of Measures, and Population Norms for the UK SF-36. Oxford: Health Services Research Unit, Department of Public Health and Primary Care, University of Oxford, Joshua Horgan Print Partnership, 1993.

32. Parker SG, Peet SM, Jagger C, et al. Measuring health status in older patients. The SF-36 in practice. Age Ageing 1998; 27:13–18.

33. Hill S, Harries U, Popay J. Is the short form 36 (SF-36) suitable for routine health outcomes assessment in health care for older people? Evidence from preliminary work in community based health services in England. J Epidemiol Commun Health 1996; 50:94–98.

34. Riemsma RP, Forbes CA, Glanville JM, et al. General health status measures for people with cognitive impairment: learning disability and acquired brain injury. Health Technol Assess 2001; 5:1–100.

35. Gwyn Seymour D, Ball AE, Russell EM, et al. Problems using health survey questionnaires in older patients with physical disabilities. The reliability and validity of the SF-36 and the effect of cognitive impairment. J Eval Clin Pract 2001; 7:411–418.

36. Kendrick AM, Trimble MR. Repertory Grid in the assessment of quality of life in patients with epilepsy. In: Trimble MR, Dodson WE, eds. Epilepsy and Quality of Life. New York: Raven Press, 1994.

37. Selai CE, Trimble MR. Adjunctive therapy in epilepsy with the new antiepileptic drugs: is it of any value? Seizure 1998; 7:417–418.

38. Selai CE, Trimble M, Rossor M, Harvey RJ. The Quality of Life Assessment Schedule (QOLAS): a new method for assessing quality of life (QOL) in dementia; In: Logsdon R, Albert S, eds. Assessing Quality of Life in Dementia. New York: Springer, 2000; 31–48.

39. Selai CE, Trimble M, Rossor M, et al. Assessing quality of life (QOL) in dementia: the feasibility and validity of the Quality of Life Assessment Schedule (QOLAS). Neuropsychol Rehab 2001; 11:219–243.

40. Folstein MF, Folstein SE, McHugh PR. 'Mini-Mental State' a practical method for grading the cognitive state of patients for the clinician. J Psychiatr Res 1975; 12:189–198.

41. O'Boyle CA. The Schedule for the Evaluation of Individual Quality of Life (SEIQOL): Administration Manual. Dublin: Royal College of Surgeons in Ireland, 1993.

42. O'Boyle CA. The Schedule for the Evaluation of Individual Quality of Life (SEIQoL). Int J Ment Health 1994; 23:3–23.

43. Meier D, Hiltbrunner B, Joyce CRB, et al. Assessment of individual quality of life in geriatric patients. Proceedings of the XVth Congress of the International Association of Gerontology. Budapest, Hungary, 1993.

44. Coen R, O'Mahony D, O'Boyle C, et al. Measuring the quality of life of dementia patients using the Schedule for the Evaluation of Individual Quality of Life. Irish J Psychol 1993; 14:154–163.

45. Scholzel-Dorenbos CJ. Measurement of quality of life in patients with dementia of Alzheimer type and their caregivers: Schedule for the Evaluation of Individual Quality of Life (SEIQoL). Tijdschr Gerontol Geriatr 2000; 31:23–26.

46. Roth M, Huppert FA, Tym E, et al. CAMDEX: the Cambridge Examination for Mental Disorders in the Elderly. Cambridge: Cambridge University Press, 1988.

47. Hickey AM, Bury G, O'Boyle CA. A new short form individual quality of life measure (SEIQoL-DW): application in a cohort of individuals with HIV/AIDS. BMJ 1996; 313: 29–33.

48. Prince PN, Gerber GJ. Measuring subjective quality of life in people with serious mental illness using the SEIQoL-DW. Qual Life Res 2001; 10:117–122.

49. Diener E, Emmons R, Larsen J, Griffin S. The Satisfaction With Life Scale. J Personality Assess 1985; 49:71–75.

50. Frisch MB. The Quality of Life Inventory. NCS Assessments, NCS Pearson Inc, Minneapolis 2001. Available at http://assessments.ncs.com/assessments/tests/qoli [accessed 4 Jan 2006].

51. Bergner M, Bobbitt RA, Kressel S, et al. The Sickness Impact Profile: conceptual formulation and methodology for the development of a health status measure. Int J Health Serv 1976; 6:393–415.

52. Bergner M, Bobbitt RA, Carter WB, et al. The Sickness Impact Profile: development and final revision of a health status measure. Med Care 1981; 19:787–805.

53. Krenz C, Larson EB, Buchner DM, et al. Characterizing patient dysfunction in Alzheimer's-type dementia. Med Care 1988; 26:453–461.

54. Teri L, McCurry SM, Buchner DM, et al. Exercise and activity level in Alzheimer's disease: a potential treatment focus. J Rehab Res Develop 1998; 35:411–419.

55. Sano M, Bell K, Cote L, et al. Double-blind parallel design pilot study of acetyl levocarnitine in patients with Alzheimer's disease. Arch Neurol 1992; 49:1137–1141.

56. Blessed G, Tomlinson BF, Roth M. The association between quantitative measures of dementia and of senile change in the cerebral grey matter of elderly subjects. Br J Psychiatry 1968; 114:797–811.

57. Gerety MB, Cornell JE, Mulrow CD, et al. The Sickness Impact Profile for Nursing Homes (SIP-NH). J Gerontol 1994; 49:M2–M8.

58. Dhanda R, Mulrow CD, Gerety MB, et al. Classifying change with the Sickness Impact Profile for Nursing Homes (SIP-NH). Aging (Milano) 1995; 7:228–233.

59. Salek MS. Development, Validation and Clinical Validation of a Health-Related Quality of Life Instrument. PhD University of Wales, Cardiff, 1990.

60. Salek MS, Thomas S, Luscombe DK, Bayer AJ. The impact of memory clinic assessment on the quality of life of patients with cognitive decline: Sensitivity of the UK Sickness Impact Profile. Pharmacy World Sci 1993; 15(suppl G):G15.

61. Salek MS, Griffith AR, Spiller C, Luscombe DK, Bayer AJ. Assessment of quality of life in patients with dementia: which measure? Pharmacy World Sci 1994; 16(suppl G): G12.

62. Yesavage JA, Brink TL, Rose TL, et al. Development and validation of a geriatric depression screening scale: a preliminary report. J Psychiatr Res 1982; 17:37–49.

63. Gerety MB, Mulrow CD, Tuley MR, et al. Development and validation of a physical performance instrument for the functionally impaired elderly: the Physical Disability Index (PDI). J Gerontol Med Sci 1993; 48:M33–M39.

64. Katz S, Ford AB, Moskowitz RW, et al. Studies of illness in the aged. The index of ADL: a standardised measure of biological and psychosocial function. JAMA 1963; 185:914–919.

65. World Health Organization. The World Health Organization Quality of Life Assessment (WHOQOL): development and general psychometric properties. Soc Sci Med 1998; 46:1569–1585.

66. Struttmann T, Fabro M, Romieu G, et al. Quality-of-life assessment in the old using the WHOQOL 100: differences between patients with senile dementia and patients with cancer. Int Psychogeriatr 1999; 11:273–279.

67. The EuroQol Group. EuroQol – a new facility for the measurement of health-related quality of life. Health Policy 1990; 16:199–208.

68. Hurst NP, Jobanputra P, Hunter M, et al. Validity of EuroQoL: a generic health status instrument in patients with rheumatoid arthritis. Br J Rheumatol 1994; 33:655–662.

69. Hollingworth W, Mackenzie R, Todd CJ, Dixon AK. Measuring changes in quality of life following magnetic resonance imaging of the knee: SF-36, EuroQoL or Rosser index? Qual Life Res 1995; 4:325–334.

70. Sculpher M, Dwyer N, Byford S, Stirrat G. Randomised trial comparing hysterectomy and transcervical endometrial resection: effect on health-related quality of life and costs two years after surgery. Br J Obstet Gynaecol 1996; 103: 142–194.

71. Coucill W, Bryan S, Bentham P, et al. EQ-5D in patients with dementia: an investigation of inter-rater agreement. Med Care 2001; 39:760–771.

72. Selai CE. Using the EuroQol EQ-5D in dementia. In: Rabin RE, Busschbach JJV, de Charro FTH, Essink-Bot ML, Bonsel GJ, eds. Proceedings of the EuroQol Plenary Meeting. Rotterdam: Erasmus University, 1997.

73. Brazier J, Jones N, Kind P. Testing the validity of the EuroQoL and comparing it with the SF-36 health survey questionnaire. Qual Life Res 1993; 2:169–180.

74. Van Agt H, Essink-Bot ML, Krabbe P, Bonsel G. Test-retest reliability of health state valuations collected with the EuroQoL questionnaire. Soc Sci Med 1994; 39:1537–1544.

75. Essink-Bot ML, Krabbe P, Bonsel G, Aaronson N. An empirical comparison of four generic health status measures: the Nottingham health profile, the medical outcomes study 36-item short-form health survey, the COOP/ WONCA charts, and the EuroQoL instrument. Med Care 1997; 35:522–537.

76. Feeny DH, Torrance GW, Furlong WJ. Health Utilities Index. In: Spilker B, ed. Quality of Life and Pharmacoeconomics in Clinical Trials, 2nd edn. Philadelphia: Lippincott-Raven, 1996: 239–252.

77. Torrance GW, Feeny DH, Furlong WJ, et al. Multi-attribute preference functions for a comprehensive health status classification system: Health Utilities Index Mark 2. Med Care 1996; 24:702.

78. Furlong W, Feeny D, Torrance GW, et al. Multiplicative Multi-Attribute Utility Function for the Health Utilities Index Mark 3 (HUI3) System: A Technical Report. McMaster University Centre for Health Economics and Policy Analysis Working Paper No. 98-11.

79. Neumann PJ, Kuntz KM, Leon J, et al. Health utilities in Alzheimer's disease: a cross-sectional study of patients and caregivers. Med Care 1999; 37:27–32.

80. Ikeda S, Yamada Y, Uemura T, Ikegami N. Health utilities of patients with Alzheimer's disease in Japan. Qual Life Res 2000; 9:1675.

81. Neumann PJ, Sandberg EA, Araki SS, et al. A comparison of HUI2 and HUI3 utility scores in Alzheimer's disease. Med Decision Making 2000; 20:413–422.

82. Morris JC. The Clinical Dementia Rating (CDR): current version and scoring rules. Neurology 1993; 34:2412.

83. Kaplan RM, Bush JW. Health-related quality of life measurement for evaluation research and policy analysis. Health Psychol 1982; 1:61–80.

84. Kaplan RM, Bush JW, Berry CC. Health status: types of validity and the Index of Well-Being. Health Serv Res 1976; 11:478–507.

85. Fanshel S, Bush JW. A Health-Status Index and its application to health-services outcomes. Op Res 1970; 18: 1021–1065.

86. Wimo A, Mattson B, Krakau I, et al. Cost-utility analysis of group living in dementia care. Int J Technol Assess Health Care 1995; 11:49–65.

87. Reisberg B, Ferris SH, de Leon MJ, Crook T. The Global Deterioration Scale for assessment of primary degenerative dementia. Am J Psychiatry 1982; 139:1136–1139.

88. Kerner DN, Patterson TL, Grant I, et al. Validity of the Quality of Well-Being Scale for patients with Alzheimer's disease. J Aging Health 1998; 10:44–61.

89. Rabins PV, Kasper JD, Kleinman L, Black BS, Patrick DP. Concepts and methods in the development of the ADRQL: an instrument for assessing health-related quality of life in persons with Alzheimer's disease. J Ment Health Aging 1999; 5:33–48.

90. Gonzalez-Salvador T, Lyketsos CG, Baker A, et al. Quality of life in dementia patients in long-term care. Int J Geriatr Psychiatry 2000; 15:181–189.

91. Salek SS, Walker MD, Bayer AJ. The community dementia quality of life profile (CDQLP): a factor analysis. Qual Life Res 1999; 8:660.

92. Walker MD, Salek SS, Bayer AJ. The reliability of the community dementia quality of life profile (CDQLP). Qual Life Res 2000; 9:329.

93. Walker MD, Salek SS, Bayer AJ. Assessing patient and carer quality of life (QOL) in dementia: validating the concept of a composite measure. Age Ageing 2001; 30(suppl 2):61.

94. Walker MD, Salek SS, Bayer AJ. The relationship between the quality of life (QOL) of dementia patients and their carers: validation of the community dementia quality of life profile (CDQLP). Age Ageing 2001; 30 (suppl 2):62.

95. Salek SS, Sharp JK, Bayer AJ, Walker MD, Luscombe DK. Quality of life measurement in Alzheimer's patients and their carers: a comparison between statutory and non-statutory care services. European Society of Clinical Pharmacy 28th European Symposium on Clinical Pharmacy: Bridging the Gaps – The Future of Clinical Pharmacy 1999; 5-A. Berlin, Germany.

96. Walker MD, Salek SS, Bayer AJ. Quality of life in community practice: assessing patient needs in dementia. European Society of Clinical Pharmacy: 2nd Spring Conference on Clinical Pharmacy 2001; 15-A. Malta.

97. Ready RE, Ott BR, Grace J, et al. The Cornell-Brown Scale for quality of life in dementia. Alzheimer Dis Assoc Disord 2002; 16:109–115.

98. Ready RE, Ott BR. Quality of life measures for dementia. Health Qual Life Outcomes 2003; 1:11–19.

99. Smith SC, Lamping DL, Banerjee S, et al. Measurement of health-related quality of life for people with dementia: development of a new instrument (DEMQOL) and an evaluation of current methodology. Health Technol Assess 2005; 9:1–93.

100. Brod M, Stewart A, Sands L, et al. The Dementia Quality of Life Rating Scale (D-QoL). Gerontologist 1996; 36(special issue 1):257.

101. Brod M, Stewart AL, Sands L, et al. Conceptualisation and measurement of quality of life in dementia: the Dementia Quality of Life instrument (DQoL). Gerontologist 1999; 39:25–35.

102. Teri L, Logsdon RG. Identifying pleasant activities for Alzheimer's disease patients: The Pleasant Events Schedule-AD. Gerontologist 1991; 31:124–127.

103. Albert SM, Castillo-Castanada C, Sano M, et al. Quality of life in patients with Alzheimer's disease as reported by patient proxies. J Am Geriatr Soc 1996; 44:1342–1347.

104. Lawton MP. Quality of life in Alzheimer's disease. Alzheimer Dis Assoc Disord 1994; 8(suppl 3):138–150.

105. Erickson P, Wilson RW, Seitz F, et al. Years of healthy life: a measure of healthy life span for Health People 2000. In: Proceedings of the 1993 Public Health Conference on Records and Statistics. Bethesda, MD: Centers for Disease Control and Prevention, 1993; 21–27.

106. Albert SM, Castillo-Castanada C, Jacobs DM, et al. Proxy-reported quality of life in Alzheimer's patients: comparison of clinical and population-based samples. J Ment Health Aging 1999; 5:47–58.

107. Albert SM, Jacobs DM, Sano M, et al. Longitudinal study of quality of life in people with advanced Alzheimer's disease. Am J Geriatr Psychiatry 2001; 9:160–168.

108. Albert SM, Marks J, Barrett V, et al. Home health care and quality of life of patients with Alzheimer's disease. Am J Prevent Med 1997; 13:63–68.

109. Stern Y, Sano M, Paulson J, et al. Modified Mini-Mental State Examination: validity and reliability. Neurology 1987; 37(suppl):179.

110. Dejong R, Osterlund OW, Roy GW. Measurement of quality of life changes in patients with Alzheimer's disease. Clin Ther 1989; 11:545–554.

111. Davis KL, Thal LJ, Gamzu ER, et al. A double-blind, placebo-controlled multicenter study of tacrine for Alzheimer's disease. N Engl J Med 1992; 327:1253–1259.

112. Farlow M, Gracon SI, Hershey LA, et al. A controlled trial of tacrine in Alzheimer's disease. JAMA 1992; 268: 2523–2529.

113. Knapp MJ, Knopman DS, Solomon PR, et al. A 30-week randomized controlled trial of high-dose tacrine in patients with Alzheimer's disease. JAMA 1994; 271:985–991.

114. Vincent SA, Harvey RJ. The ADENA Programme. Clinical Advances in Drug Development: Alzheimer's Disease Trial Design. Sevenoaks: Medpress, 1998.

115. Corey-Bloom J, Anand R, Veach J. A randomised trial evaluating the efficacy and safety of ENA 713 (rivastigmine tartrate), a new acetylcholinesterase inhibitor, in patients with mild to moderately severe Alzheimer's disease. Int J Geriatr Psychopharmacol 1998; 1:55–65.

116. Rosler M, Anand R, Cicin-Sain A, et al. Efficacy and safety of rivastigmine in patients with Alzheimer's disease: international randomised controlled trial. BMJ 1999; 318: 633–638.

117. Kumar V, Anand R, Messina J, et al. An efficacy and safety analysis of Exelon in Alzheimer's disease patients with concurrent vascular risk factors. Eur J Neurol 2000; 7: 159–169.

118. Farlow MR, Hake A, Messina J, et al. Response of patients with Alzheimer disease to rivastigmine treatment is predicted by the rate of disease progression. Arch Neurol 2001; 58:417–422.

119. Winblad B, Engedal K, Soininen H, et al. A 1-year, randomized, placebo-controlled study of donepezil in patients with mild to moderate AD. Neurology 2001; 57:489–495.

120. Wilkinson D, Murray J. Galantamine: a randomized, double-blind, dose comparison in patients with Alzheimer's disease. Int J Geriatr Psychiatry 2001; 16:852–857.

121. Gottwald MD, Rozanski RI. Rivastigmine, a brain-region selective acetylcholinesterase inhibitor for treating Alzheimer's disease: review and current status. Expert Opin Invest Drugs 1999; 8:1673–1682.

122. Birks J, Grimley Evans J, Iakovidou V, et al. Rivastigmine for Alzheimer's disease. Cochrane Database Syst Rev 2000; CD001191.

123. Qizilbash N, Whitehead A, Higgins J, et al. Cholinesterase inhibition for Alzheimer's disease: a meta-analysis of the tacrine trials. Dementia Trialists' Collaboration. JAMA 1998; 280:1777–1782.

124. Logsdon RG. Quality of life in Alzheimer's disease: implications for research. Gerontologist 1996; 36(special issue 1): 278.

125. Logsdon RG, Gibbons LE, McCurry SM, et al. Quality of life in Alzheimer's disease: patient and caregiver reports. J Ment Health Aging 1999; 5:21–32.

126. Logsdon RG, Gibbons LE, McCurry SM, Teri L. Assessing quality of life in older adults with cognitive impairment. Psychosom Med 2002; 64:510–519.

127. Hamilton M. Development of a rating scale for primary depressive illness. Br J Soc Clin Psychol 1967; 6:278–296.

128. Hamilton M. A rating scale for depression. J Neurol Neurosurg Psychiatry 1960; 23:56–62.

129. Lawton MP, Brody EM. Assessment of older people: self-maintaining and instrumental activities of daily living. Gerontologist 1969; 9:176–186.

130. Selai C, Harvey RJ, Logsdon R. Using the QOL-AD in the UK. Int J Geriatr Psychiatry 2001; 16:537–542.

131. Porzsolt F, Kojer M, Schmidl M, et al. A new instrument to describe indicators of well-being in old-old patients with severe dementia – the Vienna List. Health Qual Life Outcomes 2004; 19:10–18.

132. Richter J, Schwarz M, Eisemann M, et al. Validation of the Vienna List as a proxy measure of quality of life for geriatric rehabilitation patients. Qual Life Res 2004; 13: 1725–1735.

133. Uhlmann R, Pearlman R. Perceived quality of life and preferences for life-sustaining treatment in older adults. Arch Intern Med 1991; 151:495–497.

134. Pearlman R, Uhlmann R. Patient and physician perceptions of patient quality of life in chronic diseases. J Gerontol 1988; 43:M25–M30.

135. Pearlman RA, Uhlmann RF. Quality of life in elderly, chronically ill outpatients. J Gerontol 1991; 46:M31–M38.

136. Mezey M, Kluger M, Maislin G, et al. Life-sustaining treatment decisions by spouses of patients with Alzheimer's disease. J Am Geriatr Soc 1996; 44:144–150.

137. Byrne H, MacLean D. Quality of life: perceptions of residential care. Int J Nurs Pract 1997; 3:21–28.

138. DeLetter MC, Tully CL, Wilson JF, et al. Nursing staff perceptions of quality of life of cognitively impaired elders: instrumental development. J Appl Gerontol 1995; 14: 426–443.

139. Squire LR, Wetzel CD, Slater PC. Memory complaint after electroconvulsive therapy: assessment with a new self-rating instrument. Biol Psychiatry 1979; 14:791–801.

140. Sarao MV, Ricci C, Peri G, et al. Valutazione del livello di autonomia nelle demenze. Psich Med 1987; 3:44–46 (Italian).

141. Bottini G, Vallar G, Cappa S, et al. Oxiracetam in dementia: a double-blind, placebo-controlled study. Acta Neurol Scand 1992; 86:237–241.

142. Guinot P, Wesnes K. A quality of life scale for the elderly: validation by factor analysis. ICRS Med Sci 1985; 13: 965.

143. Wesnes K, Simmons D, Rook M, et al. A double-blind placebo-controlled trial of Tanakan in the treatment of idiopathic cognitive impairment in the elderly. Hum Psychopharmacol Clin Exp 1987; 2:159–169.

144. Yehuda S, Rabinovtz S, Carasso RL, et al. Essential fatty acids preparation (SR-3) improves Alzheimer's patients' quality of life. Int J Neurosci 1996; 87:141–149.

145. Oliver J, Huxley P, Bridges K, et al. Quality of Life and Mental Health Services. London: Routledge, 1996.

146. Godlove Mozely C, Huxley P, Sutcliffe C, et al. 'Not knowing where I am doesn't mean I don't know what I like': cognitive impairment and quality of life responses in elderley people. Int J Geriatr Psychiatry 1999; 14:776–783.

147. Parkerson GR, Broadhead WE, Tse CK. The Duke health profile. A 17-item measure of health and dysfunction. Med Care 1990; 28:1056–1072.

148. Guillemin F, Paul-Dauphin A, Virion JM, et al. The Duke health profile: a generic instrument to measure the quality of life tied to health. Sante Publique 1997; 9:35–44.

149. Novella J, Ankri J, Morrone I, et al. Evaluation of the quality of life in dementia with a generic quality of life questionnaire: the Duke health profile. Dement Geriatr Cogn Disord 2001; 12:158–166.

150. Busschbach JJ, Brouwer WB, Van der Donk A. An outline for a cost-effectiveness analysis of a drug for patients with Alzheimer's disease. Pharmacoeconomics 1998; 13:21–24.

151. Kinney J, Stephens MAP. Caregiver Hassles Scale: assessing the daily hassles of caring for a family member with dementia. Gerontologist 1989; 29:328–332.

152. Teri L, Truax P, Logsdon R, et al. Assessment of behavioural problems in dementia: the Revised Memory and Behavior Problems Checklist. Psychol Aging 1992; 7: 622–631.

153. Zarit SH, Reever KE, Bach-Peterson J. Relatives of the impaired elderly: correlates of feelings of burden. Gerontologist 1980; 20:649–655.

154. Teri L, Borson S, Kiyak HA, et al. Behavioral disturbance, cognitive dysfunction and functional skill: prevalence and relationship in Alzheimer's disease. J Am Geriatr Soc 1989; 37:109–116.

155. Mahoney FI, Barthel DW. Functional evaluation: the Barthel Index. MD State Med J 1965; 14:61–65.

156. Patterson MB, Mack JL, Neundorfer MM, et al. Assessment of functional ability in Alzheimer's disease: a review and a preliminary report on the Cleveland Scale for Activities of Daily Living. Alzheimer Dis Assoc Disord 1992; 6:145–163.

157. Spiegel R, Brunner C, Ermini-Funfschilling D, et al. A new behavioral assessment scale for geriatric out- and in-patients: the NOSGER (Nurses' Observational Scale for Geriatric Patients). J Am Geriatr Soc 1991; 39:339–347.

158. Corner L, Bond J. Quality of life (QOL) of people with dementia and their informal caregivers: involving 'customers' in the process of research. Clin Neuropsychol Assess 2000; 1:8.

159. Juniper EF, Guyatt GH, Jaeschke R. How to develop and validate a new health-related quality of life instrument. In: Spilker B, ed. Quality of Life and Pharmacoeconomics in Clinical Trials, 2nd edn. Philadelphia: Lippincott-Raven Publishers, 1996; 49–56.

160. Shulman KI, Cohen CA. Quality of life and economic aspects of community support programs for caregivers of dementia patients. Am J Geriatr Psychiatry 1993; 1:211–220.

161. Draper BM, Poulos CJ, Cole AMD, et al. A comparison of caregivers for elderly stroke and dementia victims. J Am Geriatr Soc 1992; 40:896–901.

162. Draper BM, Poulos RG, Poulos CJ, et al. Risk factors for stress in elderly caregivers. Int J Geriatr Psychiatry 1995; 11: 227–231.

163. Hinchliffe AC, Livingstone G. Carers of people with dementia: can their mental health be improved? Prim Care Psychiatry 1995; 1:249–254.

164. Mohide EA, Torrance GW, Streiner DL, et al. Measuring the well-being of family caregivers using the time trade-off technique. J Clin Epidemiol 1988; 41:475–482.

165. Kosberg JI, Cairl RE, Keller DM. Components of burden: interventive implications. Gerontologist 1990; 30:236–242.

166. Vitaliano PP, Russo J, Young HM, et al. The screen for caregiver burden. Gerontologist 1991; 31:76–83.

167. Donaldson C, Tarrier N, Burns A. The impact of the symptoms of dementia on caregivers. Br J Psychiatry 1997; 170: 62–68.

168. George LK, Gwyther LP. Caregiver well-being: a multidimensional examination of family caregivers of demented adults. Gerontologist 1986; 26:253–259.

169. Clipp EC, George LK. Dementia and cancer: a comparison of spouse caregivers. Gerontologist 1993; 33:534–541.

170. Deyo RA. The quality of life, research and care. Ann Intern Med 1991; 114:695–696.

171. Faden R, Leplege A. Assessing quality of life: moral implications for clinical practice. Med Care 1992; 30: MS166–MS175.

172. Rubenstein LV, Calkins DR, Young RT, et al. Improving patient function: a randomized trial of functional disability screening. Ann Int Med 1989; 111:836–842.

173. Long AF, Scott DL. Measuring health status and outcomes in rheumatoid arthritis within routine clinical practice. Br J Rheumatol 1994; 33:682–685.

174. Ganz PA. Impact of quality of life outcomes on clinical practice. Oncology 1995; 9(suppl 11):61–65.

175. Grudzinski AN, Hakim Z, Coons SJ, Labiner DM. Use of the QOLIE-31 in routine clinical practice. J Epilepsy 1998; 11:34–47.

176. Roizen MF, Coalson D, Hayward RS, et al. Can patients use an automated questionnaire to define their current health status? Med Care 1999; 30:MS74–MS84.

177. Velikova G, Wright EP, Smith AB, et al. Automated collection of quality of life data: a comparison of paper and computer-touchscreen questionnaires. J Clinl Oncol 1999; 17:996–1007.

178. Schwartz CE, Sprangers MAG. Methodological approaches for assessing response shift in longitudinal health-related quality-of-life research. Soc Sci Med 1999; 48:1531–1548.

179. Wilson IB. Clinical understanding and clinical implications of response shift. Soc Sci Med 1999; 48:1577–1588.

VII   Conclusion

29

Future diagnosis and management of Alzheimer's disease

Serge Gauthier, Leon L Thal and Martin N Rossor

DIAGNOSTIC ISSUES

The diagnosis of Alzheimer's disease (AD) is and will remain primarily clinical. Current diagnostic criteria (Chapter 1) and methods of assessment (Chapters 4 and 5) highlight the importance of a systematic history, physical and neurological examination, complemented by appropriate neuropsychological assessments (Chapter 6), structural (Chapter 7) and functional (Chapter 8) brain imaging studies, as well as electrophysiological (Chapter 9) and biological (Chapter 10) tests. The clinical diagnosis of AD takes time and patience, and often requires repeated visits, but all interested clinicians should be able to recognize the typical pattern of AD progression (Figure 29.1). Atypical presentations such as early appearance of aphasia, visual hallucinations or gait impairment suggest a non-AD dementia (Chapter 5) and may require a consultation in a specialized setting.

Persons with mild cognitive complaints are increasingly seeking advice as to their risk of having AD. It was fitting to add the new chapter on mild cognitive impairment (MCI) and very early stage AD (Chapter 17). The concept of MCI may lead to earlier diagnosis of AD, at a stage where there is still minimal functional impairment. An update of diagnostic criteria, particularly that of the Diagnostic and Statistical Manual and of the National and Communicative Disorders and Stroke–Alzheimer's Disease and Related Disorders Association (NINCDS-ADRDA) may now be possible, although caution is required in using MCI as a diagnosis, considering its heterogeneity and reversibility.[1]

Does apolipoprotein E (apoE) polymorphism matter? Yes in the case of amnestic MCI, where the risk of progression to a formal diagnosis of AD is greatly increased for carriers of apoE4 compared with apoE3.[2] On the other hand, current guidelines do not advocate genotyping asymptomatic persons or patients with MCI for apoE status (Chapter 27). In patients with atypical presentations of dementia, this can be considered as an optional test, since dementia

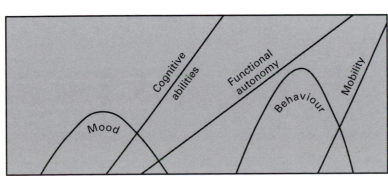

Figure 29.1 The intensity of symptoms in various domains throughout the progression of Alzheimer's disease

is more likely caused by AD in apoE4 carriers (Chapter 1).

Mixed dementias (AD with cerebrovascular features or AD with Parkinson features) are common both clinically and pathologically. Many risk factors are similar for these conditions, particularly vascular risk factors (Chapters 2 and 3), which are amenable to treatment (Table 29.1).

Finally, many asymptomatic persons come forward to their physicians with the hope of a preventive approach to AD. The assessment of risk will become more systematic (Table 29.2) as more data become available from ongoing cohort studies, and will be justified in the near future by evidence-based preventive therapies.

Table 29.1 Vascular risk factors relevant to Alzheimer's disease

- Systolic hypertension in midlife
- Diabetes mellitus
- Hypercholesterolaemia
- Atrial fibrillation
- Obesity
- Smoking

Table 29.2 Assessment of risk towards Alzheimer's disease in asymptomatic persons

- Family history
- Genetic polymorphisms (apoE)
- Biological markers (CSF total tau, β42)
- Neuropsychological tests (delayed recall)
- Neuroimaging (hippocampal volume)

NATURAL HISTORY

The natural history of AD has been well studied and can be summarized in Figure 29.2 as a sequence of disease milestones. Some of these can be a target for treatment, with good face validity and potential impact on cost of care.[3]

The progression of AD has been staged using different instruments reviewed in Chapters 12 and 15, the best known being the 7-stage Global Deterioration Scale.[4] Symptomatic domains in dementia include cognition (Chapter 14), activities of daily living (ADL; Chapter 15), mood (Chapter 13) and behaviour (Chapter 16). In many patients early changes in mood and anxiety precede the formal diagnosis of AD, with spontaneous improvement as insight about the disease is lost. Cognitive and ADL decline are relatively linear over time, whereas neuropsychiatric symptoms peak midway into the disease course and improve spontaneously through the severe stage as mobility becomes more and more impaired with emerging Parkinson-like physical signs (Figure 29.1). Knowledge of these changes over time will help the clinician plan ahead for the difficulties facing the patient and family. Some patients may progress at a faster rate than others (Chapter 11).

MANAGEMENT

A comprehensive management of AD includes an accurate diagnosis, education of the patient and family about the natural history and about available resources (Chapters 23 and 24), treatment of concomitant diseases (Chapter 21), treatment of depression and other neuropsychiatric symptoms (Chapter 22) and treatment with AD-specific medications (Chapters 18 and 19). There are ethical (Chapter 25) issues at every stage of disease, including management of the terminal stage

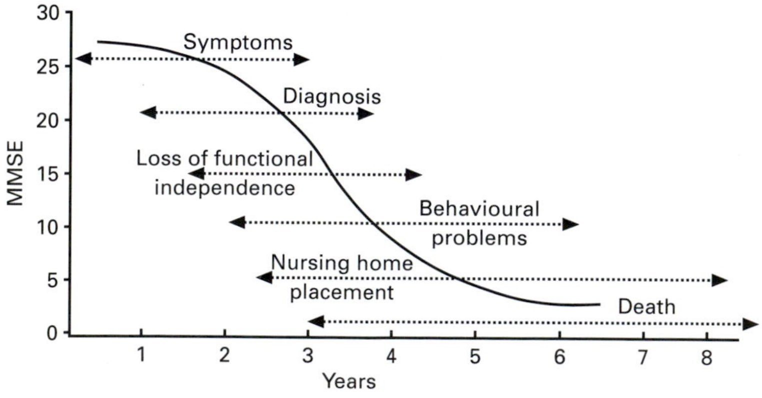

Figure 29.2 Natural history of Alzheimer's disease

(Chapter 20); loss of competency must be planned for (Chapter 26) and, although difficult to measure in AD, quality of life must be a paramount consideration in the management of this progressive condition (Chapter 28).

There has been much improvement in available symptomatic drugs over the past 10 years, with the licensing of three cholinesterase inhibitors (CIs) and of the NMDA-receptor antagonist memantine. Although 'cognitive enhancement' was the main hope for CIs as a therapeutic class, the reality that has emerged from many placebo-controlled 6-month studies and a few 1-year placebo-controlled studies is that of a small but statistically significant improvement in cognition, peaking at 3 months. The most clinically relevant finding has been the stabilization of cognitive decline with 'return to baseline' at 9 to 12 months for the actively treated groups at the higher therapeutic doses, compared with placebo treated groups who decline steadily; ADL decline is also slower in CI-treated patients. The most difficult symptomatic domain to study and to treat has been behaviour. The availability of neuropsychiatric scales such as the NPI,[5] as well as specific scales such as the Cohen-Mansfield Agitation Inventory,[6] has not yet allowed unequivocal demonstration of benefit in severe stages of AD. New methods of analysis of behaviour have been proposed,[7] and will likely be more successful in defining categories of neuropsychiatric symptoms most responsive to CIs (anxiety, hallucinations) and to memantine (agitation).

Although no drug has yet been established to delay disease progression, many attempts are underway using parallel groups over one year or longer, with the novel agent or a placebo adding to standard treatment, using outcomes known to have relatively linear changes over time such as the Clinical Dementia Rating (CDR) sum of boxes, ADAS-cog, ADCS-ADL or DAD, supplemented by volumetric brain measurements using magnetic resonance imaging (MRI) at the beginning and end of treatment. As an example, Alzhemed acting as gag-mimetic[8] is being tested in mild AD over 78 weeks, with changes from baseline to week 78 on the ADAS-cog and CDR sum of boxes as primary outcomes, and the rate of brain atrophy being calculated using MRI. Flurizan (R-flurbiprofen) is another promising anti-amyloid drug acting through inhibition of gamma-secretase, starting phase III. This design appears promising but there are uncertainties and limitations. For instance, the difference in rate of brain atrophy may be absent or opposite to expectations, with accelerated atrophy in the actively treated group, as was seen in some patients on immunotherapy. Another issue in disease modification strategies is the selection of the stage of disease where the proposed drug will be most effective. For example, numer-ous attempts at treating patients with AD in mild to moderate stages using non-steroidal anti-inflammatory drugs have failed, despite the weight of evidence from epidemiological research and the biological plausibility of an inflammatory response to β-amyloid deposition. It may be that treatment in the late presymptomatic or in the prodromal stages would be the most appropriate time. On the other hand, studies in these stages of AD would require 3 to 5 years. Alternative patient groups could be considered, such as presenilin mutation carriers or amnestic MCI with risk factors for rapid conversion to AD such as the apoε4 genotype.

In terms of which patients should participate in clinical trials, there is a discrepancy in the amount of aetiological and therapeutic research done in 'probable AD' based on NINCDS-ADRDA criteria, which exclude nearly all cases of mixed dementia and the majority of patients with mixed pathologies. There should be a broadening of inclusion criteria to include 'probable' and 'possible' AD in phase III clinical therapeutic research.

FUTURE STRATEGIES TO DELAY THE EMERGENCE OF AD

As hypotheses on the pathophysiology of AD emerge from epidemiological research in human populations, postmortem and biomarker studies in patients, and animal models, there will be a need to establish whether new therapies can delay the onset of symptoms in asymptomatic persons at varying degree of risk of AD. The prototype of trial design to establish the safety and efficacy of such therapies is the ongoing 5-year study comparing *Ginkgo biloba* to placebo in elderly subjects, with incident dementia as primary endpoint. Variations of this design may be possible, by enriching the study population with different levels of risk, such as a positive family history of AD and/or selected gene markers, although it should be remembered that any enrichment of a study population will limit the applicability of findings to the population as a whole.

It is likely that disease-modifying drugs will work best in subgroups of patients with AD, based on age of onset and genetic profile, as well as specific stages of disease. For example, amyloid suppressors may prove to be most effective in young patients where there is a predominant amyloid pathology, whereas statins may prove most useful in older patients where a vascular component to AD predominates; gag-mimetics may work best in very early stages of AD, whereas immunotherapy against amyloid will work best in mild to moderate stages.

CONCLUSIONS

We have gained a better understanding of the natural history of AD and have developed appropriate trial designs and outcomes for the various stages of this condition. There is clear benefit for the treatment of symptoms in mild to moderately severe AD using CIs and memantine. There is cautious optimism for successful disease modification using a number of agents currently under study.

Management of AD goes well beyond the use of medication, and the authors wanted this textbook to highlight the broad spectrum of issues and solutions in the long-term treatment of this condition.

REFERENCES

1. Gauthier S, Reisberg B, Zaudig M, et al. Mild Cognitive Impairment. Lancet 2006; 367:1262–1270.

2. Petersen RC, Thomas RG, Grundman M, et al. Vitamin E and donepezil for the treatment of Mild Cognitive Impairment. N Engl J Med 2005; 352:2379–2388.

3. Galasko D, Edland SD, Morris JC, et al. 'The Consortium to Establish a Registry for Alzheimer's Disease (CERAD). Part IX. Clinical milestones in patients with Alzheimer's disease followed over 3 years. Neurology 1995; 45:1451–1455.

4. Reisberg B, Ferris SH, Anand R, et al. Functional staging of dementia of the Alzheimer's type. Ann NY Acad Sci 1984; 435: 481–483.

5. Cummings JL, Mega M, Gray K, et al. The Neuropsychiatric Inventory: comprehensive assessment of psychopathology in dementia. Neurology 1994; 44:2308–2314.

6. Cohen-Mansfield J, Marx MS, Rosenthal AS. A description of agitation in a nursing home. J Gerontol 1989; 44: M77–M84.

7. Gauthier S, Wirth Y, Möbius HJ. Effects of memantine on behavioral symptoms in Alzheimer's disease patients: an analysis of the Neuropsychiatric Inventory (NPI) data of two randomized, controlled studies. Int J Geriatr Psychiatry 2005; 20:459–464.

8. Gervais F. Gag mimetics: potential to modify underlying disease process in AD. Neurobiol Aging 2004; 25(suppl 1): S11–S12.

Index

Page numbers in *italics* refer to tables and figures.